REGULATION OF PHOSPHATE AND MINERAL METABOLISM

Recent Volumes in this Series

Volume 147
INTRAOVARIAN CONTROL MECHANISMS
Edited by Cornelia P. Channing and Sheldon J. Segal

Volume 148
STRUCTURE AND FUNCTION RELATIONSHIPS IN BIOCHEMICAL SYSTEMS
Edited by Francesco Bossa, Emilia Chiancone, Alessandro Finazzi-Agrò, and Roberto Strom

Volume 149
IN VIVO IMMUNOLOGY: Histophysiology of the Lymphoid System
Edited by Paul Nieuwenhuis, A. A. van den Broek, and M. G. Hanna, Jr.

Volume 150
IMMUNOBIOLOGY OF PROTEINS AND PEPTIDES – II
Edited by M. Z. Atassi

Volume 151
REGULATION OF PHOSPHATE AND MINERAL METABOLISM
Edited by Shaul G. Massry, Joseph M. Letteri, and Eberhard Ritz

Volume 152
NEW VISTAS IN GLYCOLIPID RESEARCH
Edited by Akira Makita, Shizuo Handa, Tamotsu Taketomi, and Yoshitaka Nagai

Volume 153
UREA CYCLE DISEASES
Edited by A. Lowenthal, A. Mori, and B. Marescau

REGULATION OF PHOSPHATE AND MINERAL METABOLISM

Edited by

Shaul G. Massry

University of Southern California
Los Angeles, California

Joseph M. Letteri

State University of New York at Stony Brook and
Nassau County Medical Center
East Meadow, New York

and

Eberhard Ritz

University of Heidelberg
Heidelberg, Federal Republic of Germany

PLENUM PRESS • NEW YORK AND LONDON

Library of Congress Cataloging in Publication Data

Main entry under title:
Regulation of phosphate and mineral metabolism.

(Advances in experimental medicine and biology; v. 151)
"Proceedings of the Fifth International Workshop on Phosphate and Other Minerals, held September 23-27, 1981, in New York City, New York"—P.
Bibliography: p.
Includes index.
1. Phosphorus—Metabolism—Disorders—Congresses. 2. Phosphorus—Metabolism—Congresses. 3. Mineral metabolism—Disorders—Congresses. 4. Mineral metabolism—Congresses. I. Massry, Shaul G. II. Letteri, J. M. (Joseph M.) III. Ritz, Eberhard. IV. International Workshop on Phosphate and Other Minerals (5th: 1981: New York, N.Y.) V. Series. [DNLM: 1. Phosphates—Congresses. 2. Minerals—Congresses. W1 AD559 v. 147/ QV 285 I61 1981m]
RC632.P56M47 599.01'33 82-7602
AACR2

ISBN-13:978-1-4684-4261-8 e-ISBN-13:978-1-4684-4259-5
DOI:10.1007/978-1-4684-4259-5

Proceedings of the Fifth International Workshop on Phosphate and Other Minerals, held September 23-27, 1981, in New York City, New York

Softcover reprint of the hardcover 1st edition 1982

A Division of Plenum Publishing Corporation
233 Spring Street, New York, N.Y. 10013

TO OUR WIVES

Meira Massry
Mary Letteri
Christina Ritz

AND TO OUR CHILDREN

PREFACE

We are pleased to present to our readers the Proceedings of the Fifth International Workshop on Phosphate and Other Minerals which was held in New York City, New York, U.S.A during September 23-27, 1981. It was hosted by Joseph M. Letteri, M.D., Professor of Medicine at the State University of New York at Stonybrook School of Medicine, and Chief, Division of Nephrology, Nassau County Medical Center.

As in the previous Workshops, this meeting provided an opportunity for interested scientists from interrelated fields, including nephrology, endocrinology, physiology, biochemistry and nutrition, to get together and discuss the recent advances in the field of phosphate and mineral metabolism. There were 29 invited presentations by leading scientists and 40 oral and 90 poster presentations selected from over 250 abstracts submitted to the Organizing Committee. The Workshop was attended by 250 scientists from 14 countries including Austria, Australia, Canada, Denmark, England, France, Germany, Holland, Israel, Italy, Japan, Sweden, and the United States of America.

The Sixth International Workshop on Phosphate and Other Minerals will be held during June 24-26, 1983 in Verona, Italy. It will be hosted by Professor Giuseppe Maschio, Director, Division of Nephrology, Istituti Ospitalieri, Verona, Italy. The theme of this coming Workshop will continue to focus on the pathophysiology of phosphate homeostasis and the metabolism of other minerals.

We would like to express our thanks and gratitude for all those who have stimulated, encouraged and supported us to hold the Fifth International Workshop in New York City. This endeavor could not have been possible without the generous financial support of the National Institutes of Health, Institute of Arthritis, Diabetes, Digestive and Kidney Diseases (USA), National Kidney Foundation of New York (USA), New York Kidney Disease Institute (USA), Ciba-Geigy Pharmaceutical Company (USA), Cobe Laboratories, Inc. (USA), Gambro, Inc. (USA), Hoffman-LaRoche, Inc. (USA), Plenum Publishing Corporation (USA), S. Karger AG, Basel (Switzerland), The Cordis Dow Corporation (USA), The Proctor and Gamble Company (USA), The Upjohn Company (USA), and Travenol Laboratories, Inc. (USA).

A special tribute goes to Ms. Gracy Fick, Ms. Jeannie Scileppi, and Ms. Claire Ciaccio for their tremendous and invaluable contribution for the organization of the Workshop. Last, but not least, we would like to express our deepest appreciation for Mrs. Mary Letteri for the arrangement of the wonderful and exquisite social events during the Workshop; these were truly memorable occasions.

Shaul G. Massry
Joseph M. Letteri
Eberhard Ritz

CONTENTS

I. *RENAL HANDLING OF PHOSPHATE*

RENAL HANDLING OF PHOSPHATE

THE ADAPTIVE SYSTEM OF THE TUBULAR TRANSPORT OF PHOSPHATE

J.-P. Bonjour, J. Caverzasio, H. Fleisch,
R. Mühlbauer, and U. Troehler

Department of Pathophysiology
University of Berne
Berne, Switzerland

The present report is an attempt to review the state of our knowledge concerning the adaptation of the tubular transport of Pi in relation with the homeostasis of Pi.

DEFINITION OF ADAPTATION

According to the Webster's New World Dictionary (1), the term "adaptation" when used in biology is defined as "a change in structure or function that produces a better adjustment to environment". Therefore, adaptation of the system responsible for the renal tubular transport of inorganic phosphate (Pi) means a change in its function, i.e. an adjustment of its transport capacity. The Pi transport system in the mammalian nephron is characterized by a maximal rate at which this ion can be transferred across the tubular epithelium from lumen to blood (2). As it will be reemphasized later on, this maximal rate (Tm or max.TRPi) is not an absolute constant since it can be set at different levels according to the physiological or pathological conditions. The renal Pi transport system is essentially a saturable process with no appreciable first order component. This feature implies that Pi can completely disappear from the urine as a consequence of a very small decrement in its plasma concentration, i.e. without any change in the transport capacity at the tubular level. In such a condition, it would be inappropriate to use the term "adaptation", even though the kidney excrete a Pi-free urine.

ASSESSMENT OF OVERALL TUBULAR Pi TRANSPORT CAPACITY AND ADAPTATION

The best and only way of estimating the capacity of the tubular Pi transport system of the whole kidney is to determine the maximal net reabsorption of Pi per unit volume of glomerular filtrate under acute Pi infusion. In clinical practice an indirect estimate of the tubular Pi reabsorption capacity can be obtained by the use of a nomogram based on the relationship between the plasma concentration and the fractional excretion of Pi (3). However, in Pi depletion where the endogenous plasma Pi concentration is usually below the threshold value beyond which Pi appears in the urine, this nomogram cannot be used for estimating the tubular Pi reabsorptive capacity. Therefore, in studies concerning the tubular adaptive response to Pi restriction it is necessary to determine max.TRPi(Tm)/GFR directly by infusing acutely Pi until this value is reached.

EVIDENCE FOR ADAPTATION

That Pi can disappear from the urine in response to a restriction in the alimentary Pi supply has been known for many years (4,5, see also for review ref. 6). However, the definitive proof that this phenomenon was associated with an actual adaptation, i.e. an increase in the overall tubular capacity to reabsorb Pi was brought forward only recently (6,7) with the demonstration that this adaptation was independent of the parathyroid hormone (PTH). It has been shown that the absolute increase in max.TRPi/ml GF induced by a given Pi restriction was virtually the same in intact and chronically thyroparathyroidectomized (TPTX) rats (10). A PTH-independent adaptive increase in the tubular Pi reabsorptive capacity of the whole kidney in response to Pi restriction has been demonstrated in other mammalian species such as the pig (8), and the mouse (9). To our knowlege the demonstration of a PTH-independent change in the tubular Pi transport capacity in response to Pi deprivation in man has not been yet reported.

RENAL ADAPTATION AND Pi HOMEOSTASIS

The fact that the renal tubule can react to the amount of Pi supplied by adjusting its Pi transport capacity has some important consequence for the homeostasis of Pi. It is obvious that because of this adaptive mechanism the plasma Pi concentration will be less dependent upon variations in the amount of Pi supplied in the diet. Another homeostatic consequence of the adaptive response is related to the conservation of the Pi mobilized from body stores during the daily fasting or postabsorptive period. Indeed, in Pi deprived animals this amount of Pi which enters the extracellular compartment from body stores would be spilled in the urine without an adaptive enhancement of the tubular Pi transport capacity (11). That the adaptive system is important for Pi homeostasis will be also evoked later on in this report when the pathophysiological aspect of this topic will be presented.

ABOUT THE NECESSITY OF A PTH-INDEPENDENT REGULATION OF THE TUBULAR TRANSPORT OF Pi

As mentioned above, the tubular adaptation to Pi restriction is a PTH-independent phenomenon (6,7). PTH is essentially a calcium-regulating hormone. Since PTH stimulates the tubular reabsorption of calcium, whereas it decreases that of Pi, it is obvious that this hormone cannot cope with a situation where the availability of both Ca and Pi from the environment would vary in the same direction. Therefore, there is a necessity for a PTH-independent and specific system for regulating the tubular Pi transport capacity in order to maintain Pi homeostasis. Experimentally one can demonstrate in intact rats that decreasing both dietary Pi and Ca in the diet can be followed by either no change or an increase in the plasma level of PTH and in the excretion of nephrogenic cyclic AMP, whereas the tubular capacity to reabsorb Pi is adequately enhanced from homeostatic point of view. This finding is probably directly related to the fact that the adaptation to low Pi diet is accompanied by an inhibition of the phosphaturic action of PTH (12,13,14). Thus, PTH cannot be the unique and final controller of the tubular reabsorption of Pi.

TIME COURSE OF ADAPTATION

In our initial study in thyroparathyroidectomized (TPTX) rats (6) we were able to demonstrate that the tubular Pi adaptation of the whole kidney can be detectable 3 days after switching rats from a high to a low Pi diet. Recently, we have observed that a small but significant increase in the overall tubular capacity to reabsorb Pi can be detected in one day in either intact or TPTX rats (11). That the adaptive response could occur within hours is still unclear. In favor of this view is the fact that acute Pi infusion to intact or TPTX animals can result in a rapid fall in the absolute tubular reabsorption of Pi (15,16,17). This phenomenon might reflect an adaptation to an acute Pi loading. Alternatively change in extracellular calcium concentration (18) could account, at least in part, for this acute alteration in the renal handling of Pi. Thus, the question remains open whether this acute change is due to the same mechanism as that accounting for the long term adaptive response.

LOCALIZATION OF THE ADAPTIVE RESPONSE AT THE TUBULAR AND MEMBRANE LEVEL

Free flow micropunctures (19,20) stationary microperfusions in situ (21), perfusions of isolated tubule in vitro (22) have clearly established that the proximal tubule is an important segment of the nephron where the adaptive response to variations in the dietary Pi intake is expressed. The possibility that the distal and the collecting duct might also participate to this regulation has been suggested on the basis of data obtained by free flow micropuncture in intact and TPTX rats (19,20).

Evidence has accumulated over the last few years that the adaptive change in the transfer rate of Pi across the proximal epithelium is associated with an alteration in the sodium-dependent Pi transport system which is present in the luminal membrane. Indeed, the initial rate of the sodium-dependent Pi uptake by brush border membrane vesicles (BBMV), which reflects in most conditions the maximal velocity (Vmax) of the Pi transport system, is markedly enhanced in both intact and TPTX rats fed a low Pi diet (23,24). The same phenomenon has been also observed in other mammalian species such as mice (25), and pigs (26). However, this alteration in the transport capacity of the sodium-dependent Pi transport system of proximal BBMV does not seem to be the only mechanism whereby the entire nephron regulates Pi reabsorption (27).

ADAPTATION TO THE Pi DEMAND OF THE ORGANISM

It has been postulated (28) that the adaptive system which reacts to change in the Pi supply would also respond to variations in the Pi demand. A series of experimental data support this notion. In fact, in several situations where the Pi demand can be expected to be reduced, such as growth arrest (21), blockage of bone mineralization (28), pharmacologically-induced inhibition of protein synthesis (30), starvation (24,31) or deprivation of some essential element like magnesium (32), one can observe a PTH-independent decrease in the tubular reabsorptive Pi capacity.

PUTATIVE NATURE OF THE ADAPTIVE SYSTEM

The nature of the controlled and controlling elements of the homeostatic system which determine the adaptation of the tubular Pi transport to the Pi needs of the organism remains quite obscure. Only exclusions of some factors and speculations about others can be discussed at this stage of our present knowledge.

Controlled factor(s) (?)

Unlike the system responsible for the homeostasis of calcium, that of Pi does not seem to operate for maintaining the extracellular level of Pi at a fixed value which would be an absolute constant, whatever might be the Pi needs of the organism. Indeed, for a given Pi supply it appears that the tubular Pi transport capacity, and thereby the plasma Pi concentration, is set at different levels according to the growth and the Pi needs of the organism. Thus, some intracellular pool(s) of Pi might represent the controlled variable rather than merely the extracellular or plasma concentration of Pi per se. The identification of this (or these) pool(s) will be essential for understanding the homeostasis of Pi in relation with the adaptive response of the renal Pi transport system.

Controlling factors (?)

That there is a need for a hormonal factor which would connect this unknown controlled pool of Pi to the kidney and thereby be an essential element in the efferent limb leading to the adaptive response of the tubular transport of Pi can be, if not logically deduced, at least intuitively envisaged.

Among various candidates, parathyroid hormone, calcitonin, vitamin D metabolites; thyroxine, growth hormone and other factors secreted by the pituitary gland have been excluded (6,7,27,33,34,35).

Several attempts made in our laboratory to investigate whether the plasma or the whole blood of rats fed either low or high Pi diet could transmit, the adaptive response remained so far unsuccessful. Negative results have also been reported with regard to the presence of a low Pi diet-induced circulating factor having a direct and immediate effect on the transport of Pi of isolated proximal tubules (22).

Other attempts from our laboratory aimed at investigating whether the liver, the intestinal track or the bone could be the source of a factor affecting the tubular transport of Pi were also unsuccessful and therefore unconclusive. A recent report (36) has also provided negative results with regard to the possibility that the intestinal mucosa would be part of the sensing system responsible for the adaptive response. Despite all these negative findings, the possible existence of a hormonal factor which would be an essential controlling element of the tubular Pi adaptation mechanism remains an open and fascinating question for future research in this field.

Molecular mechanism(s) (?)

The nature of the molecular mechanism responsible for the adaptive response at the renal cellular and plasma membrane level remains also unclear at the present time. At the cellular level several studies aimed at uncovering a critical difference in the concentration of a molecule which could play a role in mediating the adaptative Pi response have provided only negative results. Indeed, measurements in the whole kidney or renal cortex of cyclic AMP, (37,38), adenylcydase activity (37) ATP, ADP, AMP, Pi, Mg (39), proteinkinase activity (38), and very recently determination of the $NADH^{+}/NAD$ ratio (40) have indicated no difference at a time when an adaptation of the Pi transport system to low Pi diet had already taken place. The only factor which appears to change with a time course similar to that of the Pi transport system is a depression in the rate of the renal gluconeogenesis (41). Whether there is a causal relationship between this alteration and the adaptive response of the tubular Pi transport system has not yet been established.

At the brush border membrane level, alkaline phosphatase has been suggested to play some role in the change in the renal Pi transport, in general (42) and more particularly in the adaptation to low Pi diet (43). However, in several studies no correlation has been found between the Pi reabsorptive capacity of the whole kidney and the alkaline phosphatase activity determined in the renal cortex, or when the Pi transport and the activity of this enzyme were measured in BBMV isolated from renal cortical slices (23,44,45).

IMPLICATIONS OF THE ADAPTIVE SYSTEM IN PATHOPHYSIOLOGY

The adaptive system of the tubular transport of Pi could be implicated in some pathophysiological situations wherein changes in the renal handling of Pi cannot be merely explained by alteration in the parathyroid hormone status.

This could be the case for instance in conditions where there is a deficiency or an excess in growth hormone, since this hormone has a strong influence on the Pi demand of the organism. It is also possible that the change in the renal handling of Pi which occurs in the course of chronic renal failure, could be due to the adaptive system (46). This possibility is discussed in another report of this symposium (Regulation mechanism of the renal phosphate handling in renal failure, by H. Fleisch, J. Caverzasio and J.-P. Bonjour). Finally, we have obtained evidence that the overall tubular Pi transport system of X-linked hypophosphatemic mice does not react to Pi restriction (47). A very recent report also suggests that in patients with this disease the tubular Pi reabsorptive capacity does not rise as in normal individuals in response to a dietary Pi restriction (48). Thus, X-linked hypophosphatemia appears to be a disease due to a defect in the adaptive system of tubular transport of Pi (47). This would imply that the homeostasis of Pi, including bone mineralization, cannot be maintained when the adaptive system of the tubular transport of Pi is impaired, thus underscoring the great importance of this system.

CONCLUSION

The adaptive system of the tubular transport of Pi appears to play a major role in the homeostasis of Pi. This system responds to variations in both the Pi supply and demand. It operates independently of parathyroid hormone and, moreover, controls very tightly the phosphaturic action of this hormone. The adaptive change in the Pi transport takes place, at least in part, along the proximal convoluted tubule. At this level, the adaptive response is accompanied by an alteration in the sodium-dependent Pi transport present in the brush border membrane. From the pathophysiological point of view, a defect in the adaptive system of the tubular transport of Pi is probably responsible for the disease X-linked hypophosphatemia. The nature of the controlled and controlling elements which determine the tubular Pi adaptation remains to be elucidated.

ACKNOWLEDGEMENTS

This work has been supported by the Swiss National Science Foundation (grant 3.824.79), and by the Ausbildungs- und Förderungsfonds der Arbeitsgemeinschaft für Osteosynthese (AO), chur, Switzerland.

REFERENCES

1. Webster's New World Dictionary of the American Language. D. B. Guraluik, ed., The World Publishing Company, Celveland and New York (1966).
2. R. F. Pitts, "Physiology of the Kidney and Body Fluids", Year Book Medical Publishers, Chicago (1968).
3. O. L. M. Bijvoet, D. B. Morgan, and P. Fourman, The assessment of phosphate reabsorption, Clin. Chim.
4. J. D. Crawford, M. M. Osborne jr., N. B. Talbot, L. M. Terry, and M. F. Morrill, The parathyroid glands and phosphorus homeostasis, J. Clin. Invest. 29:1448 (1950).

5. E. L. Chambers jr., G. S. Gordan, L. Goldman, and E. C. Reifenstein jr., Tests for hyperparathyroidism: Tubular reabsorption of phosphate, phosphate deprivation and calcium infusion, J. Clin. Endocrinol. Metab. 16:1507 (1956).
6. U. Troehler, J.-P. Bonjour, and H. Fleisch, Inorganic phosphate homeostasis. Renal adaptation to the dietary intake in intact and thyroparathyroidectomized rats. J. Clin. Invest. 57:264 (1976).
7. T. H. Steele, and H. F. DeLuca, Influence of dietary phosphorus on renal phosphate reabsorption in the parathyyroidectomized rats, J. Clin. Invest. 57:867 (1976).
8. J.-P. Bonjour, A. D. Care, and D. W. Pickard, Renal adaptation to changes in dietary phosphorus intake by thyroparathyroidectomized pigs, J. Physiol. 290:27 (1979).
9. R. C. Mühlbauer, J.-P. Bonjour, and H. Fleisch, Renal handling of phosphate (Pi) and calcium (Ca) in X-linked hypophosphatemic (HYP) mice, in: "Kidney and Body Fluids" (Vol. 11, in Advances in Physiological Sciences), Proc. 28th Int. Congress of Physiological Sciences, Budapest 1980, L. Takacs, ed., Pergamon Press, Budapest (1980).
10. J.-P. Bonjour, J. Caverzasio, H. Fleisch, R. Mühlbauer, and U. Tröhler, Renal handling of phosphate, Contr. Nephrol. 23:11 (1980).
11. U. Troehler, J.-P. Bonjour, and H. Fleisch, Plasma level and renal handling of Pi: Effect of overnight fasting with and without Pi supply, Amer. J. Physiol., in press.
12. T. H. Steele, J. L. Underwood, B. A. Stromberg, and C. A. Larmore, Renal resistance to parathyroid hormone during phosphorus deprivation, J. Clin. Invest. 58:1461 (1976).
13. J.-P. Bonjour, U. Troehler, R. Mühlbauer, C. Preston, and H. Fleisch, Is there a bone-kidney link in the homeostasis of inorganic phosphate (Pi)? in: "Phosphate Metabolism" (Vol. 81 in Advances in Experimental Medicine and Biology), Proc. 2nd Int. Workshop on Phosphate, Heidelberg 1976, S. G. Massry and E. Ritz, eds., Plenum Press, New York London (1977).
14. H. J. Gloor, J.-P. Bonjour, J. Caverzasio, and H. Fleisch, Resistance to the phosphaturic and calcemic actions of parathyroid hormone during phosphate depletion. Prevention by 1,25-dihydroxyvitamin D_3. J. Clin. Invest. 63:371 (1979).
15. A. Frick, Reabsorption of inorganic phosphate in the rat kidney: I. Saturation of transport mechanism; II. suppression of fractional phosphate reabsorption due to expansion of extracellular fluid volume, Pflügers Arch. 304:351 (1968).

16. J.-F. Boudry, U. Troehler, M. Touabi, H. Fleisch, and J.-P. Bonjour, Secretion of inorganic phosphate in the rat nephron, Clin. Sci. Mol. Med. 48:475 (1975).
17. A. Frick, and I. Durasin, Maximal reabsorptive capacity for inorganic phosphate (Tm_{Pi}) in the absence of parathyroid hormone in the rat: Decrease of the Tm_{Pi} during prolonged administration of phosphate and the role of calcium, Pflügers Arch. 377:9 (1978).
18. H. Oberleitner, R. Greger, and F. Lang, Role of calcium in the decline of phosphate reabsorption during phosphate loading in acutely thyroparathyroidectomized rats, Pflügers Arch. 374::249 (1978).
19. R. Mühlbauer, J.-P. Bonjour, and H. Fleisch, Tubular localization of the adaptation to dietary phosphate in rats, Amer. J. Physiol. 233:F342 (1977).
20. R. Mühlbauer, J.-P. Bonjour, and H. Fleisch, Tubular handling of Pi: localization of effects of 1,25(OH)$_2$D$_3$ and dietary Pi in TPTX rats, Amer. J. Physiol. 241:F123 (1981).
21. K. J. Ullrich, G. Rumrich, S. Klöss, Phosphate transport in the proximal convolution of the rat kidney. I. Tubular heterogeneity, effect of parathyroid hormone in acute and parathyroidectomized animals, and effect of phosphate diet. Pflügers Arch. 372:269 (1977).
22. P. C. Brazy, J. W. McKeown, R. H. Harris, and V. W. Dennis, Comparative effects of dietary phosphate, unilateral nephrectomy, and parathyroid hormone on phosphate transport by the rabbit proximal tubule, Kidney Int. 17:788 (1980).
23. R. Stoll, R. Kinne, H. Murer, H. Fleisch, and J.-P. Bonjour, Phosphate transport by rat renal brush border membrane vesicles: Influence of dietary phosphate, thyroparathyroidectomy, and 1,25-dihydroxyvitamin D$_3$. Pflügers Arch. 380:47 (1979).
24. S. A. Kempson, S. V. Shah, P. G. Werness, T. Berndt, P. H. Lee, L. H. Smith, F. G. Knox, and T. P. Dousa, Renal brush border membrane adaptation to phosphorus deprivation: Effects of fasting versus low-phosphorus diet, Kidney Int. 18:36 (1980).
25. H. S. Tenenhouse, and C. R. Scriver, Renal adaptation to phosphate deprivation in the Hyp mouse with X-linked hypophosphatemia, Canad. J. Biochem. 57:938 (1979).
26. P. Q. Barrett, J. M. Gertner, and H. Rasmussen, Effect of dietary phosphate on transport properties of pig renal microvillus vesicles, Amer. J. Physiol. 239:F352 (1980).

27. J. Caverzasio, J.-P. Bonjour, H. Murer, and H. Fleisch, Adaptation of renal Pi transport in young growing and adult rats: Dissociation between changes in brush border membrane vesicles (BBMV) and in whole kidney, abstract VIIIth Int. Congr. of Nephrology, Athens (1981).
28. J.-P. Bonjour, U. Troehler, C. Preston, and H. Fleisch, Parathyroid hormone and renal handling of Pi: effect of dietary Pi and diphosphonates, Amer. J. Physiol. 234:F497 (1978).
29. J. Caverzasio, J.-P. Bonjour, and H. Fleisch, Adaptation of tubular phosphate transport: Relation between phosphate requirement, as influenced by growth, and supply, in: "Phosphate and Minerals in Health and Disease" (Vol. 128, in Advances in Experimental Medicine and Biology), Proc. 4th Int. Workshop on Phosphate and Other Minerals, Strasbourg 1979, S. G. Massry, E. Ritz, and H. Jahn, eds., Plenum Press, New York and London (1980).
30. S. V. Shah, S. A. Kempson, T. E. Northrup, and T. P. Dousa, Renal adaptation to a low phosphate diet in rats, blockade by actinomycin D, J. Clin. Invest. 64:955 (1979).
31. N. Beck, S. K. Webster, and H. J. Reineck, Effect of fasting on tubular phosphorus reabsorption, Amer. J. Physiol. 237:F241 (1979).
32. H. E. Ginn, and L. L. Shanbour, Phosphaturia in magnesium-deficient rats, Amer. J. Physiol. 212:1347 (1967).
33. T. H. Steele, J. E. Engle, Y. Tanaka, R. S. Lorenc, K. L. Dudgeon, and H. F. DeLuca, Phosphatemic action of 1,25-dihydroxyvitamin D_3, Amer. J. Physiol. 229:489 (1975).
34. J.-P. Bonjour, C. Preston, and H. Fleisch, Effect of 1,25-dihydroxyvitamin D_3 on the renal handling of Pi in thyroparathyroidectomized rats, J. Clin. Invest. 60:1419 (1977).
35. D. B. N. Lee, N. Braubar, M. W. Walling, V. Silis, H. E. Carlson, R. E. Grindeland, J. W. Coburn, and C. R. Kleeman, Role of growth hormone in experimental phosphorus deprivation in the rat, Calcif. Tissue Int. 32: 105 (1980).
36. S. Moser, N. Brautbar, V. Gura, C. R. Kleeman, and S. G. Massry, On the mechanism of hypophosphaturia during acute and chronic dietary phosphate restriction, Min. Electr. Metab. 5:39 (1981).
37. N. Beck, Effects of dietary phosphorus (P) intake on renal actions of parathyroid hormone (PTH) and cyclic AMP (cAMP), Kidney Int. 10:487 (1976).

38. K. Kurokawa, W. J. Kreusser, E. Aznar, E. Sachtjen, and S. G. Massry, Effects of parathyroid hormone and calcitonin on renal cyclic AMP and protein kinase activity during phosphate depletion, Min. Electr. Metab. 4:197 (1980).
39. W. J. Kreusser, K. Kurokawa, E. Aznar, and S. G. Massry, Phosphate depletion, Min. Electr. Metab.. 5:30 (1978).
40. T. J. Berndt, F. G. Knox, and T. P. Dousa, Role of nicotine-adenine dinucleotide (NAD) in the phosphaturic response to parathryoid hormone (PTH), Kidney Int. 19:108 (1981).
41. W. J. Kreusser, C. Descoeudres, Y. Oda, and S. G. Massry, Effect of phosphate depletion on renal gluconeogenesis, Min. Electr. Metab. 3:312 (1980).
42. G. E. Plante, C. Petitclerc, T. Nawar, and R. Erian, Increased phosphaturia during inhibition of renal alkaline phosphatase, Min. Electr. Metab. 2:258 (1979).
43. S. A. Kempson, J. K. Kim, T. E. Northrup, F. G. Knox, and T. P. Dousa, Alkaline phosphatase in adaptation to low dietary phosphate intake, Amer. J. Physiol. 237:E465 (1979).
44. H. S. Tenenhouse, C. R. Scriver, and E. J. Vizel, Alkaline phosphatase activity does not mediate phosphate transport in the renal-cortical brush-border membrane, Biochem. J. 190:473 (1980).
45. B. S. Levine, A. Hodsman, K. Ho, H. F. Shaw, B. Hirayama, I. Kippin, D. B. N. Lee, and J. W. Coburn, Early renal brush border adaptation to dietary phosphorus restriction, Kidney Int. 19:113 (1981).
46. J. Caverzasio, J.P. Bonjour, H. J. Gloor, and H. Fleisch, Parathyroid hormone (PTH) is not essential for adaptation of tubular phosphate (Pi) transport to chronic renal mass reduction, in: "Hormonal Control of Calcium Metabolism", Proc. 7th Int. Conf. on Calcium Regulating Hormones, Estes Park USA, 1980, D. V. Cohn, R. V. Talmage, and J. L. Matthews, eds., Excerpta Medica, Amsterdam-Oxford-Princeton (1981).
47. R. Mühlbauer, J.-P. Bonjour, and H. Fleisch, Tubular handling of phosphate (Pi) and Ca in X-linked hypophosphatemic mice: Defective adaptation to Pi restriction associated with a renal Ca leak, in: "Hormonal Control of Calcium Metabolism", Proc. 7th Int. Conf. on Calcium Regulating Hormones, Estes Park USA, 1980, D. V. Cohn, R. V. Talmage, and J. L. Matthews, eds., Excerpta Medica, Amsterdam-Oxford-Princeton (1981).
48. K. Insogna, A. Stewart, and J. Gertner, Impaired response to acute phosphorus (P) deprivation in sex-linked hypophosphatemic rickets (HR), in: program and abstracts of the 3rd Annual Scientific Meeting of the American Society for Bone and Mineral Research, Cincinnati, p 28A, (1981).

NEPHRON SITES OF ADAPTATION TO CHANGES IN DIETARY PHOSPHATE

Franklyn G. Knox, John A. Haas and Aviad Haramati

Department of Physiology & Biophysics
Mayo Medical School
Rochester, Minnesota

Studies of the renal adaptation to changes in the dietary intake of phosphate have provided important insights into the mechanisms of regulation of phosphate transport by the renal tubule. Troehler, Bonjour and Fleisch (1) and Steele and DeLuca (2) showed that phosphate deprivation results in marked increases in phosphate transport which were independent of plasma phosphate and parathyroid hormone. Further, rats fed a low phosphate diet provide a model of resistance to the phosphaturic response to PTH (3). Whereas the expected increase in cAMP generation and hypocalciuria occur, there is no increase in phosphate excretion. Studies utilizing several different approaches support the concept that adaptive changes in phosphate transport occur in the proximal tubule. In vivo microperfusion, isolated tubule and isolated renal brush border vesicle studies of proximal tubules all illustrate enhanced phosphate transport in animals fed a low phosphate diet (4, 5, 6, 7). Micropuncture studies in dogs also show enhanced phosphate reabsorption in the proximal tubule in phosphate deprivation (8, 9). Accordingly, adaptation of proximal tubule phosphate transport is very likely. However, the contribution of this altered transport to the urinary excretion of phosphate remains controversial.

The influence of differences in dietary phosphate intake on nephron sites of phosphate transport has been reported by Muhlbauer et al (10). Although phosphate reabsorption was increased in the early portions of the proximal tubule in rats on a low phosphate diet, this difference was not significant in the late proximal tubule, suggesting that changes in the early proximal tubule were compensated in the late proximal tubule.

The major adaptation affecting urinary phosphate excretion appeared to be in the "terminal nephron" since the dietary phosphate intake markedly affected the difference in phosphate delivery between the distal tubule and the final urine. There was no net reabsorption in the low phosphate group, whereas there was a net secretion in the high phosphate group in the terminal part of the nephron. To allow for equivalent filtered loads of phosphate, all animals received a phosphate infusion in these studies. This, then, results in the apparent secretion in animals on a high phosphate diet. An alternative explanation for such apparent secretion may be a greater adaptation of deep than superficial proximal tubules. In summary, these studies suggested that the principal site of altered phosphate transport responsible for changes in urinary phosphate excretion lies in terminal nephron segments (or in greater adaptation by proximal tubules of deep nephrons than by superficial nephrons).

Lau and Eby have performed similar experiments further indicating a crucial role for "terminal" nephron segments in the adaptation to changes in dietary phosphate intake (11). It is remarkable that there was no tendency for a net adaptive response when fluid reached the early distal tubule. Subsequently, there was marked phosphate reabsorption between early and late distal reabsorptive sites and between the late distal tubule and the urine. There was no such reabsorption between the late distal tubule and the urine in animals on the high phosphate diet. Again, these differences between the late distal tubule and urine could be due to differences between superficial and deep nephron proximal tubule function.

Studies utilizing brush border membrane from dogs and rats and the isolated perfused tubules from rabbits support the concept of nephron heterogeneity of phosphate transport (12, 13). Brush border membranes from superficial cortex of animals on low phosphate diet have a greater capacity for phosphate transport than membranes from the deep cortex (12). In isolated tubules, transport rates for phosphate are higher in early than in late segments of proximal tubules when expressed per unit length and are proportionately increased in response to low phosphate diet. However, although there is no difference in phosphate transport rates between superficial and juxtamedullary nephrons per unit length, the convoluted portion is longer in juxtamedullary nephrons. The ratio of convoluted to straight portions averages 1.6 for superficial proximal tubules and 8.8 for juxtamedullary proximal tubules (14). Whether this ratio translates to a greater reabsorption by juxtamedullary nephrons remains unknown. As stated by McKeown, Brazy, and Dennis, it is therefore difficult to predict from isolated tubule studies if phosphate absorptive capacity in juxtamedullary nephrons is greater or less than in superficial ones. We agree with Valtin (15) that any final assessment of the role of either internephronal or axial heterogeneity in overall renal function requires observations obtained in vivo.

For these reasons we used in vivo micropuncture to test the hypothesis that deep and superficial nephrons respond differently to changes in dietary phosphate (16) (Figure 1). All rats were thyroparathyroidectomized to control for the effects of parathyroid hormone and calcitonin, and saline-expanded to increase flow rates in the loop of Henle. In rats fed a normal phosphate diet (0.7%), phosphate delivery from the superficial proximal tubule (as sampled from the early distal tubule) was 15 ± 4%. Phosphate delivery from the deep proximal tubule (as sampled from the tip of the loop of Henle) was 6 ± 2%. In rats fed a high phosphate diet (1.8%), fractional delivery of phosphate was 32.0 ± 6.1% from superficial proximal tubules and 15.5 ± 3.6% from deep proximal tubules. Thus, in rats fed a high phosphate diet, both superficial and deep nephrons adapted by increasing phosphate delivery. However, the adaptation was greater in superficial than in deep nephrons. In this case, urinary excretion of 27.6 ± 6.3% could be accounted for by admixture of fluid from superficial and deep proximal tubules. When fed a low phosphate diet (0.07%), fractional delivery of phosphate was 7.1 ± 2.6% from superficial proximal tubules and 9.7 ± 2.4% from deep proximal tubules. Thus, both superficial and deep proximal tubules avidly reabsorbed phosphate in low phosphate diet. However, proximal reabsorption did not account for total reabsorption since phosphate excretion was only 0.8 ± 0.2%. Accordingly, reabsorption of the remaining 7% of the filtered load of phosphate occurred in distal nephron segments.

Several studies have demonstrated distal sites of phosphate reabsorption (17, 18, 19, 20). Pastoriza-Munoz et al demonstrated distal phosphate reabsorption in the rat which was inhibited by PTH, from 13 ± 2 to 6 ± 2 pmol/min, $p<.001$ (17). We have recently confirmed these results in our laboratory. In addition, Poujeol, Jamison and de Rouffignac have concluded from microinjections into the loop of Henle that phosphate is reabsorbed by the juxtamedullary distal tubules and/or arcades connecting juxtamedullary distal tubules to the collecting system (21). Phosphate transport has been studied utilizing the isolated rabbit cortical collecting tubule (18, 22). Peraino and Suki (18) found what they consider to be significant phosphate reabsorption, whereas Dennis, Bello-Reuss and Robinson (22) concluded that there was no significant phosphate reabsorption in the cortical collecting duct. Thus, although the role of the collecting duct is somewhat equivocal, there is evidence for distal reabsorption of phosphate which may play a role in adaptation to low phosphate intakes.

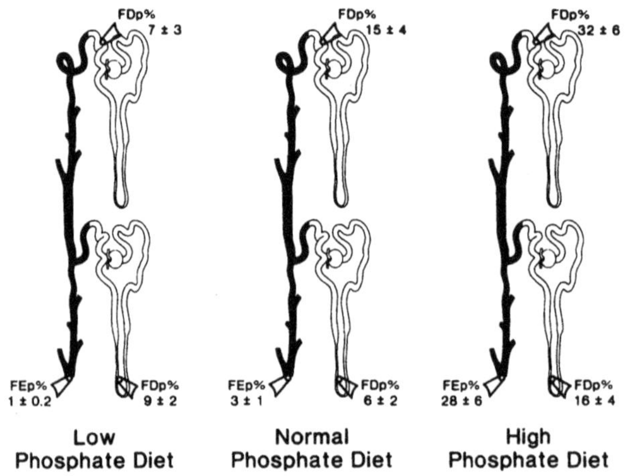

Fig. 1. Fractional delivery of phosphate from superficial and deep proximal tubules during conditions of low, normal and high phosphate diet.

Such distal sites have important implications because they might be characterized by different transport parameters, such as maximum transport capacity and affinity for the transport process, and they might be responsive to different hormones than the proximal phosphate transport site. By definition, these sites contribute to the magnitude of the final urinary excretion of phosphate and could be important regulatory sites. Nonetheless, it is clear that the proximal tubule plays a major role in adaptation to changes in the dietary intake of phosphate.

REFERENCES

1. Troehler, U., Bonjour, J-P., and Fleisch, H.: Inorganic phosphate homeostasis: Renal adaptation to the dietary intake in intact and thyroparathyroidectomized rats. J. Clin. Invest. 57:264-273, 1976.

2. Steele, T. H. and DeLuca, H. F.: Influence of dietary phosphorus on renal phosphate reabsorption in the parathyroidectomized rat. J. Clin. Invest. 57:867-874, 1976.

3. Steele, T. H.: Renal resistance to parathyroid hormone during phosphatus deprivation. J. Clin. Invest. 58:1461-1464, 1976.

4. Ullrich, K. J., Rumrich, G. and Kloss, S.: Phosphate transport in the proximal convolution of the rat kidney. I. Tubular heterogeneity, effect of parathyroid hormone in acute and chronic parathyroidectomized animals and effect of phosphate diet. Pfluegers Arch. 372:269-274, 1977.

5. Brazy, P. C., McKeown, J. W., Harris, R. H. and Dennis, V. W.: Comparative effectives of dietary phosphate, unilateral nephrectomy, and parathyroid hormone on phosphate transport by the rabbit proximal tubule. Kidney Int. 17:788-800, 1980.

6. Stoll, R., Kinne, R. and Murer, H.: Effect of dietary phosphate intake on phosphate transport by isolated rat renal brush-border vesicles. Biochem. J. 180:465-470, 1979.

7. Kempson, S. A. and Dousa, T. P.: Phosphate transport across renal cortical brush border membrane vesicles from rats stabilized on a normal, high or low phosphate diet. Life Sci. 24:881-888, 1979.

8. Wong, N. L. M., Quamme, G. A., O'Callaghan, T. J., Sutton, R. A. L. and Dirks, J. H.: Renal tubular transport in phosphate depletion: A micropuncture study. Can. J. Phys. & Pharmacol. 58:1063-1071, 1980.

9. Wen, S.-F., Boynar, J. W., Jr. and Stoll, R. W.: Effect of phosphate deprivation on renal phosphate transport in the dog. Am. J. Physiol. 234:F199-F206, 1978.

10. Muhlbauer, R. C., Bonjour, J-P. and Fleisch, H.: Tubular localization of adaptation to dietary phosphate in rats. Am. J. Physiol. 233:F342-F348, 1977.

11. Lau, K. and Eby, B.: Tubular mechanisms for the phosphaturic effects of NH_4Cl administration. Am. Soc. Neph. 13th Annual Meeting, 5A, 1980 (abstract)

12. Turner, S. T. and Dousa, T. P.: Differences in transport capacity for phosphate (Pi) of luminal brush border membrane (BBM) prepared from subcapsular (SC) and juxtamedullary (JM) cortex. Am. Soc. Neph. 14th Annual meeting, 1981 (abstract).

13. McKeown, J. W., Brazy, P. C. and Dennis, V. W.: Intrarenal heterogeneity for fluid, phosphate and glucose absorption in the rabbit. Am. J. Physiol. 237:F312-F318, 1979.

14. Woodhall, P. B., Tisher, C. C., Simonton, C. A. and Robinson, R. R.: Relationship between para-aminohippurate secretion and cellular morphology in rabbit proximal. J. Clin. Invest. 61:1320-1329, 1978.

15. Valtin, H.: Structural and functional heterogeneity of mammalian nephrons. Am. J. Physiol. 233:F491-F501, 1977.

16. Haramati, A., Haas, J. A. and F. G. Knox: Adaptation of deep and superficial nephrons to changes in dietary phosphate intake. Am. Soc. Neph. 14th Annual meeting, 1981 (abstract).

17. Pastoriza-Munoz, E., Colindres, R. E., Lassiter, W. E. and Lechene, C.: Effect of parathyroid hormone on phosphate reabsorption in rat distal convolution. Am. J. Physiol. 235:F321-F330, 1978.

18. Peraino, R. A. and Suki, W. N.: Phosphate transport by isolated rabbit cortical collecting tubule. Am. J. Physiol. 238:F358-F362, 1980.

19. Amiel, C., Kuntziger, J. and Richet, G.: Micropuncture study of handling of phosphate by proximal and distal nephron in normal and parathyroidectomized rat. Evidence for distal reabsorption. Pfluegers Arch. 317:93-109, 1970.

20. Haramati, A. and Knox, F. G.: Is phosphate reabsorbed by the distal nephron? Min. & Elect. Metab. 6:165-173, 1981.

21. Poujeol, P., Jamison, R. L. and de Rouffignac, C.: Phosphate reabsorption in juxtamedullary nephron terminal segments. Pfluegers Arch. 387:27-31, 1980.

22. Dennis, V. W., Bello-Reuss, E. and Robinson, R.: Response of phosphate transport to parathyroid hormone in segments of rabbit nephron. Am. J. Physiol. 233:F29-F38, 1977.

PHOSPHATE REABSORPTION IN THE DISTAL CONVOLUTED TUBULE

William E. Lassiter and Romulo E. Colindres

Department of Medicine, Division of Nephrology
University of North Carolina School of Medicine
Chapel Hill, North Carolina 27514

Phosphate excretion by the mammalian kidney is subject to regulation by a number of factors including, but not limited to, dietary phosphorus intake, parathyroid hormone (PTH), and extracellular volume expansion. The primary quantitative importance of the proximal tubule in this regulation is well known, but the role of more distal nephron segments has been less clearly defined. It has long been recognized that the fraction of filtered phosphate delivered to distal convolutions accessible to micropuncture on the surface of the rat kidney may exceed fractional excretion, especially in phosphate retaining states, suggesting that further phosphate reabsorption occurs in the distal tubule and/or collecting duct (1). Early microinjection studies, however, failed to reveal significant distal phosphate reabsorption (2,3). Since the composition of the final urine reflects the pooled contributions of both superficial and deep nephrons, nephron heterogeneity, with more avid reabsorption in proximal tubules of juxtamedullary nephrons, was suggested as an alternative to distal reabsorption to explain the low urinary phosphate excretion (4). These two postulated mechanisms, distal reabsorption and nephron heterogeneity, need not of course be mutually exclusive.

We have looked closely at the question of distal phosphate reabsorption, using the technique of free flow micropuncture to determine the sites and magnitude of reabsorption along superficial nephrons in the rat (5,6). The modifying effects of extracellular volume expansion and of PTH were separately evaluated, and the question whether PTH is the mediator of the response to volume expansion was also addressed. Our observations indicate that the distal convoluted tubule may play a more important role in phosphate homeostasis than has been previously appreciated.

Table 1. Kidney function during hydropenia (H) and extracellular expansion (VE). H': Sustained hydropenia (time control). FE: Fractional excretion.

Group	Phase	GFR/100 g b.w. μl · min^{-1}	Plasma PO_4 m*M*	FE PO_4, %	FE Na, %
Normal rats (n = 5)	H	459±32	2.7±0.1	21.8±2.1	0.26±0.10
	H′	428±45	2.6±0.2	20.9±1.4	0.33±0.11
p		NS	NS	NS	NS
Normal rats (n = 9)	H	432±29	2.8±0.2	18.5±0.5	0.32±0.06
	VE	459±31	2.2±0.1	26.6±2.1	4.32±0.41
p		NS	<0.001	<0.005	<0.001
TPTX rats (n = 8)	H	442±20	3.6±0.1	4.3±0.0	0.12±0.03
	H′	408±10	3.5±0.1	4.0±1.1	0.12±0.03
p		NS	NS	NS	NS
TPTX rats (n = 10)	H	372±23	3.9±0.2	1.9±0.8	0.26±0.07
	VE	405±17	3.2±0.1	1.8±0.6	4.54±0.66
p		NS	<0.01	NS	<0.001

Young adult male Sprague-Dawley rats, 190-280 g, were anesthetized with pentobarbital and prepared for micropuncture. Prior to study the animals were maintained on a standard rat diet containing 0.8% phosphorus and 1% calcium. Two groups were studied, one with parathyroid glands intact ("normal"), and the other shortly after thyroparathyroidectomy (TPTX). Completeness of parathyroid gland removal was verified by direct examination of the excised tissue and confirmed functionally by increased phosphorus and decreased calcium concentrations in the plasma, and markedly reduced urinary phosphorus excretion.

To determine the effects of volume expansion, appropriate micropuncture and clearance measurements were obtained in each animal, first during hydropenia and then after expansion with a volume of isotonic saline equivalent to 10% body weight. Extracellular volume expansion was maintained with an appropriate sustaining infusion to replace urinary losses. Function of the micropunctured kidney is summarized in Table 1. In this and all subsequent tables and figures, results are presented as mean ± SE. Fractional excretion of phosphate and sodium are shown as percent of filtered load. Plasma phosphate concentration was increased, and phosphate excretion greatly decreased in the TPTX rats, but the two groups were in other respects comparable. Renal function did not change during sustained hydropenia, confirming the stability of the animal preparation over the time course of the experiments. Volume expansion was associated with a small rise

Table 2. Tubular fluid collections from distal convolutions in normal rats.
TF: Tubular fluid. P: plasma. UF: plasma ultrafiltrate.

	Early distal convolution		Late distal convolution	
	H	VE	H	VE
$(TF/P)_{In}$ (n = 9)	5.40±0.25	3.45±0.07	12.90±1.37	6.77±0.64
p	<0.001		<0.001	
SNGFR nl · min^{-1} (n = 9)	34.4±1.0	35.4±0.9	35.0±2.8	35.2±2.1
p	NS		NS	
$(TF/UF)_{PO_4}$ (n = 9)	1.39±0.09	1.23±0.08	2.85±0.43	2.20±0.29
p	NS		NS	
$(TF/UF)_{PO_4}/(TF/P)_{In}$×100 (n = 9)	26.2±1.8	36.0±2.2	21.4±1.7	32.1±1.7
p	<0.025		<0.005	
$(TF/P)_{Na}$ (n = 9)	0.40±0.04	0.32±0.01	0.34±0.04	0.33±0.02
p	NS		NS	
$(TF/P)_{Na}/(TF/P)_{In}$×100 (n = 9)	7.7±1.0	12.5±0.5	2.8±0.3	5.5±0.9
p	<0.005		<0.025	

Table 3. Tubular fluid collections from distal convolutions in TPTX rats.

	Early distal convolution		Late distal convolution	
	H	VE	H	VE
$(TF/P)_{In}$ (n = 10)	6.82±0.94	3.81±0.30	16.08±1.42	9.13±1.04
p	<0.005		<0.001	
SNGFR nl · min^{-1} (n = 10)	32.6±2.1	34.7±2.8	27.8±3.1	29.7±3.5
p	NS		NS	
$(TF/UF)_{PO_4}$ (n = 10)	0.72±0.11	0.49±0.09	0.43±0.11	0.41±0.08
p	<0.025		NS	
$(TF/UF)_{PO_4}/TF/P)_{In}$×100 (n = 10)	12.5±2.2	13.3±2.1	3.1±0.9	5.1±1.0
p	NS		NS	
$(TF/P)_{Na}$ (n = 10)	0.41±0.03	0.44±0.03	0.36±0.02	0.36±0.03
p	NS		NS	
$(TF/P)_{Na}/(TF/P)_{In}$×100 (n = 10)	7.0±0.9	12.2±1.3	2.40±0.3	4.6±0.6
p	<0.001		<0.025	

in GFR that was not statistically significant, and a small but significant decrease in plasma phosphorus concentration in both groups. Volume expansion produced a similar degree of natriuresis in the two groups but caused phosphaturia only in the normal rats.

Table 4. Percent filtered phosphate delivered to various nephron sites during hydropenia and extracellular volume expansion. P*: Statistical significance of change induced by volume expansion at designated nephron site.

	Late proximal tubule		Early distal convolution		Late distal convolution		Pelvic urine
Normal rats							
Hydropenia (n = 9)	32.1±1.2		26.2±1.8		21.4±1.7		18.5±0.5
p		<0.01		<0.025		NS	
Volume expansion (n = 9)	44.8±2.0		36.0±2.2		32.1±1.7		26.6±2.1
p		<0.001		<0.025		<0.005	
p*	<0.001		<0.025		<0.005		<0.005
TPTX rats							
Hydropenia (n = 10)	24.3±2.7		12.5±2.0		3.1±0.9		1.9±0.8
p		<0.001		<0.005		<0.01	
Volume expansion (n = 10)	35.1±3.0		13.4±2.0		4.8±0.9		1.8±0.6
p		<0.001		<0.005		<0.025	
p*	<0.001		NS		NS		NS

Not shown here, plasma calcium concentration decreased significantly during volume expansion, from 2.29 ± 0.10 to 1.94 ± 0.08 mM in the normal, and from 2.17 ± 0.09 to 1.72 ± 0.1 mM in the TPTX rats. Although not measured, this dilutional hypocalcemia was presumably accompanied by increased PTH secretion in the normal, but not in the TPTX group.

Effects of volume expansion on distal function are summarized in Tables 2 and 3. As expected, in normal animals (Table 2) the volume of tubular fluid, which is inversely proportional to the (TF/P) inulin ratio, and sodium delivery to the early distal convolution, expressed here as percent filtered load, were both increased by volume expansion. Phosphate delivery to the distal convoluted tubule also increased, but the percent absorbed between the two distal collection sites was little changed. A different pattern was observed in TPTX rats (Table 3). Although the effects of volume expansion on salt and water delivery were similar to the normal animals, the percent filtered phosphate delivered to the early distal collection site failed to increase. As in the normals, phosphate absorption along the distal convolution was unaltered.

Changes in phosphate delivery in response to extracellular volume expansion in the presence and absence of normal parathyroid function are shown more clearly in Table 4. The last accessible proximal convolution on the surface of the kidney is included for comparison. Phosphate reabsorption in the proximal tubule is inhibited, and therefore delivery to the late proximal puncture site was increased, to a similar degree in normal and

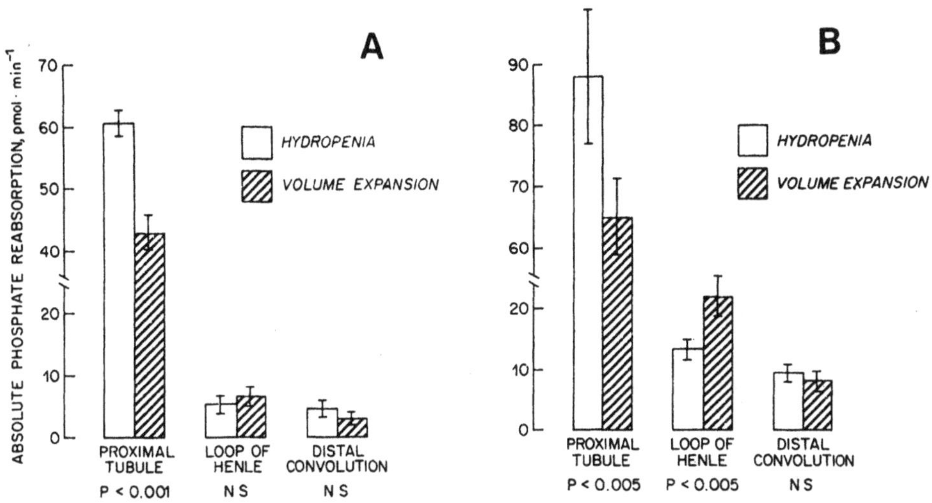

Fig. 1. Absolute magnitude of phosphate reabsorption in major nephron segments before and during extracellular volume expansion. A: normal rats. B: TPTX rats. Modified, with permission, from Pastoriza et al (6).

TPTX rats, but the increment in phosphate delivery was carried through nearly unchanged to subsequent puncture sites only in the normals. Thus volume expansion was associated with depressed reabsorption of phosphate in the proximal tubule, but with little change in more distal nephron segments in animals with normal parathyroid function. In contrast, in TPTX rats the increased phosphate delivered to the late proximal tubule was entirely reabsorbed in the loop of Henle, so that delivery to the early distal puncture site was unchanged. Phosphate reabsorption between the two distal collection sites was greater than in normal rats, but was little affected by volume expansion.

The absolute magnitude of phosphate reabsorption in each major nephron segment is illustrated in Fig. 1. In each segment the magnitude of phosphate reabsorption was greater in TPTX rats than in animals with normal parathyroid function. Nevertheless, volume expansion suppressed proximal reabsorption to a similar extent in the two groups, an effect that thus does not require the presence of PTH. In the loop of Henle, increased delivery of phosphate was accompanied by a compensatory increase in reabsorption when PTH was absent, comparable to the increased NaCl and water reabsorption that occurs with increased load in this nephron segment. In contrast, in rats with normal parathyroid

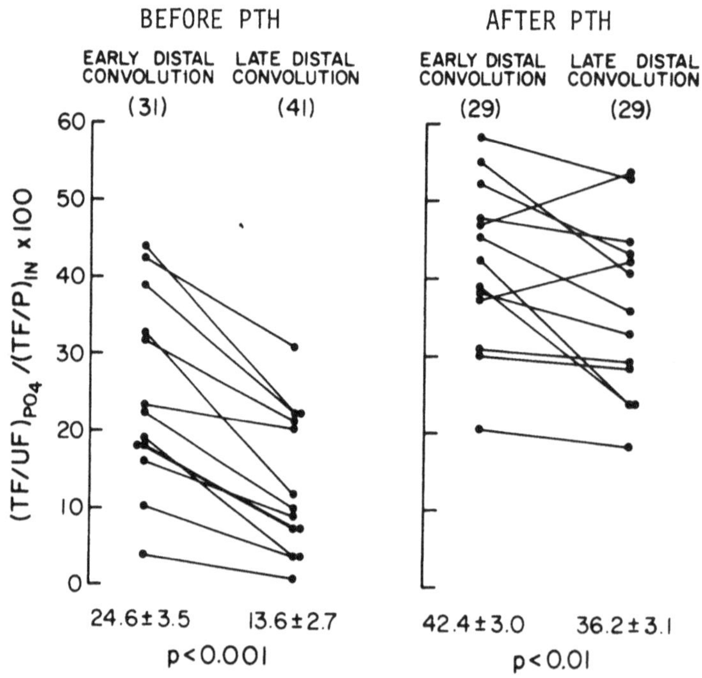

Fig. 2. Percent filtered phosphate delivered to distal convolution before and during PTH infusion in volume expanded TPTX rats. Number of collections at each site is shown in parentheses. Reproduced, with permission, from Pastoriza et al (5).

function, phosphate reabsorption in the loop failed to change in response to the increased load. Phosphate absorption along the distal convolution was little affected by volume expansion in either group.

Regardless of the state of hydration, distal phosphate reabsorption was less in normal animals than in those lacking PTH. To further document the effects of PTH on tubular function we studied TPTX rats during PTH infusion. To facilitate micropuncture, these animals were studied in a state of moderate sustained volume expansion. Time control observations demonstrated the stability of both kidney and single nephron function over the course of the experiments. Appropriate clearance measurements and micropuncture collections were made in the same animals before and during infusion of highly purified bovine PTH at a rate of 2 U/hr. Results in the 13 animals studied in this fashion are shown in Fig. 2. Each point in this figure represents mean percent phosphate delivery to the designated puncture site in an individual animal, and the lines connect early and late distal values for the same animal. Phosphate reabsorption along the distal convoluted tubule in the absence of PTH was equal to approximately 10% of the filtered load. During hormone administration phosphate delivery to the early distal convolution was increased, reflecting inhibition of reabsorption in more proximal segments, and reabsorption along the distal convolution was halved, although continuing at a rate significantly greater than zero. Phosphate excretion was greatly increased during PTH infusion, but sodium excretion did not change; thus tubular reabsorption of sodium, already suppressed in volume expansion, was not further inhibited by PTH.

The effect of PTH on the absolute magnitude of phosphate reabsorption in the various nephron segments is shown in the lower portion of Fig. 3. Reabsorption in the proximal tubule, although reduced by about 25% during PTH infusion, continued at a relatively high level, but reabsorption in the loop of Henle and the distal convolution was suppressed to less than half its former level. This effect on loop and distal phosphate absorption appears even more striking when one considers that the phosphate load to these nephron segments was greatly increased by PTH. This is shown graphically in the upper part of the figure, in which segmental reabsorption is shown as percent of the phosphate load presented to the nephron segment in question.

In order to obtain maximum separation between early and late distal collection sites, we selected distal tubules identified as either "very early" or "very late" on the basis of the tubular transit of fast green, and in most instances the early and late distal collections were from different nephrons. This is the approach usually taken in micropuncture studies because of the relative scarcity of individual nephrons that have multiple segments available for micropuncture on the surface of the kidney. It is assumed that the superficial nephrons are sufficiently homogeneous in function to permit extrapolation to the reabsorptive process in an individual nephron. To validate this assumption, we identified 9 nephrons in 4 volume-expanded TPTX rats in which successive collections could be made from two sites in the same distal tubule. These nephrons were identified by observing the passage of a tiny bolus of nigrosine dye injected into a proximal

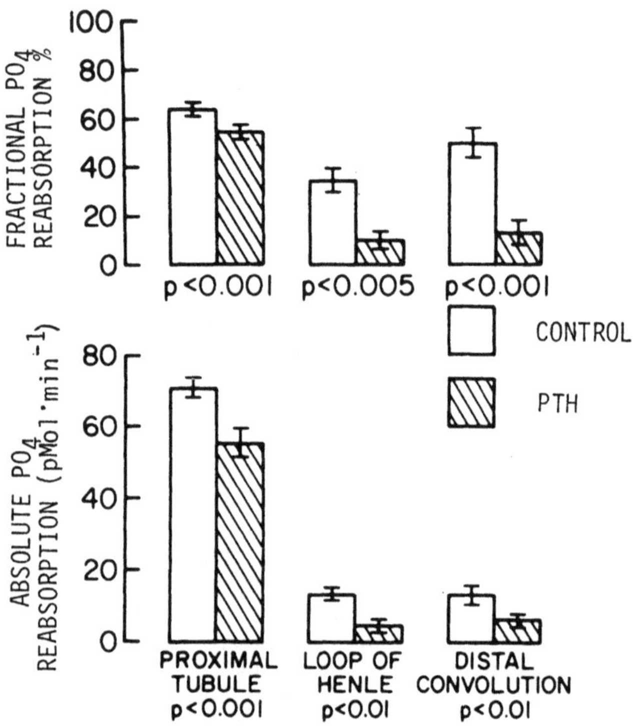

Fig. 3. Absolute and fractional phosphate reabsorption in nephron segments before and during PTH infusion in volume expanded TPTX rats. Modified, with permission, from Pastoriza et al (5).

tubule, and tubular fluid was collected first from the more distal site, so that leakage at the initial collection site could not affect tubular flow dynamics at the second. As shown in Table 5, despite the fact that in several cases the two puncture sites were relatively close together, we were able to demonstrate net phosphate reabsorption in 8 of the 9 nephrons studied. The measured reabsorption was approximately half that of the mean value observed in the other animals, but this is not surprising, since we had to be content with transit time separations

Table 5. Phosphate reabsorption in segments of individual distal convoluted tubules. Volume-expanded TPTX rats.

Tubule	Percent filtered load	pmol min^{-1}
1	3.9	6.6
2	4.6	6.0
3	-2.2	-2.7
4	1.3	2.0
5	3.4	5.5
6	7.1	8.1
7	8.7	11.0
8	7.9	10.0
9	4.9	4.0
Mean ± SE	4.4 ± 1.1	5.6 ± 1.4

as short as 10 sec., in contrast to a mean value of 30 sec. in the other studies.

To summarize our findings, we have documented the existence of phosphate reabsorption along superficial distal convoluted tubules in the rat kidney. These observations are compatible with Morel's demonstration of PTH-stimulated adenylate cyclase activity along the entire length of the distal convolution in the rat, in contrast to its absence from the early part of this segment in the rabbit (7). Although small in comparison to proximal reabsorption, phosphate reabsorption in the distal convoluted tubule is of sufficient magnitude to be physiologically significant. We believe it very likely has an important function in the homeostatic control of phosphate excretion. Phosphate reabsorption in the distal convolution, moreover, is suppressed although not abolished by PTH. Distal phosphate reabsorption is relatively insensitive to changes in extracellular volume, although its failure to increase in response to increased phosphate load during volume expansion in normal animals may have been due to a rise in circulating PTH induced by dilutional hypocalcemia. In the proximal tubule, water, sodium and phosphate reabsorption are all depressed to a similar degree by volume expansion, an effect that does not require the presence of PTH. PTH administration to volume expanded TPTX animals induces further suppression of phosphate reabsorption, but not of sodium and water. Finally, the failure of volume expansion to induce phosphaturia in TPTX animals, despite depressed proximal reabsorption, results from a load-dependent increase in phosphate reabsorption in the loop of Henle, which reduces the phosphate load presented to the distal convolution to pre-expansion levels.

We consider our evidence for phosphate reabsorption in the distal convolution to be unequivocal, but other investigators, using other techniques, have questioned its existence. As already noted, early studies failed to demonstrate reabsorption of radioactive phosphate microinjected into distal tubules (2,3). In general, microinjection studies tend to underestimate reabsorptive fluxes, since any increase in tubular flow induced by the injection will reduce apparent absorption. Recently, however, Knox, with his colleagues Greger and Lang, reported the absence of phosphate reabsorption after distal microinjection in Munich-Wistar rats, in a study in which the rate of injection was carefully controlled to prevent acceleration of flow (8). These same investigators also found no evidence of reabsorption after stop flow microperfusion (9). Although this technique has its quantitative limitations, phosphate reabsorption should have been detected had it occurred. Poujeol and de Rouffignac and their associates, likewise, failed to find distal reabsorption of phosphate after microinjection in Munich-Wistar rats. However, significant absorption, comparable to what we found in the distal convolution during free flow, was observed in two other variants of the Wistar strain, the Saclay and Bordeaux colonies (10). More recently these same investigators, in collaboration with Jamison, confirmed that phosphate reabsorption was very low after superficial distal microinjection in Munich-Wistar rats, but was large, amounting to 22% of the presented load, when the injection was made into loops of Henle of deep nephrons (11).

How can these apparently contradictory observations be reconciled? We do not believe they are due to technical artifact. Certainly some diversity of function is expected among different mammalian species and even, to a certain extent, among highly inbred strains of the same species. In most other aspects of renal physiology, however, one is struck more by the similarities than the differences between species and strains. We should like to suggest an alternative possibility, which we present as speculation, entirely without proof. Young adult Munich-Wistar rats share with immature rats of other strains two structural characteristics that make them attractive to micropuncturists. These are the persistence of superficial glomeruli visible on the surface of the kidney, and a delay in the overgrowth of renal cortex that ultimately renders the papilla inaccessible to micropuncture. Could these features of structural immaturity in the Munich-Wistar kidney reflect functional immaturity as well? The limited evidence available suggests that phosphate reabsorption in the distal portions of juxtamedullary nephrons in the Munich-Wistar rat is very similar to that which we have observed in superficial nephrons in the Sprague-Dawley (11). Since maturation occurs first in the deepest nephrons and then proceeds centrifugally towards the kidney surface, could it be that the failure of superficial distal tubules in the Munich-Wistar rat to reabsorb phosphate is a reflection of functional immaturity? A study of the effects of ageing on distal tubular function in Munich-Wistar rats and of immaturity in other strains might be revealing.

Finally, a word about nephron heterogeneity is in order. This has been suggested as a possible alternative to distal reabsorption, to explain large variations of phosphate excretion that may occur in association with relatively minor changes in reabsorption in superficial proximal tubules. Knox and his associates have presented convincing evidence that proximal tubules of juxtamedullary nephrons are more responsive than superficial nephrons to changes in homeostatic demand (4,12). Although quantitative differences undoubtedly exist, we believe that these deep nephrons will be found to respond to such interventions as PTH administration and volume expansion in a manner at least qualitatively similar to superficial nephrons. Furthermore, the observations of Poujeol, Jamison and de Rouffignac, just cited, suggest that it is reasonable to suppose that adaptive changes in phosphate reabsorption in deep nephrons might involve not only the proximal tubule but the distal nephron segments as well (11). While we do not wish to minimize the importance of nephron heterogeneity in determining the composition of the final urine, we nonetheless remain convinced that the distal convoluted tubule plays a highly significant role in phosphate homeostasis.

ACKNOWLEDGEMENT

This work was supported by NIH Grant HL02334.

REFERENCES

1. C. Amiel, H. Kuntziger, and G. Richet. Micropuncture study of handling of phosphate by proximal and distal nephron in normal and parathyroidectomized rat. Evidence for distal reabsorption. Pfluegers Arch. 317:93 (1970).
2. B. B. Staum, R. J. Hamburger, and M. Goldberg. Tracer microinjection study of renal tubular phosphate reabsorption in the rat. J. Clin. Invest. 51:2271 (1972).
3. M.G. Brunette, L. Taleb, and S. Carriere. Effect of parathyroid hormone on phosphate reabsorption along the nephron of the rat. Am. J. Physiol. 225:1076 (1973).
4. J. A. Haas, T. Berndt, and F.G. Knox. Nephron heterogeneity of phosphate reabsorption. Am. J. Physiol. 234:F287 (1978).

5. E. Pastoriza-Munoz, R. E. Colindres, W. E. Lassiter, and C. Lechene. Effect of parathyroid hormone on phosphate reabsorption in rat distal convolution. Am. J. Physiol. 235:F321 (1978).
6. E. Pastoriza-Munoz, R. E. Colindres, W. E. Lassiter, and C. Lechene. Effect of state of hydration on segmental phosphate reabsorption in rat nephron. Mineral Electrolyte Metab. 4: 246 (1980).
7. F. Morel. Site of hormone action in the mammalian nephron. Am. J. Physiol. 240:159 (1981).
8. R. Greger, F. Lang, G. Marchand, and F.G. Knox. Site of renal phosphate reabsorption. Micropuncture and microperfusion study. Pfluegers Arch. 369:111 (1977).
9. F. Lang, R. Greger, G. R. Marchand, and F. G. Knox. Stationary microperfusion study of phosphate reabsorption in proximal and distal nephron segments. Pfluegers Arch. 368:45 (1977).
10. P. Poujeol, B. Corman, C. Touvay, and C. de Rouffignac. Phosphate reabsorption in terminal nephron segments. Intrarenal heterogeneity and strain differences. Pfleugers Arch. 371: 39 (1977).
11. P. Poujeol, R. L. Jamison, and C. de Rouffignac. Phosphate reabsorption in juxtamedullary terminal nephron segments. Pfleugers Arch. 387:27 (1980).
12. F. G. Knox, J. A. Haas, T. Berndt, G. R. Marchand, and S. P. Youngblood. Phosphate transport in superficial and deep nephrons in phosphate-loaded rats. Am. J. Physiol. 233:F150 (1977).

METABOLIC ABNORMALITIES UNDERLYING THE PATHOGENESIS OF VITAMIN D RESISTANT RICKETS (VDRR)

Michele G. Brunette

Maisonneuve-Rosemont Hospital, Dept. of Pediatrics
Faculty of Medicine, Univ. of Montreal, Montreal, P.Q.

INTRODUCTION

Until recently, human investigation was the only means to study the pathogenesis of VDRR. In 1976 the discovery of a mouse model by Eicher et al facilitated the study of this disease. After five years, a substantial amount of data has accumulated, which will be summarized here.

THE SITE OF THE RENAL DEFECT

Although a defect in phosphate (Pi) transport is suspected in the intestine and bone cell, the excessive excretion of urinary Pi is probably the basis for the hypophosphatemia and the resulting symptoms.

The micropuncture studies (Giasson et al, 1977 and Cowgill et al, 1979) performed in rachitic mice, reported a major defect of Pi transport in the proximal convoluted tubule (PCT). In contrast, water and therefore Na transport, were found to be normal.

A defect in Pi transport in the PCT may result from either a curtailed inward transport through the luminal membrane or the basolateral membrane, or from a backflux of the electrolyte into the tubular lumen. As a consequence of these various possibilities, the defect may or may not modify the intracellular Pi content.

Eicher et al (1976) measured the inorganic and organic phosphorus content in cortex homogenates and found no difference between normal and rachitic mice. However, Drezner et al (1981) measured ATP as a probe of intracellular phosphate depletion and found this metabolite to be significantly decreased in diseased mice. The uptake of ^{32}Pi and its release by kidney slices are normal (Tenenhouse et al, 1978) suggesting a normal Pi movement through the basolateral membrane. In contrast, Pi transport studies through brush border membrane vesicle preparations clearly indicate a defect in rachitic mice, thus explaining the low ATP intracellular concentration.

Are the regulatory mechanisms of Pi transport preserved in VDRR? The finding of a brush border membrane defect does not establish its primary or secondary nature. However, it is plausible that a primary defect would curtail the normal response of this membrane to the physiological regulatory mechanisms.

Several studies (Tenenhouse and Scriver 1979, Mulbauer et al 1980, and Insogna et al 1981) indicate that the mechanisms of Pi saving in a phosphate depletion situation is intact in VDRR. Not only does the fractional excretion of Pi fall from 57% to 1.4% but also the Tm value increases in the same manner as in normal animals, but at lower levels. As in normal mice the information is transmitted to the brush border which reporduces in vitro the increased Pi uptake observed in vivo, following a low Pi diet.

In VDRR man the tubular response to exogenous PTH is curtailed. It has been proposed that the brush border membrane possesses two types of Pi transport, one of which, sensitive to PTH is absent in VDRR. This is probably not the case, since according to Cowgill et al (1979) and our laboratory (unpublished data), VDRR mice respond normally to parathyroidectomy by increasing Pi reabsorption in the same way as normal mice.

PLASMA PTH AND NUCLEOTIDE METABOLISM IN VDRR

The PTH level has been repeatedly measured in man and mice. In man, the results are contradictory; levels were found to be either normal or slightly increased (Arnaud et al 1971, Lewy et al 1972, and Reitz and Weinstein, 1973). In mice, Eicher et al (1976) and Cowgill et al (1979) reported normal or low normal levels. In any case, the hyperphosphaturia is not related to hyperparathyroidism.

Aside from the observations of a normal or almost normal PTH plasma level, and a well preserved response to parathyroidectomy, an abnormal nucleotide metabolism has been consistently reported in this disease. The absolute urinary excretion of cAMP was found to be high by Tenenhouse et al (1978) and by Meyer et al (1980b). However, the tissue adenylate cyclase response to PTH is significantly decreased (Cowgill et al, 1979). In a microdissection study (Brunette et al, 1979) we found that this defect was localized in the proximal convoluted tubule (PCT). In the distal convoluted tubule the adenylate cyclase response to PTH is normal but the response to calcitonin (CT) is sevenfold increased, an observation which may explain the consistent finding of an increased basal urinary cAMP excretion.

VITAMIN D METABOLISM IN VDRR

Because vitamin D also influences Pi transport through the PCT, its metabolism in VDRR was studied by several authors. In man and mouse, the basal plasma levels of $25OHD_3$ are normal (Haddad et al 1972, Meyer et al 1978). The basal level of $1,25(OH)_2D_3$ is also normal despite chronic phosphate depletion (Insogna, 1981). However, when the rachitic man or mouse is further depleted in phosphate by diet, the concentration of this metabolite falls (Insogna et al, 1981) or becomes undetectable (Meyer et al, 1980). This abnormality corresponds specifically to an incorrect response to phosphate deficiency, since calcium deficiency in rachitic mice yields to a normal increase of the metabolite. This curtailed response to phosphate deficiency may be an explanation for the decreased vitamin D_3 turnover observed in man by Avioli et al (1967). Low plasma levels of $24,25(OH)_2D_3$ has been recently reported by Meyer et al (1981), a finding which is interesting since this hormone is suspected to influence Pi transport through the bone cell.

Finally, alkaline phosphatase activity in the brush border membrane is decreased by 20% (Brunette et al, 1981). This low enzyme activity is unexpected if one considers the state of phosphate depletion in these rachitic animals.

COMMENT

Data are accumulating concerning the metabolic abnormalities accompanying the renal Pi transport defect in VDRR. None of them, however, can be considered to be at the origin of the disease. Positive findings concern the brush border membrane capacity of transporting Pi, nucleotide metabolism, vitamin D metabolism, and alkaline phosphatase activity in the brush border membrane. Let us discuss these positive findings, as well as the negative ones, on a schematic representation of factors which are known to influence Pi transport through the proximal tubule (Figure 1).

The Na linked transport of Pi through the brush border membrane is curtailed, but until the discovery of the exact molecular disease the primary or secondary nature of this disorder cannot be established.

The adenylate cyclase response to PTH is low in the PCT, a phenomenon which must be considered as secondary, because a primary defect would yield an increased Pi transport, rather than the contrary.

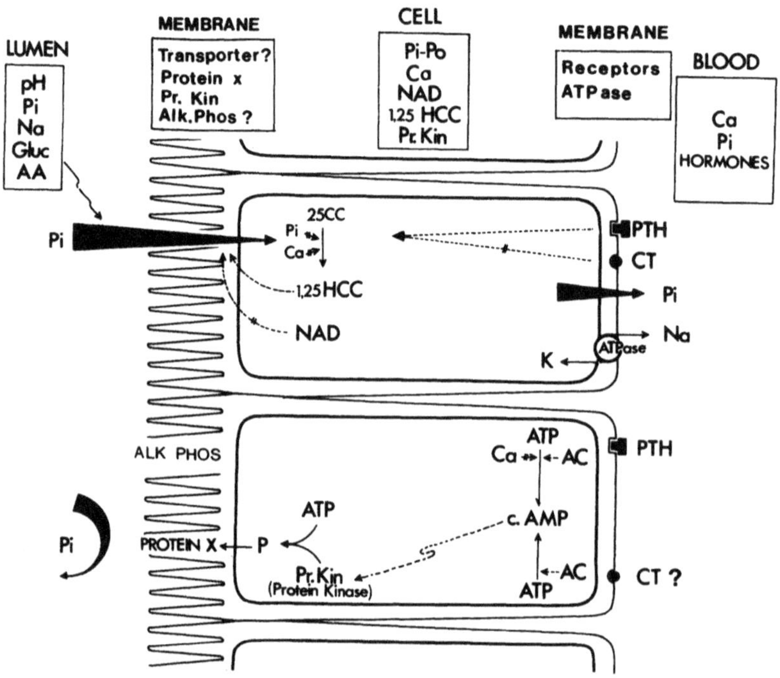

Figure 1. Factors regulating phosphate transport through the proximal tubule.

The adenylate cyclase response to CT in the distal tubule is exaggerated. However, the major or only site of the transport defect is proximal, thus minimizing this hypersensitivity to CT as a role in the pathogenesis of the disease.

The decreased response of adenylate cyclase to PTH stimulation, and the increased response of this enzyme to CT are not accompanied by any abnormal levels of tissue cAMP (Cowgill et al, 1979). It is, therefore, possible that cAMP catabolism is modified in this disease. Plasma calcitonin level has never been reported in the literature. It might be of value for the interpretation of these data.

The response of $1,25(OH)_2D_3$ to phosphate depletion is abnormally low but, here again, this is not at the origin of the disease which would resemble the well known entity of the pseudocarential rickets.

Finally, alkaline phosphatase activity is diminished. The exact role of this enzyme in Pi transport is unknown, but recent data suggests that inhibition of this enzyme in brush border vesicle preparations does not influence Pi transport through these vesicles, thus denying any direct role of this enzyme in this transport.

Negative findings do not really contribute to our understanding of the disease. The brush border membrane maintains its capacity of adaptation to phosphate depletion, and the total kidney response to PTX is also intact. The integrity of these mechanisms is compatible with a quantitative rather than a qualitative problem of a Pi transporter or with an extrarenal cause of phosphaturia.

Many other factors influencing Pi transport in the kidney were also found to be normal in VDRR, such as amino acid, glucose, bicarbonate and Na+ transport, which eliminates these substrate transport defects as causes of the disease.

There is no consensus about Pi transport in the gut in VDRR. Stickler (1963) and Short et al (1973) utilizing two different techniques concluded that a phosphate transport defect occurs in gut. However, Glorieux et al (1976) did not consistently find a significant decrease of ^{33}P uptake in human biopsies, nor did they confirm the conclusion of O'Doherty et al (1977) who reported a lack of response to $1,25(OH)_2D_3$ in mice.

Finally, in bone, Glorieux et al (1980) and Marie et al (1981) described two fundamental lesions: rickets and osteomalacia. Treatment with phosphate supplement improves rickets and treatment with $1,25(OH)_2D_3$ improves the osteomalacia. But the necessity of utilizing high doses of $1,25(OH)_2D_3$, despite the correction of plasma phosphate suggests a primary transport defect at the level of the osteoblast.

CONCLUSION AND PROSPECTIVE

Data concerning VDRR are accumulating but many links are missing and the origin of the disease is still unknown. Many fields of investigation in and outside the kidney should be undertaken; the modification of the brush border membrane should be identified, the intracellular electrolyte distribution, the redox system should be studied. The modulation of 1,25 and $24,25(OH)_2D_3$ synthesis, the catabolism of cAMP should be further studied. Calcitonin should be measured. However, those efforts may hit the obstacle of our lack of knowledge of the normal steps of the pathology of the Pi transport. It is likely that the understanding of the pathogenesis of this disease will closely follow progress in the basic understanding of the normal physiology of membrane transport.

REFERENCES

Arnaud, C., Glorieux, F., and Scriver, C., 1971, Serum parathyroid hormone in X-linked hypophoshatemia, Sciences, 1973:845-847.

Avioli, V., Williams, T.F., Lund, J., and DeLuca, H.F., 1967, Metabolism of vitamin D_3 ^3H in vitamin D resistant rickets and familial hypophosphatemia, J. Clin. Invest., 46:1907-1915.

Brunette, M.G., Chabardes, D., Imbert-Teboul, M., Clique, A., Montegut, M., Morel, F., 1979, Hormone sensitive adenylate cyclase along the nephron of genetically hypophosphatemic mice, Kidney Int., 15:357-369.

Brunette, M.G., Chan, M., Lebrun, M., 1981, Phosphatase activity along the nephron of mice with hypophosphatemic vitamin D resistant rickets, Kidney Int., In Press.

Cowgill, L.D., Goldfarb, S., Lau, K., Slatopolsky, E., and Agus, Z.S., 1979, Evidence for an intrinsic renal tubular defect in mice with genetic hypophosphatemic rickets, J. Clin. Invest., 63:1203-1210.

Drezner, M.K., Holmes, E.W., and Sabina, R.L., 1981, Evidence for phosphate deficiency in the X-linked hyp-mouse kidney: observations paradoxical to normal serum $1,25(OH)_2D_3$ levels, Am. Soc. Bone and Minerals, Annual Meetings, Cincinnati, (Abstract).

Eicher, E.M., Southard, J.L., Scriver, C.R., and Glorieux, F., 1976, Hypophosphatemia: mouse model for human familial hypophosphatemic (vitamin D resistant) rickets, Proc. Natl. Acad. Sci. USA, 73:4667-4671.

Giasson, S.C., Brunette, M.G., Danan, G., Vigneault, N., and Carriere, S., 1977, Micropuncture study of renal phosphorus transport in hypophosphatemic vitamin D resistant rickets mice. Pflugers Arch., 371:33-38.

Glorieux, F.H., Morin, C.L., Travers, R., Delvin, E.E., Poirier, R., 1976, Intestinal phosphate transport in familial hypophosphatemic rickets, Pediat. Res., 10:691-696.

Glorieux, F.H., Marie, P.J., Pettifor, J.M., Delvin, E.E., 1980, Bone response to phosphate salts, ergocalciferol and calcitrol in hypophosphatemic vitamin D resistant rickets, New Engl. J. Med., 303:1023-1031.

Haddad, J.G., Chyu, K.J., Hahn, T.J., and Stamp, T.C.B., 1973, Serum concentrations of 25 hydroxy vitamin D in sex-linked hypophosphatemic vitamin D-resistant rickets, J. Lab. Clin. Med., 81:22.

Isogna, K., Stewart, A., and Gertner, J., 1981, Impaired response to acute phosphorus deprivation in sex-linked hypophosphatemic rickets, Am. Soc. for Bone and Minerals, Annual Meeting, Cincinnati.

Lewy, J.E., Cabana, E.C., Repetto, H.A., Canterbury, J.M., and Reiss, E., 1972, Serum parathyroid hormone in hypophosphatemic vitamin D resistant rickets. J. Pediat., 81:294-300.

Marie, P.J., Travers, R., Glorieux, F.H., 1981, Healting of rickets with phosphate supplementation in the hypophosphatemic male mouse, J. Clin. Invest., 67:911-914.

Meyer, R.A., Gray, R.W., Meyer, M.H., 1980a, Abnormal vitamin D metabolism in the X-linked hypophosphatemic mouse, Endocrinology, 107:1577-1581.

Meyer, R.A., Gray, R.W., Kiebza, K., and Mish, P.M., 1980b, Altered vitamin D, cyclic nucleotide and trace mineral metabolism, E. Ritz and H. Jahn Eds., Phosphate and Minerals in Health and Disease, Plenum Press, New York, 351-359.

Meyer, R.A., Meyer, M.H., and Gray, R.W., 1981, Metabolites of vitamin D in X-linked hypophosphatemic mice, Am. Soc. for Bone and Minerals, Annual Meeting, Cincinnati, (Abstract 22A).

Mulbauer, R., Bonjour, J.P., and Fleisch, H., 1980, Tubular handling of phosphate and Ca in X-linked hypophosphatemic mice: defective adaptation to Pi restriction associated with a renal Ca leak, VII International Conference on Ca Regulating Hormones, Estes Park, Colorado.

O'Doherty, P.J.A., DeLuca, H.F., and Eicher, E.M., 1977, Lack of effect of vitamin D and its metabolites on intestinal phosphate transport in familial hypophosphatemia of mice, Endocrinology, 101: 1325-1330.

Reitz, R.E., and Weinstein, R.L., 1973, Parathyroid hormone secretion in familial vitamin D resistant rickets, 1973, N.E. J. Med., 289: 941-945.

Short, E., Binder, H.J., Rosenberg, L.E., 1973, Familial hypophosphatemic rickets: defective transport of inorganic phosphate by intestinal mucosa, Science, 179:700-702.

Stickler, G.B., 1963, External calcium and phosphorus balances in vitamin D. resistant rickets, J. Pediat., 63:942.

Tenenhouse, H.S., Scriver, C.R., McInnes, R.R., Glorieux, F.H., 1978, Renal handling of phosphate in vivo and in vitro by the X-linked hypophosphatemic male mouse: Evidence for a defect in the brush border membrane, Kidney Int., 14:236-244.

Tenenhouse, H.S., and Scriver, C.R., 1979, Renal brush border membrane adaptation to phosphorus deprivation in the Hyp/Y mouse, Nature, 281:225-227.

RELATIONSHIP BETWEEN PLASMA PHOSPHATE AND RENAL HANDLING OF PHOSPHATE: STUDIES WITH LOW PHOSPHATE DIET AND NICOTINAMIDE

Aviad Haramati and Franklyn G. Knox

Department of Physiology & Biophysics
Mayo Medical School
Rochester, Minnesota

Acute intravenous infusions of phosphate have been used to study the relationship between plasma phosphate concentration and renal phosphate excretion (1 - 10). Animals maintained on a normal intake of phosphorus (0.8 - 1.2%) respond to acute phosphate infusions with phosphate excretions ranging from 60 - 90% of the filtered load (5, 7, 9). The high phosphate excretions are not only the result of increases in tubular load exceeding the reabsorptive capacity, but recent studies indicate that at high plasma phosphate concentrations (induced by prolonged intravenous phosphate infusions) the maximal transport rate actually declines (3, 4, 6, 9-11).

The reasons for the decrease in reabsorption are not readily apparent. The fall of phosphate reabsorption occurs in thyroparathyroidectomized (TPTX) as well as in intact animals and is therefore independent of parathyroid hormone (6, 9, 10, 12). Other factors such as volume, acid base status and plasma potassium have also been ruled out as playing central roles in this effect (12). In separate studies, Frick and Durasin (9) and Oberleithner et al (10) found that if the hypocalcemia associated with phosphate infusion is corrected by infusion of calcium, the fall in phosphate reabsorption can be attenuated. Thus, it was proposed that hypocalcemia may mediate the decrease in phosphate transport (9, 10, 12).

As mentioned earlier, most of the studies just described examined the renal effects of phosphate infusions in animals maintained on a normal phosphate diet. However, the influence of diet on renal phosphate handling is so pronounced that dietary intake of phosphate is now recognized to be an important, if not primary, regulator of renal phosphate excretion (11, 14). Therefore, the effects of changes in dietary intake of phosphate on the renal response to phosphate infusions needs to be evaluated. It might be argued that, since the tubular adaptation to dietary phosphate intake occurs at times without changes in plasma phosphate, the adaptation is independent of plasma phosphate and would therefore not respond to increases in plasma phosphate by phosphate infusions. On the other hand, it is possible that the infusion of phosphate results not only in increases in plasma phosphate, but also in changes of other factors that may modulate phosphate excretion. Indeed, previous studies examining this question have yielded somewhat conflicting results.

Steele and DeLuca (8) demonstrated that in rats maintained on a diet containing 1.0% phosphorus for two weeks and subsequently acutely TPTX, the infusion of 7.5 μmol/min of phosphate increased fractional phosphate excretion from a baseline of 1% to 23% at 2 hours post-infusion. However, in rats on a lower phosphorus diet (0.02%), the increase in fractional phosphate excretion in response to the same protocol was significantly less, from a baseline of 0.2% to 9%. These experiments were repeated in animals chronically TPTX (48 hr) with no change in fractional phosphate excretion of 0.2%. In contrast, Troehler et al (7) found that the infusion of 7 μmol/min of phosphate resulted in significant increases in phosphate excretion in chronically TPTX rats fed either a low (0.2%) or normal phosphorus diet (1.2%). Although the increase in fractional phosphate excretion from 0.12% to 65% in rats fed a low phosphorus diet was less than that seen in the normal diet from 2.5% to 76%, the widely different phosphate excretions obtained in low phosphate diet in both these studies, 0.2% vs. 65%, makes it difficult to conclude whether phosphate infusions are phosphaturic in phosphate deprivation.

Consequently, in the first series of experiments, we sought to re-examine the effect of adaptation to a low phosphate diet on the renal response to acute phosphate infusions. Clearance experiments were performed in six rats fed a low phosphate diet (0.07%) for 4 days prior to the experiment. Previous balance studies in our laboratory have demonstrated that by day 3 on this diet the urine is essentially phosphate-free. The animals underwent acute TPTX on the day of the experiment, and allowed 2 hours to recover from surgery and to attain steady state. Following a control clearance period, phosphate was infused at progressively increasing rates of 1, 2 and 3 μmol/min.

In response to phosphate infusion, plasma phosphate concentration increased in a stepwise fashion from a control value of 2.26 ± .23 mM to a final value of 4.91 ± .14 mM. However, fractional phosphate excretion remained unchanged throughout the phosphate infusions (Figure 1). These findings concur with results obtained by Steele and DeLuca (8) as described earlier. It is possible that part of the discrepancy between these observations and those reported by Troehler et al (7) may relate to different dietary regimens. Troehler et al utilized a diet (0.2%) which, although it resulted in lower phosphate excretions compared to normal (1.2%) or high (1.8%) phosphate diets, was perhaps not sufficient to induce a condition of phosphate deprivation characterized by a resistance to the phosphaturic effects of acute phosphate infusions.

In a second series of experiments we tested whether pretreatment with nicotinamide (NiAm) will reverse the resistance of phosphate-deprived rats to phosphate infusion. The rationale for these experiments stems from recent studies proposing an important role of nicotinamide adenine dinucleotide (NAD) as an intracellular regulator of renal phosphate transport (15 - 17). We previously reported that NiAm treatment increased renal cortical NAD content and restored the phosphaturic response to PTH, calcitonin and dibutyryl cAMP in rats fed a low phosphate diet (16, 18). The present series was conducted to determine whether NiAm pretreatment will reverse the resistance to the phosphaturic effects of a non-hormonal stimulus, namely, phosphate infusions. The experiments were performed in 6 acutely TPTX rats fed a low phosphate diet (0.07%) and injected with NiAm (1 g/kg) 2 hours prior to anesthesia. The subsequent experimental protocol was identical to the first series.

As in the earlier group, plasma phosphate concentration increased progressively in response to phosphate infusions, from a control value of 2.50 ± .16 mM to a value of 4.28 ± .20 mM during the final phosphate infusion. However, in contrast to the control rats, fractional phosphate excretion in NiAm-treated rats increased steadily from a control excretion of 2.2 + 1.7% to 20.4 ± 4.0% at 3 μmol/min (Figure 1). It is not likely that the effects of NiAm pretreatment were related to the decline in plasma calcium since values changed similarly in response to phosphate infusion in both groups (from 1.89 ± .08 mM to 1.24 ± .03 mM in control rats versus 1.85 ± 0.7mM to 1.30 ± .05mM in NiAm-treated rats).

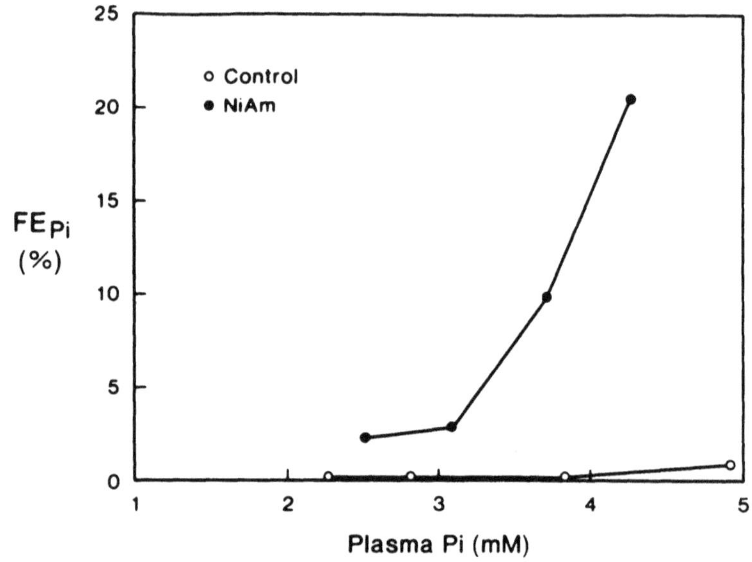

Figure 1.

The results of these studies are summarized in figure 1 depicting the relationship between phosphate excretion and plasma phosphate concentration. During phosphate deprivation, acute increases in plasma phosphate do not lead to a phosphaturia. Pretreatment with NiAm increases baseline phosphate excretion which is not related to plasma phosphate concentration. However, phosphate infusions which raise plasma phosphate >3.0 mM evoke a phosphaturic response. These studies are consistent with the hypothesis proposed by Dousa and colleagues (15, 17) which postulates that NAD is an important modulator of renal phosphate transport.

ACKNOWLEDGEMENTS

The authors gratefully acknowledge the contributions of Michael Baldwin and Jeffrey Postlewaite to these studies, during their participation in the Student Interim program of the Mayo Medical School.

We thank Theresa Berndt, Rita Glasscock, John Haas and Marcy Onsgard for their technical assistance, and June M. Hanke for providing secretarial assistance.

These studies were supported by AM 19715, AM 07013 and the Mayo Foundation.

REFERENCES

1. Pitts, R. F. and R. S. Alexander. The renal reabsorptive mechanism for inorganic phosphate in normal and acidotic dogs. Am. J. Physiol. 142:648-662, 1944.
2. Hogben, C. A. M. and J. L. Bollman. Renal reabsorption of phosphate: Normal and thyroparathyroidectomized dog. Am. J. Physiol. 164:670-681, 1951.
3. Frick, A. Reabsorption of inorganic phosphate in the rat kidney I. Saturation of transport mechanism. II. Suppression of fractional phosphate reabsorption due to expansion of extracellular fluid volume. Pfluegers Arch. 304:351-364, 1968.
4. LeGrimellec, C., N. Roinel and F. Morel. Simultaneous Mg, Ca, P. K. Na and Cl analysis in rat tubular fluid. IV. During acute phosphate plasma loading. Pfluegers Arch. 346:189-204, 1974.
5. Boudry, J. F., U. Troehler, M. Touabi, H. Fleisch and J.-P. Bonjour. Secretion of inorganic phosphate in the rat nephron. Clin. Sci. Mol. Med. 48:475-489, 1975.
6. Engle, J. E. and T. H. Steele. Renal phosphate reabsorption in the rat: Effect of inhibitors. Kidney Int. 8:98-104, 1975.
7. Troehler, U., J.-P. Bonjour and H. Fleisch. Inorganic phosphate homeostasis. Renal adaptation to the dietary intake in intact and thyroparathyroidectomized rats. J. Clin. Invest. 57:264-273, 1976.
8. Steele, J. H. and H. F. DeLuca. Influence of dietary phosphorus on renal phosphate reabsorption in the parathyroidectomized rat. J. Clin. Invest. 57:867-874, 1976.
9. Frick, A. and I. Durasin. Maximal reabsorptive capacity for inorganic phosphate (TM_{Pi}) in the absence of parathyroid hormone in the rat: Decrease of the TM_{Pi} during prolonged administration of phosphate and the role of calcium. Pfluegers Arch. 377:9-14, 1978.
10. Oberleithner, H., R. Greger and F. Lang. Role of calcium in the decline of phosphate reabsorption during phosphate loading in acutely thyroparathyroidectomized rats. Pfluegers Arch. 374:249-254, 1978.
11. Thompson, D. D. and H. H. Hiatt. Effects of phosphate loading and depletion on the renal excretion and reabsorption of inorganic phosphate. J. Clin. Invest. 36:566-572, 1957.
12. Lang, G., H. Oberleithner, R. Greger and P. Deetjen. Factors involved in the altered phosphate reabsorption during phosphate loading in thyroparathyroidectomized rats. Adv. Exp. Med. Biol. 103:81-86, 1978.
13. Lang. F. Renal handling of calcium and phosphate. Klin. Wochenschr. 58:985-1003, 1980.

14. Sutton, R. A. L. and J. H. Dirks. Renal handling of calcium, phosphate and magnesium. IN: The Kidney, B. M. Brenner and F. C. Rector, eds., Saunders, Chapt. 12, pp. 551-618, 1981.
15. Kempson, S. A., G. Colon-Otero, S.-Y. L. Ou, S. T. Turner and T. P. Dousa. Possible role of nicotinamide adenine dinucleotide as an intracellular regulator of renal transport of phosphate in the rat. J. Clin. Invest. 67:1347-1360, 1981.
16. Berndt, T. J., F. G. Knox and T. P. Dousa. Role of nicotine-adenine dinucleotide (NAD) in the phosphaturic response to parathyroid hormone (PTH). Kidney Int. 19:108, 1981 (Abstract).
17. Dousa, T. P. and S. A. Kempson. Regulation of renal brush border membrane transport of phosphate. Min. & Elect. Metab. 1981 (in press).
18. Berndt, T. J., F. G. Knox, S. A. Kempson and T. P. Dousa. Nicotinamide adenine dinucleotide and renal response to parathyroid hormone. Endocrinology 108:2005-2007, 1981.

PROTEIN PHOSPHORYLATION IN PROXIMAL TUBULAR BRUSH-BORDER MEMBRANES

Jürg Biber, Vito Scalera and Heini Murer

Institute of Physiology, University of Zurich, Zurich
Switzerland

Many processes of the living cell are currently believed to be finally regulated via the phosphorylation status of some of the proteins involved, whereby such phosphorylation processes can be influenced by various factors, e.g. cAMP and/or Ca^{2+}-ions (1).

For proximal tubular transport of inorganic phosphate evidence is obtained for a cAMP-dependent regulation of the sodium dependent phosphate transport mechanism located in the brush border membrane. It has been shown that an acute infusion or injection of parathyroid hormone or dibutyryl-cAMP leads to a decrease in the sodium dependent phosphate reabsorption (2,3). Interestingly, brush border membrane vesicles isolated from parathyroid hormone treated or dibutyryl-cAMP infused animals show also reduced sodium-dependent phosphate transport activity as compared to vesicles isolated from control animals (4). A first evidence for a protein phosphorylation mediated action of parathyroid hormone has been obtained by showing a parathyroid hormone dependent change in phosphorylation of rat kidney cortical proteins (5).

As the parathyroid hormone effect seems to be retained - at least in terms of transport functions - at the level of the isolated brush border membrane, there might be a reasonable chance to test more directly a possible role of protein phosphorylation as a final event in parathyroid hormone dependent alteration in sodium dependent phosphate transport.

In order to study the phosphorylation of the membrane proteins of the brush border and the basal-lateral membrane of the renal proximal tubular epithelial cell, a system is described in this contribution which allows an analysis of the phosphorylation of these membranes under "physiological" conditions, starting with an incubation of cortical kidney slices. The experiments presented represent only a characterization of the system without attempting to document specific alterations.

METHODS

Cortex slices from rat kidneys (male wistar, 200 gr.) were cut into small pieces. Cortex from half a kidney was then incubated in 3 ml of a minimal essential medium (GIBCO 78-5217) to which was added $CaCl_2$ (2 mmoles/l), L-lactate (5 mmoles/l) and $NAHCO_3$ (25 mmoles/l). The incubation was performed at 37° C under a continuous stream of 95% O_2 / 5% CO_2 in a shaking water bath at about 100 cycles per min. ^{32}P-orthophosphate was added up to 50 μCi/ml, which resulted in a free concentration of phosphate of 0,1 mmoles/l. At the end of the incubation period brush border and basal-lateral membranes were prepared as follows:

Brush border membranes were prepared by a Mg/EGTA precipitation method (6) in a buffer of 300 mmoles/l mannitol, 5 mmoles/l EGTA and 30 mmoles/l Tris-HCl (pH 7.2). Starting from one slice, enough brush border membranes could be obtained for the subsequent analysis. Starting from one kidney, baso-lateral membranes were prepared according to Heidrich et al. (7). After a mild homogenization a heavy microsomal fraction was obtained, which was further separated by free-flow electrophoresis (Desaga FF48).

Protein phosphorylation was analyzed by SDS-polyacrylamidgel-electrophoresis according to Laemmli (8) on 8,4% gels. Membranes were denaturated by boiling for 2 min in a Tris-buffer (pH 6,8) containing 2% SDS and 25% β-mercaptoethanol. Gel-electrophoresis was calibrated using molecular weight standards from Pharmacia. Autoradiography was performed on Kodak X-ray films (X-omat, SO-282) at - 80° C. Protein was determined according to Bradford (9) using the Bio Rad reagent.

RESULTS AND DISCUSSION

When rat kidney cortex slices were incubated for various times, total incorporation of ^{32}P into the brush border membrane phospholipids and proteins increases almost linearly over a period of 3

Table 1. Incorporation of ^{32}P into brush border membranes from proximal tubules

time of incubation min.	total incorporation of ^{32}P cpm/mg protein	incorporation of ^{32}P into	
		the lipids* %	the proteins* %
10	120'000	16	35
30	236'000	45	65
60	400'000	100	100
90	560'000	145	95
120	650'000	215	112
150	792'000	300	100

Brush border membranes were prepared after an incubation of cortex slices as described in Methods. The lipids were separated from the proteins by chromatography on Sephadex LH-60, equilibrated with EtOH: 80% HCOOH = 4 : 1 (v/v). Brush border membranes were solubilized in the same solvent system by shaking for one minute.
*The data are given in percentages of the value obtained after an incubation of 1 hour. [100% in the lipids = 240'000 cpm/mg protein; 100% in the proteins = 160'000 cpm/mg protein]. The data represent the mean of at least two experiments.

hours (Table 1). In order to analyze the incorporation of ^{32}P into the proteins and the lipids separately, brush border membranes were solubilized in EtOH/80% HCOOH = 4 : 1 (v/v) and separated by chromatography on Sephadex LH-60. This quantitative separation of the lipids and the proteins showed, that the incorporation of ^{32}P into the protein fraction reaches a plateau after an incubation period of 60 min and that this phosphorylation status is stable at least for the next two hours. However, the incorporation of ^{32}P into the lipid fraction increases almost linearly over the total incubation period (Table 1). That the metabolic activity of the cell is a prerequisite for the incorporation of ^{32}P into the brush border membranes is indicated as follows: i) When ^{32}P was added to a homogenate of cortex slices, which has been incubated in the absence of ^{32}P, no radioactivity could be detected in the brush border membrane fraction. ii) Metabolic inhibitors like KCN, FCCP and dinitrophenol prevented the incorporation of ^{32}P into the brush border membrane to a large extent (Table 2).

Table 2. Effect of metabolic inhibitors on the incorporation of ^{32}P in the brush border membranes

Inhibitor	Total incorporation of ^{32}P cpm/mg protein	%
no addition	92076	100
1 mM KCN	53404	58
5 mM dinitrophenole	21177	23
FCCP (3 μg/ml)	23019	25

Brush border protein phosphorylation was further analyzed by SDS polyacrylamide-gelelectrophoresis and subsequent autoradiography (Fig. 1). Most of the polypeptides stained by Coomassie-Blue could also be detected by autoradiography. That this phosphorylation pattern represents ^{32}P bound to the polypeptides is documented as follows: i) The ^{32}P-pattern of the protein fraction after Sephadex LH-60 chromatography is almost identical to the original one (not shown); and ii) after ^{32}P was added to denaturated but unlabeled brush border membranes no unspecifically bound radioactivity could be detected on the gels (not shown). Furthermore, it could be shown, that most of the ^{32}P bound to the polypeptides is linked to threonine and/or serine residues (not shown).

In addition, brush border membrane vesicles were also phosphorylated by γ-^{32}P-ATP. Since brush border membranes are obtained as closed and right side out vesicles (10), phosphorylation of the brush border membrane at the cytoplasmic surface is only possible if ATP is able to traverse the membrane. In the experiment shown in Fig. 1 (C + D) phosphorylation by γ-^{32}P-ATP was performed in the presence of 0,1% saponine as detergent. The phosphorylation pattern obtained by the use of γ-^{32}P-ATP under these conditions turned out to be similar to the one obtained by the in vitro incubation of the slices. In the absence of the detergent however, only two polypeptides of similar molecular weights were phosphorylated, corresponding to the alkaline phosphatase (11). These results indicate that most of the acceptor sites for ^{32}P are located at the cytoplasmic surface of the brush border membrane. These sites are certainly also accessible under the in vitro conditions.

The small differences in the phosphorylation pattern as observed by the two different phosphorylation procedures, might indicate the problems in performing such experiments. The differences can be due to several factors, e.g. dephosphorylation during mem-

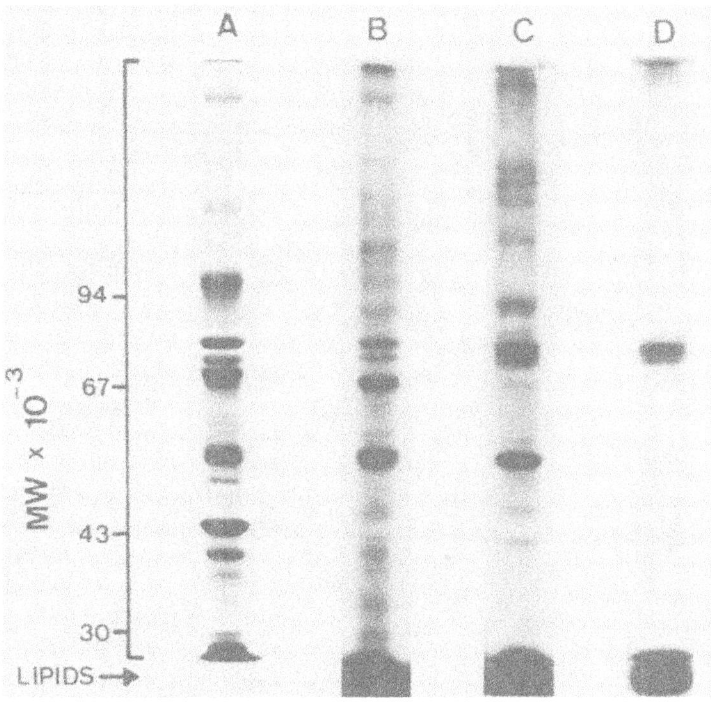

Fig. 1. Phosphorylation patterns of brush border membranes from rat renal cortex. Brush border membranes were labeled in vitro by incubation of slices with ^{32}P-orthophosphate [B] and by γ-^{32}P-ATP in the presence of 0,1% saponine [C] or in the absence of saponine [D]. Phosphorylation by 20 µmoles/l γ-^{32}P-ATP (10 µCi) was performed in 50 mmoles/l mannitol, 10 mmoles/l Tris-HCL (pH 7.5) and 5 mmoles/l $MgCl_2$ for 30 s at room-temperature. The reaction was stopped by denaturating the membranes as described in Methods. Gel-electrophoresis was performed on (8,4 x 2,7)-gels. [A]: Coomassie-Blue staining.

brane isolation or different organization of the membrane proteins due to a given isolation procedure.

In order to study regulation mechanisms of transepithelial transport processes, basal-lateral membranes have also to be considered. Therefore basal-lateral membranes from the proximal tubule were purified as well and analyzed by gelelectrophoresis. Fig. 2. shows the polypeptide pattern and the phosphorylation patterns of the NaK-ATPase rich fractions (basal-

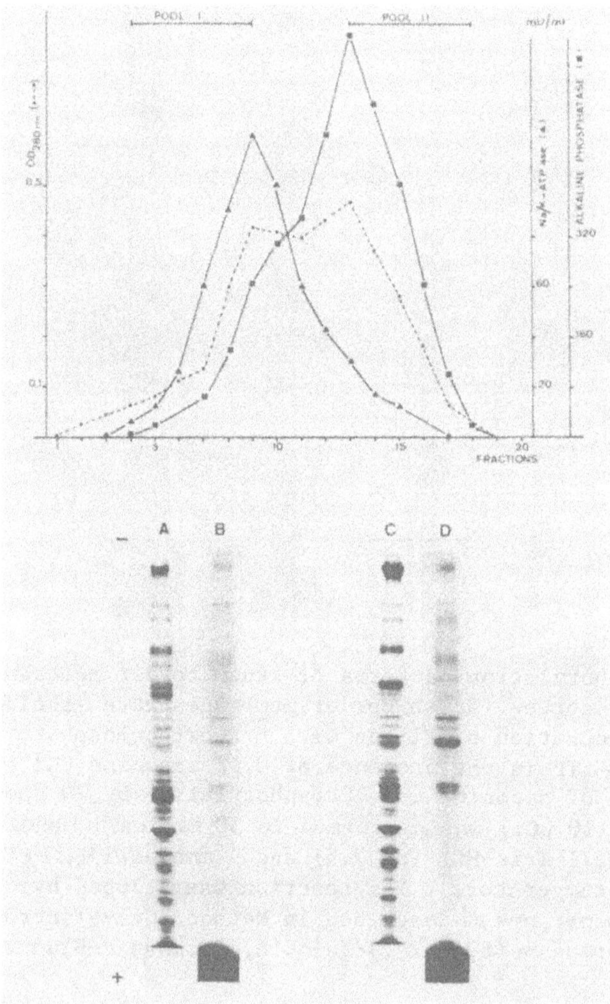

Fig. 2. Phosphorylation patterns of brush border and basal-lateral membranes separated by free-flow electrophoresis. Membranes were isolated from cortex slices of one kidney incubated in vitro with ^{32}P-orthophosphate. Na/K-ATPase rich fractions (pool I) and alkaline phosphatase rich fractions (pool II) were analyzed by SDS-polyacrylamide-gelelectrophoresis. A, C: Coomassie Blue staining; B,D: Autoradiography.

lateral membranes) and the alkaline phosphatase rich fractions (brush border membranes)after separation by free flow electrophoresis Although a separation of the two membranes was obtained, the polypeptide pattern as well as the phosphorylation pattern of the brush border and the basal-lateral membranes were not strikingly different*. In general however, less protein bound ^{32}P could be detected in the basal-lateral membrane fraction, as juged by gel-electrophoresis.

In addition, it is shown that the phosphorylation pattern of the brush border membranes prepared by free-flow electrophoresis is similar to that of brush border membranes prepared by the Mg/EGTA-method (compare Fig. 1 and 2). Optimistically, this can be taken as an evidence that the isolation procedure, its buffer composition and its length respectively, do not alter the phosphorylation pattern of the membrane, i.e. that dephosphorylation does not induce a significant alteration of the physiological pattern of phosphorylated proteins. This is further supported by the finding, that an incubation at 37° C for 1 hour of brush border membranes phosphorylated by the slice procedure is unable to alter the phosphorylation pattern.

In summary, a well defined in vitro system is described, which allows the study of the phosphorylation of the proteins of the plasmamembrane (brush border and basolateral membranes) of the rat proximal tubule under "physiological" conditions. This approach should allow us in future experiments to answer the question, whether an altered membrane protein phosphorylation pattern correlates with a parathyroid hormone induced alteration of phosphate transport. It should, however, be emphasized that an altered phosphorylation pattern will not represent a direct experimental proof for an involvement of membrane protein phosphorylation in parathyroid hormone action on phosphate transport. Certainly, a more difficult task will be represented by correlating (causal relation) membrane phosphorylation and altered phosphate transport.

ACKNOWLEGMENTS

This work was supported by the Swiss National Science Foundation, Grant No. 3.452.079.

---

*The question whether the similar phosphorylation pattern observed in basal-lateral membranes is due to cross-contamination by brush border membranes is now under further investigation.

REFERENCES

1. P. Greengard, Phosphorylated proteins as physiological effectors, Science 199: 146 (1978).
2. K.J. Ullrich, G. Rumrich and S. Klöss, Phosphate transport in the proximal convolution of rat kidney. I. Tubular heterogeneity, effect of parathyroid hormone in acute and chronic pharathyroid ectomized animals and effect of phosphate diet. Pflügers Arch. 372: 269 (1977).
3. K. Lau, S. Goldfarb and M. Goldberg, The effects of parathyroid hormone on renal phosphate handling, in: "Renal Handling of Phosphate," S.G. Massry and H. Fleisch, ed., Plenum Press (1980).
4. C. Evers, H. Murer and R. Kinne, Effect of parathyroid hormone on the transport properties of isolated renal brush border vesicles, Biochem. J. 172: 49 (1978).
5. D. Ausiello, J. Handler and J. Orloff, Effect of parathyroid hormone and cyclic AMP on protein phosphorylation in rabbit kidney cortex, Biochim. Biophys. Acta 451: 372 (1976).
6. J. Biber, B. Stieger, W. Haase and H. Murer, A high yield preparation for rat kidney brush border membranes; different behaviour of lysosomal markers, Biochim. Biophys. Acta, in press.
7. H.-G. Heidrich, R. Kinne, E. Kinne-Saffran and K. Hannig, The polarity of the proximal tubule cell in rat kidney, J. of Cell Biology 54: 232 (1972).
8. U.K. Laemmli, Cleavage of structural proteins during the assembly of the head of bacteriophage T_4, Nature 227: 680 (1970).
9. M.M. Bradford, A rapid and sensitive method for the quantitation of microgram quantities of protein utilizing the principle of protein-dye binding, Anal. Biochem. 72: 248 (1976).
10. W. Haase, A. Schäfer, H. Murer and R. Kinne, Studies on the orientation of brush border membrane vesicles, Biochem. J. 172: 57 (1978).
11. H.R. De Jonge, W.E.J.M. Ghijsen and C.H. van Os, Phosphorylation intermediates of Ca^{++}-ATPase and alkaline phosphatase in plasma membranes from rat duodenal epithelium, Biochim. Biophys. Acta, in press.

POSSIBLE RELATIONSHIP OF GLUCONEOGENESIS TO MODULATION OF PHOSPHATE TRANSPORT IN THE PROXIMAL TUBULE

Thomas P. Dousa

Nephrology Research Laboratories
Mayo Clinic and Foundation
Rochester, MN

The renal cortex, specifically the proximal tubule (1-3), is the only tissue besides the liver capable of synthesizing glucose from smaller carbon fragments. Contribution of renal gluconeogenesis (GNG) to the maintenance of blood glucose homeostasis is relatively minor, in comparison with GNG in the liver (4). Numerous studies in the past have shown that the rate of renal GNG changes in response to a variety of hormonal or pharmacologic stimuli and in various pathophysiologic situations (4,5). Whether and how the GNG pathway in renal proximal tubules relates to specific functions of this segment of the nephron remains unknown. Recent observations from our laboratory (6,7) taken together with reports by other investigators in the past, led us to propose a hypothesis (Fig. 1) according to which the rate of GNG in the cells of proximal tubules might modulate the rate of phosphate (Pi) reabsorption from luminal fluid across the epithelium of the proximal tubules (7,8,9).

A key link between GNG and regulation of proximal tubular transport of Pi is nicotinamide adenine dinucleotide (NAD), a compound which is known to serve as a coenzyme of many dehydrogenases. Our recent studies suggest that the NAD, namely the oxidized form (NAD^+) in cytoplasm of tubular cells may modulate the uptake of Pi from the tubular fluid across luminal brush border membrane (BBM) (6). NAD added _in vitro_ to isolated renal BBM vesicles specifically inhibited Na^+ gradient-dependent ($Na^+_o > Na^+_i$) uptake of Pi. _In vivo_ administration of the NAD precursor, nicotinamide, resulted in profound phosphaturia, increase in renal cortical NAD^+ (6), and a specific inhibition of Na^+ gradient-dependent transport of Pi across BBM (6). Administration of nicotinamide is a complex pharmacologic maneuver which increases NAD^+ by increasing NAD^+

synthesis and by inhibiting its enzymatic breakdown (10). Total tissue content of NAD (NAD^+ plus the reduced form, NADH), [NAD^+ + NADH], also increases in response to nicotinamide (6). The question then arose whether physiologic stimuli may increase the content of NAD^+ in renal cells, which would then cause inhibition of proximal tubular Pi transport via the proposed mechanism, which involves NAD^+-BBM interactions (6,8,9).

First, it should be realized that in cells of parenchymal organs (10) including kidney (6), most of total cellular NAD is found in cytoplasm and only a smaller portion is sequestered in cellular organelles, mainly in mitochondria; the inner mitochondrial membrane is virtually impermeable for NAD (11,12). The cytoplasmic pool of NAD, which is in immediate contact with BBM, is therefore primarily relevant to the proposed regulatory system.

Furthermore, total NAD present in the cytoplasmic pool is compartmentalized by binding (12) on soluble cytoplasmic proteins and taken together, consists of free NAD^+, bound NAD^+, free NADH and bound NADH (11,12). It has been shown that NADH binds on cytoplasmic proteins--virtually all these proteins are various cytoplasmic dehydrogenases (12)--with an affinity about 100 x higher than that of NAD^+ (12,13,14). It therefore can be assumed that under the ambient condition in cytoplasm most of NADH is

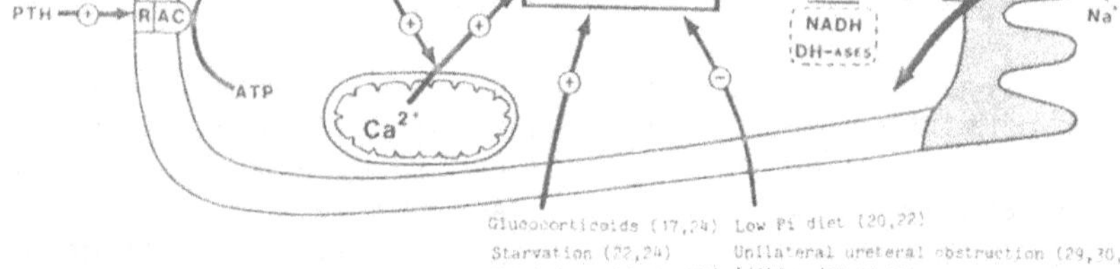

Fig. 1. Scheme of "GNG-NAD-BBM" hypothesis on modulation of Pi transport in proximal tubule by phsiologic or pathohysiologic (———>) or pharmacologic (- - - ->) factors. ⊕ denotes stimulation; ⊖ denotes inhibition; PTH, parathyroid hormone; ATP, adenosine 5'-triphosphate; cAMP, cyclic AMP; Ca^{2+}, calcium; R, receptor for PTH; AC, adenylate cyclase; NAD^+, oxidized NAD; NADH, reduced NAD; DH-ases, cytoplasmic dehydrogenases using NAD^+/NADH as co-enzyme system (NADH-binding proteins).

sequested by binding on dehydrogenases (12), while most NAD^+ is in the free form. This compartmentalization by binding is reflected in findings which show that while the ratio total NAD^+/total NADH is about 2:1, the ratio of free NAD^+/free NADH, determined indirectly using a redox metabolite indicator method (15), is more than 100 x higher (11; also our unpublished results). From these considerations it follows that the biochemical processes which oxidize the cytoplasmic NADH to NAD^+, result in conversion of the protein-bound form of NADH to free NAD^+, and NAD^+ may be then available for interaction with BBM. There is no indication to date that the effect of NAD to inhibit BBM transport of Pi depends on its redox properties (6,9). Our recent in vitro studies have shown that BBM isolated from rat kidney cortex binds NAD^+ with a high degree of specificity and two sets of NAD binding sites were identified; the low affinity binding site ($K_D = 2.2 \times 10^{-3}$ M NAD^+) and high affinity site ($K_D = 2.2 \times 10^{-5}$ M NAD^+) (16). The high affinity BBM-binding sites can bind NAD^+ in concentrations which may be expected to prevail in cytoplasm, and BBM could thus compete for NAD^+ with binding sites of cytosolic proteins (13,16).

Considering numerous metabolic processes present in the cytoplasm of proximal renal tubular cells, the GNG pathway appears to be uniquely suited for control of cytoplasmic NAD^+ levels (9). NADH is oxidized to NAD^+ at the glyceraldehyde-3-phosphate dehydrogenase (GADP) step of GNG pathway (4,7). Therefore, enhancement of the GNG rate may be expected to increase levels of cytoplasmic free NAD^+, by conversion from NADH. It is of particular interest that some hormonal and metabolic factors known to decrease Pi reabsorption in proximal tubules were found, in biochemical studies, also to stimulate renal GNG. The rate of GNG can be altered in principle either by change in the supply of GNG substrates, by increased synthesis of key "pacemaker" enzymes, or by direct activation of key GNG enzymes, e.g. by Ca^{2+} (5). The question then arises whether changes in the rate of renal GNG can cause predicted changes in NAD^+ level--this problem has not been addressed in the past. Using both in vivo and in vitro approaches, we recently explored whether changes in the rate of GNG alter the tissue level of NAD^+ in the expected direction (7,17,18).

In the in vitro study on rat renal cortical slices the rate of GNG was altered by increased supply of GNG substrates or by inhibitors which block GNG at specific enzymatic steps (7). We found that with incubation of tissue in the presence of 10 mM α-ketoglutarate, the rate of GNG (assessed as glucose production) was enhanced, and also tissue level of NAD^+ was significantly increased. Addition of 3-mercaptopicolinic acid, a compound reported to inhibit phosphoenolpyruvate carboxykinase (PEP-CK), inhibited both the rate of GNG and accumulation of NAD^+. When the rate of glucose formation was increased by the supply of another substrate, 10 mM L-glutamate, NAD^+ content again significantly increased. The addition of quinolinic acid, a compound reported to inhibit glutamate deaminase and to a lesser degree PEP-CK, blunted both GNG and the enhancement of tissue NAD^+. It is noteworthy that in the presence of the above mentioned changes in the rate of GNG and in NAD^+ levels, the content of ATP measured in the same tissue was not changed at all (7). This feature may suggest that if changes in ATP metabolism occurred, i.e. increased the supply of ATP for GNG (19), these changes were either quantitatively small, or that ATP biosynthesis and catabolism were in balance. When NAD^+ was measured after incubation with or without substrate supply (L-glutamate) and tissue then fractionated, the increase of NAD^+ was found in cytosol only; no significant change was detected in the particulate fraction (100,000 x g pellet) of homogenate. When the effect of the addition of 10 mM α-ketoglutarate and 10 mM fructose, as substrates for GNG were compared, incubation with both substrates enhanced glucose formation but only the incubation with α-ketoglutarate was associated with a significant increase in tissue NAD^+ (S. A. Kempson, unpublished observation). This differential effect of two substrates is likely due to the fact that fructose enters GNG pathway distal to a GADP step and, therefore, does not contribute directly to conversion of NADH to NAD^+ by GADP (7).

To explore whether an increase in the rate of renal GNG also has a similar effect on NAD^+ in renal cortical tissue _in vivo_, several known stimuli of renal GNG (4,5) were studied in rats stabilized on low Pi diet (LPD). In this nutritional state renal reabsorption of Pi is maximized, Na^+-dependent uptake of Pi by renal BBM is enhanced (9) and renal GNG is blunted (20). When rats stabilized on LPD and treated for two days with i.p. injection of glucocorticoids were examined, we found that GNG was enhanced, total NAD level [NAD^+ + NADH] in renal cortex was not changed, but the ratio of NAD^+/NADH significantly increased, thus suggesting the shift of bound NADH to free NAD^+ (17; Turner and Dousa, unpublished results). Infusion of PTH to glucocorticoid-treated animals fed LPD further enhanced the rate of GNG, and increased the NAD^+/NADH ratio, without changes of total NAD (18; also Czekalski, et al, in preparation). In rats stabilized on LPD, administration of glucocorticoids resulted in phosphaturia (17,18) which was further enhanced by administration of PTH (18). Phosphaturia was associated with a specific decrease in BBM uptake capacity for Pi (17). Dr. Kempson examined the effect of metabolic acidosis, induced in rats stabilized on LPD by loading with NH_4Cl (21), with use of analogous experimental setting as in studies on glucocorticoids. Metabolic acidosis in LPD rats caused an increase in the rate of renal GNG, increase of NAD^+/NADH ratio (but no change in total NAD) and marked phosphaturia, associated with inhibition of BBM transport of Pi (21). Finally, starvation superimposed in animals already stabilized previously on LPD, reverses renal retention of Pi (22) and restores responsiveness to PTH (23). In a state of starvation superimposed on LPD, the previously depressed GNG was enhanced along with phosphaturia (24).

Parathyroid hormone (PTH) is to date the most extensively studied extrarenal phosphaturic hormone. The effects of PTH on renal Pi excretion could be well explained according to the proposed GNG-NAD-BBM hypothesis (6,8,9). PTH stimulates GNG both in vitro (25) and in vivo (24), and cAMP mimicks PTH effects. We found that infusion of PTH enhances the NAD^+/NADH ratio without changes in total NAD or ATP content of cortical tissue, along with eliciting phosphaturia (26). Administration of PTH was shown in other studies to decrease selectively BBM uptake of Pi (27,28). All these pieces of evidence, taken together, suggest that indeed PTH may cause phosphaturia via the proposed GNG-NAD-BBM mechanism (9).

It is interesting to note that in some conditions associated with reduction in the rate of renal GNG, renal excretion of Pi is diminished. First, a decreased rate of GNG in the renal cortex and increased renal Pi reabsorption were observed in animals stabilized on LPD (20). Likewise, decreased GNG and reduced Pi excretion was found in the kidneys of animals after release of unilateral ureteral obstruction (29-31). Furthermore, administration of lithium which decreased urinary Pi excretion (32) and blunted phosphaturic effect of PTH (33) was recently reported to lower renal GNG (34). Finally, insulin, a hormone that increases renal tubular reabsorption of Pi (35), was shown to inhibit renal GNG (36) and to increase BBM uptake of Pi (37). Interestingly, in an insulinopenic diabetes mellitus, renal GNG is enhanced (4,5).

Caveat emptor! While the findings recounted above in principle agree with the proposed "GNG-NAD-BBM" hypothesis (Fig. 1), caution should be voiced against oversimplified and premature conclusions as well as undue generalization. First, it should be stressed that the proposed cellular modulation via "GNG-NAD-BBM" mechanism may not necessarily be applicable to all regulations of proximal Pi transport. Biochemical analysis of GNG pathway in relation to the NAD^+/NADH system has so far been conducted only in whole renal cortex, not yet in specific tubular segments. Using even rather simple macroanatomic subdivision of cortex to layers, it has been shown that the rate of GNG differs in various zones of cortex (1). Also, the capacity of BBM for Na^+-dependent Pi uptake differs in membranes prepared from superficial and juxtamedullary zones of cortical tissue (38). Moreover, intracellular localization of GNG differs between mammalian species. In rat proximal tubules GNG is almost exclusively localized in cytoplasm, but in species such as rabbit, man, or dog, a substantial portion of GNG pathway is also located in mitochondria (39). Only cytoplasmic GNG is likely to influence directly NAD^+ available for interaction with BBM. While the highest activity of the major "pacemaker" enzyme of GNG, the PEP-CK was found in early proximal convoluted tubules

(2,3), the rate of GNG from pyruvate in intact tubules was highest in proximal straight tubule (1). Therefore, all major components of the proposed cellular regulatory system, and their relationships, ought to be ultimately investigated in specific segments (and subsegments) of proximal tubules and, for comparison, also in other (distal) tubular segments. Besides obvious changes in the major components of the system, such as concentration of free NAD^+ in cytoplasm or rate of GNG, other factors may play a role. For example, the affinity of BBM for NAD^+ (16), coupling between the rate of GNG and the rate of NAD^+ generation (7)--or modulatory actions of calcium at several points of GNG (40)--all these aspects conceivably could be affected by hormonal, pharmacologic, or metabolic factors and contribute to overall cellular response. Finally, the cytoplasmic free NAD^+ may be conceivably influenced not only by reactions which are part of the GNG pathway, but also by other cytoplasmic dehydrogenases and/or by enzymes which synthetize and catabolize NAD^+, such as NAD-glycohydrolase (10). For all these and other reasons, everybody should be acutely aware that "GNG-NAD-BBM" scheme is at the present time a working hypothesis. Its validity, exclusiveness, and general applicability to specific tubular segments, in nephrons of various mammalian species, needs to be meticulously scrutinized in future studies.

While the conclusions about applicability of the "GNG-NAD-BBM" hypothesis should remain guarded at the present time, the hypothesis is remarkably attractive. It may explain the complete cellular chain of regulatory events for some hormones (PTH, insulin) and also mutual interactions between hormonal (PTH) and complex metabolic (dietary Pi) stimuli which all contribute to regulation of single transport system--reabsorption of Pi in proximal tubules.

Acknowledgements: This work was supported by USPHS grants AM-16105 and AM-19715 and by the Mayo Foundation. Mrs. Bonnie Becker provided excellent secretarial assistance. Studies on this topic from our laboratory were carried out in close collaboration with Drs. Kempson and Turner, Ms. J. Braun, Mrs. R. Holets, visiting scientist Dr. Czekalski, and with Dr. Knox and his associates. Dr. Kempson's present address is Renal and Electrolyte Division, University of Pittsburgh, Pittsburgh, PA.

REFERENCES

1. A. Maleque, H. Endou, C. Koseki, and F. Sakai, Nephron heterogeneity: Gluconeogenesis from pyruvate in rabbit nephron, Febs Lett. 116:154 (1980).
2. A. Vandewalle, G. Wirthensohn, H-G. Heidrich, and W. Guder, Distribution of hexokinase and phosphoenolpyruvate carboxykinase along the rabbit nephron, Am. J. Physiol. 240:F492 (1981).

3. H. B. Burch, R. G. Narins, C. Chu, S. Fagioli, S. Choi, W. McCarthy, and O. H. Lowry, Distribution along the rat nephron of three enzymes of gluconeogenesis in acidosis and starvation, Am. J. Physiol. 235:F246 (1978).
4. C. I. Pogson, D. Longshaw, A. Roobol, S. A. Smith, and G. A. O. Alleyne, Phosphoenolpyruvate carboxykinase and renal gluconeogenesis, in: "Gluconeogenesis: Its Regulation in Mammalian Species," R. W. Hanson and M. A. Mehlman, ed., John Wiley & Sons, New York, pp. 335-368 (1976).
5. J. J. Cohen, and D. M. Kamm, Renal metabolism relation to renal function, in: "The Kidney," B. M. Brenner and F. C. Rector, Jr., ed., W. B. Saunders Co., Philadelphia, pp. 144-248 (1981).
6. S. A. Kempson, G. Colon-Otero, S-Y. L. Ou, S. T. Turner, and T. P. Dousa, Possible role of nicotinamide adenine dinucleotide as an intracellular regulator of renal transport of phosphate in the rat, J. Clin. Invest. 67:1347 (1981).
7. S. Y. L. Ou, S. A. Kempson, and T. P. Dousa, Relationship between rate of gluconeogenesis and content of nicotinamide adenine dinucleotide in renal cortex, Life Sci. 29:1195-1202 (1981).
8. T. P. Dousa, and S. A. Kempson, Role of nicotinamide adenine dinucleotide (NAD) in control of proximal renal tubular phosphate transport, in: "Urolithiasis Clinical and Basic Research," L. H. Smith, W. G. Robertson, and B. Finlayson, ed., Plenum Press, New York (1981).
9. T. P. Dousa, and S. A. Kempson, Regulation of renal brush border membrane transport of phosphate, Mineral Electrolyte Metab. vol. 6 in press (1981).
10. N. O. Kaplan, The pyridine coenzymes. in: "The Enyzmes," P. D. Boyer, H. Lardy, and K. Myrback, ed., Academic Press, Inc., New York, pp. 39-56 (1960).
11. M. E. Tischler, D. Friedrichs, K. Coll, and J. R. Williamson, Pyridine nucleotide distributions and enzyme mass action ratios in hepatocytes from fed and starved rats. Arch. Biochem. Biophys. 184:222 (1977).
12. T. Bucher, and H. Sies, Mitochondrial and cytosolic redox states in perfused rat liver: Methods and problems in metabolic compartmentation. in: "Use of Isolated Liver Cells and Kidney Tubules in Metabolic Studies," J. M. Tager, H. D. Soling, and J. R. Williamson, ed., North Holland Publishing Co., Amsterdam, pp. 41-64 (1976).
13. K. Daziel, Kinetics and mechanism of nicotinamide-nucleotide-linked dehydrogenases, in: "The Enzymes," P. D. Boyer, ed., Academic Press, New York, pp. 1-66 (1975).
14. S. Subramanian and P. D. Ross, Thermodynamics of binding of oxidized and reduced nicotinamide adenine dinucleotides, adenosine 5'-diphosphoribase and 5'-iodosalycilate to dehydrogenases, Biochemistry 17:2192 (1978).

15. K. S. Gumaa, P. McLean, and A. L. Greenbaum, Compartmentation in relation to metabolic control in liver, in: "Essays in Biochemistry," P. N. Campbell, and F. Dickens, ed., Academic Press, London, 7:39-85 (1971)
16. J. L. Braun, B. A. Jackson, and T. P. Dousa, Interaction of nicotinamide adenine dinucleotide (NAD) with renal cortical brush border membranes (BBM). Clin. Res.:in press (1981).
17. S. T. Turner, T. A. Haugen, and T. P. Dousa, Mechanism of phosphaturia induced by glucocorticoids (GCD) in rats adapted to low phosphate diet (LPD), Clin. Res. 29:556A (1981).
18. S. Czekalski, M. Onsgard, T. J. Berndt, R. Holets, T. P. Dousa, and F. G. Knox, Phosphaturia and restoration of the phosphaturic response to parathyroid hormone (PTH) by glucocorticoid treatment in rats fed low phosphate diet (LPD), Clin. Res. 29:553A (1981).
19. R. C. Haynes, Jr., Mitochondrial metabolism in hormonal stimulation of gluconeogenesis, in: "The Regulation of Carbohydrate Formation and Utilization in Mammals, C. M. Veneziale, ed., University Press, Baltimore, pp. 345-362 (1981).
20. W. J. Kreusser, C. Descoeudres, Y. Oda, S. G. Massry, and K. Kurokawa, Effect of phosphate depletion on renal gluconeogenesis, Mineral Electrolyte Metab. 3:312 (1980).
21. S. A. Kempson, Renal brush border membrane adaptation to low phosphate diet: Effect of metabolic acidosis, The American Society of Nephrology 14th Annual Meeting, in press (1981).
22. S. A. Kempson, S. V. Shah, P. G. Werness, T. Berndt, P. H. Lee, L. H. Smith, F. G. Knox, and T. P. Dousa, Renal brush border membrane adaptation to phosphorus deprivation: Effects of fasting versus low-phosphorus diet. Kidney Int. 18:36 (1980).
23. N. Beck, S. K. Webster, and H. J. Reineck, Effect of fasting on tubular phosphorus reabsorption, Am. J. Physiol. 237:F241 (1979).
24. S. Czekalski, S. T. Turner, M. Onsgard, F. G. Knox, and T. P. Dousa, Reversal of renal adaptation to low phosphate diet (LPD) by stimulation of renal gluconeogenesis (GNG). Proceedings VIIIth International Congress of Nephrology, Athens, Greece, June, RM-034, p. 61 (1981).
25. H. Rasmussen, D. B. P. Goodman, N. Friedmann, N. E. Allen, and K. Kurokawa, Ionic control of metabolism, in: "Handbook of Physiology," G. D. Aurbach, ed., Am. Physiol. Soc., pp. 225-264 (1976).
26. T. J. Berndt, F. G. Knox, S. A. Kempson, and T. P. Dousa, Nicotinamide adenine dinucleotide and renal response to parathyroid hormone. Endocrinology 108:2005 (1981).

27. R. Kinne, W. Berner, N. Hoffman, and H. Murer, Phosphate transport by isolated renal and intestinal plasma membranes, Adv. Exp. Med. Biol. 81:265 (1976).
28. M. R. Hammerman, I. E. Karl and K. A. Hruska, Regulation of canine renal vesicle Pi transport by growth hormone and parathyroid hormone, Biochim. Biophys. Acta 603:322 (1980).
29. M. L. Purkerson, D. B. Rolf, L. R. Chase, E. Slatopolsky, and S. Klahr, Tubular reabsorption of phosphate after release of complete ureteral obstruction in the rat, Kidney Int. 5:326 (1974).
30. J. Blondin, M. D. Purkerson, D. Rolf, A. C. Schoolwerth, and S. Klahr, Renal functions and metabolism after relief of unilateral ureteral obstruction. Proc. Soc. Exp. Biol. Med. 150:71 (1975).
31. H. Nito, C. Descoeudres, K. Kurokawa, and S. G. Massry, Effect of unilateral ureteral obstruction on renal cell metabolism and function, J. Lab. Clin. Med. 91:60 (1978).
32. S. Angielski, L. Pempkowiak, P. Gmaj, A. Hoppe, and C. Nowicka, The effect of maleate and lithium on renal function and metabolism, in: "Current Problems in Clinical Biochemistry: Renal Metabolism in Relation to Renal Function," U. Schmidt and U. C. Dubach, ed., Hans Huber Publishers, Bern, pp. 142-152 (1976).
33. S. Angielski and M. Szczepanska, Restoration of the phosphaturic effect of parathyroid hormone in lithium-treated rats, in: "Current Problems in Clinical Biochemistry: Biochemical Nephrology, W. G. Guder and U. Schmidt, ed., Hans Huber Publishers, Bern, pp. 463-471 (1978).
34. S. Angielski, K. Drewnowska, A. Ryboczynska, M. Szczepanska, and J. Stepinski, Renal metabolism of citrate and oxoglutarate in lithium-treated rats, in: Proceedings, 8th International Congress of Neprology, Athens, Greece, W. Zurukzoglu, M. Papadimitriou, M. Pyrpasopoulos, M. Sion, C. Zamboulis, S. Karger, Basal, pp. 807-813 (1981).
35. A. Nizet, P. Lefebvre, A. Luyckx, and J. Crabbe, Hormones and non-specific humoral factors in the interferences between sodium, glucose and phosphate handling by dog kidney, in: "Current Problems in Clinical Biochemistry: Renal Metabolism in Relation to Renal Function," U. Schmidt and U. C. Dubach, ed., Hans Huber Publishers, Bern, pp. 262-271 (1976).
36. J. A. Lupianez, K. N. Dileepan, and S. R. Wagle, Interrelationship of somatostatin, insulin, and calcium in the control of gluconeogenesis in kidney cortex slices, Biochem. Biophys. Res. Comm. 90:1153 (1979).
37. T. E. Northrup, Insulin (INS) induced increases in phosphate (Pi) transport across renal luminal brush border membranes (LBBM), Fed. Proc. 40:462 (1981).

38. S. T. Turner and T. P. Dousa, Differences in transport capacity of phosphate (Pi) of luminal brush border membrane (BBM) prepared from subcapsular (SC) and juxtamedullary (JM) cortex. Abstr. of 14th Annual Meeting of the American Society of Nephrology, 1981, Washington, D.C., November, 1981, in press.
39. M. Watford, P. Vinay, G. Lemieux, and A. Gougoux, Inhibition of renal gluconeogenesis and phosphoenopyruvate carboxykinase activity by 3-mercaptopicolinic acid: studies in rat, guinea pig, dog, rabbit, and man, Can. J. Biochem. 58:440 (1980).
40. H. Rasmussen and D. Waisman, The messenger function of calcium in endocrine systems, in: "Biochemical Actions of Hormones, Vol. VIII, G. Litmach, ed., Academic Press, New York, pp. 2-117 (1981).

INTERACTIONS BETWEEN PHOSPHATE TRANSPORT AND OXIDATIVE METABOLISM IN THE RABBIT PROXIMAL TUBULE

P.C. Brazy, S.R. Gullans, L.J. Mandel and V.W. Dennis

Duke University Medical Center
Durham, North Carolina

INTRODUCTION

In proximal renal tubules, inorganic phosphate is both a transported solute and a substrate for intracellular metabolism. While these two functions may involve separate pools of phosphate, it is more likely that there is some interaction between phosphate transport and the metabolic processes which use inorganic phosphate. Within the proximal tubular cell, several types of metabolic processes involve inorganic phosphate. Glycolysis and oxidative phosphorylation utilize inorganic phosphate in the production of ATP. On the other hand, gluconeogenesis and the sodium-potassium ATPase hydrolyze ATP to generate inorganic phosphate. Furthermore, the intracellular concentration of inorganic phosphate may contribute to the phosphorylation potential, i.e. [ATP]/[ADP]·[Pi], which regulates the rates of these metabolic processes.

The objective of the present study was to examine the relationship of one aspect of intracellular metabolism, oxidative phosphorylation, to phosphate transport in proximal renal tubules. Our approach was to inhibit or stimulate oxidative metabolism and to determine the effect of each maneuver on specific transport processes. The data indicate that phosphate transport in proximal convoluted tubules is closely coupled to the rate of oxidative phosphorylation.

METHODS

Two basic methods were used to study transport and

metabolism in renal tubules. 1. Transport studies. Proximal convoluted tubules from rabbit kidney were isolated and perfused by previously described techniques.[1] These tubules were perfused with a physiological fluid that resembled an ultrafiltrate of rabbit serum. The bathing medium was either commercial rabbit serum or the perfusion fluid plus 6 g/dl defatted albumin or 3 g/dl dialyzed dextran (40,000 mol. wt.). Lumen-to-bath fluxes of phosphate and glucose were measured with radioisotopes. Fluid absorption rates (Jv) were measured with a water marker, radiolabelled iothalamate. 2. Metabolic studies. Oxygen consumption rates were measured in suspensions of cortical tubules from rabbit kidney. Separated tubules were prepared by a collagenase infusion of the kidney by previously described techniques.[2] These tubules were then suspended in a physiological fluid containing dextran. The final concentration of tubules was 3-5 mg tubular protein per ml. Suspensions were placed in a closed chamber where the oxygen tension was monitored as a function of time with a Clark electrode. The slope of this plot reflected the oxygen consumption rate which was normalized per mg tubular protein in the suspension. Data are expressed as a mean $\pm$ SE for a number of tubules or suspensions examined. Each tubule or suspension served as its own control prior to the addition of the test substance.

RESULTS

Effects of Arsenate

Arsenate is an inorganic analogue of phosphate in many transport and enzyme systems. In renal brush-border membranes, arsenate is a competitive inhibitor of phosphate uptake.[3] In the intact epithelium, however, the primary action of arsenate is as an uncoupler of oxidative phosphorylation.[4] We examined the effects of arsenate on tubular transport function to determine the relationship of specific transport processes to mitochondrial function. It should be noted that arsenate is a relatively weak uncoupler of oxidative phosphorylation. The addition of 1 mM arsenate to suspensions of cortical tubules incresed oxygen consumption rates by 20.5 $\pm$ 2.9 percent. Thus, this concentration of arsenate may be expected to cause only a partial reduction in mitochondrial production of ATP.

The effects of arsenate on tubular transport were examined in isolated, perfused proximal connvoluted tubules. The addition of arsenate to only the bathing medium had no effect on tubular function. The addition of 1 mM arsenate to the luminal fluid significantly reduced transport processes. Therefore, arsenate must enter the tubular cell across the brush-border membrane. The pattern of arsenate-induced inhibitions of transport was unusual.

For example, the phosphate absorptive flux was reduced to 42% of its control value (7.87 $\pm$ 2.43 to 3.30 $\pm$ 1.23 pmol/mm·min; N,6); the glucose absorptive flux was reduced slightly to 85% of its control rate (82.7 + 4.3 to 70.2 $\pm$ 3.9 pmol/mm·min; N,5); and the fluid absorption rate was reduced to 50% of its control value (1.18 $\pm$ 0.12 to 0.59 $\pm$ 0.08 nl/mm·min; N,8). This pattern of inhibition is quite different from the global inhibition of solute transport that occurs with ouabain.[5,6] This difference may reflect the relationship between mitochondrial function and transport, or the uniqueness of arsenate-induced inhibitions. Therefore, we examined the effects of another uncoupler of oxidative phosphorylation, m-chlorocarbonyl cyanide phenylhydrazone (CCCP).

Effects of CCCP

CCCP is a potent uncoupler of mitochondrial oxidative phosphorylation. At a concentration of 10^{-6}M in the medium, CCCP increased oxygen consumption rates by 51.2 $\pm$ 2.3 percent. This response was twice as great as that of 1mM arsenate. In isolated, perfused proximal convoluted tubules the addition of CCCP (10^{-6}M in the bathing medium) caused profound inhibitions of transport in a pattern that was similar to the effects of arsenate. That is, phosphate absorption was reduced to 24% of its control value (7.00 $\pm$ 2.15 to 1.70 $\pm$ 0.50 pmol/mm·min; N,6); fluid absorption was reduced to 28% of its control rate (1.22 $\pm$ 0.16 to 0.34 $\pm$ 0.05 nl/mm·min; N,8); and glucose absorption was reduced to 57% of its control (79.6 $\pm$ 5.2 to 45.2 $\pm$ 3.9 pmol/mm·min; N,4). Therefore, the data with CCCP are qualitatively the same as the arsenate data. Together, these results indicate that inhibition of oxidative phosphorylation causes proportional decreases in phosphate and fluid absorption. This inhibition does not affect all transported solutes which are handled significantly by the proximal tubule because glucose transport was reduced to a lesser extent than phosphate transport. These data suggest that intracellular factors related to mitochondrial respiration might regulate phosphate transport. We examined this possibility further by stimulating mitochondrial respiration with succinate.

Effect of Succinate

Succinate is a metabolic substrate that readily enters renal tubules and stimulates mitochondrial respiration. Succinate stimulates oxygen consumption by increasing the flow of electrons through a flavoprotein linked dehydrogenase. Increasing oxygen consumption in this way bypasses the first phosphorylation step, so the rate of ATP production may not increase in proportion to the increases in oxygen consumption rate. In suspensions of rabbit cortical tubules, the addition of sodium succinate (1mM) to the bathing medium increased oxygen consumption rates by 30.4 ± 2.7 percent. In perfused proximal convoluted tubules, succinate (1mM) stimulated solute transport. Phosphate absorption rates increased by 29% (4.22 ± 1.15 to 5.43 ± 1.18 pmol/mm·min; $P<0.01$; N,6). Glucose transport increased by 12% (47.7 ± 2.0 to 53.4 ± 0.9 pmol/mm·min; $P<0.02$; N,4). Fluid absorption rates were unchanged (0.98 ± 0.08 to 1.06 ± 0.08 nl/ mm·min; $P<0.30$; N,8). These data indicate that phosphate transport rates can reflect increases in the rate of mitochondrial respiration as well as decreases. Phosphate transport rates reflect these alterations in intracellular metabolism to a greater extent than either fluid absorption or glucose transport. These data provide additional evidence for the presence of an interaction between phosphate transport and mitochondrial respiration.

DISCUSSION

The present studies indicate that phosphate transport in the proximal convoluted tubule has a unique relationship to oxidative phosphorylation. Inhibitors of oxidative phosphorylation, like arsenate and CCCP, decrease phosphate transport to a greater extent than glucose transport and to a similar extent to net sodium absorption. In addition, stimulation of oxidative metabolism by succinate increases phosphate transport with little or no effect on glucose and net sodium absorption. These data indicate the presence of an interrelationship between phosphate transport and oxidative metabolism, but they do not define the mechanism of this interaction.

The simplest explanation for this interaction is that some component of intracellular phosphate regulates phosphate transport. The present data may be explained as follows: Inhibition of oxidative metabolism increases the intracellular content of inorganic phosphate.[7] This accumulation of intracellular phosphate would impose a concentration gradient that might decrease phosphate uptake into the cell. Therefore, phosphate transport would be inhibited to a greater extent than other transport processes which depend on the availability of ATP or the sodium gradient. In the other case, a stimulation of oxidative phosphorylation may reduce the intracellular content of inorganic phosphate and thereby provide a more favorable phosphate gradient which would increase phosphate transport selectively. This explanation assumes that these experimental conditions do not alter other metabolic processes which involve inorganic phospahte.

There are numerous other explanations for these data. Recent studies by Kempson et al[8] have suggested another interaction between phosphate transport and cellular metabolism. Their studies showed that the metabolic cofactor, NAD, inhibits phosphate uptake by brush-border membrane vesicles. This observation raises the possibility that changes in cellular metabolism might regulate phosphate entry via changes in cytoplasmic NAD. In the intact epithelium, NAD is produced by gluconeogenesis. This metabolic process also generates inorganic phosphate from ATP. Therefore, an alteration in gluconeogenesis may be associated with an alteration in the intracellular content of phosphate and the activity of other phosphate involving processes.

In summary, this study describes a close coupling of phosphate transport and oxidative phosphorylation in the proximal renal tubule. The mechanism of this coupling is uncertain and potentially could involve a number of metabolic processes within the cell.

REFERENCES

1. V. W. Dennis and P. C. Brazy, Sodium, phosphate, glucose, bicarbonate and alanine interactions in the isolated proximal convoluted tubule of the rabbit kidney, J. Clin. Invest. 62:387 (1978).
2. R. S. Balaban, S. P. Soltoff, J. M. Storey and L. J. Mandel, Improved renal cortical tubule suspension. Spectrophotometric study of oxygen delivery, Am. J. Physiol. 238:F50 (1980).
3. N. Hoffmann, M. Thees and R. Kinne, Phosphate transport by isolated renal brush border vesicles, Pfluegers Arch. 362:147 (1976).
4. P. C. Brazy, R. S. Balaban, S. R. Gullans, L. J. Mandel and V. W. Dennis, Inhibition of renal metabolism. Relative effects of arsenate on sodium, phosphate and glucose transport by the rabbit proximal tubule, J. Clin. Invest. 66:1211 (1980).
5. V. W. Dennis, P. B. Woodhall and R. R. Robinson, Characteristics of phosphate transport in isolated proximal renal tubule, Am. J. Physiol. 231:979 (1976).
6. P. C. Brazy and V. W. Dennis, Characteristics of glucose-phlorizin interactions in isolated proximal tubules, Am. J. Physiol. 234:F279 (1978).
7. D. F. Wilson, M. Erecinska, C. Drown and I. A. Silver, Effect of oxygen tension on cellular energetics, Am. J. Physiol. 233:C135 (1977).
8. S. A. Kempson, G. Colon-Otero, L. Ou, S. T. Turner and T. P. Dousa, Possible role of NAD as an intracellular regulator of renal transport of phosphate in the rat, J. Clin. Invest. 67:1347 (1981).

ABNORMAL TUBULAR Pi ADAPTATION TO DIETARY Pi RESTRICTION AND DECREASED CALCIUM REABSORPTION IN X-LINKED HYPOPHOSPHATEMIC (HYP) MICE

R.C. Mühlbauer, J.-P. Bonjour and H. Fleisch

Department of Pathophysiology
University of Berne
Berne, Switzerland

The renal transport of Pi is under a powerful parathyroid hormone-independent adaptation mechanism (1,2). It has been suggested (3) that this adaptation mechanism could be defective in X-linked hypophosphatemia, a disease characterized by vitamin D-resistant rickets and decreased tubular reabsorption of Pi (4).

HYP mice first described by Eicher et al. (5) are considered as animal model of the human X-linked hypophosphatemic rickets. In a recent study (6) we have tested the hypothesis whether the renal leak of Pi might be caused by a defect in the adaptation mechanism which adjusts the renal handling of Pi according to the dietary Pi intake. Male HYP mice (HYP/Y) and normal littermates (+/Y) were submitted to high (0.75 %) or low (0.25 %) phosphorus diets for periods varying between 1 and 20 days. Then the urinary fractional excretion of Pi (FEPi) at endogenous plasma Pi $[Pi]_{Pl}$ was measured. Furthermore, Pi excretion was measured in all animals at increasing $[Pi]_{Pl}$ during an acute Pi infusion. The overall tubular Pi transport capacity was assessed by determining the maximal net Pi reabsorption per unit volume of glomerular filtrate (max. TRPi/ml GF). As shown in the upper panels of Fig. 1, in both +/Y and HYP/Y mice a dramatic fall in FEPi was observed already after 1 day of Pi restriction. In the left lower panel the progressive and marked enhancement of max.TRPi/ml GF beyond the first day of feeding low Pi diet in +/Y mice is shown. The results obtained in HYP/Y mice are depicted in the right lower panel. In sharp contrast it can be seen that HYP/Y mice are unable to increase significantly their

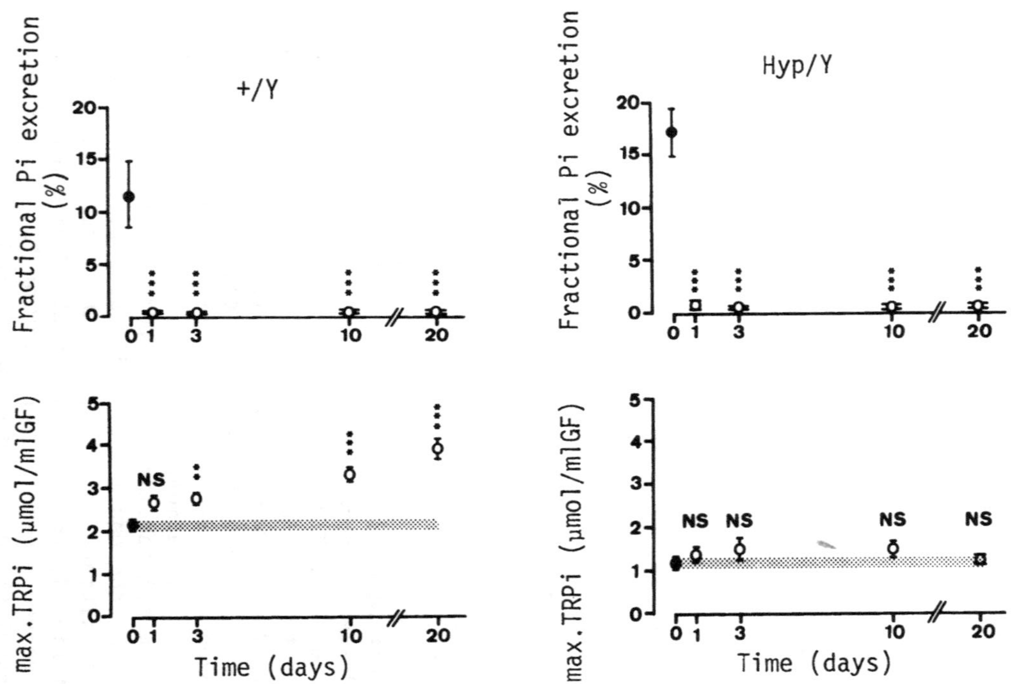

Fig. 1. Upper panels: Fractional excretion of phosphate in control +/Y (left) and hypo-phospatemic HYP/Y (right) mice fed either a high (●) or a low (O) phosphate diet for various periods of time.
Lower panels: Maximal phosphate reabsorption per ml GF in +/Y (left) and HYP/Y (right) mice fed low (O) phosphate diet for various periods of time. (●) and dotted lines indicate the values obtained in animals fed the high phosphate diet.
The values represent means + SEM. NS = not significantly different, ** $p < 0.01$, *** $p < 0.001$ as compared to the corresponding high phosphate group. Adapted from (6).

max.TRPi/ml GF when fed low Pi diet for up to 20 days. Even challenging HYP/Y mice with a very low Pi diet (0.03 %) for 10 days did not lead to a significant increment of the reabsorptive capacity for Pi (6). In chronically thyroparathyroidectomized (TPTX) animals 10 days of low Pi diet stimulated conspicuously max. TRPi/ml GF in +/Y mice, whereas the same regimen did not significantly change the Pi reabsorptive capacity of HYP/Y counterparts (6).

Thus, the normal adaptive response which is reflected by a progressive and marked enhancement in max.TRPi/ml GF after the first day of Pi restriction is not observed in intact or TPTX HYP/Y mice.

In a second study we have investigated by renal clearance studies whether the reduced concentration of plasma calcium observed (5,7,8,9,10,11,12) in male hypophosphatemic (HYP/Y) mice compared with normal littermates (+/Y) could be due, at least in part, to a decrease in the overall tubular capacity to reabsorb calcium. The results indicate that HYP/Y mice have a decrease in the tubular capacity to reabsorb calcium. This decrease appears to be related to the phosphate status of the animals, since it is much more pronounced when the animals are fed a low phosphorus diet. The decrement in the tubular reabsorption and plasma concentration of calcium in HYP/Y mice is not accompnied by an augmentation in the absolute urinary excretion of calcium. It is associated with an increase in the urinary excretion of cyclic AMP in agreement with previous works (13,14). Furthermore, removal of the thyroparathyroid glands leads to much larger fall in the plasma concentration of calcium in HYP/Y than in +/Y mice.

In conclusion, the results of this study strongly suggest that murine X-linked hypophosphatemia is a disease with a defect in the mechanism responsible for the adaptation of the tubular Pi transport system to Pi restriction. This abnormality is associated with a decrease in the tubular calcium reabsorption which appears to be related to the degree of Pi depletion. Despite the reduced tubular reabsorptive capacity for calcium, there was no apparent increase in the mobilization of calcium from intestinal and body sources as reflected by the absence of an augmentation in the absolute amount of calcium excreted in the urine. These findings could account for a propensity to hypocalcemia which would be partially compensated by secondary hyperparathyroidism. This compensation could explain the increase in urinary cyclic AMP excretion and the exaggerated hypocalcemic response to removal of the parathyroid glands observed in murine X-linked hypophosphatemia.

ACKNOWLEDGEMENTS

This work has been supported by the Swiss National Science Foundation (grant 3.824.79) and by the Ausbildungs- und Förderungsfonds der Arbeitsgemeinschaft für Osteosynthese (AO), Chur, Switzerland.

REFERENCES

1. U. Tröhler, J.-P. Bonjour, and H. Fleisch, Inorganic phosphate homeostasis. Renal adaptation to the dietary intake in intact and thyroparathyroidectomized rats, J. Clin. Invest. 57:264 (1976).
2. T. H. Steele, and H. F. DeLuca, Influence of dietary phosphorus on renal phosphate reabsorption in the parathyroidectomized rat, J. Clin. Invest. 57:867 (1976).
3. J.-P. Bonjour, and H. Fleisch, Tubular adaptation to the supply and requirement of phosphate, in: "Renal Handling of Phosphate", S. G. Massry and H. Fleisch, eds., Plenum Publishing Company, New York (1980).
4. R. W. Chesney, Tubular defects in phosphate reabsorption in clinical medicine, in: "Renal Handling of Phosphate", S. G. Massry and H. Fleisch, eds., Plenum Publishing Company, New York (1980).
5. E. M. Eicher, J. L. Southard, C. R. Scriver, and F. H. Glorieux, Hypophosphatemia: Mouse model for human familial hypophosphatemic (vitamin D-resistant) rickets, Proc. Natl. Acad. Sci. USA 73:4667 (1976).
6. R. C. Mühlbauer, J.-P. Bonjour, and H. Fleisch, Abnormal tubular adaptation to dietary phosphorus restriction in X-linked hypophosphatemic mice, Amer. J. Physiol., to be published.
7. H. S. Tenenhouse, and C. R. Scriver, Renal adaptation to phosphate deprivation in the hyp mouse with X-linked hypophosphatemia, Can. J. Biochem. 57:938 (1979).
8. R. A. Meyer, Jr., R. W. Gray, and M. H. Meyer, Abnormal vitamin D metabolism in the X-linked hypophosphatemic mouse, Endocrinology, 107:1577 (1980).
9. P. J. A. O'Doherty, H. F. DeLuca, and E. M. Eicher, Intestinal calcium and phosphate transport in genetic hypophosphatemic mice, Biochem. Biophys. Res. Commun. 71:617 (1976).
10. P. J. A. O'Doherty, H. F. DeLuca, and E. M. Eicher, Lack of effect of Vitamin D and its metabolites on intestinal phosphate transport in familial hypophosphatemia of mice, Endocrinology 101:1325 (1977).
11. W. G. Beamer, M. C. Wilson, and H. F. DeLuca, Successful treatment of genetically hypophosphatemic mice by 1 α-hydroxyvitamin D_3 but not 1,25-dihydroxyvitamin D_3, Endocrinology 106:1949 (1980).

12. R. Mühlbauer, J.-P. Bonjour, and H. Fleisch, Tubular handling of phosphate (Pi) and Ca in X-linked hypophosphatemic mice: Defective adaptation to Pi restriction associated with a renal Ca leak, in: "Hormonal control of calcium metabolism", Proc. 7th Int. Conf. on Calcium Regulating Hormones, Estes Park, USA, 1980, D. V. Cohn, R. V. Talmage, and J. Les Matthews, eds, Excerpta Medica, Amsterdam-Oxford-Princeton (1981).
13. H. S. Tenenhouse, C. R. Scriver, R. R. McInnes, and F- H. Glorieux, Renal handling of phosphate in vivo and in vitro by the X-linked hypophosphatemic male mouse: Evidence for a defect in the brush border membrane, Kidney Int. 14:236 (1978).
14. R. A. Meyer, Jr., R. W. Gray, G. M. Kiebzak, and P. M. Mish, Altered vitamin D, cyclic nucleotide and trace mineral metabolism in the X-linked hypophosphatemic mouse, in: "Phosphate and Minerals in Health and Disease" (Vol. 128, in Advances in Experimental Medicine and Biology) Proceedings 4th Int. Workshop on Phosphate and Other Minerals, S.G. Massry, E. Ritz, and H.Jahn, eds., Plenum Press, New York and London (1980)

RENAL Pi TRANSPORT IN YOUNG GROWING AND ADULT RATS: COMPARATIVE STUDIES IN BRUSH BORDER MEMBRANE VESICLES (BBMV) AND IN WHOLE KIDNEY

J. Caverzasio, J.-P. Bonjour, H. Murer
and H. Fleisch
Institute of Pathophysiology
University of Berne
Berne, Switzerland

The question where and how the renal transport of inorganic phosphate (Pi) is regulated has been the subject of numerous investigations over the last few years. In this regard, the discovery of a sodium-dependent Pi transport system in the brush border membranes of the renal cortex (1) has been of particular interest. It gave rise to the question of whether the Pi transfer rate determined by this system across the luminal membrane of the proximal tubule would be the only limited and regulated step of the overall net tubular Pi reabsorption. Therefore we have been particularly interested in studying the relationship between alterations in the overall tubular Pi reabsorptive capacity and changes in the Pi transport at the level of brush border membrane vesicles (BBMV) of the renal cortex of rats. In this investigation the alterations in the renal handling of Pi were provoked by variation in dietary Pi, removal of the parathyroid gland, chronic administration of either 1,25-dihydroxyvitamin D_3 to thyroparathyroidectomized animals or the diphosphonate ethane-1-hydroxy-1,1-diphosphonate (2,3). Analysis of these experiments (2,3,4) revealed an impressive correlation between the initial rate of the sodium-dependent Pi uptake by BBMV of renal cortex and the tubular Pi transport capacity of the whole kidney, as assessed by measuring the maximal net Pi reabsorption per unit volume of glomerular filtrate (max.TRPi/ml GFR). Such a correlation suggested that the transfer rate across the luminal membrane of the proximal tubule represents the key process in the overall tubular regulation of the transport of Pi. However, free-flow micropuncture data indicated that other tubular segments localized beyond the proximal tubule may also participate in this regulation (5,6,7,8). In the present communication we present situations wherein the sodium-dependent Pi uptake by BBMV does not always vary in parallel with changes observed in the whole kidney.

Thus we have observed that max. TRPi/ml GF is markedly lower in adult than in young growing rats fed either low (0.2 %) or normal (0.8 %) phosphorus diet (9). Studies with BBMV indicate, however, that it is only under the low phosphorus diet that the Pi uptake is depressed in adult as compared to young animals. Other clearance experiments have also shown that in contrast to the conspicuous adaptive change observed in young growing rats, max. TRPi/ml GF is not significantly enhanced in adult rats submitted to a low phosphorus diet (0.2 %) for 8 days (9). Studies with BBMV indicate, however, that after this period of reduced Pi supply, the Pi uptake is significantly enhanced in adult as in young rats.

In conclusion, these experiments demonstrate that the Pi transport in BBMV does not appear to change commensurately with that of the whole kidney in all circumstances. These results therefore strongly suggest that the regulation of the transfer rate of Pi across the renal epithelium probably involves other additional modulating factors than merely the sodium-dependent transport system localized in the luminal membrane of the proximal tubule. Thus, it is possible that at the level of the proximal tubule, changes in the driving forces or in the Pi transfer across the baselateral membrane could participate to the determination of the overall transepithelial transfer rate. Finally, other segments than the proximal tubule could also play a non-negligeable role in the regulation of the renal handling of Pi.

ACKNOWLEDGEMENTS

This work has been supported by the Swiss National Science Foundation (3.824.79), and the Ausbildungs- und Förderungsfonds der Arbeitsgemeinschaft für Osteosynthese (AO), Chur, Switzerland.

REFERENCES

1. N. Hoffmann, M. Thees, and R. Kinne, Phosphate transport by isolated renal brush border vesicles, Pflügers Arch. 362:147 (1976)

2. R. Stoll, R. Kinne, H. Murer, H. Fleisch, and J.-P. Bonjour, Phosphate transport by rat renal brush border membrane vesicles: Influence of dietary phosphate, thyroparathyroidectomy, and 1,25-dihydroxyvitamin D_3, Pflügers Arch. 380:47 (1979).
3. R. Stoll, H. Murer, H. Fleisch, and J.-P. Bonjour, Effect of diphosphonate treatment on phosphate transport by renal brush border vesicles, Amer. J. Physiol. 239:F13 (1980).
4. J.-P. Bonjour, J. Caverzasio, H. Fleisch, R. Mühlbauer, and U. Tröhler, Renal handling of phosphate. Contr. Nephrol. 23:11 (1980).
5. R. C. Mühlbauer, J.-P. Bonjour, and H. Fleisch, Tubular localization of the adaptation to dietary phosphate in rats, Amer. J. Physiol. 233:F342 (1977).
6. R. C. Mühlbauer, J.-P. Bonjour, and H. Fleisch, Chronic thyroparathyroidectomy and tubular handling of phosphate: Increased reabsorption in late but not in early proximal tubule, Pflügers Arch. 388:185 (1980).
7. R. C. Mühlbauer, J.-P. Bonjour, and H. Fleisch, Tubular handling of phosphate along the nephron of thyroparathyroidectomized rats injected with ethane-1-hydroxy-1,1-diphosphonate, Clin. Sci. 60:171 (1981).
8. R. C. Mühlbauer, J.-P. Bonjour, and H. Fleisch, Tubular handling of Pi: localization of effects of $1,25(OH)_2D_3$ and dietary Pi in TPTX rats, Amer. J. Physiol. 241:F123 (1981).
9. J. Caverzasio, J.-P. Bonjour, H. Murer, and H. Fleisch, Adaptation of renal Pi transport in young growing and adult rats: Dissociation between changes in brush border membrane vesicles (BBMV) and in whole kidney, in: abstracts 8th Internat. Congr. of Nephrology, Athens, CA-079 (1981).

DIFFERENCE IN RENAL TUBULAR TRANSPORT EFFECTS OF 1-34 and 1-84 PARATHYROID HORMONE (PTH)

J.B. Puschett, J. McGowan, J. Fragola, T.C. Chen, M. Rosenblatt, and H. Keutmann

University of Pittsburgh School of Medicine, Pittsburgh PA, and Endocrine Unit, Massachusetts General Hospital Boston, MA

It has recently been established that the fragment of parathyroid hormone (PTH) consisting of the first 34 amino acids at the amino terminus possesses biological activity similar to that demonstrated by the native, 1-84 hormone molecule. In particular, the 1-34 fragment has been shown to be capable of inducing hypercalcemia and phosphaturia in vivo, and can stimulate the adenylate cyclase system in vitro.[1-3] The characteristic acute effects of PTH on the kidney are the production of a marked phosphaturia associated with either a decline or no change in calcium excretion.[4] Although data detailing the effects of 1-34 PTH on phosphate excretion are available in the literature, the effect of the fragment on calcium transport has not been studied. We therefore compared the action of 1-34 and 1-84 PTH on calcium excretion in acute clearance studies performed in the dog.

Female mongrel dogs underwent thyroparathyroidectomy at least 48 hrs. and usually 72 hrs. to 1 week prior to study. Thyroid hormone was replaced. Inulin and p-aminohippurate (PAH) were begun and a 60 min. equilibration period was accomplished. Following the procurement of control phase blood and urine collections, the animals were divided into one of three experimental protocols. They received either synthetic bovine 1-34 PTH or naturally occurring bovine 1-84 PTH in doses of .5-1.0 μg/kg./hr. for two hours, or else were infused only with saline in similar volumes to those employed for the hormone. The latter group served as time controls. In some of the 1-34 studies, the substituted compound 8,18 norleucine, 34-tyrosine amide was utilized.

No changes in phosphate or calcium excretion occurred in the control dogs from control to experimental phase of the studies. The 1-84 and 1-34 hormone preparation produced equivalent increments in percentage phosphate excretion of about 19% of filtered load. However, their actions on calcium excretion were strikingly different. Whereas the infusion of the 1-84 preparation resulted in no alteration in calcium excretion, the 1-34 fragment was actually calciuric. The percentage of filtered calcium excreted tripled after infusion of the 1-34 hormone.

In none of the three groups of animals were there any changes in glomerular filtration rate, effective renal plasma flow or serum ultrafilterable calcium which could have accounted for the calcium or phosphate excretion results obtained. Furthermore, both hormone preparations were active in vitro in stimulating the adenylate cyclase system, in our hands. We conclude from these experiments that the first 34 amino acids of the amino terminal portion of the PTH molecule are sufficient for the hormone to inhibit phosphate transport. However, in order for PTH to produce its characteristic effects on calcium excretion, the entire 84 amino acids seem to be required. Furthermore, this difference in the effects of the two hormone preparations on calcium excretion does not appear to be mediated by variations in the response of the adenylate cyclase system to the hormone. Studies are currently underway to determine the mechanism(s) of this difference in the renal tubular effects of the two hormone molecules.

REFERENCES

1. J.T. Potts, Jr., G.W. Tregear, H.T. Keutmann, H.D. Niall, R. Sauer, L.J. Deftos, G.F. Dawson, M.L. Hogen, and G.D. Aurbach, Synthesis of a biologically active N-terminal tetratriacontapeptide of parathyroid hormone, Proc. Natl. Acad. Sci. USA 68:63 (1981).
2. G.W. Tregear, J. Van Rietschoten, E. Greene, H.T. Keutmann, H.D. Niall, B. Reit, J.A. Parsons, and J.T. Potts, Jr., Bovine parathyroid hormone: minimum chain length of synthetic peptide required for biological activity, Endocrinology 93:1349 (1973).
3. F.G. Knox and C. Lechene, Distal site of action of parathyroid hormone on phosphate reabsorption, Am. J. Physiol. 229:1556 (1975).
4. J.B. Puschett, Renal tubular effects of parathyroid hormone: an update, Clin. Orthop. 135:249 (1978).

1,25-DIHYDROXYCHOLECALCIFEROL (CALCITRIOL): EFFECT ON PHOSPHATE (PO_4) ABSORPTION BY ISOLATED PARS RECTA

Robert A. Peraino and Wadi N. Suki

Baylor College of Medicine & The Methodist Hospital
Houston, Texas

INTRODUCTION

Phosphate handling by the kidney is influenced by a number of factors including extracellular fluid volume, plasma calcium concentration, bicarbonate administration, parathyroid hormone, and dietary phosphate balance. Vitamin D metabolites have also been demonstrated to augment renal phosphate absorption in the presence and absence of PTH (1-6). Bonjour, Preston and Fleisch have demonstrated that calcitriol increases phosphate excretion in the thyroparathyroidectomized rat (7), and Gloor, Bonjour, Caverzasio and Fleisch demonstrated that calcitriol prevents the renal resistance to the phosphaturic response to PTH during phosphate depletion (8). These investigators localized the site of action of calcitriol to the proximal convoluted tubule and beyond the point of micropuncture in the distal tubule in the rat (9).

The purpose of the present study was to examine the renal tubule effect of calcitriol using the technique of in vitro perfusion of isolated rabbit tubule segments. Because an effect of PTH to inhibit phosphate absorption by the isolated pars recta of the rabbit has been demonstrated, we chose to examine this nephron segment.

METHODS

Segments of superficial and juxtamedullary pars recta were isolated from female New Zealand white rabbits fed a normal diet containing adequate amounts of calcium and 6 I.U. cholecalciferol per gram of diet. Segments were bathed and perfused with an artificial solution simulating glomerular filtrate without protein in the bath. Four

Groups of tubules were studied.

Group I: Segments of superficial and juxtamedullary pars recta were perfused with the artificial solution to which was added propylene glycol, the vehicle for calcitriol. After waiting 30 minutes, tubule fluid collections were obtained. The bath and perfusate were then changed to ones containing calcitriol, 10 nM, and collections obtained after waiting at least 30 minutes.

Group II: Segments were perfused with the artificial solution and collections obtained during the control period. For the experimental period, the bath and perfusate were changed to ones containing 8-bromo-cAMP, 10 uM, and collections obtained.

Groups III: Segments were perfused and bathed with the artificial solution containing 8-bromo-cAMP during the control period. For the experimental period calcitriol, either 10 nM or 50 pM, was added to bath and perfusate in the presence of the cAMP.

Groups IV: Segments were perfused and bathed with the artificial solution containing calcitriol, 10 nM, during the control period. For the experimental period synthetic bovine (1-34) PTH was added to the bath to give a final concentration of 0.2 U/ml, while the calcitriol was continued.

The rate of fluid absorption was measured with tritiated inulin in the perfusate only; unidirectional lumen to bath phosphate absorption was measured with 32-P in the perfusate only; the potential difference at the perfusion end of the tubule segment was monitored by standard techniques. Tubule segments were perfused at 10 - 25 nl/min.

RESULTS

Neither calcitriol alone (Group I) nor 8-bromo-cAMP alone (Group II) affected the rate of fluid absorption, lumen to bath phosphate flux, nor the potential difference in either superficial or juxtamedullary pars rectae. When calcitriol was superimposed on 8-bromo-cAMP, however, a 50% inhibition of lumen to bath phosphate flux was demonstrated in both anatomic segments of the proximal straight tubule. No changes in rate of fluid absorption or potential difference were observed with the cyclic nucleotide plus calcitriol. When synthetic bovine (1-34) PTH was superimposed upon calcitriol, the rate of fluid absorption was decreased 30%. However, no changes in lumen to bath phosphate flux or potential difference were observed. Additionally, no differences in lumen to bath phosphate flux were observed when superficial segments were compared to juxtamedullary tubules.

The results of these studies demonstrate that there is no internephron heterogeneity for phosphate transport by the rabbit pars recta; that, in the presence of cyclic AMP, calcitriol inhibits phosphate absorption without changes in fluid absorption or potential difference. Thus phosphate transport in part may be by an active mechanism and that calcitriol may be a modulator of cyclic AMP action. In addition, the failure of PTH to inhibit phosphate flux in the presence of calcitriol suggests that the vitamin D metabolite may be an inhibitor of PTH action upon the pars recta of the rabbit.

1. Puschett, J.B., Morony, J., and Kurnick, W.S., 1972, Evidence for a direct action of cholecalciferol and 25-hydroxycholecalciferol on the renal transport of phosphate, sodium, and calcium, J. Clin. Invest., 51:373.
2. Puschett, J.B., Beck, W.S., Jr., and Jelonek, A., 1975, Parathyroid hormone and 25-hydroxyvitamin D3: Synergistic and antagonistic effects on renal phosphate transport, Science, 190:473.
3. Puschett, J.B., Beck, W.S., Jr., Jelonek, A., and Fernandez, P.C., 1974, Study of the renal tubular interactions of thyrocalcitonin, cyclic adenosine 3',5'-monophosphate, 25-hydroxycholecalciferol, and calcium ion, J. Clin. Invest., 53:756.
4. Costanzo, L.S., Sheehe, P.R., and Weiner, I.M., 1974, Renal actions of vitamin D in D-deficient rats, Amer. J. Physiol., 226:1490.
5. Popovtzer, M.M., Robinette, J.B., DeLuca, H.F., and Holick, M.D., 1974, The acute effect of 25-hydroxycholecalciferol on renal handling of phosphorus. Evidence for a parathyroid hormone-dependent mechanism, J. Clin. Invest., 53:913.
6. Puschett, J.B., Fernandez, P.C., Bolye, I.T., Gray, R.W., Omdahl, J.L., and DeLuca, H.F., 1972, The acute renal tubular effects of 1,25 dihydroxycholecalciferol, Proc. Soc. Exp. Biol. Med., 141:379.
7. Bonjour, J-P., Preston, C., and Fleisch, H., 1977, Effect of 1,25-dihydroxyvitamin D3 on the renal handling of Pi in thyroparathyroidectomized rats, J. Clin. Invest., 60:1419.
8. Gloor, H.J., Bonjour, J-P., Caverzasio, J., and Fleisch, H., 1979, Resistance to the phosphaturic and calcemic actions of parathyroid hormone during phosphate depletion. Prevention by 1,25-dihydroxyvitamin D3, J. Clin. Invest., 63:371.
9. Muhlbauer, R.C., Bonjour, J-P., and Fleisch, H., 1981, Tubular handling of Pi: localization of effects of $1,25(OH)_2D_3$ and dietary Pi in TPTX rats, Amer. J. Physiol., 241:F123.

IN VIVO AND *IN VITRO* EFFECTS OF VITAMIN D_3 [1,25-$(OH)_2D_3$] ON THE UPTAKE OF PHOSPHATE BY ISOLATED CHICK KIDNEY CELLS

Bertram Sacktor, Linda Cheng and C. Tony Liang

National Institute on Aging, National Institutes of Health, Baltimore City Hospitals, Baltimore, MD 21224

INTRODUCTION

Harrison and Harrison[1] first proposed that vitamin D acts as an important regulator of phosphate homeostasis. Since then, it has has been demonstrated that the active form of the vitamin, 1,25-dihydroxycholecalciferol [1,25-$(OH)_2D_3$], enhances, by an unknown mechanism, the intestinal absorption of phosphate[2,3]. The effect of 1,25-$(OH)_2D_3$ on the reabsorption of phosphate in the kidney is less clear. In some studies, infusion of the vitamin has been found to decrease phosphate excretion[4,5], whereas in other investigations 1,25-$(OH)_2D_3$ has been reported to be phosphaturic[6] or without effect on urinary phosphate[7]. Some of the difficulties in resolving the apparent discrepancies stem, in part, from the complex interactions in the *in vivo* animal of the vitamin D metabolic and phosphate transport systems with various regulatory factors, including parathyroid hormone and other endocrines, dietary status, and calcium[8,9]. This prompted us to initiate studies on a simpler model system, namely, the isolated renal cell. In this report we will examine the effects of 1,25-$(OH)_2D_3$ on the uptake of phosphate by these isolated cells; first, after the vitamin is administered to a D-deficient chick *in vivo*, and second, when 1,25-$(OH)_2D_3$ is incubated with the cells *in vitro*.

METHODS

One day old White Leghorn cockerels were kept in a darkened room for 19 to 24 days and maintained on a Vitamin D-deficient diet (Teklab Test Diet TD 75007, Madison, WI), containing 0.6% phosphorus and 0.6% calcium. The chicks had free access to deionized water.

The 1,25-$(OH)_2D_3$-treated birds were given orally 1 μg of the vitamin dissolved in 200 μl of propylene glycol.

Chick renal cells were isolated by a collagenase-hyaluronidase procedure[10], that was recently modified and described in detail[11]. The final preparation of cells, suspended in a medium containing 280 mM mannitol, 10 mM Hepes-KOH buffer, pH 7.2, 2.5 mM glutamine, 0.5 mM β-hydroxybutyrate, and 1 mM mannose, consisted almost exclusively of single cells or clusters of 2 to 5 cells, with an occasional small tubular fragment of 5 to 12 cells. The average yield was 4 x 10^7 cells/g of tissue. The isolated cells excluded trypan blue essentially completely, suggesting that the plasma membrane remained intact after the collagenase-hyaluronidase preparative procedure. The metabolic state of the cells from D-deficient animals, reflected in terms of oxygen consumption in the presence of endogenous and exogenous substrates and uncouplers of oxidative phosphorylation, were recently reported[11]. It was found that the renal cells, as isolated, did not exhibit evidence of metabolic impairment; rather they retained the properties characteristic of metabolically active and functionally intact cells. No significant difference was found in the oxygen uptake of cells from D-deficient chicks and cells from 1,25-$(OH)_2D_3$-repleted animals[11].

Uptake of $[^{32}P]$-phosphate and $[^{14}C]$-α-methylglucoside by the isolated cells were measured by a centrifugation method reported previously[11]. Briefly, a 100 μl aliquot of the cell suspension, about 1.6 x 10^6 cells representing about 0.5 mg of protein, was pre-equilibrated at 37°C. Uptake was initiated with the addition of 100 μl of a medium comprised of 140 mM NaCl or KCl, 10 mM Hepes-KOH buffer, pH 7.2, and either 0.2 mM $[^{32}P]$-phosphate or 0.1 mM $[^{14}C]$-α-methylglucoside. Uptake was terminated by removing 180 μl of the reaction mixture and adding the aliquot to a centrifuge tube containing 1 ml of ice-cold stopping solution containing 124 mM NaCl, 10 mM Na_2HAsO_4 and 1 mM Hepes-KOH buffer, pH 7.2. The cells were centrifuged for 1 min, the supernatant discarded, and the pellet washed with an additional 1 ml of stopping solution. The cells were pelleted, solubilized with alkali, and the radioactivity taken up countered. Uptakes were linear with respect to cell number and protein within the range used in these experiments.

When determining the uptakes of $[^{32}P]$-phosphate and $[^{14}C]$-α-methylglucoside by cells that were pre-incubated with 1,25-$(OH)_2D_3$ *in vitro*, the isolated cells were resuspended in McCoy's medium. To each ml of cell suspension 50 μl of fresh serum from vitamin D-deficient chicks were added. After 5 min at room temperature, 5 μl of 1,25-$(OH)_2D_3$ in ethanol, or ethanol alone, were added. The cells were then pre-incubated for 2.5 hrs at 37°C. Afterwards, the cells were collected by centrifugation and washed twice with a medium containing 280 mM mannitol, 10 mM Hepes-KOH buffer, pH 7.2,

2.5 mM glutamine, 0.5 mM β-hydroxybutyrate, and 1 mM mannose. Uptakes of [^{32}P]-phosphate and [^{14}C]-α-methylglucoside were carried out as described above.

RESULTS

The uptakes of [^{32}P]-phosphate and [^{14}C]-α-methylglucoside by cells from D-deficient chicks are described in Fig. 1. The presence of 70 mM NaCl in the extracellular medium markedly enhanced the uptakes of both labeled substrates. At 1 min, the uptake of phosphate was 10- to 20-times greater with Na^+ than with K^+ in the medium. The stimulation of the uptake of the sugar by Na^+ was 4- to 8-fold. At concentrations of 0.1 mM phosphate and 0.05 mM α-methylglucoside the uptake of phosphate was about 20-times that of the sugar. Accumulation of radioactivity was not linear with time, however, even at the earliest measured time points. Nevertheless, for comparative purposes, the uptakes of phosphate at 1 min and α-methylglucoside at 2 min were used in this study to approximate

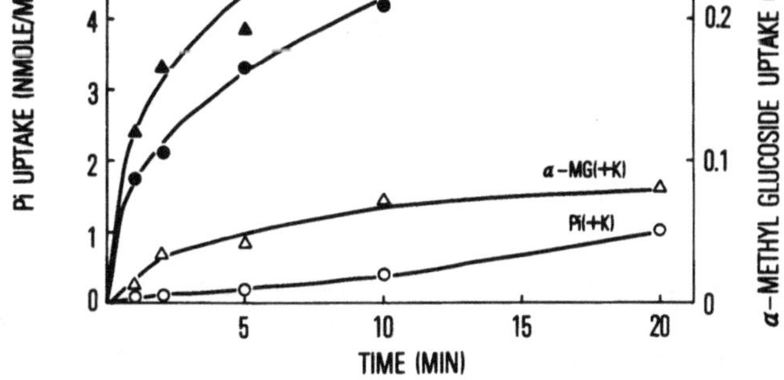

Fig. 1. The uptakes of phosphate and α-methylglucoside by renal cells isolated from D-deficient chicks. The extracellular medium contained 70 mM NaCl or KCl. (Data are from Liang *et al.*[11]).

roughly initial rates. The uptake of phosphate by the isolated renal cells was a saturable transport process. In the presence of 70 mM Na^+ in the incubation medium the apparent K_m for the system was 0.19 mM phosphate and the V_{max} was 5 nmol/min·mg cell protein.

The effects of 1,25-$(OH)_2D_3$ repletion of D-deficient chicks on the uptake of phosphate and α-methylglucoside by the renal cells are shown in Fig. 2. The animals were given 1 μg of 1,25-$(OH)_2D_3$ orally. Control animals received only the vehicle solution. Three hrs later, the cells were isolated and the uptakes of the metabolites by the repleted and deficient cells were compared. Na^+-dependent phosphate uptake by cells from 1,25-$(OH)_2D_3$-treated chicks was increased by about 60%, 2.00 ± 0.13 compared to 1.26 ± 0.13 nmol/min·mg protein ($0.005<P>0.01$). Only the Na^+-dependent uptake was enhanced; phosphate uptake in the presence of extracellular K^+ was unchanged. Repletion with 1,25-$(OH)_2D_3$ had no significant effect on the uptake of α-methylglucoside in the presence or absence of Na^+.

This early response to the injection of 1,25-$(OH)_2D_3$ *in vivo* preceded significant measurable changes in serum levels of phosphorus and calcium. The concentrations of phosphorus in the serum of D-deficient and 3 hr-repleted animals were essentially identical, 3.55 ± 0.27 and 3.64 ± 0.52 mg/dl, respectively. The serum concentrations of calcium in D-deficient and 3 hr-repleted chicks did not differ significantly, 6.93 ± 0.23 and 7.40 ± 0.27 mg/dl, respectively.

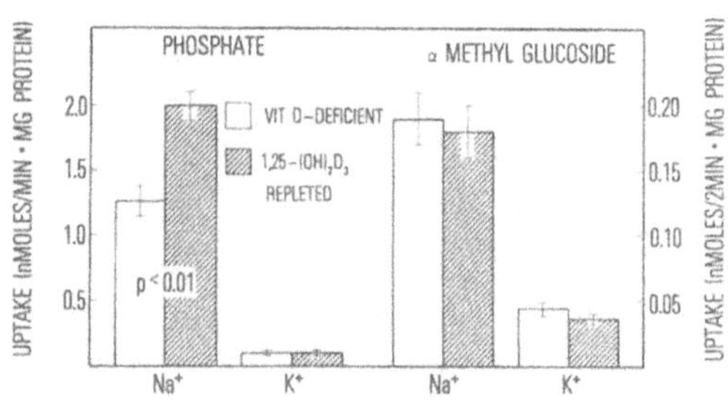

Fig. 2. The effects of 1,25-$(OH)_2D_3$ administered *in vivo* to D-deficient chicks on the uptake of phosphate and α-methylglucoside by isolated renal cells. (Data are from Liang *et al.*[11]).

The preceding experiment showed that the uptake of phosphate by isolated renal cells reflected the vitamin D status of the chick from which the cells were derived. This suggests that the isolated cell may represent an appropriate model to study the mechanism by which 1,25-$(OH)_2D_3$ influences phosphate transport. The utility of the model becomes evident additionally from our experiments which demonstrate that 1,25-$(OH)_2D_3$ incubated with the cells, *in vitro*, affects phosphate uptake. Fig. 3 shows that when cells obtained from D-deficient chicks were pre-incubated, *in vitro*, with 1,25-$(OH)_2D_3$ for 2.5 hrs and then initial rates of phosphate uptake determined a significant increase in uptake was found. Again, only Na^+-dependent phosphate uptake was enhanced; uptake was unaffected in the presence of extracellular K^+, substituting for Na^+, in the medium (data not shown). Other experiments (not illustrated) showed that the action of 1,25-$(OH)_2D_3$ was specific for phosphate since the uptakes of α-methylglucoside in the presence and absence of Na^+ were not

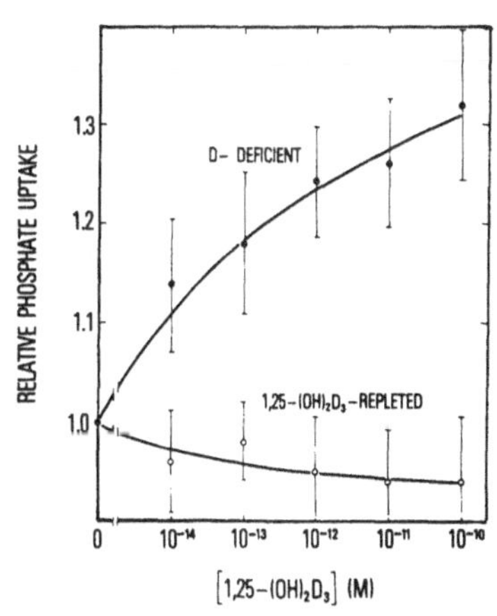

Fig. 3. The effects of the concentration of 1,25-$(OH)_2D_3$ pre-incubated with isolated renal cells from D-deficient and 1,25-$(OH)_2D_3$-repleted chicks on the uptake of phosphate by these cells.

altered by these concentrations of the vitamin.

Fig. 3 shows that the stimulatory effect of 1,25-$(OH)_2D_3$ on phosphate uptake was dependent on the concentration of the vitamin. A concentration as low as 10^{-14} M enhanced the uptake by about 15%. At the physiological concentration of 1,25-$(OH)_2D_3$, approximately 10^{-10}M, uptake was increased by 30%. Higher concentrations of 1,25-$(OH)_2D_3$ in the incubation medium did not stimulate uptake further.

In contrast to the increase in phosphate uptake found when 1,25-$(OH)_2D_3$ was incubated, *in vitro*, with cells from D-deficient animals, Fig. 3 shows that the vitamin did not enhance uptake when incubated with cells derived from chicks injected with the vitamin 3 hrs previously. In fact, a slight inhibition, perhaps of questionable statistical significance, was found. Thus, renal cells from D-deficient animals differed from cells from 1,25-$(OH)_2D_3$-repleted animals in their *in vitro* response to 1,25-$(OH)_2D_3$. This finding suggests that once stimulation of phosphate uptake was induced by 1,25-$(OH)_2D_3$, as was the case when the vitamin was administered 3 hours earlier to the D-deficient animal, the cell became refractory to further stimulation by the vitamin.

In the preceding experiment, increases in phosphate uptake by cells from D-deficient animals were found after the isolated cells were pre-incubated with 1,25-$(OH)_2D_3$ for 2.5 hrs. Stimulation of phosphate uptake was measurable after a pre-incubation period of only 1 hr (Fig. 4). However, the maximal response required at

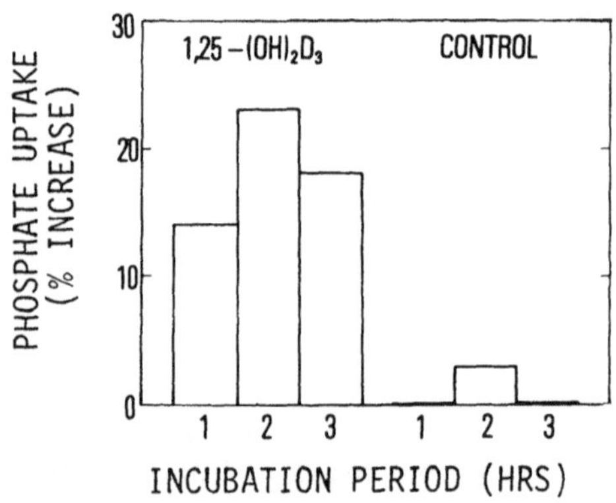

Fig. 4. The effect of time of pre-incubation of 1,25-$(OH)_2D_3$ with isolated renal cells on the cellular uptake of phosphate.

least 2 hrs. This finding suggests that an interim period of time was necessary between the exposure of the cells to the vitamin-inducer and the maximal response, expressed by an enhancement in phosphate uptake. This requirement for a lag-period was consistent with the results from other experiments showing that the 1,25-$(OH)_2D_3$-induced increase in phosphate uptake could be blocked by actinomycin D or cycloheximide.

The specificity of 1,25-$(OH)_2D_3$ in stimulating, *in vitro*, phosphate uptake is shown in Fig. 5. Cholecalciferol, (vitamin D_3) was essentially inactive at a concentration as high as 10^{-7}M. 24,25-$(OH)_2D_3$ showed slight activity in inducing the increase in phosphate uptake, but only at a concentration of 10^{-10} M, 4-orders of magnitude greater than found for 1,25-$(OH)_2D_3$. 1-$(OH)D_3$ was effective in stimulating phosphate uptake. However, 100-times the concentration of 1-$(OH)D_3$ was needed relative to 1,25-$(OH)_2D_3$. At very high concentrations, 25-$(OH)D_3$ also effected an increase in phosphate uptake. Whether this stimulation was a direct response to 25-$(OH)D_3$ or required the conversion of 25-$(OH)D_3$ to 1,25-$(OH)_2D_3$ by the renal cells during the pre-incubated period was not ascertained.

When the isolated renal cells were incubated with $[^3H]$-1,25-$(OH)_2D_3$ it was found that the labeled vitamin was taken up by the cells. For example, in a 2 ml incubation mixture containing

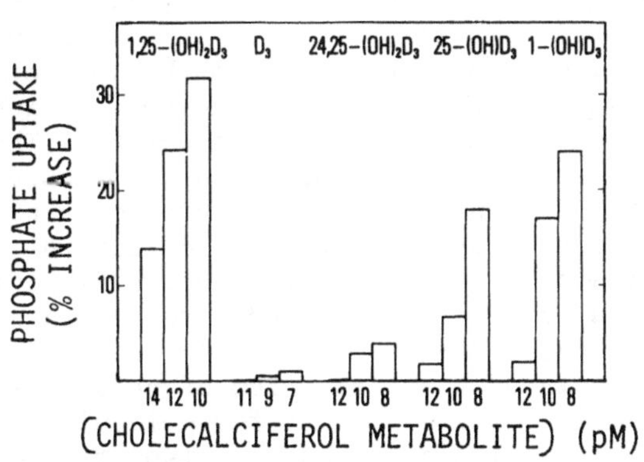

Fig. 5. The specificity of 1,25-$(OH)_2D_3$ in stimulating, *in vitro*, phosphate uptake by isolated renal cells.

3×10^7 cells and 4×10^{-11}M 1,25-$(OH)_2D_3$, 15% of the total label, or 1.25×10^{-14} moles of 1,25-$(OH)_2D_3$ was taken up in 2.5 hrs. It could be calculated that the average uptake per cell was 4.1×10^{-22} moles, indicating an average uptake of about 250 molecules of 1,25-$(OH)_2D_3$ per cell. This value was likely to be an overestimation of the amount of 1,25-$(OH)_2D_3$ actually needed to induce the phosphate transport response since in this experiment the concentration of 1,25-$(OH)_2D_3$ in the mixture was far greater than that required to demonstrate an effect. It is not unreasonable to suggest that induction could have been initiated by the uptake of as little as one or at most very few molecules of 1,25-$(OH)_2D_3$ per cell.

SUMMARY

The uptake of phosphate and α-methylglucoside by renal cells isolated from vitamin D-deficient and 1,25-$(OH)_2D_3$-repleted chicks were stimulated markedly by the presence of Na^+ in the extracellular medium. Three hrs after 1,25-$(OH)_2D_3$ was injected into D-deficient chicks the Na^+-dependent phosphate uptake by the isolated cells had increased 60%. Phosphate uptake in the presence of K^+ in the extracellular medium and α-methylglucoside uptake in the presence and absence of Na^+ were unaltered. When cells obtained from D-deficient animals were pre-incubated, *in vitro*, with 1,25-$(OH)_2D_3$, the cells showed an increased rate of Na^+-dependent phosphate uptake. The stimulation of phosphate uptake was dependent on the concentration of 1,25-$(OH)_2D_3$; a concentration as low as 10^{-14} increased the rate of uptake by 15%. Cells derived from chicks injected with the vitamin 3 hrs previously showed no enhanced uptake when they were pre-incubated with 1,25-$(OH)_2D_3$. This finding suggests that once stimulation of phosphate uptake was induced by 1,25-$(OH)_2D_3$ the cell became refractory to further stimulation by the vitamin. A lag-period of about 2 hrs was found between the initiation of exposure of the cells to the vitamin and the maximal response of the cell, expressed as an increase in phosphate uptake. The 1,25-$(OH)_2D_3$-induced increase in phosphate uptake could be blocked by inhibitors of protein synthesis. The enhancement of phosphate uptake was specific for 1,25-$(OH)_2D_3$. Cholecalciferol (Vitamin D_3) and other metabolites of D_3 were either inactive or active at concentrations several orders of magnitude greater than 1,25-$(OH)_2D_3$. When incubated with $[^3H]$-1,25-$(OH)_2D_3$, renal cells take up the vitamin. It was calculated that induction of phosphate uptake was initiated by the average uptake of very few molecules of 1,25-$(OH)_2D_3$ per cell. These findings indicate that the isolated renal cell represents an excellent model to study the mechanism by which 1,25-$(OH)_2D_3$ regulates phosphate transport in the kidney.

REFERENCES

1. H. E. Harrison and H. C. Harrison, Transfer of Ca^{45} across the intestinal wall *in vitro* in relation to the action of vitamin D and cortisol, *Am. J. Physiol.* 192:265 (1960).
2. S. Kowarski and D. Schachter, Effects of vitamin D on phosphate transport and incorporation into mucosal constituents of rat intestinal mucosa, *J. Biol. Chem.* 244:221 (1969).
3. T. C. Chen, L. Castillo, M. Korycka-Dahl and H. F. DeLuca, Role of vitamin D metabolites in phosphate transport of rat intestine, *J. Nutr.* 104:1056 (1974).
4. J. B. Puschett, P. C. Fernandez, I. T. Boyle, R. W. Gray, J. L. Omdahl and H. F. DeLuca, The acute renal tubular effects of 1,25-dihydroxycholecalciferol (36781), *Proc. Soc. Exp. Biol. Med.* 141:379 (1972).
5. M. M. Popovtzer, J. B. Robinette, H. F. DeLuca and M. F. Holick, The acute effect of 25-hydroxycholecalciferol on renal handling of phosphorus, *J. Clin. Invest.* 53:913 (1974).
6. J.-P. Bonjour, C. Preston and H. Fleisch, Effect of 1,25-dihydroxyvitamin D_3 on the renal handling of P_i in thyroparathyroidectomized rats, *J. Clin. Invest.* 60:1419 (1977).
7. T. H. Steele, J. E. Engle, Y. Tanaka, R. S. Lorenc, K. L. Dudgeon and H. F. DeLuca, Phosphatemic action of 1,25-dihydroxyvitamin D_3, *Am. J. Physiol.* 229:489 (1975).
8. H. F. DeLuca, The Vitamin D system in the regulation of calcium and phosphorus metabolism, *Nutr. Rev.* 37:161 (1979).
9. F. G. Knox, A. Hoppe, S. A. Kempson, S. V. Shah and T. P. Dousa, Cellular mechanisms of phosphate transport, in: "Renal Handling of Phosphate," S. G. Massry and H. Fleisch, eds., Plenum Publ. Corp., New York (1980).
10. H. L. Henry, Regulation of the hydroxylation of 25-hydroxyvitamin D_3 *in vivo* and in primary cultures of chick kidney cells, *J. Biol. Chem.* 254:2722 (1979).
11. C. T. Liang, J. Barnes, L. Cheng, R. Balakir and B. Sacktor, Effects of 1,25-dihydroxy vitamin D_3 administered *in vivo* to D-deficient chicks on the uptake of phosphate by isolated renal cells, *Am. J. Physiol.*, submitted.

POTASSIUM IMBALANCE AND PHOSPHATE RENAL HANDLING: A MICROPUNCTURE STUDY

Ph. Jaeger, B. Karlmark, J.Ph. Bonjour*, and G. Giebisch

Department of Physiology, Yale University
New Haven, CT 06510

INTRODUCTION

In order to study the relationship between potassium excretion and that of the main urinary buffer, i.e. phosphate, rat micropuncture experiments were carried out. The effects of acute potassium loading and chronic potassium depletion on phosphate transport along superficial nephrons were evaluated: marked antiphosphaturia was observed in both conditions. Whereas an impaired renal response to parathyroid hormone (PTH) in potassium depletion had already been described (1) it was not known whether such a mechanism might be involved in acute hyperkalemia. Hence, in an additional series of clearance experiments during acute hyperkalemia, the effect of parathyroidectomy on the potassium-induced reduction of phosphate excretion was also assessed.

METHODS

Three groups of white rats were studied. One group of controls receiving 135 mmol/ℓ NaCl intravenously at a rate of 3 ml/h, one group of acutely K-loaded animals (135 mmol/ℓ KCl) and one group of chronically K-depleted rats (fed for 5-7 weeks a K-free diet). Details of the preparation of the animals for clearance and free-flow micropuncutre experiments are described in another paper (2).

* Department of Pathophysiology, University of Bern, Switzerland

Late proximal, early distal and late distal fluid was analyzed for Na, K, inulin, pH and titratable acid (TA). TA was obtained by titrating microsamples, using a glass pH-electrode system for pH-measurements, and an antimony system for addition of OH ions (3). P_i (inorganic phosphate) in blood and urine was measured with a colorimetric method. P_i in tubular fluid was derived by calculation from the TA value, using the Henderson-Hasselbalch equation for a phosphate buffer system. This approach has been found to be valid provided the other urinary buffers which have a pKa close to the titration range are present at low physiological concentrations (mainly uric acid:pKa 5, 8 and creatinine:Pka 4, 65) (4).

The role of PTH in the K-related effects was assessed in a group of animals receiving either NaCl or KCl and which had been thyroparathyroidectomized (TPTX) 10 days before the experiment. In these clearance experiments no phosphate was added to the NaCl or KCl infusion solution during the first clearance period of 30 min; then sodium phosphate was added at concentrations of 15 (2nd period), 30 (3rd period) and 45 mmol/ℓ (4th period).

Results were compared with those obtained in the corresponding group of intact animals. Details on technical preparation for TPTX, on criteria of adequacy of this operation, and on L-thyroxine substitution have been given in another paper (5).

RESULTS

Plasma K^+ was elevated in K-rats (7.91 ± 0.34 mM.ℓ, mean ± SEM) and lowered in low K-rats (1.90 ± 0.10), as compared with controls (3.91 ± 0.14). Plasma P_i was comparable in the three groups: in controls it was 2.55 ± 0.12, in the K-group 2.32 ± 0.11 whereas in low K-rats it was 2.48 ± 0.17 mmol/ℓ. Although GFR and urine flow rates were not significantly different in these groups it is noteworthy that the filtered phosphate load was slightly lower in the K-group.

Kaliuresis markedly increased in K-rats, and was absent in low K-rats. Natriuresis was blunted in both groups. Acute hyperkalemia depressed phosphaturia by 45%; chronic hypokalemia depressed this parameter by 52%. pH in blood, urine and tubular fluid did not change after acute hyperkalemia, but was significantly increased after chronic potassium depletion (2). Fig. 1 shows the progression of P_i loads along superficial nephrons in the three experimental conditions; it also depicts the participation of the collecting duct system of each group. In <u>controls</u>,

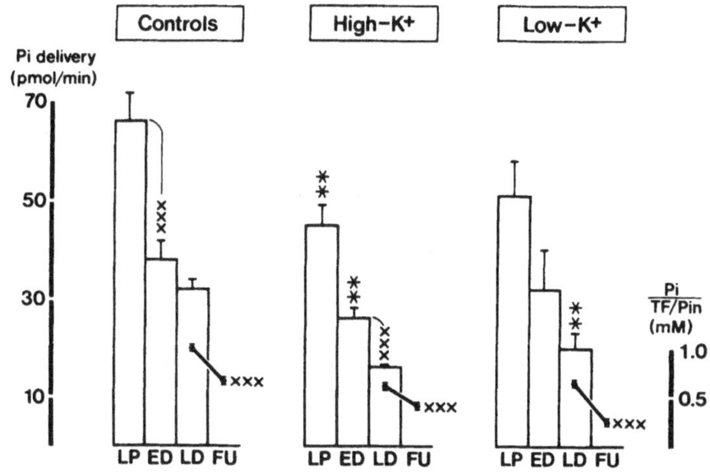

Figure 1.

Renal phosphate handling in control, acutely K-loaded and chronically K-depleted rats. Open bars represent P_i deliveries along superficial nephrons in three experimental groups. Values were derived from measurements of titratable acid. To evaluate whether the amount of P_i delivered to the late distal tubules could fully account for the respective urinary excretion rates, phosphate concentrations were divided by the TF/P inulin ratios (dots). LP = late proximal; ED = early distal; LD = late distal; FU = final urine. Values shown are $\bar{X} \pm$ SEM. For statistical analysis, * refers to a comparison with the corresponding nephron segment of the control group and X to a comparison between two successive sites of superficial nephrons. X or *: $p < 0.05$; XX or **: $p < 0.01$; XXX or ***: $p < 0.0025$.

significant net reabsorption of phosphate could be detected along the Henle's loop as well as along the collecting duct system, but not along the superficial distal tubule. In high K-rats P_i reabsorption along the proximal tubule was accentuated as compared with controls. In addition, further loss of P_i occurred along both the superficial distal tubule and along the collecting duct system. In low K-rats, the amount of P_i delivered to the late proximal tubule was not significantly different from that obtained in control condition. However, whereas the amount of P_i delivered to the early distal tubule was also not significantly different from controls, P_i delivery to the late distal tubule was significantly lower in low K-rats versus controls: this suggests participation of the distal tubule to the drop in phosphaturia observed in these rats. In addition, further loss of P_i could be detected between late distal tubule and final urine: this indicates that in K-depleted animals, the collecting duct system also participates in the final regulation of phosphate excretion. An alternative explanation is that this effect, observed in each group, reflects heterogeneity between deep and superficial nephrons.

Results from experiments performed in phosphate loaded intact animals demonstrate that the decrement in phosphaturia observed after acute hyperkalemia was maintained even when the filtered P_i-load was kept identical to that of controls; in addition we observed during K-loading a significant enhancement of both the mean tubular reabsorption of P_i (TRP_i) in the four clearance periods (2.39 ± 0.07 vs 1.98 ± 0.06 µmol/ml glomerular filtrates (GF), $p < 0.0025$), as well as of the maximum TRP_i (2.54 ± 0.06 vs 2.31 ± 0.06 µmol/ml GF, $p < 0.05$). In contrast, in TPTX animals, the decrement in phosphaturia after acute hyperkalemia was blunted, the mean TRP_i for the four clearance periods being identical in both K-groups and controls (3.19 ± 0.05 vs 3.17 ± 0.11 µmol/ml GF). The maximum TRP_i values (3.44 ± 0.07 vs 3.59 ± 0.13 µmol/ml GF) were also not significantly different from each other.

DISCUSSION

These studies confirm that in control conditions P_i reabsorption occurs mainly in the proximal tubule; no significant P_i reabsorption could be detected along the distal tubule, but was apparent along the collecting duct system, although this effect could be the reflection of nephron heterogeneity. When potassium metabolism is primarily disturbed the capacity of the distal tubule to increase phosphate reabsorption is unmasked.

In the high K and low K condition different mechanisms might be involved to account for this activation of P_i transport. We have shown that the drop in phosphaturia observed after acute hyperkalemia is blunted in TPTX animals: this suggests either depression of PTH secretion or decreased renal sensitivity to PTH. In addition, insulin secretion is known to be stimulated by an acute K load (6), and this hormone has been shown to be antiphosphaturic, at least at the level of the proximal tubule (7). Furthermore, cell alkalinization has been observed in muscle after K-loading (8). If this were also to occur in renal tubule cells such a mechanism could be involved in the observed stimulation of phosphate reabsorption. Indeed, Knox et al. have recently suggested that cellular alkalinization might be a common denominator for many phosphate transport activating processes (9). Finally, changes in luminal pH, in distal Na-delivery and in transepithelial PD are to be considered as potential mechanisms, but our micropuncture studies have not provided support for the notion that they might be critically involved in the K-induced alterations of distal tubular phosphate transports.

A decreased sensitivity to PTH has also been described in case of chronic potassium depletion (1) and could be involved in the reduced phosphate excretion observed in this condition. We have observed an alkalinization of tubular fluid pH in K-depletion and this factors is known to influence renal phosphate transport (10). Finally, Na retention was observed in our experiments along the terminal nephron in low K-rats. Possibly this could affect distal tubular phosphate transport if a cotransport system were present.

REFERENCES

1. N. Beck, and B.B. Davies. Impaired renal response to parathyroid hormone in potassium depletion. Am. J. Physiol. 228: 179 (1975).

2. B. Karlmark, Ph. Jaeger, and G. Giebisch. Luminal buffer transport in the rat cortical tubule: relationship to potassium metabolism. Am. J. Physiol. (submitted).

3. B. Karlmark, Ph. Jaeger, H. Fein, and G. Giebisch. Coulometric acid-base titration in nanoliter samples with glass and antimony electrodes. Am. J. Physiol. (in press).

4. Ph. Jaeger, B. Karlmark, B. Stanton, R.G. Kirk, and G. Giebisch. Micropuncture study of distal tubular activation of phosphate reabsorption in the rat. Advances in Exp. Med. and Biol. 128: 77 (1980). Phosphate and minerals in health and disease. S.G. Massry, E. Ritz and H. Jahn, editors.

5. J.P. Bonjour, C. Preston, and H. Fleisch. Effect of 1,25-dihydroxyvitamin D3 on the renal handling of P_i in thyroparathyroidectomized rats. J. Clin. Invest. 60: 1419 (1977).

6. R.G. Dluhy, L. Axelrod, and G.M. Williams. Serum immunoreactive insulin and growth hormone response to potassium infusion in normal man. J. Appl. Physiol. 33: 22 (1972).

7. R.A. DeFronzo, M. Goldberg, and Z. Agus. The effect of glucose and insulin on renal electrolyte transport. J. Clin. Invest. 58: 83 (1976).

8. S. Adler, and D.S. Fraley. Potassium and intracellular pH. Kidney Int. 11: 433 (1977).

9. F.G. Knox, A. Hoppe, S.A. Kempson, S.V. Shah, and P.P. Dousa. Cellular mechanisms of phosphate transport. In: Renal Handling of Phosphate (Massry & Fleisch, editors). New York, Plenum, p. 79 (1980).

10. N. Bank, and G. Malnic. Effect of urinary alkalinization on renal phosphate reabsorption. In: Renal Handling of Phosphate (Massry & Fleisch, editors). New York, Plenum, p. 209 (1980).

RENAL HANDLING OF DIVALENT CATIONS AND PHOSPHATE DURING WATER IMMERSION IN THE AWAKE DOG

J.C. Ayus, J.P. Frommer, G. Eknoyan, W.N. Suki

Baylor College of Medicine
Houston, TX 77030

INTRODUCTION

Previous studies in the human have failed to show any effects of head-out water immersion on serum parathyroid hormone (PTH) concentration, serum ionized calcium concentration (Ca^{++}) or urinary phosphate excretion (UPO_4V) (2). No studies have been reported on the effects of water immersion on the renal handling of phosphate and divalent cations in animals. Thus, the present experiments were designed to characterize the effects of head-out water immersion on the urinary excretion of phosphate (UPO_4V), calcium ($U_{Ca}V$), and magnesium ($U_{Mg}V$) in the awake dog.

METHODS AND RESULTS

Experiments were carried out in 53 awake female mongrel dogs weighing between 13 and 19 kg. Food was withheld for 18 hours prior to the experiments but the dogs were allowed free access to water. All animals were trained to stand still in the water tank, immersed to the neck, on at least three occassions prior to the experiment. Surgery was performed at 8:30 AM on the experimental day, and consisted of the insertion of a jugular, femoral artery and femoral vein catheters under local anesthesia. A bladder catheter was also inserted. All animals received 5 mg of deoxycorticosterone acetate in oil, intramuscularly, at 9:00 AM.

The dogs were then placed in the empty tank, and after a 60 minute equilibration period, the experiment was begun. Urine was collected anaerobically every hour, and the samples were refrigerated until analysis. Arterial blood samples were obtained anaerobically, in a heparinized syringe, in the middle of each hourly period. They were analyzed for pH and pCO_2, and immediately centrifuged thereafter. The plasma was refrigerated until analysis. Calcium magnesium and phosphorus were determined by methods previously described (1). Arterial pH was determined on an IL pH/ pCO_2 meter.

The experimental protocol consisted of an initial two hours control period, after which the tank was filled with warm water until the animal was immersed to the neck, at a temperature previously determined. This was followed by a two hour immersion period, followed by a recovery period of one hour.

Three groups of dogs were studied. Group I consisted of 19 dogs which served as time-controls and were observed from 10 AM to 4 PM. Group II conisted of 22 dogs, in which the experiment was performed between 10 AM and 4 PM, and were immersed to the neck in water at a temperature of $36.0 \pm 0.5^{\circ}C$. Group III consisted of 12 dogs, in which the experiment was performed between 4 PM and 10 PM. Each dog in this group served as his own time-control two days prior to water immersion. Six dogs in this group were immersed at a bath temperature of $36.0 \pm 0.5^{\circ}C$, and the remaining six, at a bath temperature of $33.0 \pm 0.5^{\circ}C$. Since no significant differences were found between both groups, their results are reported together.

All values are expressed as the mean± standard error of the mean (SEM), and the statistical significantce of differences between periods was assessed using Student's t-test for paired and unpaired observations when two means were compared, and using analysis of variance when more than two means were compared.

Figures 1 and 2 illustrate the fact that head out water immersion failed to alter the spontaneous diurnal pattern of UPO_4V. As shown in Figure 1, UPO_4V was increasing spontaneously at the time of day when immersion was performed in Group II. Figure 2 shows that water immersion did not alter the spontaneous decrease in UPO_4V in the evening (Group III).

Table I depicts the effect of head-out water immersion on $U_{Ca}V$ and $U_{Mg}V$ in all groups. As shown in the table, water immersion failed to alter the urinary excretion of both calcium and magnesium in Group II. However, when immerson was performed in the evening (Group III), the maneuver induced a significant increase in $U_{Ca}V$ and $U_{Mg}V$. Plasma concentration of PO_4, Ca, and Mg, or arterial pH, did not change with immersion in any of the experimental groups.

DISCUSSION

Preliminary studies from our laboratory have indicated that water immersion induces central hypervolemia in the awake dog (3). Thus, this maneuver, is a very useful tool in the study of the effects of volume expansion on the renal handling of PO_4, Ca

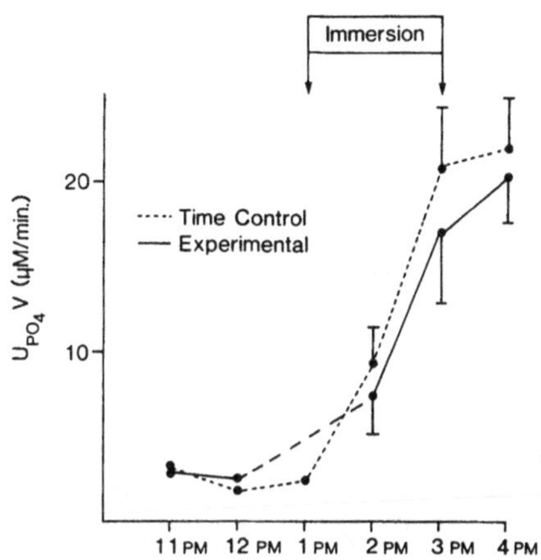

Figure 1. Effect of head-out water immersion UPO_4V in Group I and Group II. Immersion failed to alter the spontaneous diurnal pattern of UPO_4V.

and Mg. Studies in the human show that head-out water immersion does not alter serum PTH or serum ionized calcium levels, nor does it affect UPO_4V, (2). The effect of water immersion on the renal handling of PO_4, Ca and Mg have not been previously studied in the dog. Our results agree with the findings in the human, in that water immersion fails to alter the circadian pattern of

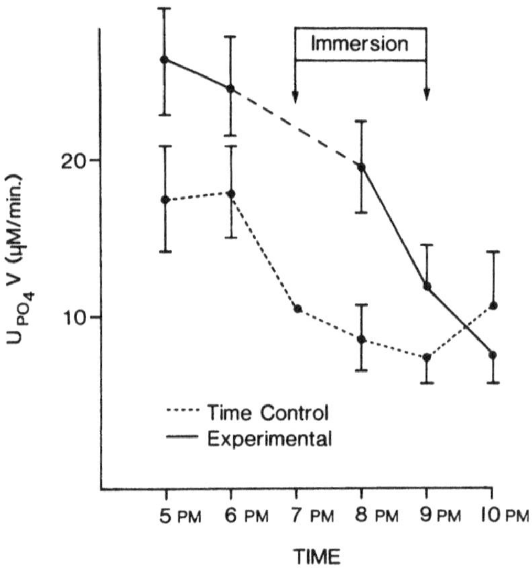

Figure 2. Effect of head-out water immersion on UPO_4V in Group III. These dogs served as their own time-controls. Immersion did not alter the decreasing pattern of UPO_4V.

UPO_4V. Moreover, addtional data on these dogs, presented elsewhere, show that head-out immersion does not alter the spontaneous diurnal pattern of urinary sodium ($U_{Na}V$) or potassium (U_KV) excretion (3). This information suggests that head-out water immersion does not appear to have much of an effect on the proximal tubule in the awake dog. Head-out water immersion induced a significant increase in $U_{Ca}V$ and $U_{Mg}V$ in Group III. $U_{Na}V$ did not change in this group (3), thus, urinary calcium excretion was dissociated from $U_{Na}V$ under these experimental circumstances. Since calcium transport in the proximal tubule in general, parallels sodium transport in proximal tubule (4), a dissociation of $U_{Ca}V$ from $U_{Na}V$ suggests that calcium transport is being altered in the distal segments of the nephron. The fact that $U_{Mg}V$ also increased with immersion in Group III, coupled with fact that the main tubular site for magnesium transport seems to be the loop of Henle, also argues in favor of the contention that immersion alters Ca and Mg handling either in the loop of Henle, or in the distal segments of the nephron (5). Experimental studies in which serum calcium and magnesium are elevated, suggest that a distal common pathway of reabsorption for both these cations may exist (6,7).

The exact mechanism for the increase in $U_{Ca}V$ and $U_{Mg}V$ during water immersion observed in group III, cannot be determined from the present study. However, this mechanism seems unrelated to PTH action, or acid-base changes, since UPO_4V and arterial pH did not change.

The failure of head-out water immersion to affect $U_{Ca}V$ and $U_{Mg}V$ when the maneuver was performed between 1 PM and 3 PM (Group II) is likely due to the overriding effect of PTH. Indeed, studies from our laboratory (Frommer and Ayus, unpublished observations), and the present study, show that UPO_4V and $UHCO_3V$ are on the rise, while $U_{Ca}V$ and $U_{Mg}V$ are decreasing between 1 PM and 3 PM. This is compatible with increasing PTH action on the kidney (8). A circadian rhythm for PTH has been demonstrated in the human (9,10). Our study suggests that this also may occur in the awake dog. PTH-induced increase in the tubular reabsorption of calcium and magnesium between 1 PM and 3 PM may have been responsible for the lack of effect of head-out water immersion on $U_{Ca}V$ and $U_{Mg}V$ in group II.

Table I. EFFECTS OF HEAD-OUT WATER IMMERSION ON $U_{Ca}V$ AND U_{Mg} V IN THE AWAKE DOG

	U_{Ca} V μM/min					U_{Mg} V μM/min				
Group I: Time Control; 10 AM to 4 PM (N=19)										
	C		I		R	C		I		R
Mean ±	0.28		0.21		0.14	1.00		0.83		0.58
SEM	0.06		0.02		0.02	0.17		0.08		0.08
P		NS		NS			NS		NS	
Group II: Immersion; 10 AM to 4 PM (N=22)										
	C		I		R	C		I		R
Mean ±	0.41		0.32		0.15	0.92		1.21		0.54
SEM	0.07		0.05		0.02	0.21		0.17		0.08
P		NS		<0.05			NS		<0.05	
Group III: Time Control; 4 PM to 10 PM (N=12)										
	C		I		R	C		I		R
Mean ±	0.17		0.15		0.17	0.32		0.24		0.32
SEM	0.05		0.04		0.05	0.09		0.05		0.12
P		NS		NS			NS		NS	
Group III: Immersion; 4 PM to 10 PM (N=12)										
	C		I		R	C		I		R
Mean ±	0.20		0.50		0.31	0.39		0.91		0.40
SEM	0.06		0.07		0.06	0.06		0.24		0.08
P		<0.005		<0.005			<0.05		<0.05	

C=Control; I=Immersion; R=Recovery

REFERENCES

1. C.S. Hebert, D. Rouse, G. Eknoyan, M. Martinez-Maldonado, W.N. Suki, Decreased phosphate reabsorption by volume expansion in the dog, Kidney Int. 2:247-252, 1972.

2. M. Epstein, D.S. Pins, W. Silvers, R. Loutzenhiser, J.M. Canterbury, E. Reiss, Failure of water immersion to influence parathyroid hormone secretion and renal phosphate handling in normal man, J. Lab. Clin. Med 87:218-226, 1976.

3. J.P. Frommer, W.N. Suki, J.C. Ayus, Head-out water immersion does not induce natriuresis in the awake dog. Kidney Int. 19:240, 1981, (Abstract).

4. W.N. Suki and D. Rouse, Mechanisms of calcium transport, Mineral Electrolyte Metab. 5:175-182, 1981.

5. G.A. Quamme and J.H. Dirks, Magnesium transport in the nephron, Am. J. Physiol 239:F393-F401, 1980.

6. S.G. Massry, J.J. Ahumada, J.W. Coburn and C.R. Kleeman. Effect of $MgCl_2$ infusion on urinary Ca and Na during reduction in their filtered loads. Am. J. Physiol 219:881-885, 1970.

7. S.G. Massry, J.W. Coburn and C.R. Kleeman, Renal handling of magnesium in the dog. Am. J. Physiol 216:1460-1467, 1969.

8. R.A.L. Sutton and J.H. Dirks, Renal handling of calcium, phosphate and magnesium. B.M. Brenner and F.C. Rector (eds.), The Kidney, (W.B. Saunders, Philadelphia, PA) 1981, p. 566.

9. W. Jubiz, J.M. Canterbury, E. Reiss, and F.H. Tyler, Circadian rhythm in serum parathyroid hormone concentration in human subjects: correlation with serum calcium, albumin, and growth hormone levels, J. Clin. Invest, 51:2040-2046, 1972.

10. G.H. Mudge, W.O. Berndt and H. Valtin, Tubular transport of urea, glucose phosphate, uric acid, sulfate and thiosulfate, In Orloff J, Berliner RW (eds.): Handbook of Physiology: Renal Physiology, (Williams & Wilkins Co, Baltimre) 1973, p. 609-610.

THE EFFECTS OF CALCIUM ON ADH ACTION IN CORTICAL COLLECTING TUBULES PERFUSED *IN VITRO*

Stanley Goldfarb

Renal Electrolyte Section
Hospital of the University of Pennsylvania
Philadelphia, Pennsylvania

INTRODUCTION

The effects of calcium on ADH action have been the object of intense study for 20 years (1). Extreme elevations in serosal calcium (Ca^{++}) concentration (10 mM) have been shown to block ADH-induced water flow in the toad urinary bladder (1,2). To test the effects of smaller elevations of calcium level on ADH action in a mammalian system, studies were performed in the ADH responsive cortical collecting tubule, "light" segment (3).

RESULTS

Eight tubules were perfused in an artificial ultrafiltrate of plasma with calcium level of 1.25 mM. A 150 mOsm/kg gradient was applied across the tubule. Water flow (Jv) was .03±.15 nl/mm/min prior to ADH exposure. After 25 μu/ml ADH, Jv rose to 1.56±.6 nl/mm/min and hydraulic conductivity (Lp) rose to 123±22 cm/sec atm x 10^7. Seven tubules were exposed to similar conditions but bath calcium level was raised to 3.75 mM. In these tubules, Jv was 0.003±.06 nl/mm/min prior to ADH and rose to 2.96±.60 nl/mm/min, ($p < .05$ vs control) following ADH as Lp rose to 286±62 cm/sec atm x 10^7 ($p < .05$ vs control).

DISCUSSION

The results of these experiments suggest that raising bath calcium level by 3 fold leads to a marked increase in the hydroosmotic action of ADH. These data strongly suggest that the polyuria seen in a variety of hypercalcemic conditions is not due to a direct tubular antagonism of ADH induced water transport but rather is mediated by changes in medullary solute accumulation. The mechanism of the stimulatory effect of calcium is unknown but the current findings are consonant with recent studies which show that ionophore A23187 stimulates, and the calcium blocking agent, verapamil, reduces ADH-dependent water flow.

REFERENCES

1. M.J. Peterson and I.S. Edelman, Calcium inhibition of the action of vasopressin on the urinary bladder of the toad. J. Clin. Invest. 43: 583 (1964).
2. W.P. Argy, Jr., J.S. Handler, and J. Orloff, Ca^{++} and Mg^{++} effects on toad bladder response to cyclic AMP, theophylline and ADH analogues. Am. J. Physiol. 213: 803 (1965).
3. M. Imbert, D. Chabardes, M. Montegut, A. Clique, and F. Morel, Vasopressin dependent adenylate cyclase in single segments of rabbit kidney tubule. Pflugers Arch. 357: 173 (1975).

PHOSPHATE METABOLISM IN HEALTH AND DISEASE

THE CREATINE-CREATINE PHOSPHATE SHUTTLE FOR ENERGY TRANSPORT - COMPARTMENTATION OF CREATINE PHOSPHOKINASE IN MUSCLE

Susan Erickson-Viitanen, Paul Geiger, W.C.T. Yang and Samuel P. Bessman

Department of Pharmacology and Nutrition
University of Southern California School of Medicine
Los Angeles, CA 90033

INTRODUCTION

There are two viewpoints regarding the role of the enzyme creatine phosphokinase (CPK), which catalyzes the reversible transphosphorylation of creatine and adenine nucleotides in energy transport. The classical viewpoint (Fig. 1) regards CPK as a near equilibrium enzyme buffering cytosolic changes in nucleotide concentration (1,2), with creatine phosphate representing a reservoir of high energy phosphate equivalents (3) and with regulation of energy production relegated to the adenine nucleotides whether in the form of energy charge (4), adenylate phosphate potential (5,6), or ATP/ADP ratio (7). The second viewpoint places CPK and its products, creatine and creatine phosphate, in the central role of energy transport (8-11). The evidence for the latter viewpoint has come about from several diverse lines of reasoning (reviewed in 9). Jacobs et al discovered a distinct isoenzyme of CPK bound to mitochondria in 1964 (12). The significance of this mitochondrial bound form of CPK was studied by Bessman and Fonyo (13) in pigeon breast mitochondria where the possibility of feedback regulation of respiration through production of acceptor creatine was suggested, in accordance with Bessman's earlier observation on the insulin-like effect of exercise in diabetics (14). Such a role for CPK was extended to cardiac muscle as well (15). During the 1970's, isoenzymes of CPK were localized to sites of energy utilization in muscle including myofibrils (16), sarcoplasmic reticulum (17), and plasma membrane (18). At the same time it was becoming apparent that a large proportion of the cellular adenine nucleotides were compartmentalized so as to be largely unavailable for effective regulation of energy production and utilization (19,20), such that muscle function was really correlated with the content of creatine phosphate (reviewed in 11). Thus, biochemical, physiological and clinical lines of experimental thought have led to the proposal that the regulation and transport of energy in muscle is carried out via a creatine-creatine phosphate "shuttle" as diagrammed in Figure 2.

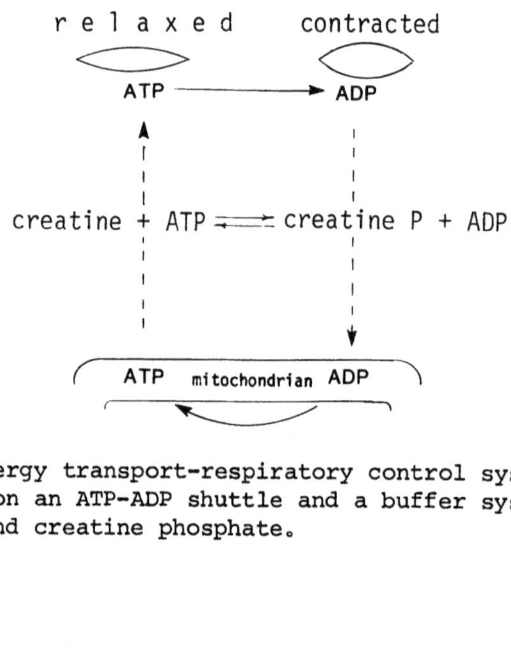

Fig. 1. The energy transport-respiratory control system of muscle based on an ATP-ADP shuttle and a buffer system of creatine and creatine phosphate.

Perhaps the most important postulate of this proposed shuttle system is that the localization of CPK isoenzymes within mitochondria and myofibrils (Fig. 2) bears functional significance to ATP generating and utilizing reactions. There is extensive kinetic evidence to suggest that mitochondrial ATP synthesis is coupled to creatine phosphate synthesis in an efficient manner (13,15,21,22),

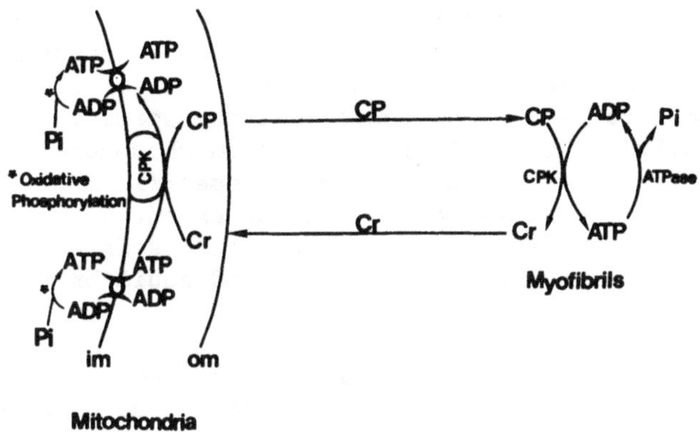

Fig. 2. Schematic view of a creatine-creatine phosphate shuttle for energy transport. Abbreviations: Cr, creatine; CP, creatine phosphate; im, inner mitochondrial membrane; om, outer mitochondrial membrane.

and the kinetic constants of myofibrillar CPK and ATPase reactions are such that efficient rephosphorylation of ADP from creatine phosphate likely occurs at this site (18,23). The questions we posed concerned the closeness of the reaction of mitochondrial CPK to the sites on the mitochondrion which deliver ATP, and the closeness of myofibrillar CPK to the sites on the myofibril where ATP is hydrolyzed (Fig. 2). To study these interactions, we labeled various components of the nucleotide requiring reactions of isolated mitochondria and myofibrils and followed the radioactivity of the phosphorylated intermediates formed over short incubation periods before isotopic equilibrium was achieved.

EXPERIMENTAL METHODS

Mitochondria from rabbit ventricle or rat hind leg muscle were isolated by differential centrifugation after mechanical disruption of tissue. Individual reactions were carried out essentially as described earlier (24) using 0.5 to 1.0 mg mitochondrial protein and 0.05 to 0.70 mM ATP. Reactions were initiated by addition of creatine and isotope, and terminated with perchloric acid after short time intervals (0,5,10 seconds) so that the specific activity changes were virtually linear, and to prevent product inhibition of CPK (22). Reactions were carried out with either labeled inorganic phosphate (^{33}Pi) or γ-labeled ATP ([γ-^{32}P]-ATP) as isotopic precursor.

Isolated myofibrils contain both ATPase and CPK activities (18,23). In the absence of an ATP regenerating system, e.g., lack of creatine phosphate, an initially gamma-labeled pool of ATP will decrease in size as the ATP is hydrolyzed, at a constant specific activity. In the presence of creatine phosphate, regeneration of ATP via CPK maintains the pool size, but the specific activity of ATP is gradually diluted with the unlabeled phosphate of creatine phosphate. Therefore, measurement of Pi specific activity relative to that of ATP gives an indication of the extent to which creatine phosphate-derived ATP is utilized by the ATPase in a "direct" or "coupled" manner, i.e., prior to mixing and equilibration of the 2 ATP pools.

The contents and specific activities of phosphorylated intermediates in various incubations are measured simultaneously on extracts of reactions terminated with $HClO_4$ via the automated phosphate analyzer developed by Bessman (25). Complete details of preparation of mitochondria and myofibrils, incubation conditions and analysis of compounds is given elsewhere (26,27).

RESULTS AND DISCUSSION

Compartmentation of Mitochondrial CPK

A quantitative statement defining the proportion of creatine phosphate synthesis directly linked to oxidative phosphorylation was derived on the basis of consideration of two ATP pools; that present in the medium, and that synthesized de novo and exported from the mitochondrial matrix into the intermembrane space where the active site of CPK is located (22,28). Under the experimental conditions employed (linear creatine phosphate synthesis), the specific activity of nascent creatine phosphate formed in a given interval of time can be written as the sum of fractional contributions from medium and intermembrane space pools of ATP. The small amount of endogenous nucleotide contained in isolated mitochondria (7.50 ± 0.5 nmol/mg, n=6) and internal compartmentation of this nucleotide within the matrix (29) hinder direct measurement of the de novo synthesized ATP pool directly. However, the extremely rapid rate of phosphate transport into mitochondria (30) and its incorporation into exported ATP (29) suggested that the specific activity of newly synthesized mitochondrial ATP could be approximated to that of inorganic phosphate. Therefore, an estimate of the apparent mitochondrial contribution to creatine phosphate synthesis was written as:

$$\text{\% Apparent Mitochondrial Contribution} = \frac{SA(CP)_{5-10} - SA(ATP)_{5-10}}{SA(Pi)_{5-10} - SA(ATP)_{5-10}}$$

where SA(CP) is the specific activity of nascent creatine phosphate formed between 5 and 10 seconds, and SA(ATP) and SA(Pi) are the

TABLE 1

COMPARTMENTATION OF CREATINE PHOSPHOKINASE IN MITOCHONDRIA

Source of Mitochondria	N	(ATP) µM	MITOCHONDRIAL CONTRIBUTION	
			Nascent CP %	Nascent G6P
Rabbit Heart	3	399±20	7.00±0.57	-
	6	69±4	24.30±4.30	-2.92±1.5
Rat skeletal Muscle	3	332±18	1.11±1.60	-
	6	70±2	19.62±1.50	-

average ATP and Pi specific activities, respectively, for this time interval as determined from specific activity versus time profiles. This reaction interval was chosen to allow for equilibration of the added isotope with the preexisting pool, while still being early enough that total equilibration of all phosphate molecules did not occur.

Table 1 shows the results of studies carried out with rabbit heart or rat skeletal muscle mitochondria at 2 levels of total ATP. It can be seen that for both sources of mitochondria, the extent of this measured compartmentation effect depends on the external ATP concentration. When external ATP is relatively large, the apparent contribution by mitochondrial ATP is small, whereas apparent contributions increase at lower total nucleotide levels. At the lowest ATP concentration tested (40 µM), nearly 40% of the creatine phosphate synthesis appears to derive from mitochondrially synthesized ATP (26). This concentration dependence reflects the competition between medium and newly exported ATP for the ATP binding site of CPK. Our direct measurement of concentration-dependent compartmentation is similar to the concentration-effect curve indirectly derived by kinetic measurements and computer simulation by Saks and coworkers for rat heart (21).

Table 1 also shows a comparison between the apparent contributions to nascent creatine phosphate versus nascent glucose-6-phosphate synthesized by added yeast hexokinase. This experiment was designed to directly test our method of analysis for possible artifact. One to two Units of yeast hexokinase were added to reaction vessels along with rabbit heart mitochondria. It was reasoned that product glucose-6-phosphate synthesized by this external kinase would exclusively reflect the medium ATP environment. As expected, the specific activity of newly formed glucose-6-

TABLE 2

INFLUENCE OF RESPIRATION ON OBSERVED K_m FOR ATP

Reaction System	Observed K_m ATP (μM)
Respiring Heart Mitochondria	90
Inhibited Heart Mitochondria Plus PEP and Pyruvate Kinase	131
Respiring Skeletal Muscle Mitochondria	76

phosphate was very close to that of the average ATP for the reaction interval. The small negative number derived from the contribution equation (see above) indicates that our method slightly underestimates the degree of compartmentation.

We also verified the extent of apparent compartmentation through independent means; measurement of the observed K_m for ATP of CPK under various conditions. Saks and coworkers have reported a 5- to 10-fold difference in the observed K_m value for ATP when respiring versus inhibited rat heart mitochondrial preparations were compared (22). Table 2 shows that the difference in rabbit heart is not as great (about 1.5-fold); more importantly however, solution of the kinetic equation for creatine phosphate synthesis (21) using the K_m values defined, results in apparent respiration-linked velocity enhancement that is in quantitative agreement with the extent of observed compartmentation measured by the isotope technique.

As there is only one true K_m for a given enzyme-substrate complex, the apparent decrease in the K_m for ATP could indicate that there is a local higher concentration or "microenvironment" of ATP present within the intermembrane space surrounding the bound CPK when oxidative phosphorylation is operating. This is consistent with either a direct physical interaction between CPK and the adenine nucleotide translocase molecules (21,22), or a diffusion limitation to nucleotide created by the location of CPK between the outer and inner mitochondrial membranes. In either case, the compartment is not a closed system; e.g., direct utilization of de novo synthesized ATP is subject to competition by external nucleotide in a concentration dependent manner. Clearly, however, such a compartmentation effect would insure efficient creatine phosphate synthesis over a wide range of free external nucleotide levels. The ultimate physiological significance of the compartment awaits accurate determination of the levels of free nucleotide that exist near the mitochondrial membranes under various metabolic states associated with the contraction-relaxation cycle in heart and skeletal muscle.

Compartmentation of Myofibrillar CPK

Saks et al (23) showed that the observed K_m values for ATP for myofibrillar ATPase and for creatine liberation coupled to ATPase activity were coincident, implying that the CPK reaction could respond to and in essence be controlled by myofibrillar ATPase. Likewise, with constant ATP concentration, the rate of the coupled reaction was shown to depend on the concentration of creatine phosphate (18). Such reciprocal control suggests that myofibrillar ATPase and CPK are compartmented in such a way that nucleotide produced from one of the enzymes is very efficiently utilized by the other so that the net products of the coupled system are creatine and inorganic phosphate.

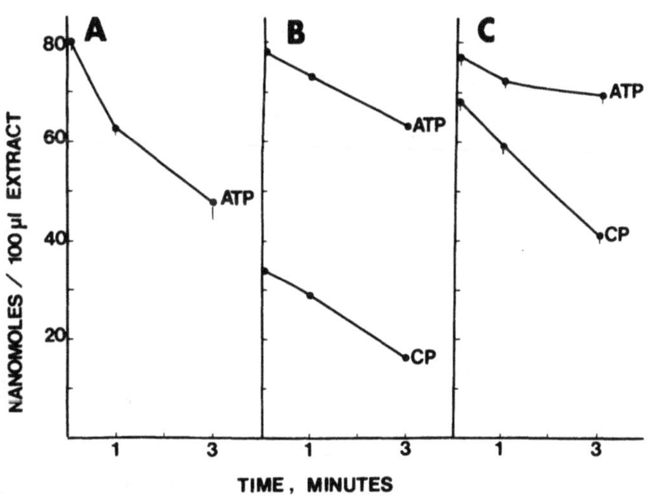

Fig. 3. Effect of creatine phosphate on ATP levels in isolated myofibrils. Values shown correspond to 1/20 of the original reaction volume.

A: 1.5 mM ATP (initial concentration)

B: 1.5 mM ATP plus 0.8 mM creatine phosphate

C: 1.5 mM ATP plus 1.4 mM creatine phosphate

Values represent mean ± S.E.M. for 3 to 5 preparations of myofibrils. For "B" values are averages from 2 preparations where the individual values differed by less than 6%.

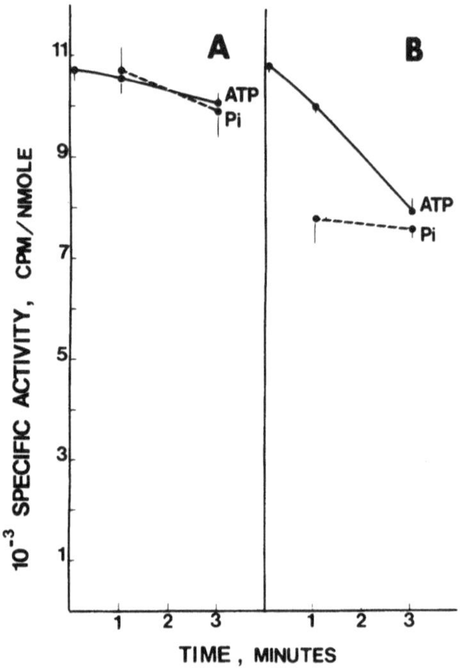

Fig. 4. Specific activities of ATP and Pi in isolated myofibrils in the presence of [γ-^{32}P]-ATP.
A: 1.5 mM ATP
B: 1.5 mM ATP plus 1.4 mM creatine phosphate
Values represent mean ± S.E.M. for 3-5 preparations of myofibrils, after normalizing for the starting ATP specific activity.

Studies in which the ability of creatine phosphate-generated ATP to be utilized by the myofibrillar ATPase as measured by the isotope technique are illustrated in Figures 3 and 4. (See also ref. 27). Figure 3 shows that myofibrils isolated from rabbit cardiac muscle contain CPK activity as evidenced by the decrease in creatine phosphate levels with time. Increasing the added quantity of creatine phosphate led to decreased net hydrolysis of ATP as expected.

Figure 4, panel A, shows a control experiment in which net ATP hydrolysis in the absence of ATP regenerating ability was allowed to occur. As expected, the result of net hydrolysis of initially labeled ATP is formation of product Pi of identical specific activity. Panel B shows the specific activity profiles of ATP and Pi when unlabeled creatine phosphate was included in the reaction mixture. The specific activity of the Pi was much lower than expected from the decreasing ATP specific activity, i.e., as with mitochondrial incubations, the specific activity of product can be compared to the average specific activity of precursor over a given reaction interval. It thus appeared that a portion of the Pi measured had come from *de novo* synthesized unlabeled ATP, as catalyzed by myofibrillar CPK. The extent of this apparent compartmentation can be calculated (27); more than one-fourth of the Pi formed in the first minute appears to have been derived from CPK-catalyzed ATP synthesis. The next reaction interval shows less of the direct nucleotide transfer, presumably because of the lower rate of ATP production by CPK, as the substrate, creatine phosphate, concentration decreases (Fig. 3).

These findings lead to the conclusion that myofibrillar ATPase and CPK are coupled, such that the ATP generated from creatine phosphate via CPK has "special access" to the myofibrillar ATPase (27). Within this compartment of CPK, myofibrillar ATPase and nucleotide, the transfer of energy can be regulated by both the level of ATPase activity and the available concentration of creatine phosphate (18,31,32).

These results indicate that both mitochondrial and myofibrillar isoenzymes of creatine phosphokinase have special interactions with ATP synthesis and utilization reactions that we have called compartmentation. The localization of the isoenzymes themselves, within the rather structured environment of myofibrils and mitochondrial membranes thus leads to the maintenance of metabolic compartments of nucleotide. Further study of such compartments in both normal and pathologically distressed tissue should enhance our knowledge of transport of energy in muscle as well as offer insight into the mechanisms by which the transport system may be affected in certain disease states.

REFERENCES

1. J.R. Williamson, Mitochondrial function in the heart, *Ann. Rev. Physiol.* 41:485 (1979).
2. R.A. Altshuld and G.P. Brierly, Interaction between the creatine kinase of heart mitochondria and oxidative phosphorylation, *J. Molec. Cell. Cardiol.* 9:875 (1977).
3. E.A. Newsholme and C. Start, "Regulation in Metabolism", John Wiley and Sons, New York (1973).
4. D.E. Atkinson, "Cellular Energy Metabolism and its Regulation", Academic Press, New York (1977).
5. M. Erecinska, R.L. Veech and D.F. Wilson, Thermodynamic relationships between the oxidation-reduction reactions and the ATP synthesis in suspensions of isolated pigeon heart mitochondria. *Arch. Biochem. Biophys.* 160:412 (1974).

6. K. Nishiki, M. Erecinska and D.F. Wilson, Energy relationships between cytosolic metabolism and mitochondrial respiration in rat heart, Am. J. Physiol. 234:C73 (1978).
7. E.J. Davis and W.I.A. Davis-van Thienen, Control of mitochondrial metabolism by the ATP/ADP ratio, Biochem. Biophys. Res. Commun. 83:1260 (1978).
8. S.P. Bessman, Hexokinase acceptor theory of insulin action, new evidence, Israel J. Med. Sci. 8:344 (1972).
9. S.P. Bessman and P.J. Geiger, Transport of energy in muscle: the phosphorylcreatine shuttle, Science 211:448 (1981).
10. W.E. Jacobus, Myocardial energy transport, current concepts of the problem, in: "Heart Creatine Kinase, the Integration of Isoenzymes for Energy Distribution", W.E. Jacobus and J.S. Ingwall, eds., Williams and Wilkins, Maryland (1980).
11. M. Seraydarian, The correlation of creatine phosphate with muscle function, in: "Heart Creatine Kinase, the Integration of Isoenzymes for Energy Distribution", W.E. Jacobus and J.S. Ingwall, eds., Williams and Wilkins, Maryland (1980).
12. H. Jacobs, H.W. Heldt and M. Klingenberg, High activity of creatine kinase in mitochondria from muscle and brain and evidence for a separate mitochondrial isoenzyme for creatine kinase, Biochem. Biophys. Res. Commun. 16:516 (1964).
13. S.P. Bessman and A. Fonyo, The possible role of the mitochondrial bound creatine kinase in regulation of mitochondrial respiration, Biochem. Biophys. Res. Commun. 22:597 (1966).
14. a) S.P. Bessman, A contribution to the mechanism of diabetes mellitus, in: "Fat Metabolism", V. Najjar, ed., Johns Hopkins Press, Maryland (1954). b) S.P. Bessman, Diabetes mellitus: observations, theoretical and practical, J. Pediatr. 56:191 (1960). c) S.P. Bessman, A molecular basis for the mechanism of insulin action, Am. J. Med. 40:740 (1966).
15. W.E. Jacobus and A.L. Lehninger, Creatine kinase of rat heart mitochondria. Coupling of creatine phosphorylation to electron transport. J. Biol. Chem. 248:4803 (1973).
16. D.C. Turner, T. Walliman and H.M. Eppenberger, A protein that binds specifically to the M-line of skeletal muscle is identified as the muscle forms of creatine kinase. Proc. Natl. Acad. Sci. 70:702 (1973).
17. W.E. Jacobus and R.J. Baskin, Cardiac creatine kinase (MM) bound to isolated sarcoplasmic reticulum. Circulation 50: 111 (1974).
18. V.A. Saks, N.V. Lipina, G.B. Chernousova, V.G. Sharov, V.N. Smirnov, E.I. Chasov and R. Grosse, Functional coupling of isoenzyme MM of creatine phosphokinase with Mg-ATPase of myofibrils and Na,K-ATPase of plasma membrane of heart cells. Biokhimiya 41:2099 (1976).

19. S. Gudbjarnason, P. Mathes and K.G. Ravens, Functional compartmentation of ATP and creatine phosphate in heart muscle. J. Molec. Cell. Cardiol. 1:325 (1970).
20. R.L. Nunnally and D.P. Hollis, Adenosine triphosphate compartmentation in living hearts, a phosphorous NMR saturation transfer study, Biochemistry 18:3641 (1979).
21. V.A. Saks, N.V. Lipina, V.N. Smirnov and E.I. Chazov, The functional coupling between mitochondrial creatine phosphokinase and ATP-ADP translocase: Kinetic evidence, Arch. Biochem. Biophys. 173:34 (1976).
22. V.A. Saks, V.V. Kupriyanov, G.V. Elizarova and W.E. Jacobus, Studies of energy transport in heart cells, the importance of creatine kinase localization for the coupling of mitochondrial phosphorylcreatine production to oxidative phosphorylation. J. Biol. Chem. 255:755 (1980).
23. V.A. Saks, G.B. Chernousova, R. Vetter, V.N. Smirnov and E.I. Chasov, Kinetic properties and the functional role of particulate MM-isoenzyme of creatine phosphokinase bound to heart muscle myofibrils, FEBS Letters 62:293 (1976).
24. W.C.T. Yang, P.J. Geiger, S.P. Bessman and B. Borrebaek, Formation of creatine phosphate from creatine and ^{32}P-labeled ATP by isolated rabbit heart mitochondria. Biochem. Biophys. Res. Commun. 76:882 (1977).
25. P.J. Geiger, S. Ahn and S.P. Bessman, Separation and automated analysis of phosphorylated intermediates, in: "Methods in Carbohydrate Chemistry", R. Whistler, ed. Vol. 8, Academic Press, New York (1980).
26. S. Erickson-Viitanen, Ph.D. Dissertation, University of Southern California (1981).
27. S.P. Bessman, W.C.T. Yang, P.J. Geiger and S. Erickson-Viitanen, Intimate coupling of creatine phosphokinase and myofibrillar adenosinetriphosphatase. Biochem. Biophys. Res. Commun. 96:1414 (1980).
28. H.R. Scholte, P.J. Weijers and E.M. Wit-Peeters, The localization of mitochondrial creatine kinase and its use for the determination of the sidedness of submitochondrial particles, Biochim. Biophys. Acta 291:764 (1973).
29. P.V. Vignais, Molecular and physiological aspects of adenine nucleotide transport in mitochondria. Biochim. Biophys. Acta 456:1 (1976).
30. W.A. Coty and P.L. Pedersen, Phosphate transport in rat liver mitochondria. Kinetics and energy requirements, J. Biol. Chem. 249:2593 (1974).
31. M.W. Seraydarian and B.C. Abbott, The role of the creatine phosphocreatine system in muscle. J. Molec. Cell. Cardiol. 8:741 (1976).
32. V.A. Saks, L.V. Rosenshtraukh, V.N. Smirnov and E.I. Chasov, Role of creatine phosphokinase in cellular function and metabolism, Can. J. Physiol. Pharmacol. 56:691 (1978).

HORMONAL REGULATION OF PHOSPHATE TRANSPORT IN THE DIFFERENTIATING CHICK SMALL INTESTINE

Heide Sing Cross and Meinrad Peterlik

Department of General and Experimental Pathology
University of Vienna, Austria

INTRODUCTION

The intestine is the prime target organ of vitamin D where the sterol, by virtue of its active metabolite 1,25-dihydroxyvitamin D_3, promotes calcium and inorganic phosphate (P_i) absorption (for review see Wasserman, 1981).

An organ culture system of embryonic chick small intestine (Corradino, 1973a) has proven very useful to study the mode of action of vitamin D: when maintained in organ culture the embryonic intestine, being devoid of any vitamin D compound (Moriuchi and DeLuca, 1974), responds to biologically active vitamin D steroids without further metabolism (Corradino, 1973b). It has been shown (Peterlik, 1978) that in this system P_i uptake is mediated by an active Na^+-dependent transport mechanism which is sensitive to vitamin D_3. The sterol induces P_i as well as calcium transport by gene activation in a mode comparable to that of other steroid hormones (Corradino, 1973c; Peterlik, 1978).

In earlier stages of embryonic development around day 15, the intestinal epithelium consists of a uniform population of undifferentiated absorptive cells. Further differentiation proceeds along two ways: a small fraction of cells differentiates into non-absorptive cells, while the majority undergoes gradual development into fully differentiated columnar cells (Overton and Shoup, 1964; Cheng and Leblond, 1974). We reasoned, therefore, that embryonic small intestine cultured at various stages of development could be used to answer the question if, and in what manner, P_i uptake - as a response of the intestine towards vitamin D - is affected by different levels of differentiation. Attempts

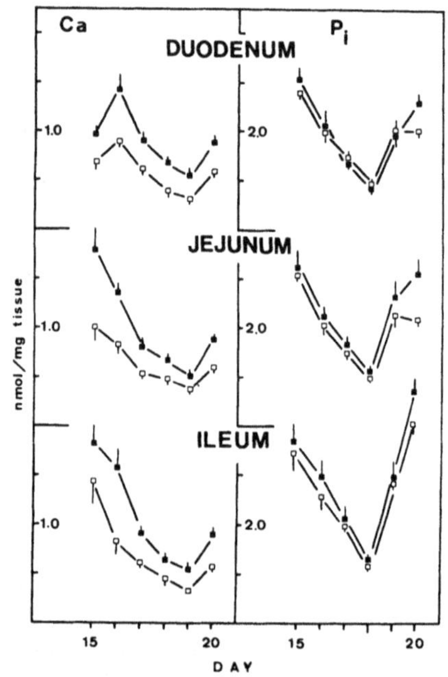

Fig. 1 Vitamin D effect on basal Ca (left) and P_i transport (right) in embryonic intestine. ■ 26 µM vitamin D_3. □ vitamin D_3-free controls. Culture period 48 h. Data are means ± S.E. (vertical bars) from at least 12 determinations. Significance of difference (at least at $P < 0.05$ level): Ca transport: day 15-20; P_i transport: day 20 only.

were also made to influence a differentiation-related effect of the sterol on P_i transport by other hormones, viz. insulin.

In this study, duodenum, jejunum and ileum from embryonic chicks at different stages of development (day 15-20) was cultured in serum-free McCoy's 5A mod. medium. Concentration of vitamin D_3 in the culture medium was 26 µM when not mentioned otherwise. Insulin concentration was 1.0 µM. P_i and Ca transport was determined as tissue accumulation of radiotracers as detailed previously (Corradino, 1973a; Peterlik, 1978).

VITAMIN D SENSITIVITY OF THE DIFFERENTIATING CHICK SMALL INTESTINE

Developmental Pattern of Intestinal P_i and Ca Transport

Figure 1 illustrates basal, i.e. vitamin D-independent, and vitamin D-induced P_i and Ca transport in different segments of the small intestine. P_i accumulation in all segments decreases markedly from day 15 to day 18 - this tendency is dramatically reversed just prior to hatching. A similar, though more moderate decline in basal transport of Ca during embryonic maturation can also be observed.

Most importantly, P_i uptake cannot be induced significantly before day 20 of embryonic life, whereas Ca uptake can be raised by addition of vitamin D_3 at least from day 15 on. This suggests that also immature intestinal epithelial cells are basically sensitive towards vitamin D, though induction of a particular transport system, like P_i, may require an advanced stage of differentiation.

Regional Differences in Vitamin D_3 Induction of P_i Transport

Unlike basal Ca transport which is uniform throughout the entire embryonic small intestine (Fig. 1), vitamin D-independent P_i accumulation in different segments of day 20 small intestine obviously increases in the proximal-to-distal direction (Table 1). In vitamin D_3-treated segments P_i uptake in general is higher than in vitamin D-free controls. However, only the proximal parts of the duodenum and jejunum exhibit a significant increase in contrast to the respective distal portions of these segments. The ileum over its total length displays a slight but statistically significant increase in P_i transport. The highest relative increment due to vitamin D was observed in the proximal half of the jejunum (Table 1). Thus, this segment was used exclusively in all subsequent experiments on P_i transport in embryonic chick intestine.

Table 1. Response to Vitamin D_3 of Different Regions of Embryonic Small Intestine (Day 20)

Addition to culture medium	Inorganic phosphate uptake (nmol/mg tissue)					
	Duodenum		Jejunum		Ileum	
	prox.	dist.	prox.	dist.	prox.	dist.
None	2.28 $\pm$0.21	2.43 $\pm$0.24	2.37 $\pm$0.15	3.00 $\pm$0.12	4.36 $\pm$0.28	3.87 $\pm$0.26
Vitamin D_3	3.04* $\pm$0.33	2.82 $\pm$0.24	3.32* $\pm$0.17	3.21 $\pm$0.18	4.81* $\pm$0.36	4.66* $\pm$0.30

For data pairing, hemisegments were prepared by longitudinal section of the respective part of the intestine. Data are means $\pm$ S.E. from 8 hemisegments. Asterisk indicates significant difference from vitamin D_3-free controls at least at $P < 0.05$ level (paired _t_-test). Culture time: 48 h.

Table 2. Dose-Response Relationship and Time Course of Vitamin D_3 and 1,25-Dihydroxyvitamin D_3 Action

Culture time (hours)	Inorganic phosphate transport Sterol concentration in culture medium							
	Vitamin D_3 (µM)				1,25-Dihydroxyvitamin D_3 (nM)			
	0.026	2.6	26	260	6.2	62	100	120
12	n.d.	n.d.	109 $\pm$ 10	n.d.	n.d.	n.d.	109 $\pm$ 7	n.d.
24	n.d.	n.d.	122* $\pm$ 4	n.d.	n.d.	n.d.	124* $\pm$ 10	n.d.
48	114 $\pm$ 7	117* $\pm$ 4	142* $\pm$ 6	142* $\pm$ 9	110 $\pm$ 6	134* $\pm$ 7	139* $\pm$ 13	148* $\pm$ 13

Data are means $\pm$ S.E. from at least 12 determinations and are expressed as "percent of vitamin D-free control (100%)"; n.d., not determined. Asterisk indicates significant increase over controls (at least at $P < 0.05$ level).

Characteristics of Vitamin D Action on P_i Transport in Embryonic Jejunum

Addition of either vitamin D_3 or 1,25-dihydroxyvitamin D_3 to the medium results in a steady increase in P_i transporting capacity of the 20 day old proximal jejunum when cultured over 48 hours, with a significant rise above control levels after 24 hours (Table 2). Thus, there is no difference in the time course of P_i transport induction by vitamin D_3 or its active metabolite.

However, there is a striking difference in the effectiveness of the sterols. A dose-response study (Table 2) reveals that maximal levels of P_i transport can be induced either by 26 µM vitamin D_3 or 100 nM 1,25-dihydroxyvitamin D_3. Apparently the dihydroxy-compound is 260 times more effective than vitamin D_3.

Addition of the transcriptional inhibitor actinomycin D (5.5 µg/ml culture medium, 18 h) to 24 h cultures reduces basal P_i uptake to 65 % of controls and, in addition, prevents the induction of P_i transport by either sterol (data not shown). This indicates that gene activation is probably involved in elevation of the intestinal P_i transport system by both vitamin D compounds.

The combined data suggest that either vitamin D_3 or 1,25-dihydroxyvitamin D_3, at appropriate dose levels, can be indiscriminately used for studying vitamin D effects on P_i transport by embryonic intestine.

THE EFFECT OF INSULIN ON P_i UPTAKE

In view of the well known promotion of differentiation by insulin (Menard and Malo, 1979) it was attempted to influence the differentiation-dependent block on vitamin D induction of P_i transport by addition of this hormone to cultures of embryonic chick jejunum. In the course of this study, the action of insulin on intestinal P_i transport could be separated into an early effect, which permits induction of P_i transport in an otherwise non-responsive epithelium (Table 3), and a late effect on basal, vitamin D-independent P_i uptake (Table 4).

Insulin Facilitates an Effect of Vitamin D on P_i Uptake

Immature (day 18) jejunum does not respond to vitamin D by induction of P_i transport (Fig. 1). When insulin is added for 6 hours at the end of a 48 h culture period it does not change P_i uptake either. However, insulin allows induction of P_i transport by vitamin D (Table 3) to levels as achieved by the sterol alone in mature intestinal epithelium **(Table 2).** The effective insulin concentration in this steroid-peptide hormone interaction is between 0.01-1.0 µM. An increase in P_i transport can already be observed after 30 min. Half-maximal levels are reached approximately after 2 h (data not shown). This permissive effect of insulin on vitamin D induction of P_i uptake can be completely abolished by addition of the transcriptional inhibitor actinomycin D (Table 3).

The facilitating effect of insulin on vitamin D action can be observed in 20 day old mature epithelium as well. Vitamin D induction of P_i uptake does not reach significant levels before 24 h of culture (Table 2), however in conjunction with insulin this is already achieved after 12 h culture (Table 3). P_i uptake induced by vitamin D_3 after 48 h (Table 2) is not further enhanced by insulin (not shown).

Table 3. Early Action of Insulin: Permissive Effect on Vitamin D_3-Induction of P_i Uptake

Embryonic development (day)	Addition to culture medium			P_i uptake
	Vit.D	Insulin	Act.D	(% of Control)
	-	-	-	100 ± 2
	-	-	+	72 ± 2
	-	+	-	105 ± 3
18	+	-	-	102 ± 2
	+	-	+	73 ± 3
	+	+	-	130 ± 4*
	+	+	+	79 ± 5
	-	-	-	100 ± 4
20	-	+	-	99 ± 5
	+	-	-	104 ± 5
	+	+	-	116 ± 5*

Day 18 jejuna were cultured for 48 h. Act. D: actinomycin D (5.5 µg/ml culture medium) was added for last 24 h of culture. Day 20 jejuna were cultured for 12 h. Insulin was added 6 h before termination of the culture. Data are means ± S.E. from at least 12 determinations. Asterisk indicates significant increase over controls (at least at $P < 0.05$ level).

A Vitamin D-Independent Effect of Insulin on P_i Uptake

When present over prolonged culture periods (up to 48 h), insulin itself influences P_i uptake by embryonic intestine: Dependent on the degree of differentiation the peptide hormone activates or decreases vitamin D-independent P_i transport (Table 4).

In mature 20 day jejuna insulin produces a 22 % increase in P_i uptake above basal levels (Table 4). This is in contrast to Ca uptake, where, under identical culture conditions, insulin does not have any effect whatsoever (not shown). Actinomycin D inhibits this augmentation, suggesting that, as in the case of vitamin D induction of P_i uptake, interaction with the genetic information is required. The failure to observe an additive effect in the presence of both hormones (Table 4) suggests the induction of an identical P_i transport system.

Table 4. Late Effect of Insulin on Vitamin D-Independent P_i Uptake

Embryonic development (day)	Addition to culture medium Vit.D_3	Insulin	Act.D	P_i Uptake (% of Control)
18	-	-	-	100 $\pm$ 4
	-	+	-	75 $\pm$ 2*
	+	-	-	95 $\pm$ 6
	+	+	-	78 $\pm$ 3*
20	-	-	-	100 $\pm$ 3
	-	-	+	73 $\pm$ 3
	-	+	-	122 $\pm$ 4*
	-	+	+	79 $\pm$ 5
	+	-	-	138 $\pm$ 6*
	+	-	+	73 $\pm$ 9
	+	+	-	136 $\pm$ 6*
	+	+	+	88 $\pm$ 6

Culture time 48 h. Insulin was added at beginning of culture period. Act. D: actinomycin D (5.5 μg/ml culture medium) was added for last 24 h of culture. Data are means $\pm$ S. E. from at least 12 determinations. Asterisk marks significant change in P_i uptake induced by either hormone (at least at $P < 0.05$ level).

In contrast to its stimulatory action on P_i transport in mature embryonic intestinal epithelium insulin depresses uptake in less differentiated day 18 intestine by 30 % - regardless whether vitamin D is present in the culture medium or not (Table 4).

GLUCAGON AND CYCLIC NUCLEOTIDES

Glucagon (1.0 µM) added for 48 h to cultures of mature day 20 proximal jejunum was without effect either on basal P_i uptake or on the vitamin D_3-induced increment (not shown).

Cyclic nucleotides are often implicated as mediators in the complex action of insulin. However, dibutyryl-cAMP or dibutyryl-cGMP (0.8 mM), when added to cultures of embryonic jejunum instead of insulin, did not mimick any action of the hormone on intestinal P_i uptake. It is concluded therefore that neither the fast interaction of insulin with vitamin D to induce P_i transport, nor its late effect on vitamin D-independent P_i uptake is mediated by cyclic nucleotides.

CONCLUSIONS

The expression of vitamin D action on Ca or P_i transport in embryonic chick small intestine requires different levels of differentiation. Though immature epithelium responds to vitamin D by an increase in Ca uptake and, thus, proves that undifferentiated intestinal cells are intrinsically sensitive to vitamin D, a high degree of differentiation is necessary for vitamin D induction of P_i transport. Since this effect is the consequence of gene activation by the steroid hormone, a differentiation-linked block of this step or of subsequent protein synthetic and post-translational processes could be responsible for the observed failure of vitamin D to induce P_i transport in immature epithelium.

To overcome this inhibition, advanced differentiation and/or additional hormonal factors may be required. In fact, insulin in a fast and transcription-dependent step, allows the response of the P_i uptake system to vitamin D in immature tissue. Beyond this permissive effect, insulin itself influences vitamin D-independent P_i transport: Depression of P_i uptake in less differentiated intestine is turned into stimulation during late embryonic development. It is conceivable, therefore, that this slow action of insulin, whose mediators are not yet known, is a consequence of the proteohormone's possible effect on intestinal maturation.

ACKNOWLEDGEMENTS

These investigations were supported by Grant No. 3031 of the Fonds zur Förderung der wissenschaftlichen Forschung in Österreich. Synthetic 1,25-dihydroxyvitamin D_3 was kindly provided by Dr. Milan Uskoković, Hoffmann-LaRoche, Inc., Nutley, N.J. The expert technical assistance of Peter Wyskovsky and Andreas Köck is thankfully acknowledged.

REFERENCES

Cheng, H., and Leblond, C.P., 1974, Origin, differentiation and renewal of the four main epithelial cell types in the mouse small intestine, Am. J. Anat., 141:461.

Corradino, R. A., 1973a, Embryonic chick intestine in organ culture: A unique system for the study of the intestinal calcium absorptive mechanism, J. Cell Biol., 58:64.

Corradino, R. A., 1973b, Embryonic chick intestine in organ culture: Response to vitamin D_3 and its metabolites, Science, 179:402.

Corradino, R. A., 1973c, 1,25-Dihydroxycholecalciferol: Inhibition of action in organ-cultured intestine by actinomycin D and α-amanitin, Nature, 243:41.

Menard, D., and Malo, C., 1979, Insulin-evoked precocious appearance of intestinal sucrase activity in suckling mice, Dev. Biol., 69:661.

Moriuchi, S., and DeLuca, H. F., 1974, Metabolism of vitamin D_3 in the chick embryo, Arch. Biochem. Biophys., 164:165.

Overton, J., and Shoup, J., 1964, Fine structure of cell surface specializations in the maturing duodenal mucosa of the chick, J. Cell Biol., 21:75.

Peterlik, M., 1978, Phosphate transport by embryonic chick duodenum: Stimulation by vitamin D_3, Biochim. Biophys. Acta, 514:164.

Wasserman, R. H., 1981, Intestinal absorption of calcium and phosphorus, Fed. Proc., 40:68.

MEASUREMENT OF INTRACELLULAR INORGANIC PHOSPHATE IN HUMAN BLOOD RED CELLS, LEUCOCYTES AND PLATELETS

A. Noorwali, C.J. Preston, A. Challa, R.G.G. Russell

Dept. of Human Metabolism & Clinical Biochemistry
University of Sheffield Medical School, Beech Hill
Road, Sheffield, S10 2RX UK

INTRODUCTION

Inorganic phosphate (Pi) has long been known to play an important role in biological systems. It is essential for structural integrity of cells, for example, as a constituent of membrane phospholipids. It is also involved in a host of anabolic and catabolic processes. In glycolysis, Pi participates in the degradation of glucose and synthesis of ATP. Pi has an important role in the regulation of the activity of many enzyme systems involved in energy-transforming reactions. In erythrocytes, through its regulation of the levels of 2,3-DPG (2,3-diphosphoglycerate) and ATP, Pi is indirectly involved in the delivery of oxygen to tissues (1). In urine, Pi is the major buffer system. In hypophosphatemic states, phosphate deficiency leads to many metabolic disturbances, including myopathy, haemolysis and impaired phagocytosis (2).

In clinical disorders where phosphate metabolism is changed, only the extracellular Pi (plasma Pi) has been studied in detail and there have been very few studies of intracellular Pi in different tissues.

We have therefore developed methods for the specific measurement of intracellular phosphate. We have previously devised a method for erythrocytes and we have now extended the studies to other accessible human cells, i.e. leucocytes and platelets. Comparison between values in erythrocytes and other cell types are of interest since they provide insight into the subcellular distribution of phosphate; thus, red cells contain only cytosol and no organelles, whereas white cells are nucleated and contain organelles such as mitochondria, as do platelets.

The method we use for measuring Pi in red cells, leucocytes and platelets is based on the phosphate method of Hall (3) and is specific for Pi.

The investigation of intracellular metabolism requires studies of the major metabolic compartments within the cell. These include, in the case of Pi, the extramitochondrial compartment. We have adapted a rapid cell lysis technique based on the use of digitonin in order to allow tissue fractionation, as described by Zuurendonk & Tager (4), to be applied to studies of subcellular localisation of Pi and ATP in platelets and leucocytes.

METHODS

Venous blood samples were collected from normal volunteers or patients after an overnight fast and were kept on ice until assayed. Inorganic phosphate (Pi) and nucleotides in red blood cells, platelets and leucocytes, were measured in the same blood sample.

Extraction of Pi from human blood cells

1. RED BLOOD CELLS

A 1 ml sample of whole blood and of heparinised plasma was deproteinised by precipitation with 2 ml of ice cold 1.0 M perchloric acid and spun at 3000 x g for 15 mins at $4^{o}C$. 1.5 ml of the supernatant was neutralised with 0.25 ml of a mixture of 3.5 M potassium hydroxide + 0.5 M imidazole to prevent hydrolysis of organic phosphates. A sample of whole blood was taken for measurement of the haematocrit, which was used as a measure of the red cell volume.

2. LEUCOCYTES

10 ml of whole blood was added to a tube containing 1.1 ml of 3.8% sodium citrate and centrifuged at 150 x g for 10 mins at $4^{o}C$ to produce platelet-rich plasma. This was removed and used for the determination of Pi in platelets (see below). To three volumes of the remaining buffy coat and red cell layer was added one volume of 6% Dextran (MW=256,000 Daltons) in normal saline. This was mixed and allowed to sediment for 45 mins at $4^{o}C$. The leucocyte-rich supernatant layer was removed from the sedimented red blood cells and a portion centrifuged at 800 x g for 5 mins at $4^{o}C$ to produce a leucocyte-poor supernatant.

0.5 ml of the leucocyte-rich and poor supernatants were deproteinised with 1.0 ml ice cold 1M perchloric acid. The tubes were centrifuged at 3000 x g for 10 mins at $4^{o}C$ and 1.2 ml of the supernatants neutralised with 0.2 ml potassium hydroxide + imidazole (3.87 M KOH + 0.8 M imidazole). The neutralised extracts were spun at 1000 x g for 1 min at 4°C.

3. PLATELETS

A portion of the platelet-rich plasma (PRP) obtained during the preparation of leucocytes was centrifuged at 1500 x g for 10 mins at 4°C to produce platelet-poor plasma (PPP). The PRP and PPP samples were deproteinised and neutralised as for the leucocytes.

ANALYSIS OF INORGANIC PHOSPHATE

To 0.5 ml of the neutralised extracts was added an equal volume of acid molybdate solution (prepared as 5.7 ml 5% ammonium molybdate + 2.0 ml conc. HCl + 1.3 ml distilled water). The resulting phosphomolybdate complex was extracted into 1.0 ml isobutanol : petroleum ether (4:1) by shaking. The tubes were spun at 1000 x g for 1 minute and 2 x 0.25 ml of the upper layer was pipetted into tubes. To this was added 1.25 ml of absolute ethanol and 25 µl stannous chloride solution (4% w/v $SnCl_2$ in 0.5 M HCl), mixed and a further 1.25 ml ethanol added. The blue product formed was measured at 725 nm in a spectrophotometer. A standard curve was set up by substituting 0.5 ml of Pi standard solutions (0-3mM) for the neutralised extract in the assay.

MEASUREMENT OF PLATELET AND LEUCOCYTE VOLUME

The method used was based upon the distribution of tritium labelled water (^3H_2O) and ^{14}C inulin inside and outside the cells. ^3H-labelled H_2O was assumed to distribute throughout the intracellular and extracellular water space whereas ^{14}C-inulin was assumed to remain outside the cells.

To 0.5 ml of the leucocyte-rich layer of PRP was added 0.25 µCi ^3H_2O and 0.05 µCi ^{14}C inulin and the mixture incubated for 10 minutes at 37°C. The tubes were centrifuged at 1500 x g for 10 minutes at room temperature, the supernatant discarded and the pellet resuspended in 0.5 ml isotonic saline. Standards were prepared in exactly the same way except that the tubes either contained ^3H_2O or ^{14}C inulin alone.

100 µl aliquots of sample or standard were taken up in 5 ml of scintillant solution and the radioactivity counted with counting channels set optimally for ^3H and ^{14}C.

The phosphate content was calculated from the difference between Pi values in whole blood and plasma for red cells, taking haematocrit as the measure of cell volume. For white cells and platelets the difference in phosphate concentrations in the cell-rich and cell-poor suspension was calculated and the concentration within the cells expressed in terms of cell water as based on the distribition of ^3H_2O relative to ^{14}C-inulin.

Subcellular fractionation

The digitonin-lysis technique offers a method for the rapid and almost complete separation of cytosol from particulate fractions. Digitonin is a glycoside with a high affinity for free cholesterol with which it forms stable complexes. Since in general, plasma membranes contain more free cholesterol than membranes of other cell organelles, specific disruption of plasma membranes may be induced (4).

For measurement of Pi in the cytosol and particulate fractions the following procedure was used.

Freshly drawn venous blood was collected into tubes containing 3.8% trisodium citrate and centrifuged at 150 x g for 10 min at $4^{o}C$. The platelets were isolated by repeated centrifugation and resuspension in EDTA-containing tris buffer.

Leucocytes prepared by the Dextran method described above were isolated by centrifugation at 400 x g for 5 min and resuspended in Krebs Ringer buffer containing 3 mM EDTA.

In an Eppendorf microfuge centrifuge tube, the following gradient was established:- Lower layer; 100 μl of 10% glycerol (for determination of enzyme activities); middle layer; 250 μl of a 3:2 (vol/vol) mixture of dibutyl phthalate and dinonyl phthalate. For Pi and adenine nucleotide measurements. the lower layer was replaced by 200 μl perchloric acid (2M). 50 μl of digitonin suspension was added in various concentrations (see results) to 1 ml of cell suspension and shaken in an Eppendorf mixer for 10-15 sec., then 1 ml of the mixture was layered gently on the top of the phthalate layer. The tube was centrifuged for 45-60 sec at 10,000 x g in an Eppendorf microfuge centrifuge. The upper layer and lower layer were separated and analysed. The whole procedure was performed at $4^{o}C$ in a cold room.

For measurement of Pi in the cytosol fraction, 0.5 ml of the top layer at the end of the centrifugation was added to 1 ml cold PCA (1M). The perchloric acid extracts of the cytosol and particulate fraction were neutralised with the KOH/Imidazole buffer and the Pi was measured as described for red blood cells.

Subcellular markers

To monitor the extent of cell lysis during digitonin treatment, as well as the contamination of the cytosol with other subcellular components due to the effect of digitonin on other membranes, several markers were used. Lactic dehydrogenase was used as a cytosol marker. Glutamate dehydrogenase (GIDH), N-acetyl-β-D-glucosaminidase (NAGA) and ^{14}C-serotonin were used as markers for mitochondrial matrix, hydrolase vesicles lysosomes, and dense granules in platelets respectively.

Marker enzymes were assyed in both the cytosol and the particulate fractions.

Measurement of Nucleotides

The nucleotides, adenosine triphosphate and adenosine diphosphate, were measured in neutralised perchloric extracts of the whole cells and in the cytosol and particulate fractions by High Pressure Liquid Chromatography (HPLC). The HPLC method used a reverse phase C_{18} column with 0.125 M ammonium dihydrogen orthophosphate at pH 5.0 as the mobile phase and detection of the nucleotides at 254 nm.

RESULTS

The standard curve for measurement of Pi was linear up to 3 mmol/L. Addition of phosphate-containing organic compounds (ATP, hexose phosphates, etc) which may be present in human blood, did not interfere with the method. When ^{32}P-pyrophosphate was added to the assay there were no detectable counts in the isobutanol layer, which illustrates the great selectivity of the extraction method for Pi. Results from 14 normal plasma values showed a coefficient of variation for the assay of 4%. Interassay variation for measurement of Pi in platelets and leucocytes from 14 normal subjects were 5.8 and 5.0% respectively. Intrassay variation for erythrocyte, platelet and leucocyte Pi measurements were 5.7%, 4.6% and 4.1% respectively.

Concentrations of Pi and nucleotides in normal plasma as well as in all three cell types are shown in Table 1.

Table 1. Concentrations of Pi and nucleotide found in normal persons

	Pi *mM/L	ATP mM/L	ADP mM/L	ATP/ADP
Plasma	1.09 ± 0.03	-	-	-
Red cells	0.78 ± 0.04	1.58 ± 0.04	-	-
White cells	2.01 ± 0.05	2.22 ± 0.13	0.94 ± 0.09	2.36
Platelets	4.12 ± 0.08	3.07 ± 0.12	2.12 ± 0.07	1.44

n = 14

*mM/L of total cell volume for red cells and of cell water volume for leucocytes and platelets.

Data are presented as the mean ± SE.

Concentrations of Pi in red cells was less than in the corresponding plasma, whereas leucocyte Pi was twice the plasma concentration, and platelet Pi four times that of plasma. Nucleotide concentration in platelets were higher than those of leucocytes and red cells. Some of the nucleotides found in platelets are stored in the dense granules (5). ADP, which is present in larger concentrations in the granules of platelets than other nucleotides, probably accounts for the lower total ATP/ADP ratio in platelets.

Incubation of platelets with increasing concentrations of digitonin induced differential leakage of LDH, ^{14}C-serotonin and N-AGaAse (Fig.1). At a platelet count of 4 x 10^{-5} cells/µl, 90% of total LDH activity was liberated at 0.14 mM digitonin whereas much higher digitonin concentrations were required for liberating ^{14}C serotonin and N-AGAase (about 1 mM) and GIDH (3-4 mM). This enabled isolation of the LDH-containing cell compartment (cytosol) with minimal contamination by lysosomes (15% based on N-AGAase activity), electron dense granules (10%, ^{14}C-serotonin) and mitochondrial matrix (0.4%, GIDH activity). Optimal separation was obtained after 15 sec incubation; longer incubation increased the leakage of granular components.

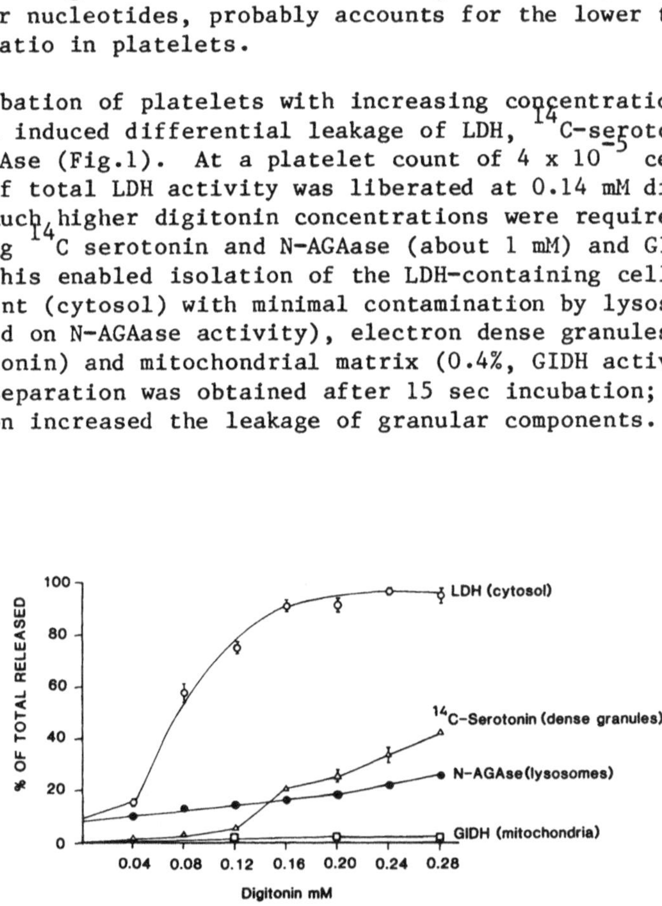

Fig.1.Release of LDH, NAGAase and ^{14}C-serotonin into supernatant of digitonin-treated platelets at increasing digitonin concentration. Leakage of GIDH was below 1%. Data are means of 3 experiments ±SE.

Relationship between platelet number and digitonin-induced leakage of LDH

In this experiment different concentrations of platelets i.e. platelet suspensions with different cell numbers were incubated with increasing concentrations of digitonin. LDH leakage was tested in the supernatants. The dose-dependence of leakage induced by digitonin was measured for each population (Fig. 2a). The minimal amount of digitonin causing more than 90%. Leakage of LDH was linearly related to cell number (Fig.2b).

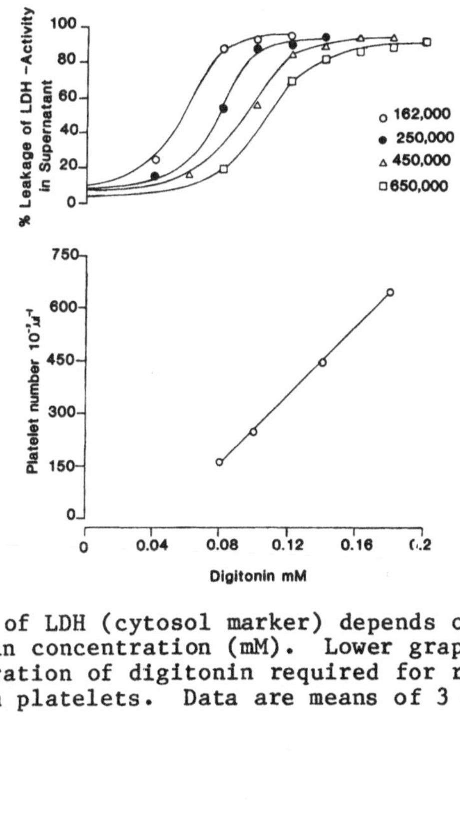

Fig.2.Release of LDH (cytosol marker) depends on platelet number digitonin concentration (mM). Lower graph shows concentration of digitonin required for release of 90% of LDH from platelets. Data are means of 3 experiments.

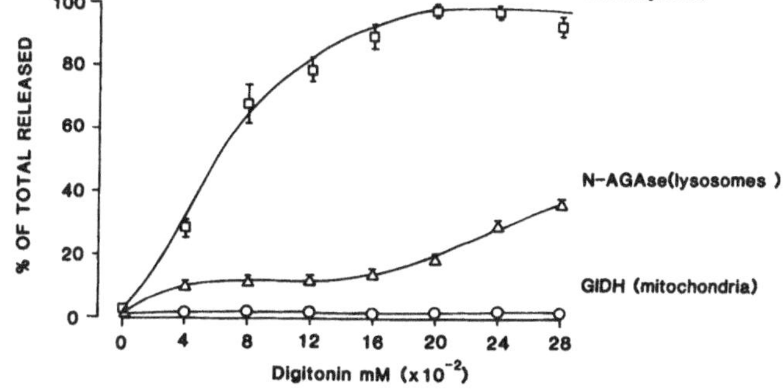

Fig.3.Release of LDH and N-AGAase after treating leucocytes with increasing concentrations of a digitonin. Leakage of GIDH was below 1%. Data are means of 3 experiments ±SEM.

Table 2. Pi, nucleotides and subcellular markers in platelet fractions, obtained by digitonin-induced cell lysis

	Total Intracellular µmoles/10^{11} platelets	Cytosol µmoles/10^{11} platelets	Particulate fraction µmoles/10^{11} platelets
Pi	10.27 ± 0.48	6.10 ± 0.24	3.83 ± 0.25
ATP	7.03 ± 0.33	5.57 ± 0.31	2.01 ± 0.05
ADP	4.14 ± 0.46	0.95 ± 0.13	3.13 ± 0.34
ATP+ADP	11.17	6.52	5.14
Ratio of ATP/ADP	1.69	5.83	0.64
	Percentage distribution of subcellular markers		
LDH	100	91.7 ± 1.3	undetectable
5HT	100	0.5	85.0 ± 7.0
GIDH	100	0.0	90.0
NAGA	100	5.7 ± 1.3	96.4 ± 0.9

Data are means of 3 experiments ± SE.

Table 3. Pi, nucleotides, and subcellular markers in leucocyte fractions, obtained by digitonin-induced cell lysis

	Total Intracellular concentration µmoles/10^9	Cytosol µmoles/10^9 leucocytes	Particulate fraction µmoles/10^9 leucocytes
Pi	5.04 ± 0.18	3.82 ± 0.13	0.856 ± 0.12
ATP	3.92 ± 0.12	3.56 ± 0.13	0.183 ± 0.40
ADP	1.32 ± 0.07	0.78 ± 0.07	0.417 ± 0.05
ATP+ADP	5.25	4.34	0.6
Ratio of ATP/ADP	2.97	4.55	0.44
	Percentage distribition of subcellular markers		
LDH	100	91.9 ± 2.2	0 -
GIDH	100	0 -	91.2 ± 2.3
NAGA	100	2	94

Data are means of 3 experiments ± SE

Values of LDH, GIDH and NAGA are % of total.

Platelet suspensions from 3 normal subjects were treated with appropriate concentrations of digitonin. Pi and nucleotides as well as the subcellular markers were measured in both cytosol and particulate fractions. Table 2 shows the amount of Pi and adenine nucleotides in intact platelets, and in the cytosol and particulate fractions obtained after digitonin treatment. About 40% of Pi and 45% of the sum of ATP plus ADP were found in the particulate fraction. The ATP/ADP ratio was about 6 in the cytosol and about 0.6 in the pellet fraction. The latter ratio indicates that most of the ADP probably comes from the electron dense granules. The ATP/ADP ration of 0.6 in particulate fractions of platelets is close to the ratio of 0.6-1.1 that was measured extracellularly after thrombin treatment (5).

Incubation of leucocytes with digitonin at increasing concentrations induced differential release of LDH and NAGA (see Fig.3). 90% of total LDH activity was liberated at 0.16 mM digitonin whereas much higher digitonin concentrations were required for liberating GIDH and NAGAase. This enabled isolation of cytosol with minimal contamination by lysosomes (10%, based on NAGAase activity) and mitochondrial matrix (0.6%, GIDH activity).

Leucocytes suspensions from 3 normal subjects were treated with appropriate concentrations of digitonin. Pi and nucleotides as well as the subcellular markers were measured in both cytosol and particulate fractions. Table 3 shows the amount of Pi and adenine nucleotides in intact leucocytes, and in the cytosol and particulate fractions. About 75% of Pi and 80% of the sum of ATP + ADP were found in the cytosol fraction. The ATP/ADP ratio was about 4.5 in the cytosol and 0.4 in the particulate fraction.

SUMMARY

The measurement of Pi in red blood cells, leucocytes, platelets and plasma by this method is both highly selective and sensitive for Pi. Whereas the ratio of intracellular to extracellular Pi is less than 1 in red cells, it is about 4 in platelets and about 2 in leucocytes. In platelets, where there are storage granules, the nucleotide levels are higher than in red cells or leucocytes. Cell lysis by digitonin proved to be a reliable technique for the rapid and efficient separation of cytosol from the particulate fraction. The isolation of cytosol with minimal contamination by lysosomes, electron dense granules and mitochondrial matrix depended on the use of appropriate concentration of digitonin. There was a linear relationship between platelet number and digitonin concentration which induced leakage of 90% of the LDH. In platelets about half of the Pi and 50% of the total ATP + ADP were found in the particulate fractions. In leucocytes most of the Pi and the bulk of nucleotides are present in the cytosol. These findings indicate the presence of at least two pools of nucleotides in platelets and leucocytes, and suggests that the inorganic phosphate in cytosol is at a higher concentration than outside the cells, implying a concentration gradient across the plasma membrane.

REFERENCES

1. M.A. Lichtman, D.R. Miller, J. Cohen et al: Reduced red cell glycolysis, 2,3-diphosphoglycerate and adenosine triphosphate concentration, and increased hemoglobin oxygen affinity caused by hypophosphatemia. Ann.Intern.Med. 74: 562-568, 1971.
2. P.R. Craddock, Y. Yawata, L. Van Santen et al: Acquired phagocyte dysfunction: A complication of the hypophosphatemia of parenteral hyperalimentation. N.Engl.J.Med. 290: 1403, 1974.
3. R.J. Hall: An improved method for the micro determination of inorganic phosphate in small volumes of biological fluids. J.of Med.Lab.Technology. 20: 97-103, 1963.
4. P.F. Zuurendonck, F.M. Tager: Rapid separation of particulate components and soluble cytoplasm of isolated rat-liver cells. Biochimica et Biophysica Acta. 333, 393-399, 1974.
5. H. Holmsen, H.J. Day and E. Storm: Adenine nucleotide metabolism of blood platelets. VI Subcellular localisation of nucleotide pools with different functions in the platelet release reaction. Biochemica et Biophysica Acta. 186, 254-266, 1969.

INTRACELLULAR INORGANIC PHOSPHATE AND ATP LEVELS IN HUMAN BLOOD ERYTHROCYTES, LEUCOCYTES AND PLATELETS IN NORMAL SUBJECTS AND IN DISEASES ASSOCIATED WITH ALTERED PHOSPHATE METABOLISM

C.J.Preston, A.Noorwali, A.Challa, A.D. Paterson, D.J. Beard, J.A. Kanis, R.G.G. Russell

Dept. of Human Metabolism & Clinical Biochemistry
University of Sheffield Medical School,Beech Hill Road, Sheffield, S10 2RX UK

INTRODUCTION

Phosphorus plays an important role in a variety of biological systems. It occurs in structural components such as phospholipids, and in other important cellular constituents, eg, nucleic acids, nucleotides, proteins, sugars etc. It is involved in the regulation of many metabolic pathways(1).

In man about 80% of total body phosphorus is in bone and the remainder associated with soft tissues where it is a major intracellular anion. Although the majority of intracellular phosphorus is present in organic compounds, the relatively minor inorganic pool is critical since it influences many metabolic processes, such as the generation of nucleotide triphosphates (ATP etc).

The plasma phosphate concentration in man is under physiological control, the level being largely determined by the tubular reabsorptive capacity of the kidney(2), which in turn is influenced by hormones such as parathyroid hormone, growth hormone, etc.

There are however many diseases in man in which the plasma phosphate concentration is altered(3), and although there has been great interest in phosphate homeostasis in recent years little work has been done on corresponding intracellular levels and their changes in disease states.

We have therefore measured intracellular concentrations of inorganic phosphate(Pi) and ATP in a variety of diseases using specific methods and applied them to readily accessible human tissues namely red blood cells, leucocytes and platelets.

METHOD

The methods developed for measuring Pi and ATP in the blood cells are described elsewhere in these proceedings. (Measurement of intracellular inorganic phosphate in human blood cells, A. Noorwali et al, this volume).

COLLECTION OF BLOOD SAMPLES

Venous blood samples collected from normal volunteers or patients after an overnight fast were kept on ice until assayed, Pi and ATP in the various cell types were assayed in the same sample.

RESULTS

Table 1 shows the absolute normal ranges for Pi and ATP in whole cell extracts obtained in a group of 14 normal subjects whose ages ranged from 22-40 years.

Table 1

Intracellular Pi and ATP in normal subjects.

Cell	Pi mmol/l	ATP mmol/l
Red blood cells	0.6-0.95	1.3-1.9
Leucocytes	1.7-2.4	1.5-2.9
Platelets	3.7-4.5	2.3-3.6

Results expressed as per litre of red cell volume, and per litre intracellular water for platelets and leucocytes.

Paget's disease

During treatment with the bisphosphonate, EHDP, at doses of 20mg/Kg/day, there is a rise in plasma phosphate which has been shown to be due to an increase in renal tubular reabsorption (4). Intracellular Pi values measured in four patients after two weeks therapy with EHDP were not significantly different from the pretreatment values even though the plasma phosphate doubled (Fig.1). There was also no change in the intracellular ATP values measured in all cell types.

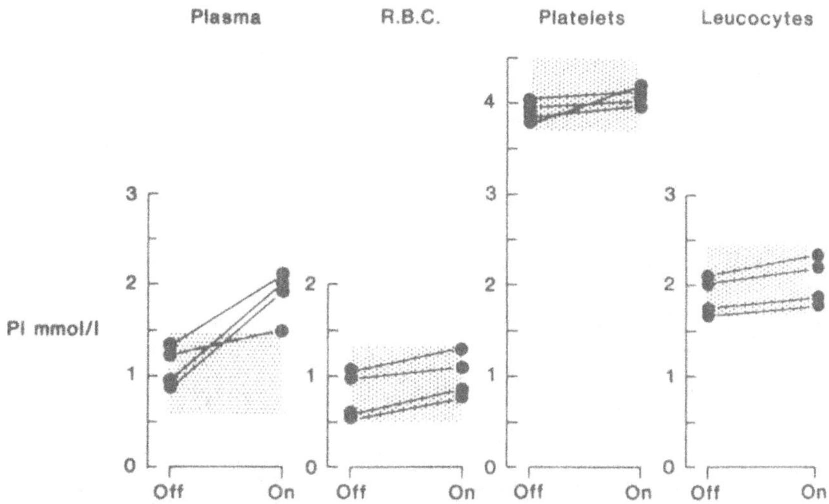

Fig. 1. Inorganic phosphate in 4 patients with Paget's disease before and after two weeks treatment with EHDP (20mg/Kg/day).
Shaded area is the normal range.

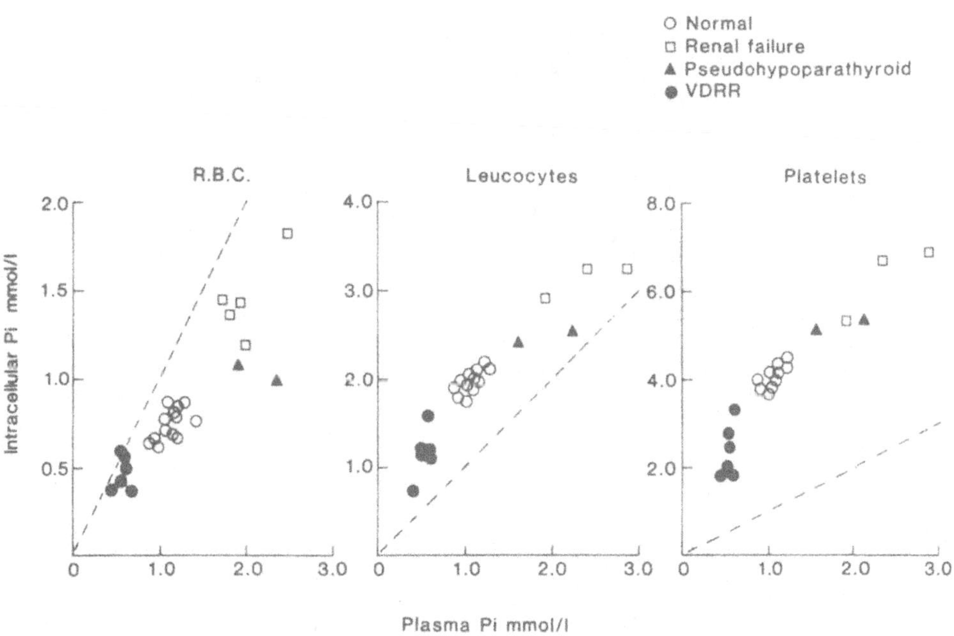

Fig. 2. Plasma phosphate versus intracellular Pi in normal subjects and in patients with high or low plasma phosphate.
Dotted line shows line of equality.

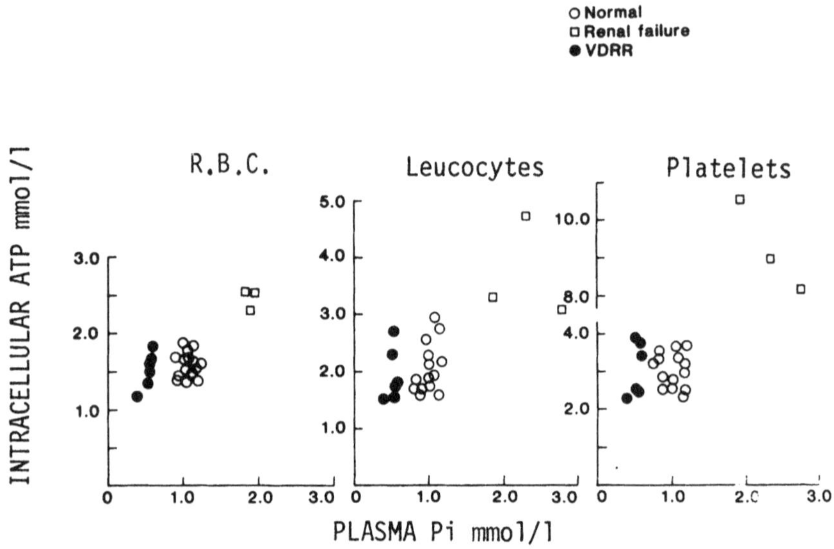

Fig. 3. Plasma phosphate versus intracellular ATP in normal subjects and patients with high and low plasma phosphates.

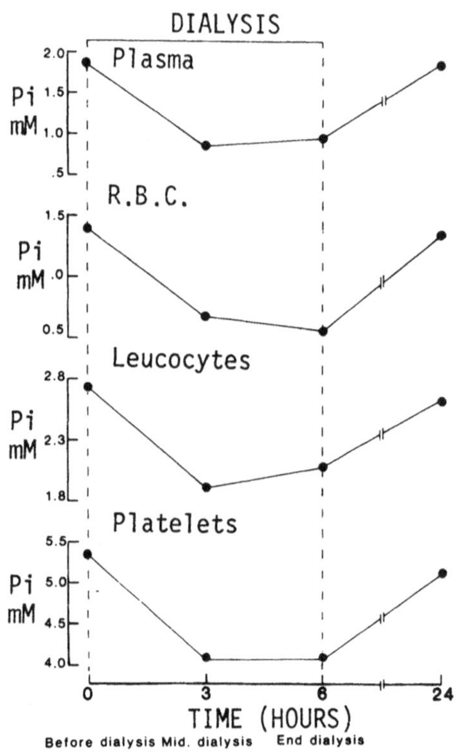

Fig. 4. Effect of haemodialysis on changes in plasma phosphate and intracellular Pi.

Renal failure

When compared to normal subjects, patients with chronic renal failure who had elevated plasma phosphate levels all exhibited raised intracellular concentrations of Pi (Fig.2) and ATP (Fig.3) in all the cell types studied.

During haemodialysis of one of these patients the fall in plasma phosphate was mirrored by a fall in Pi in red blood cells leucocytes and platelets, such that the values fell into the normal range (Fig. 4). However intracellular values measured 24 hours after haemodialysis had finished had all returned to baseline levels.

Vitamin D resistant rickets

Six patients with hypophosphataemic (Vitamin D resistant) rickets (VDRR) were studied. All had low plasma phosphate but normal plasma calcium values. None had muscle weakness or other renal tubular abnormalities (Table 2).

Intracellular Pi values measured in these patients were about half that observed in our normal subjects (Fig.2). In contrast, ATP levels were maintained within the normal range even though the plasma and intracellular Pi values were low (Fig 3).

Table 2

Vitamin D resistant Rickets (VDRR)

Patient	Sex	Age	Clinical details
1. D.G.	M	16	Familial
2. M.G.	F	47	" (Mother of D.G)
3. P.G.	F	19	"
4. M.G.	M	21	"
5. R.H.	F	5	"
6. J.M.	M	32	Adult onset

Renal tubular acidosis

Figure 5 illustrates the changes in Pi before and during the treatment of a patient with renal tubular acidosis. The plasma phosphate on admission to hospital was at the lower end of the normal range and the intracellular Pi concentrations below

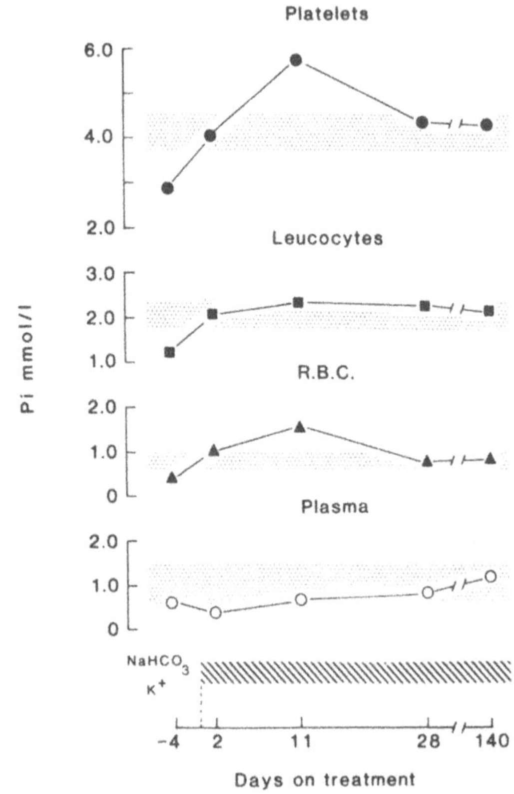

Fig. 5. Plasma phosphate and intracellular Pi changes in a patient with renal tubular acidosis.

our normal range. Two days after beginning treatment with bicarbonate and potassium, the plasma phosphate fell slightly and this was accompanied by a rise in the intracellular Pi such that by the eleventh day of treatment the intracellular Pi values were raised above the upper normal limit. At this time her muscle strength, initially week, had improved markedly. Samples assayed at 28 days and again at 4 months after treatment started were all within the normal range.

Intracellular ATP concentrations, which were initially near the lower end of the normal range, fell during treatment and only returned to normal when the plasma and intracellular Pi values had returned to normal (Fig. 6).

SUMMARY

Red blood cells, leucocytes and platelets show changes in their intracellular Pi levels according to the prevailing level

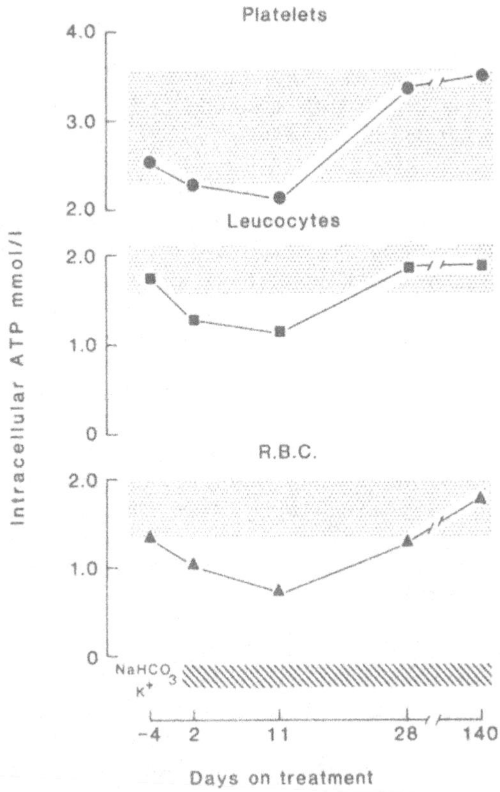

Fig. 6. Intracellular ATP concentrations in a patient with renal tubular acidosis.

of plasma phosphate both in normal subjects and in a variety of diseases. In the red blood cell the intracellular to extracellular Pi ratio is less than unity. Leucocytes and platelets, on the other hand, exhibit ratios that are above unity. This is probably due to intracellular compartmentalisation of phosphate within cell organelles such as mitochondria.

The study performed during haemodialysis clearly shows that a reduction in plasma phosphate is accompanied by a similar change in the intracellular Pi concentration, such that the intra: extracellular ratio remained essentially unaltered. However there was no change in the concentration of ATP in the cells, which has also been reported by other workers. (5).

In the patients with Paget's disease treated with EHDP the distribution of Pi was markedly altered. Although the plasma phosphate rose the expected rise in intracellular Pi did not occur. The underlying mechanism causing this lack of a response in the cells remains to be elucidated.

There was a marked dissociation between the plasma and intracellular Pi values in the patient with renal tubular acidosis during treatment, perhaps reflecting the importance of pH in determining the distribution of phosphate across biological membranes. Intracellular Pi values rose sharply during treatment and this was accompanied by a transient fall in plasma phosphate.

Blood pH levels are known to affect phosphate influx into cells, a rise in pH increases glycolysis and promotes phosphate uptake by the cell(6). Thus the rise in intracellular Pi observed in this patient during bicarbonate therapy to correct the acidosis may be explained by a rise in blood pH. However increasing the glycolytic rate of cells should lead to a rise in ATP levels, which in this case did not occur, the levels actually falling below the normal range.

Although the patients with Vitamin D resistant rickets showed the expected reduced intracellular Pi concentrations they were able to maintain their intracellular ATP levels in the normal range. If this observation is also true for ATP levels in muscle cells this may account for the lack of an obvious muscle weakness in these patients.

REFERENCES

1. E.A.Newsholme and C. Start. Regulation in metabolism. John Wiley. London (1973).

2. O.L.M.Bijvoet. Relation of plasma phosphate concentration to tubular reabsorption of phosphate. Clinical Science. 37: 23-36 (1969).

3. J.P.Knockel. The pathophysiology and clinical characteristics of severe hypophosphataemia. Archives of Internal Medicine. 137: 203-220. (1977).

4. R.J.Walton, R.G.G.Russell and R.Smith. Changes in the renal and extrarenal handling of phosphate induced by etidronate (EHDP) in man. Clinical Science and Molecular Medicine. 49: 45-56, (1975).

5. M.A.Lichtman, M.S.Murphy, B.J.Byer and R.B.Freeman. Haemoglobin affinity for oxygen in chronic renal disease: the effects of haemodialysis. Blood, 43: 417-424, (1974).

6. M.E.Mostellar and E.P.Tuttle. Effect of alkylosis on plasma concentration and urinary excretion of inorganic phosphate in man. Journal of Clinical Investigation, 43: 138-148, (1964).

PREVENTION OF PHOSPHATE INDUCED PROGRESSION OF EXPERIMENTAL UREMIA BY 3-PHOSPHOCITRIC ACID

W. Gordon Walker, Luis Gimenez, William P. Tew and Judith A. Hermann

O'Neill Laboratories - Department of Medicine
Johns Hopkins University School of Medicine
Baltimore, Maryland 21205

Excess dietary phosphate produces progressive increase in calcium content of the kidney and also leads to progressive deterioration of renal function[1-3]. The important variables responsible for determination of both the rate of deposition of calcium and loss of renal function are the quantity of dietary phosphate, the amount of functioning renal tissue and the level of parathyroid activity[3,4]. Given sufficient reduction in the size of the functioning renal mass, progressive deposition of calcium can be demonstrated in the kidney of animals maintained on a diet of normal phosphate content[5]. The histologic changes associated with these progressive calcium deposits provide convincing evidence of the structural damage produced, apparently resulting from cellular damage associated with calcium phosphate deposition [3,6].

The study of Ibels, et al. showed that normal dietary phosphate intake could produce progressive renal damage in the rat remnant kidney model and that this damage could be prevented when such animals were maintained on a very low phosphate diet[5]. While the extent to which dietary phosphorus plays a role in determining the rate of progression of renal failure in the various clinical entities leading to end stage renal disease remains to be defined, the experimental evidence deocumenting the severity of phosphate nephrotoxicity is sufficiently impressive that a vigorous search for ways of modifying this mechanism of renal damage appears warranted. Haut and associates examined the effect of di-sodium-ethane-1-diphosphonate (EHDP) upon phosphate nephrotoxicity and noted a reduction in severity of histologic changes in the EHDP treated animals after six weeks but failed to demonstrate significant differences in renal function between animals so treated and a comparable group with remnant kidney receiving a diet containing three percent phosphate without such treatment[6].

Tew and associates[7] synthesized 3-Phosphocitric acid, a compound proposed as a naturally occurring inhibitor of calcium phosphate precipitation[8], and demonstrated that it successfully inhibits both precipitation and crystallization in vitro and in vivo. We have reported preliminary evidence indicating that this compound is effective in preventing renal calcification and in preventing the phosphate induced renal damage in the rat remnant kidney model[9,10]. Some of the findings of this study relevant to the phosphate induced renal damage are presented below.

METHODS AND MATERIALS

Production of Remnant Kidney Model of Renal Insufficiency

Male Sprague-Dawley rats weighing between 250 and 300 grams were subjected to right nephrectomy through a right flank incision under nembutal-ether anesthesia. Following closure of the right flank incision, a partial left nephrectomy was achieved by exposing, ligating and removing successively the upper and lower poles, leaving the middle third of the left kidney intact as the functioning segment. After removal of the capsule, the right kidney was weighed and weight of the total renal mass estimated as twice the weight of the right kidney[11]. Since the weights of the right and left kidney do not differ by more than three percent[11], the upper and lower segments of the left kidney were weighed separately and weight of the remaining functioning remnant taken as the difference between weight right kidney and the total weights of upper and lower thirds of left kidney. This estimated weight was compared to measured weight of the remnant at sacrifice to yield a measure of hypertrophy.

All animals were allowed two weeks to recover from surgery, and then were randomized into three groups:

Control Group (n=5)

These animals received a synthetic diet consisting of 8% fat, 20% protein and 72% carbohydrate and containing 17.7 mmols of calcium and 18.8 mmols of phosphorus plus 1 mg of vitamin A and 300 I.U. of vitamin D per 100 grams of chow[12]. Food intake of 19 grams of food per rat per day in this control group provided an average phosphate intake of 3.6 mmols per day.

Phosphate-Fed Group (n=12)

Received the same diet as the control group, adjusted to contain 71 mmols of phosphate/100 gms diet by addition of Na2HPO4. Food intake averaged 16.9 grams/rat/day, providing an estimate of phosphorus intake of 12 mmols/day.

Phosphocitrate Treated (n=15)

Animals were treated identically to the phosphate-fed group but also received 50 μmols of 3-Phosphocitric acid given intraperitoneally daily. Food intake averaged 19.7 gms/day in these animals, providing a phosphorus intake of 14 mmols/day.

Each week all animals were weighed and total food and water intake determined for one twenty-four hour period. Blood was taken for creatinine determination before surgery, immediately after surgery and at approximately biweekly intervals after the experiment was begun.

All animals were anesthetized and sacrificed by exsanguination after 28 days on the specially prepared diet and approximately 40 days after surgery. Following sacrifice renal tissue was taken for staining with hematoxylin-eosin and Von Kossa's stain, respectively, and for tissue [Ca] determinations. Histologic changes were evaluated and quantified by a pathologist who had no knowledge of the prior treatment of the animals. The increase in renal mass was expressed as percentage increase in weight based upon the estimate of the original weight of the remaining remnant ((final kidney weight less original weight estimate/original weight estimate)x100). Renal weights and renal [Ca] were also determined on six normal rats of comparable weight and age but not operated upon.

Creatinine was measured by a modification of the Bonsnes and Taussky method[13], calcium by atomic absorption spectrometry and phosphate by a modification of the method of Fiske and SubbaRow[14]. Statistical comparisons between the groups were based upon the use of Student's non-paired "t" test.

RESULTS

The quantity of renal tissue remaining immediately after nephrectomy was estimated to range between 30 and 33 percent of the original mass of renal tissue in each of the three groups (Table 1). No significant differences in residual renal mass between the three groups could be demonstrated by this estimate. During the initial two weeks following surgery when all groups were maintained on the standard diet with normal phosphate intake, the serum creatinine which measured $0.87 \pm .07$ mg/dl (mean value for all animals±SEM) declined to $0.64 \pm .06$ mg/dl ($p < .001$), for the entire group just before randomization and initiation of phosphate feeding. Thereafter the serum creatinine behaved differently in the three groups as illustrated in Figure 1. The phosphate fed group receiving no phosphocitrate exhibited the higher serum creatinine values at sacrifice ($p < .003$). Also shown are data on 6 normal rats of the same age and

Table I
QUANTITY OF RENAL TISSUE REMOVED

	1. BODY WT. AT SURGERY	2. WT. OF EXCISED RIGHT KIDNEY	3. WT. OF REMOVED TISSUE FROM LEFT KIDNEY	4. TOTAL WT. OF REMOVED KIDNEY TISSUE	5. ESTIMATED WT. OF REMAINING KIDNEY TISSUE*
CONTROL (C) n=5	280.4±6.1	1.254±.1	.4708±.06	1.725±.15	.7835±.006 (31.3%)
PHOSPHATE-FED (U) n=12	283.25±5.8	1.275±.08	.4320±.04	1.706±.1	.8425±.08 (32.8%)
PHOSPHATE-FED + PHOSPHOCITRATE (T) n=15	279.6±.08	1.244±.05	.4910±.02	1.736±.05	.7532±.04 (30.1%)

All values expressed as MEAN±SEM

* Values from this column=2XColumn2 - Column 4.

C=nephrectomy plus standard diet.

U=nephrectomy plus 12 mmol/phosphate/day

T=nephrectomy plus 14 mmol/phosphate/day plus 50μmol/phosphocitrate/day

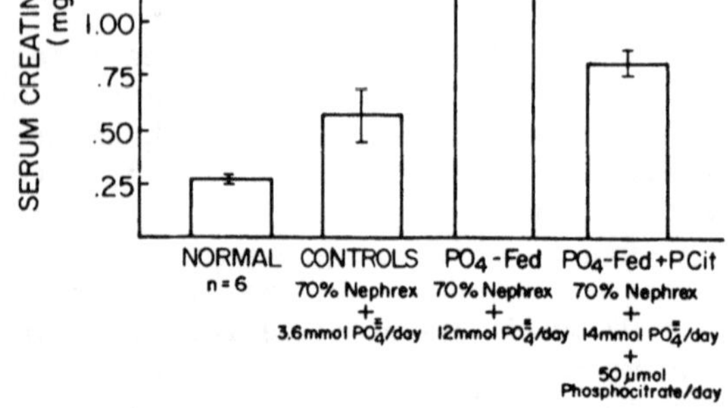

Fig. 1. Serum creatinine values at the time of sacrifice. The bar labeled normal represents values (mean±SEM) for creatinine in normal animals not operated upon. Other groups are as identified in text.

weight that were not operated on. The animals which were nephrectomized and then maintained on a normal diet exhibited higher creatinine values than did the normal control. There was no significant difference in mean creatinine values at sacrifice between this control group maintained on normal diet after surgery and the phosphate-fed group that received daily phosphocitrate injections.

The phosphate-fed group that received no phosphocitrate treatment exhibited the greatest increase in mass of the renal remnant despite the fact that this group also had the poorest renal function. The percentage increase in mass exhibited by the phosphate-fed animals treated with phosphocitrate did not differ from the control partially nephrectomized group maintained on a normal phosphate intake. Also shown in Table II are data on serum [Ca] and serum [P]. Of great interest is the finding that the calcium + phosphate product in the phosphocitrate treated group exceeded 95 $(mg/dl)^2$ and despite this abnormally high product, the drug was remarkably effective in preventing renal functional deterioration as well as nephrocalcinosis.

Table II

Data from Three Groups at Sacrifice

	CONTROL n=5	PHOSPHATE FED n=12	PHOSPHATE FED + PHOSPHOCITRATE n=15
REMNANT KIDNEY WT.	1.43±.05	2.43±.28	1.47±.08
% KIDNEY HYPERTROPHY	86.7%	194.3%	99.5%
SERUM CREATININE	.61±.13	1.86±.23	.81±.07
SERUM CALCIUM	10.13±.24	6.02±.65	7.39±.41
SERUM PHOSPHORUS	7.41±.6	16.9±1.9	12.9±1.2

Figure 2 represents the data on renal calcium content for each group. The calcium content of the kidneys in the phosphate-fed animals is nearly 80-fold greater than values from controls on a

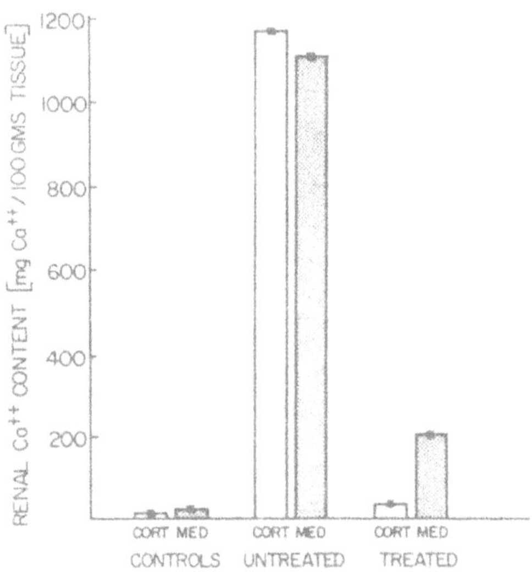

Fig. 2. Renal calcium content. No significant difference was observed between cortical and medullary calcium content in the control animals who received a normal phosphate diet after partial nephrectomy. Animals receiving high phosphate intake only exhibited a marked and highly significant increase in both cortical and medullary calcium content in the kidney remnant. In contrast, the animals receiving increased phosphate intake plus phosphocitrate showed no significant increase in cortical calcium and only a modest rise in medullary calcium.

normal diet. In contrast, the phosphocitrate treated rats exhibit renal [Ca] values that are on average only twice as great as the control. Differences between phosphate-fed animals receiving phosphocitrate and those receiving phosphate alone were highly significant ($p<.001$). Despite this marked increase in calcium content, the contribution of the increased calcium content to the increase in renal mass exhibited by the phosphate-fed group was insignificant, the total calcium mass of the kidney remnant representing only 3 percent of the weight increase.

These functional differences were associated with equally striking histological differences as shown in Figure 3A and B. The renal parenchyma in the animals fed phosphate only showed severe damage, exhibiting extensive interstitial nephritis, marked tubular dilatation and extensive calcification. In contrast, the control group and the group treated with phosphocitrate showed very little distortion of the normal architecture. This remarkable difference

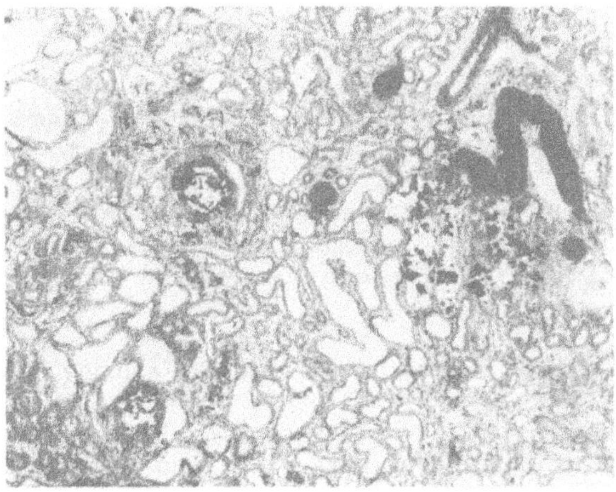

Fig. 3A. Effects of 4 weeks of excessive phosphate intake. Marked tubular dilatation, extensive calcium deposits within the tubules and interstices, extensive interstitial inflammation and scarring are evident.

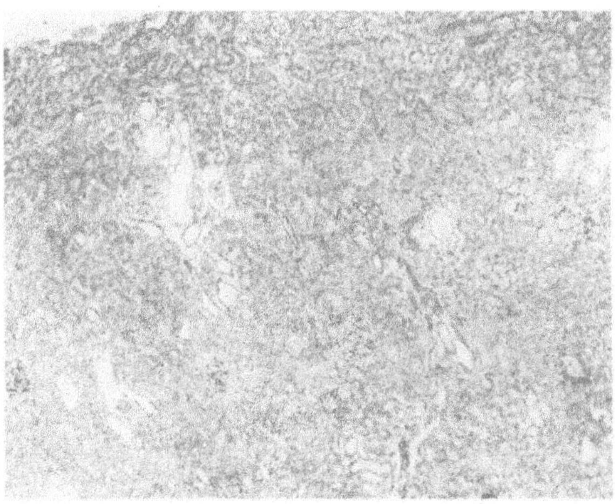

Fig. 3B. Phosphocitrate treatment. Renal architecture is much more nearly normal and no calcification is seen. No interstitial inflammation or scarring is evident in this section. Renal function in this group was correspondingly better as described in the text.

in histological change between the phosphate-fed animals receiving phosphocitrate and those receiving phosphate alone, plus the higher creatinine values in the latter group, indicate that the much larger increase in mass exhibited by this group did not result in the achievement of functionally superior compensatory hypertrophy.

DISCUSSION

These studies demonstrate that phosphocitrate can prevent the renal damage produced by phosphate in the remnant kidney model of renal insufficiency in the rat. This protective effect is exerted despite the fact that marked hyperphosphatemia persists and the calcium x phosphate product remains high in the animals receiving phosphocitric acid during the four week period of high phosphate intake.

Both histological and chemical evidence support the view that the severe renal damage exhibited by the phosphate fed animals in the present experimental series was due to progressive deposition of calcium phosphate in the renal parenchyma and the associated interstitial nephritis which it produced. The nephrotoxic effect of increased dietary phosphate intake has been well established, beginning with the careful work of MacKay and Oliver[1]. Renal damage is related to the quantity of phosphate ingested as well as the total functioning renal mass[2,3,4,15]. Necrosis of cells followed by calcification in the areas of necrosis have been described in the proximal convoluted tubule with similar changes also being seen in the loop of Henle and elsewhere[1,3,15]. Depending upon the dose and route of administration, calcification of basement membranes surrounding proximal convoluted tubules in the outer and inner cortex, glomeruli, and outer medulla are often associated with calcification of intraluminal casts as well as extensive interstitial inflammation. As in the present study, previous reports have identified increased calcium content associated with these changes and it would appear that calcium phosphate precipitation is most likely the initial event leading to progressive renal damage and loss of function. Hence a plausible explanation for the mechanism of action of 3-Phosphocitric acid in the present study is that it prevented the precipitation and crystallization of calcium phosphate, thereby preventing progression of renal impairment. It is of interest that this inhibitory effect appears to have been sustained despite a very high Ca x P product (Table II).

The mechanism whereby 3-Phosphocitric acid prevents progression of renal damage in these animals is most likely related to its ability to inhibit precipitation and crystallization of calcium phosphate[7]. Phosphocitrate has been proposed as a naturally occurring inhibitor of biologic calcification found in urine and mitochondrial preparations[8,16]. Although existence of this substance as a naturally occurring compound in living tissue has not been unequivocally proven, Tew et al. have synthesized the compound and have shown that it acts as an extremely powerful inhibitor of calcium phosphate precipitation from metastable solutions as well as an inhibitor of the accompanying growth of hydroxyapatite crystals[7]. Preliminary observations in our laboratory have also indicated that the compound is active in vivo in preventing deposition of calcium phosphate in tissues under a variety of abnormal situations predisposing to biologic calcification[9,10].

The exact mechanism whereby phosphocitrate exerts this action remains to be clarified, but it has been demonstrated that phosphocitrate becomes bound to microcrystals of calcium phosphate, thereby preventing crystal growth and facilitating crystal dissolution in the process of exerting its inhibitory action[7]. This incorporation into the calcium phosphate lattice creates a steric hindrance that prevents further crystal growth. It would appear from the present experiments that it is sufficiently successful at preventing crystal growth that it prevents the expected nephrocalcinosis and the attendant interstitial inflammation that produces such marked renal damage.

The studies reported here provide clear evidence that phosphocitrate is effective in preventing the deposition of calcium phosphate in the kidney and in preserving renal function at least in the rat remnant model of renal insufficiency. Whether it is of comparable benefit in retarding or arresting renal damage in other forms of progressive experimental renal disease remains to be determined. Similarly it is not known whether administration for longer periods can be safely undertaken; this must await more detailed toxicologic studies. Nevertheless this compound appears promising as a therapeutic agent which could arrest or retard the rate of progression in at least one form of experimental renal disease and thus merits further study in this and other forms of experimental renal disease. Further study is also necessary to define the metabolism, pharmacology and toxicity of phosphocitrate.

REFERENCES

1. E. M. MacKay, and J. Oliver, Renal damage following the ingestion of a diet containing an excess of inorganic phosphate, J. Exp. Med. 61:319 (1935).
2. A. M. Pappenheimer, The effect of experimental reduction of kidney substance upon the parathyroid glands and skeletal tissue, J. Exp. Med. 64:965 (1936).
3. J. Craig, Observations on the kidney after phosphate loading in the rat, Arch. Pathol. 68:306 (1959).
4. P. Haase, Parathyroid stimulation in phosphate-induced nephrocalcinosis, J. Ant. 125:299 (1978).
5. L. S. Ibels, A. C. Alfrey, L. L. Haut, and W. E. Huffer, Preservation of function in experimental renal disease by dietary restriction of phosphate, N. Engl. J. Med. 298:122 (1978).
6. L. L. Haut, A. C. Alfrey, S. Guggenheim, B. Buddington, and N. Schrier, Renal toxicity of phosphates in rats, Kidney Int. 17:722 (1980).

7. W. P. Tew, C. Mahle, J. Benavides, J. E. Howard, and A. L. Lehninger, Synthesis and characterization of phosphocitric acid, a potent inhibitor of hydroxyapatite crystal growth, Biochemistry 19:1983 (1980).
8. J. E. Howard, Studies on urinary stone formation: A saga of clinical investigation, Johns Hopkins Med. J. 139:239 (1976).
9. W. P. Tew, C. D. Malis, and W. G. Walker, The effects of phosphocitrate on experimentally induced nephrocalcinosis, Kidney Int. 19:117 (1981).
10. L. Gimenez, W. P. Tew, J. A. Hermann, and W. G. Walker, Prevention of phosphate-induced renal insufficiency by phosphocitrate, Kidney Int. 19:110 (1981).
11. J. M. Kaufman, H. J. DiMeola, N. J. Siegel, B. Lytton, M. Kashgarian, and J. P. Hayslett, Compensatory adaptation of structure and function following progressive renal ablation, Kidney Int. 6:10 (1974).
12. H. E. Harrison, and H. C. Harrison, Inhibition of urine citrate excretion and the production of renal calcinosis in the rat by acetazoleamide administration, J. Clin. Invest. 34:1662 (1955).
13. J. F. Van Pilsum, Determination of creatinine and related guanidinium compounds, in: "Methods of Biochemical Analysis," D. Glick, ed., Interscience Publishers, New York 7:193 (1959).
14. C. H. Fiske, and Y. Subbarow, The colorimetric determination of phosphorus, J. Biol. Chem. 66:375 (1925).
15. D. McFarlane, Experimental phosphate nephritis in the rat, J. Pathol. 52:17 (1941).

PHOSPHATE HOMEOSTASIS IN CIMETIDINE TREATED UREMIC DOGS

Allan I. Jacob, George Gavellas, Janet M. Canterbury,
Phillip W. Lambert, Jacques J. Bourgoignie

Department of Medicine, University of Miami School of
Medicine, Miami, Florida 33101

INTRODUCTION

More than a decade ago, a secondary hyperparathyroidism (HPTH) was postulated to be directed at the maintenance of phosphate homeostasis in chronic uremia (1). Each decrement in glomerular filtration rate would be associated with transient hyperphosphatemia, hypocalcemia and an increase in PTH secretion. Secondary HPTH would cause phosphaturia and restore phosphate balance, thereby normalizing serum phosphate and calcium levels. As renal function deteriorates, phosphate balance would be maintained at the expense of increasingly severe HPTH.

We recently reported that cimetidine, a histamine H_2 antagonist, decreased circulating concentrations of immunoreactive parathyroid hormone (iPTH) by 75% in a group of hemodialysis patients, without associated changes in serum ionized calcium or phosphorus concentrations (2). After discontinuation of the drug, hyperparathyroidism returned. In the chronically uremic dog, infusion of cimetidine is associated with a significant decrease in circulating iPTH at the fifth hour of administration of the drug (3). This inhibition occurs without changes in serum ionized calcium or phosphorus, urinary excretion of sodium, potassium, calcium, or phosphate. We have recently reported detailed observations on the effect of prolonged cimetidine therapy in chronically uremic dogs (4). Cimetidine was effective in decreasing circulating iPTH by 75% in our dogs with a remnant kidney and chronic renal insufficiency. Reduction of iPTH was evident despite the persistence of those factors that lead to secondary hyperparathyroidism, i.e. a decrease in renal function and maintance of a normal phosphate intake. The reversal of secondary hyperparathyroidism in these dogs presents an opportunity to examine the role of PTH in phosphate homeostasis in uremia. A detailed description of cimetidine effects on iPTH and calcium balance in uremic dogs has been described (4). This report will present the effect of cimetidine therapy on phosphate homeostasis.

METHODS

Seven adult, female, mongrel dogs weighing 15 to 18 kg. were studied. Renal insufficiency was induced by ligation of the majority of the branches of the renal artery on one side followed 2 weeks later by contralateral nephrectomy. After a period of stabilization varying from 12-18 months the dogs were studied under metabolic conditions described previously. In brief, after a period of adjustment in metabolic cages, control observation was made for 1 week. Five dogs then received cimetidine in tablet form for 20 weeks. The tablets were placed in the pharynx and swallowing was assured by observation. Three dogs received 300 mg. daily and 2 received 300 mg. twice daily. Two dogs served as controls and did not receive cimetidine. All dogs remained in metabolic cages for 4 additional consecutive weeks during which the experimental observations were made. The dogs were then removed from the cages and placed in runs for 7 weeks. The same amount of diet was offered daily. The dogs were then returned to cages for further balance studies on week 12. Cimetidine treatment was then continued for a total of 20 weeks. Fourteen weeks after discontinuation of cimetidine the dogs were restudied in the balance cages.

The dogs ate Purina High Protein dog meal (Ralston Purina Co., St. Louis, Mo.) containing 1.6 gm calcium, 0.950 gm phosphorus, 0.150 gm magnesium and 176 units of vitamin D per 100 gm diet. Three-hundred grams of the diet were offered daily while the dogs were in the cages. Blood samples were obtained anarobically three times a week during balance studies at 10:00 a.m. from an anterior limb vein before changing the food. Samples were analyzed for ionized calcium, phosphorus, iPTH and creatinine. Blood samples were also obtained during the 20th week of therapy and 7, 14, and 20-30 weeks after discontinuation of cimetidine.

Fifteen to twenty weeks after beginning cimetidine therapy, a 500 mg oral phosphate load was given. On the day of the experiment the animals were studied awake standing in a supporting sling, after a 15 hour fast. They had free access to water until the time of the experiment. A urinary catheter was inserted into the bladder for quantitative urine collection. Venous catheters were placed in the inferior vena cava through a hind limb for infusion and blood sampling. After injection of a priming dose of creatinine, a solution of 2.5% dextrose in water containing creatinine was infused at a rate of 0.3 mg/min. After a 60 minute period of equilbration, three 20 minute control clearance periods were obtained. Thereafter, 500 mg of phosphorus was administered by oral gastric tube as a neutral sodium phosphate solution in a volume of 50 ml. Immediately after the 50 ml of phosphorus was administered, 5 one hour experimental clearance periods were obtained. At the end of each period the bladder was washed with 30 ml of sterile water to insure complete urine collection. At the mid-point of each period a sample of blood was drawn anarobically.

Formal 72 hour metabolic balances were performed during the control first, second, third, fourth, and twelfth week of treatment and 14 weeks after discontinuation of treatment. Twenty-four hour urines were collected during the balance study and analyzed for calcium, phosphorus, and creatinine. Carmine red dye was given via orogastric tube on Mondays and Thursdays and all stool passed between the appearance of marker was collected. Stool was prepared for analysis as described previously (4). Total calcium concentration was measured in all samples by atomic absorption. Phosphorus and creatinine were measured by Auto Analyzer and ionized calcium was measured with a selective ion flow through electrode. Serum iPTH was assayed by methods previously described in great detail (5).

Serum collected from the 5 cimetidine treated dogs during the control week and 20th week of therapy was pooled, concentrated and chromatographed on a Bio-Gel P-10 column to separate the different immunoreactive molecular species of circulating iPTH (5). Plasma 25(OH)D, 24,25$(OH)_2$D and 1,25$(OH)_2$D were measured by methodology previously reported (6). The data were analyzed by the Prophet computer system. Statistical analysis used two-way analysis of variance and Dunnet's multiple range test and are expressed as mean ± SEM.

RESULTS

The values for iPTH, serum calcium, serum phosphorus, GFR and fractional excretion of phosphorus are presented in Table 1. The creatinine clearance ranged from 5.5-16.1 ml/min. Fasting ionized calcium was within the range seen for normal dogs ingesting a similar diet in our laboratory. Serum phosphorus ranged from 3.8-9.0 mg/dl. All dogs were hyperparathyroid before treatment and the mean iPTH value was 536±67 ulEq/ml (normal, 10-70 ulEq/ml) for the 5 dogs. HPTH is a consistent finding in chronically uremic dogs. The fall in iPTH after cimetidine was progressive and by the 20th week of therapy iPTH had fallen to 155±30 ulEq/ml ($P<0.01$). In 2 dogs iPTH values fell to within the normal range. In contrast, iPTH values in the 2 untreated control uremic dogs remained constant (not shown in Table). When cimetidine was discontinued, iPTH returned to pretreatment levels in an unpredictable pattern. In 2 dogs iPTH remained suppressed for 14 weeks after discontinu-

Table 1. EFFECT OF CIMETIDINE THERAPY IN CHRONICALLY UREMIC DOGS*

	CONTROL	Wk4	Wk 12	Wk 20	Wk 14 POST D/C
iPTH (ulEq/ml)	536±67	377±54**	219±25**	155±30**	251±55**
S_{Ca+2} (meq/l)	2.67±.04	2.70±.03	2.75±.03	2.71±.03	2.69±.04
Sp (mg/dl)	5.7±.9	4.5±.6**	4.8±.5	3.4±.2**	5.4±.4***
GFR (ml/min)	11.5±1.9	12.6±2.0	13.6±1.8	16.4±2.4	13±1.2
FE_{PO_4} (%)	45±10	54±11	56±8	——	46±7

*All values except week 20 obtained during metabolic balances. The normal range for iPTH is 10-70 ulEq/ml.
**P<.05 vs. control wk ***P<.05 vs. wk 20

ing the drug. However, iPTH returned to near baseline levels in all dogs by 20 weeks.

Pooled samples of serum obtained during the control and 20th week of therapy were fractionated by gel filtration and the eluates assayed for immunoreactivity. The decrease in iPTH was associated with a decrease in all the immunoreactive species. This indicates that the decrease is circulating iPTH during cimetidine therapy was secondary to less hormone secretion from the parathyroid glands rather than modifications in peripheral hormone metabolism.

Serum ionized calcium did not change throughout the study period. However there was a progressive decrease in serum phosphorus from 5.7±0.9 mg/dl during the control week to 4.5±0.5 mg/dl during the 3rd and 4th week and 3.4±0.2 mg/dl by the 20th week of cimetidine therapy. Fourteen weeks after withdrawal of cimetidine serum phosphorus returned to 5.4±0.4 mg/dl (P<.05).

Metabolic balance studies revealed that during cimetidine therapy calcium balance became positive (Figure 1). Negative calcium balance is a consistent feature in chronically uremic man (7) and dogs (8) and is due to fecal calcium losses. During the first four weeks after initiation of cimetidine therapy the mean change in calcium balance was +550±259 and +674±334 mg/72 hours, respectively. These changes reached borderline significance (0.05<P<0.1). During the 12th week of cimetidine, calcium balance was positive in all 5 dogs and increased by 1,509±518 mg/72 hours (P<.05). In contrast calcium balance remained negative in the control dogs.

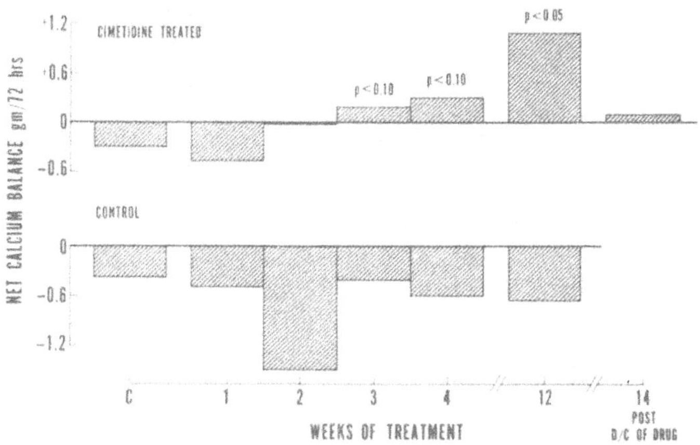

Figure 1. Mean calcium balance in five chronically uremic dogs before, during and after cimetidine treatment. The two control dogs remained in negative calcium balance.

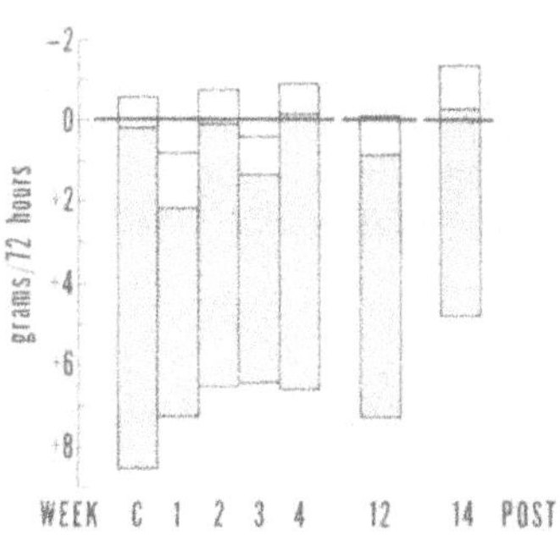

Figure 2. Phosphorus balance in a chronically uremic dog before, during and after cimetidine treatment. Downward excursions represent intake. The closed and open regions describe fecal and urine output, respectively.

Circulating concentrations of 25(OH)D, 24,25$(OH)_2$D and 1,25 $(OH)_2$D were measured before and after cimetidine therapy. Serum 25(OH)D increased insignificantly from 31.2±7.6 ng/ml before therapy to 35.3±6 ng/ml after therapy. However, 1,25$(OH)_2$D increased in all treated dogs by a mean of 55% from 33.4±4.3 pg/ml before therapy to 51.8±2.4 pg/ml after therapy ($P<.01$). 24,25$(OH)_2$D decreased concomitantly from 2.4±0.3 ng/ml to 1.9±0.2 ng/ml ($P<.05$).

Despite dramatic reductions in circulating iPTH levels, fractional excretion of phosphate did not change (Table 1). During the control week fractional excretion of phosphate was 44.6±9.4% and remained unchanged for the duration of cimetidine treatment. After twelve weeks of cimetidine treatment, fractional excretion of phosphorus was 55.9±7.9%, not significantly different from the control observation. Furthermore, phosphorus balance did not change during cimetidine therapy (Figure 2). Both net intestinal phosphorus absorption and urinary phosphorus excretion were unchanged.

The increase in serum phosphorus concentration after a 500 mg oral phosphate load, (Figure 3) was similar to untreated uremic hyperparathyroid dogs (9). The mean serum phosphorus concentration was 3.4±.3 mg/dl before phosphate and increased to a maxium of 7.2±.2 mg/dl during the 3rd hour after the phosphate load. These changes are compared to the change in serum phosphorus after a identical challenge in normal dogs and uremic dogs not treated with cimetidine. The phosphatemia in uremic dogs is greater than that observed in normal dogs ($P<.02$). However, the uremic dogs treated with cimetidine, despite marked reduction in serum iPTH levels, manifested phosphatemia similar to the uremic dogs. Furthermore, the normal dogs excreted 300±25 mg phosphorus during 5 hours after the phosphate load. The uremic and uremic-cimetidine treated dogs excreted less phosphorus, 137±16 mg and 168±22 mg respectively (P .05). Thus the reversal of secondary hyperparathyroidism was not associated with an exaggerated phosphatemic response to or an impaired excretion of oral phosphate load.

DISCUSSION

Studies with parathyroid slices from normal bovine glands, (10) and isolated dispersed cells from human adenomatous glands (11) have shown that histamine stimulates cAMP production and PTH release. These effects are blocked by cimetidine. Circulating iPTH in normal subjects acutely decreases with cimetidine infusion and returns to control levels when the infusion is terminated (10). Histamine may therefore play a role in normal parathyroid physiology and hyperparathyroid conditions. Stimulation of PTH secretion by hypocalcemia and B-agonists is felt to be secondary to activation of adenylate cyclase. It is possible that parathyroid gland adenylate cyclase may be histamine sensitive, a characteristic of cardiac (12) and gastric adenylate cyclase (13). In addition, our

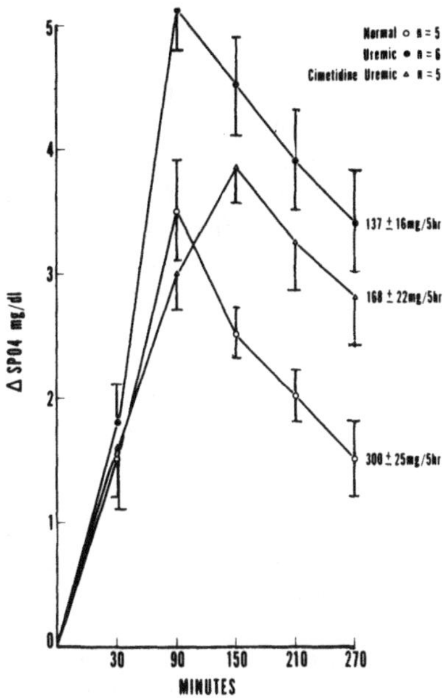

Figure 3. Change in serum phosphorus concentration (mg/dl) after a 500 mg oral phosphate load. The control values in each group were: normal-3.8±0.2, uremic-4.9±0.3, cimetidine uremic-3.4±.3. The total phosphorus excreted in each group is listed at each curve. The data in normal and uremic dogs is taken from previous studies in our laboratory (9) using the identical protocol.

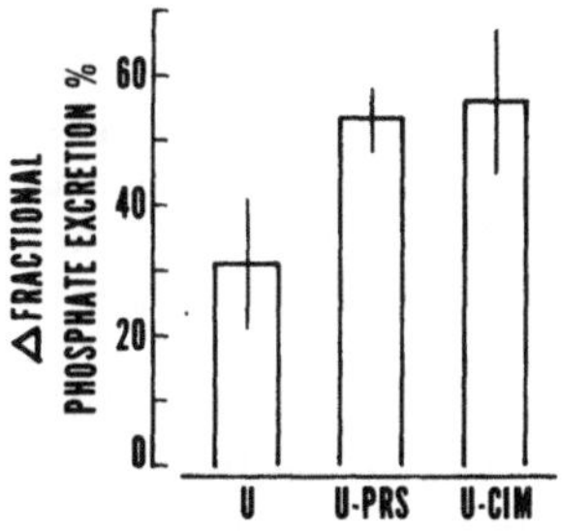

Figure 4. Maximal increase in FE_{PO4} (%) during a 500 mg oral phosphate load in uremic dogs (U), uremic dogs fed a phosphorus restricted diet (U-PRS), and cimetidine treated uremic dogs (U-CIM). The control values for FE_{PO4} in each group were: U-50±5, U-PRS-8±5, U-CIM-17±10.

findings suggest that non-ionic forces, such as histamine, contribute to uremic hyperparathyroidism.

The mechanisms responsible for the decrease in serum phosphorus concentration during cometidine therapy are unclear. Decreased intestinal absorption or increased renal losses did not contribute to the change in serum phosphorus. After 3 weeks of cimetidine treatment, serum phosphorus had decreased significantly, but net intestinal absorption and urinary excretion of phosphorus varied inconsistently from the control week. These observations exclude primary changes in phosphorus balance as operative and evoke shifts of phosphorus within body compartments as a tangible explanation. The decreased concentration of iPTH after cimetidine may have caused less phosphorus loss from bone thereby decreasing serum phosphorus. The changes in D-metabolites may have been secondary to the decrease in serum phosphate concentration, an important modulator of renal 1α-and 24-hydroxylase activities (14). The increase in 1,25 $(OH)_2D$ concentration probably accounts for the net positive calcium balance during cimetidine therapy.

During the oral phosphate load the fractional phosphate excretion in cimetidine treated dogs increased by 56±12% (Figure 4). In contrast, the increase in uremic dogs under identical conditions (9) is only 29±4%. Furthermore, the increase in FE_{PO4} in uremic dogs rendered euparathyroid by phosphorus restriction, 53±4%, is similar to the increase observed in our dogs. The enhanced renal response suggests that cimetidine suppressed biologically active PTH, thereby exposing more binding sites to PTH released during phosphorus loading.

If phosphorus intake and enteric absorption remain constant as renal function declines, there is a progressive increase in the fractional excretion of phosphate allowing for the continued maintenance of external balance (15). The maintenance of equality between intake and output of phosphorus is associated with a progressive rise in PTH levels (1). If phosphorus intake is reduced in exact proportion to the reduction in GFR, the need for an increase in the fractional excretion of phosphate is obviated and the PTH levels remain within the normal range (16). It has been suggested that the rise in circulating PTH levels plays a central role in the increasing rate of phosphorus excretion per nephron (1). Our data suggests that the adaptation in the remaining nephrons and the increased fractional phosphate excretion can occur despite marked attenuation of secondary hyperparathyroidism. This does not imply that parathyroid hormone is not necessary for phosphorus excretion, but does suggest that phosphate homeostasis can be maintained in chronic renal failure in the absence of an increased PTH secretion. Swenson et al. have shown that phosphate homeostasis may be maintained in parathyroidectomized uremic dogs given vitamin D, although a direct effect of vitamin D on renal phosphate handling in uremia was not excluded (17). Our data indicate that chronic phosphate homeostasis does not change in uremic dogs despite a marked reduction of iPTH. In fact, iPTH during cimetidine treatment was normal in two of the five dogs. Phosphate balance and fractional phosphate excretion did not change. Moreover, the acute response to a phosphate load in the cimetidine-treated dogs was not impaired and in fact was similar to animals with chronic renal insufficiency and corrected secondary hyperparathyroidism. It is also of note that the PTH immunoassay used in the present study is that which was utilized in the original observations used to describe the "trade-off" hypothesis (1). If the elevated iPTH in that investigation relates to phosphate homeostasis in chronic renal failure, our observations dissociate these phenomoenon.

ACKNOWLEDGEMENTS

We gratefully acknowledge the secretarial assistance of Ms. Robin Brown.

REFERENCES

1. Slatopolsky, E., Caglar, J.P., Pennell, J.P., Taggart, D.D., Canterbury, J.M., Reiss, E., Bricker, N.S.: On the pathogenesis of hyperparathyroidism in chronic experimental renal insufficiency in the dog. J. Clin. Invest. 50:492-499, 1971.
2. Jacob, A.I., Lanier, D., Canterbury, J.M., Bourgoignie, J.J.: Cimetidine suppression of circulating parathyroid hormone in uremia. N. Engl. J. Med. 302:671-674, 1980.
3. Bourgoignie, J.J., Jacob, A.I., Gavellas, G., Canterbury, J.M.: Effects of cimetidine on parathyroid hormone in chronic uremia, in "Phosphate and Minerals in Health and Disease (1980)" Massry, S.G., Ritz, E., John, H., eds., Plenum Publishing Corp. New York.
4. Jacob, A.I., Canterbury, J.M., Gavellas, G., Lambert, P.W., Bourgoignie, J.J.: Reversal of secondary hyperparathyroidism by cimetidine in chronically uremic dogs. J. Clin. Invest. 67:1753-1760, 1981.
5. Canterbury, J.M., Reiss, E.: Multiple immunoreative molecular forms of parathyroid hormone in human serum. Proc. Soc. Exp. Biol. Med. 140:1393-1398, 1972.
6. Lambert, P.W., Taft, D.A., Hodgson, S.F., Lindmark, E.A., Witwach, B.J., Roos, B.A. An improved method for the measurement of $1,25(OH)_2D$ in human plasma. Endocr. Res. Commun. 5:293-310, 1979.
7. Liu, S.H., Chu, H.I.: Studies of calcium and phosphorus metabolism with special reference to the pathogenesis and effect of dihydrotachysterol (AT 10) and iron. Medicine 22:103-161, 1943.
8. Canterbury, J.M., Gavellas, G., Bourgoignie, J.J., Reiss, E.: Metabolic consequences of oral administration of 24,25-

dihydroxycholecalciferol to uremic dogs. J. Clin. Invest. 65:571-576, 1980.

9. Kaplan, M.A., Canterbury, J.M., Gavellas, G., Jaffe, D., Bourgoignie, J.J., Reiss, E., Bricker, N.S.: Interrelations between phosphorus, calcium, parathyroid hormone, and renal phosphate excretion in response to an oral phosphorous load in normal and uremic dogs. Kid. Inter. 14:207-214, 1978.
10. Williams, G.A., Longley, R.S., Bowser, E.N., et al.: Parathyroid hormone secretion in normal man and in primary hyperparathyroidism: role of histamine H_2 receptors. J. Clin. Endo. Metab. 52:122-127, 1981.
11. Brown, E.M.: Histamine receptors in dispersed parathyroid cells from pathological human parathyroid tissue. J. Clin. Endo. Metab. 51:1325-1329, 1980.
12. Levey, G.S., Klein, I.: Solubolized myocardial adenylate cyclase. Restoration of histamine responsiveness by phosphatidylserine. J. Clin. Invest. 51:1578-1582, 1972.
13. Dousa, T.P., Code, C.T.: Effect of histamine and its methyl derivatives in cyclic AMP metabolism in gastric mucosa and its blockade by an H_2-receptor antagonist. J. Clin. Invest. 53:334-337, 1974.
14. Tanaka, Y., DeLuca, H.F.: The control of 25-hydroxyvitamin D metabolism by inorganic phosphorus. Arch. Biochem. Biophys. 145:566-574, 1973.
15. Slatopolsky, E., Robson, A.M., Elkan, I., Bricker, N.S.: Control of phosphate excretion in uremic man. J. Clin. Invest. 47:1864-1874, 1968.
16. Slatopolsky, E., Caglar, S., Gradowski, L., Canterbury, J.M., Reiss, E., Bricker, N.S.: On the prevention of secondary hyperparathyroidism in experimental chronic renal disease using proportional reduction of dietary phosphorus intake. Kidney Int. 2:147-151, 1972.
17. Swenson, R.S., Weisinger, J.R., Ruggeri, J.L. Reaven, G.M.: Evidence that parathyroid hormone is not required for phosphate homeostasis in renal failure. Metabolism 24:199-204, 1975.

REGULATION OF PHOSPHATE EXCRETION BY THE DISEASED KIDNEY: THE INTRINSIC PROXIMAL TUBULAR ADAPTATION

Norimoto Yanagawa, Patty Yeung, Walter Trizna
and Leon G. Fine

Division of Nephrology
Department of Medicine
UCLA School of Medicine
Center for the Health Sciences
Los Angeles, California 90024

The maintenance of phosphate homeostasis in chronic renal failure has been ascribed to PTH-dependent[1-4] and PTH-independent mechanisms[5-9]. While the phosphaturic effect of elevated PTH levels undoubtedly plays an important role in modulating tubular phosphate reabsorption as nephrons are progressively destroyed, there is equally impressive evidence that intrinsic adaptations in tubular transport may occur independently of biologically active PTH levels. Such adaptations would include changes in the basal rate of phosphate transport and in the sensitivity and responsiveness of the renal tubule to PTH.

In order to examine the nature of these adaptations, we have performed in vitro studies on isolated perfused superficial proximal straight tubules (PST) obtained from rabbits with remnant kidneys. The obvious advantage of using this system is that the luminal and peritubular environment of the tubule can be precisely controlled and accurate dose-response relationships obtained.

Experimental Groups

Four groups of adult rabbits were studied: 1) normal rabbits, 2) uremic rabbits with remnant kidneys on a normal phosphorus diet (ad lib P intake), 3) uremic rabbits given a diet adjusted to maintain urinary phosphorus excretion at the same level as in normal rabbits (controlled P intake) and 4) uremic rabbits on a high phosphorus diet. (Table 1) Since a radioimmunoassay for PTH has not been developed for the rabbit, we evaluated biologically-active PTH in the serum of the four groups of animals using a bioassay procedure. Sera from the three uremic groups were compared with normal sera by measuring their inhibitory effect on lumen-to-bath phosphate flux in isolated perfused PSTs. Using this assay uremic rabbits on an ad lib and a controlled phosphorus diet were found to be euparathyroid whereas uremic rabbits on a high phosphorus diet were hyperparathyroid.

PTH Sensitivity and Responsiveness of the Uremic Proximal Tubule

The sensitivity of the PST to PTH was assessed *in vitro* by measuring the inhibition of lumen-to-bath phosphate flux by PTH in a dose-response fashion. A left- or right-shift of the dose-response curve is defined as a change in sensitivity to the hormone. A change in the maximal inhibitory effect of the hormone is defined as a change in responsiveness. As may be seen in Fig. 1, PTH sensitivity was altered in both uremic groups and was dependent upon the phosphate intake and/or the *in vivo* PTH status of the animals. In the euparathyroid-uremic PSTs, half-maximal inhibition was achieved at a bath PTH concentration one order of magnitude lower than in the normal PSTs indicating an increased sensitivity. In contrast, PTH sensitivity was decreased by an order of magnitude in the hyperparathyroid uremic PSTs.

In order to assess whether the altered sensitivity represented an adaptation at the receptor-adenylate cyclase level or at a post-cAMP step,the dose response to dibutyryl cAMP was evaluated over a concentration range of 10^{-8}M to 10^{-5}M. No differences in responsiveness or sensitivity to dibutyryl cAMP were detected between the three experimental groups.

Basal Rates of Phosphate Flux Across Isolated Perfused PSTs

The intrinsic rate of phosphate and fluid reabsorption by isolated perfused PSTs was studied in a bath of normal rabbit serum. Phosphate flux from lumen-to-bath Jp-lb, and bath-to-lumen, Jp-bl was measured using ^{32}P. Net volume flux, Jv, was measured simultaneously. The mean±SE values for each experimental group are shown in Table 2. Jp-net was increased above normal only in the uremic euparathyroid group on an ad lib diet due to an increase in Jp-lb. This presumably reflects a direct dietary influence since euparathyroid animals on a controlled P intake did not have this adaptation. In contrast, Jv was significantly increased in all uremic groups. This

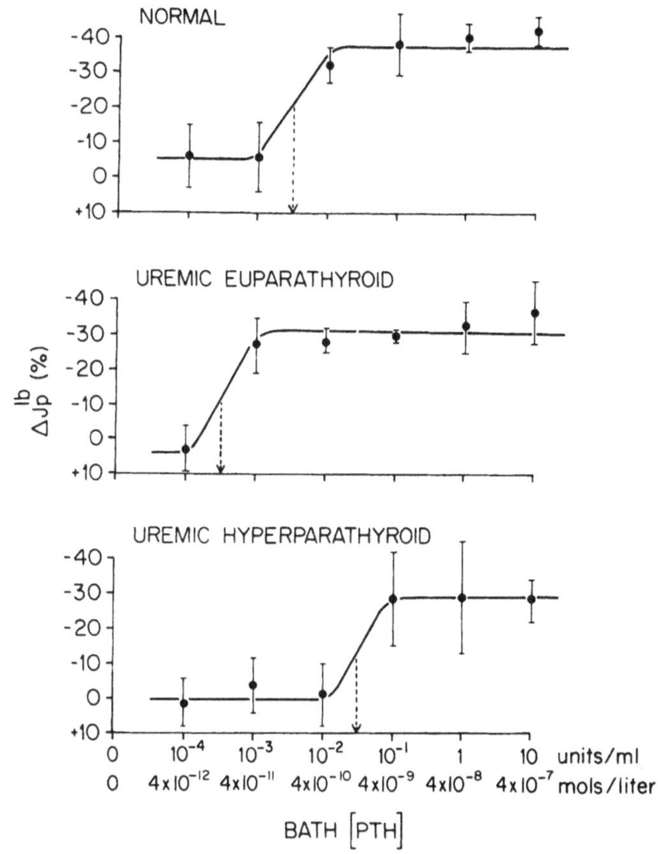

Figure 1. Dose-response relationship between bath bPTH (1-34) concentration and percent inhibition of lumen-to-bath phosphate flux (Jp-lb) in isolated perfused proximal straight tubules from normal and uremic rabbits. The approximate half-maximal inhibitory concentration of PTH is shown by the broken arrow. (Mean±SE).

TABLE 1. Glomerular Filtration Rate and Urinary Phosphate and Cyclic AMP Excretion Rates in Normal and Uremic Rabbits.

	C_{Cr} (ml/min)	S_{Ca} (mg/dl)	S_P (mg/dl)	U_{cAMP}/GFR (nmol/min)
NORMAL (N=15)	10.58 ±1.43	13.9 ±0.3	5.4 ±0.9	0.03 ±0.002
UREMIC EUPARATHYROID AD LIB P INTAKE (N=12)	2.60 ±0.45	14.7 ±2.8	5.1 ±.95	0.30* ±0.1
UREMIC EUPARATHYROID CONTROLLED P INTAKE (N=6)	2.05* ±0.20	14.3 ±1.6	5.7 ±0.8	- -
UREMIC HYPERPARATHYROID (N=12)	2.53* ±0.65	12.7 ±1.4	8.2 ±0.5	0.48* ±0.12

MEAN± SE
*p<0.05 vs NORMAL

TABLE 2. Phosphate (Jp) and Volume (Jv) Fluxes in Superficial Proximal Straight Tubules of Normal and Uremic Rabbits.

	Jp			Jv
	1 -> b	b -> 1	Net	(nl/mm/min)
	(a) Normal Rabbits			
Mean	4.39	0.80	3.68	0.45
±SE	±0.40	±0.18	±0.48	±0.07
	(b) Uremic Euparathyroid Rabbits-Ad Lib P Intake			
Mean	10.43*	2.71	7.71*	0.97*
±SE	±0.96	±0.68	±0.59	±0.13
	(c) Uremic Euparathyroid Rabbits - Controlled P Intake			
Mean	4.92	1.20	3.50	0.83*
±SE	±0.63	±0.60	±0.95	±0.21
	(d) Uremic Hyperparathyroid Rabbits			
Mean	6.39*	1.94	4.59	1.04*
±SE	±0.66	±0.36	±0.70	±0.21

*: $p<0.05$ vs Normal
1 -> b lumen-to-bath; b -> l bath-to-lumen.

dissociation between Jp-net and Jv indicates that changes in Jp-net are adaptations induced by specific homeostatic requirements rather than being intrinsic, fixed properties of the hypertrophied remnant kidney tubules.

Conclusions

These studies demonstrate that intrinsic adaptations in phosphate transport occur in the proximal tubules of remnant kidneys. When studied in a normal milieu, the basal rate of phosphate transport increases only if the animal's phosphate absorption is low. In addition there is an alteration in the PTH-sensitivity of the proximal tubule which is a cellular event which occurs prior to the formation of cAMP. The increased PTH sensitivity of the euparathyroid uremic kidney may explains why urinary cAMP excretion is increased above normal in this group of animals despite the fact that biologically active PTH levels are normal. (Table I)

The data are strongly suggestive of an alteration in proximal tubular function at the level of the PTH receptor. An increase in receptor number (or affinity) would explain the increased sensitivity to PTH. Whether or not this occurs as a global phenomenon associated with compensatory hypertrophy is not clear. High circulating PTH levels appear to decrease the sensitivity of the nephron to the hormone presumably by a process of "down-regulation" or persistent receptor occupancy. The unchanged maximal response to PTH and the normal dose-response to dibutyryl cAMP suggest that post-receptor-cyclase cellular events are intact.

These studies serve to highlight the fact that the uremic state is associated both with intrinsic tubular adaptations and with altered circulating PTH levels. It appears as if the intrinsic adaptations of tubular function may be induced by or linked to the steady-state circulating PTH levels and dietary phosphorus intake and dietary phosphorus intake in such a way that the renal effects of PTH are actually regulated at the level of the end-organ[10].

REFERENCES

1. E. Slatopolsky, L. Gradowska, C. Kashensant, R., Keltner, C. Male, and N.S. Bricker, The control of phosphate excretion in uremia. J Clin Invest 45:672-677 (1966).

2. E. Slatopolsky, M. Robson, I. Elkan, and N.S. Bricker, Control of phosphate excretion in uremic man. J Clin Invest 47:1865-1847 (1968).
3. E. Slatopolsky, S. Caglar, J.P. Pennell, D.D. Taggart, J.M. Canterbury, E. Reiss, and N.S. Bricker, On the pathogenesis of hyperparathyroidism in experimental chronic renal disease using "proportional reduction" of dietary phosphorus intake. Kidney Int 2:147-151 (1971).
4. E. Slatopolsky, S. Caglar, L. Gradowska, J.M. Canterbury, E. Reiss, and N.S. Bricker, On the prevention of secondary hyperparathyroidism in experimental chronic renal disease using "proportional reduction" of dietary phosphorus intake. Kidney Int 2:147-151 (1972).
5. M.M. Popovtzer, W.F. Penggera, M.P. Hutt, J. Robinette, C.G. Halgrimson, and T.E. Starzl, Serum parathyroid hormone levels and renal handling of phosphorus in patients with chronic renal diseases. J Clin Endocrinol Metab 35:213-218 (1972).
6 R.S. Swensen, J.R. Weisinger, J.L. Rubberi, and G.M. Rearen, Evidence that parathyroid hormone is not required for phosphate homeostasis in renal failure. Metabolism 24:199-204 (1975).
7. M.S. Christensen, J. Brochner-Mortensen, L. Tougaard, E. Sornsen, and P. Rodbro, Minor influence of parathyroid hormone on fractional tubular reabsorption of phosphate in chronic renal failure, in: "Phosphate Metabolism" S.G. Massry and E. Ritz, eds., Plenum Press, New York. (1977).
8. S. Fotino, Phosphate excretion in chronic renal failure: Evidence for a mechanism other than circulatory parathyroid hormone. Clin Nephrol 8:499-503 (1977).
9. N. Loreau, J.P. Cosyns, C. Lepreuz, and R. Ardaillou, Renal adenylate cyclase calcitonin receptors and phosphate excretion in rats immunized against tubular basement membrane, in: "Phosphate Metabolism" S.G. Massry, and E. Ritz, eds., Plenum Press, New York, (1977).
10. L.G. Fine, Regulation of phosphate excretion by the diseased kidney: Reabsorption sites and hormone-receptor interactions. Mineral Electrolyte Metab 6:308-315 (1981).

PARATHYROID HORMONE RESISTANCE IN RENAL ALLOGRAFT RECIPIENTS

M. Kleerekoper, R.S. Bernstein, C. Cruz, N.W. Levin, A.M. Parfitt

Department of Medicine
Henry Ford Hospital
Detroit, MI., USA

Hypophosphatemia is common after renal transplantation and has been variously ascribed to persistent hyperparathyroidism, to tubular damage from rejection, or to the effect of corticosteroid or immunosuppressive therapy (1-3). To learn more about the mechanisms, we measured TmP/GFR, nephrogenous cyclic AMP (NcAMP) and immunoreactive PTH in 25 renal transplant patients with stable renal function (Ccr$\geqslant$70 ml/min/1.73 m^2,$\geqslant$6 months post-transplant), 21 healthy control subjects and 5 uninephrectomized renal transplant donors. On the basis of the parathyroid function tests, we divided the patients into three groups. In Group 1 (5 patients) serum calcium, NcAMP and PTH were all normal; these patients had resolved hyperparathyroidism. In Group 2 (6 patients) serum calcium, NcAMP and PTH were all raised; these patients had persistent hypercalcemic hyperparathyroidism. In Group 3 (14 patients) serum calcium was normal but either NcAMP or iPTH or both were raised; these patients had persistent normocalcemic hyperparathyroidism. These three groups did not differ significantly in duration of graft survival, creatinine clearance, type or dose of immunosuppressive therapy, or serum levels of vitamin D metabolites.

The Group 1 patients with resolved hyperparathyroidism were compared with the normal controls and the uninephrectomized donors. These three groups did not differ significantly in serum calcium, PTH or NcAMP. The two groups with only one kidney did not differ significantly in any of the five measurements. Compared to normal subjects, both groups had, as expected, a significantly lower creatinine clearance, but in addition had lower values for serum phosphate and TmP/GFR (table). This indicates that the presence

of only a single kidney, whether this is the individual's own kidney or someone else's kidney, is associated with a significant depression of tubular reabsorption which is unrelated to parathyroid hormone (4).

The Group 2 patients with persistent hypercalcemic hyperparathyroidism were compared with patients with primary hyperparathyroidism matched for creatinine clearance, PTH and NcAMP. There were no significant differences in serum calcium or serum phosphate, but the transplant patients with only one kidney had a significantly lower mean value for TmP/GFR than the patients with primary hyperparathyroidism (table). Comparison of five groups of subjects indicate that hyperparathyroidism reduces TmP/GFR by about 1.3 mg/dl, with or without a single kidney, and a single kidney reduces TmP/GFR by about 0.7 mg/dl, with or without hyperparathyroidism. This indicates that the single kidney effect on phosphate reabsorption is mediated by a separate PTH-independent mechanism.

Some of the Group 3 patients with persistent normocalcemic hyperparathyroidism were compared with individually matched patients with primary hyperparathyroidism. The matching was possible for the transplant patients who had increases in both PTH and NcAMP and in patients who had increases in NcAMP but not in PTH. A further sub-group with normal NcAMP and raised PTH could not be included in the matching because this combination was observed in only one of more than 100 patients with primary hyperparathyroidism. Despite equivalent degrees of hyperparathyroidism, the transplant patients not only failed to show hypercalcemia, but the mean values for both serum phosphate and TmP/GFR were not lower than in the primary hyperparathyroid patients (table 1). Unlike all the other patients with a single kidney, the post-transplant patients in this group failed to show the expected additive effects of a single kidney and of hyperparathyroidism on phosphate reabsorption. We have therefore identified a substantial group of renal transplant recipients who have persistent hyperparathyroidism and at least partial resistance to both the hypercalcemic and the phosphaturic effects of endogenous PTH. We suggest that in these patients the target cell resistance to PTH characteristic of the uremic state fails to be completely reversed by renal transplantation (5).

Summary and Conclusions

1. Post-transplant hypophosphatemia is due to the separate and additive effects of persistent hyperparathyroidism and of a single kidney. Graft rejection, immunosuppressive and corticosteroid therapy appeared not to be important.

2. A substantial minority of renal transplant patients with persistent hyperparathyroidism displayed some resistance to both the hypercalcemic and the hypophosphatemic effects of endogenous PTH.

Table 1. Mean values for TmP/GFR in three groups of renal transplant patients, and various control groups. HPT - hyperparathyroidism.

Group	n	TmP/GFR mg/dl ±SD	P vs N <	P vs PHPT <
Normal subjects (N)	21	3.35±0.44	-	-
Uninephrectomized donors	5	2.65±0.62	0.01	-
Group 1 (resolved HPT)	5	2.72±0.31	0.01	-
Group 2 (Hypercalcemic HPT)	6	1.39±0.15	0.001	0.01
Primary HPT	16	2.06±0.43	0.001	-
Group 3 (normocalcemic HPT)	10	2.13±0.49	0.001	NS

REFERENCES

1. H.N. Ward, R.C. Pabico, B.A. McKenna and R.B. Freeman, The The renal handling of phosphate by renal transplant patients: correlation with serum parathyroid hormone, cyclic 3',5' - adenosine monophosphate urinary excretion, and allograft function, Adv. Exp. Med. Biol. 81:173 (1977).
2. N.D. Vaziri, R.E. Nellans, R.M. Brueggemann, C.H. Barton and D.C. Martin. Renal tubular dysfunction in transplanted kidneys. Southern Med. J. 72:530 (1979).
3. M. Garabedian, C. Silve, D. Levy, A. Bourdeau, A. Ulmann, M. Broyer and S. Balsan, Chronic hypophosphatemia in kidney transplanted children and young adults, Adv. Med. Biol 128:249, (1980).
4. R.C. Pabico, B.A. McKenna and R.B. Freeman, Renal function before and after unilateral nephrectomy in renal donors, Kidney Int. 8:166 (1975).
5. S.G. Massry, J.W. Coburn, D.B.N. Lee, J. Jowsey, C.R. Kleeman, Skeletal resistance to parathyroid hormone in renal failure. Ann. Intern. Med. 78:357 (1973).

HYPOPHOSPHATEMIA AND PHOSPHATE DEPLETION

MODELS OF HYPOPHOSPHATEMIA AND PHOSPHATE DEPLETION

James P. Knochel

University of Texas
Southwestern Medical
School, Dallas, Texas

One objective of scientific investigation in medicine is to elucidate the specific cause and mechanisms of tissue injury or dysfunction in a specific disease state. Since most of us attending this meeting are concerned with human disease and physiology, and since animals often respond differently to disease-producing factors than man, it follows that human subjects or their materials should be utilized for scientific investigation whenever possible. When this is not possible the investigator must resort to either experimental animals, their components or in vitro simulators in hope of providing an inferential solution to the human problem. Of equal importance, in the search for appropriate models of human disease, zealous efforts should be made to select an animal that responds to interventions or injurious agents in a manner similar to that of man.

Most modern studies examining the effects of experimentally-induced phosphorus depletion and hypophosphatemia have been conducted on five species. These include man, rats, dogs, chickens, and pigs. In addition, discovery of the hypophosphatemic mouse has provided an exceptional model for study of the disease resembling vitamin D resistant rickets or osteomalacia in man.

Since my particular field of interest has been related to the systemic and the muscular effects of phosphorus deficiency and hypophosphatemia, I will confine the remainder of my remarks to these topics.

A number of studies conducted in the 1920's and the 1930's firmly established the critical role of phosphorus in growth and nutrition of dairy animals (1-3). Short term phosphorus deprivation in cattle caused anorexia, weight loss, declining milk production, and abnormalities in reproduction. When phosphorus was deprived for long periods of time, animals displayed muscular weakness, stiffness, swelling of joints, and soft bones. Also noted were a marked increase in susceptibility to infection, and early death due to a variety of causes. Horses grazing on phosphorus-depleted pastures became smaller and smaller during successive generations and eventually adult animals were the size of ponies (4).

The effects of soil phosphate depletion on farm animals was noted in France during and after WWII because phosphate fertilizers were not available to replenish losses incident to crop harvests. Although the problem of phosphorus depletion from soil is well understood, the issue is becoming important once again. Based upon current predictions, there is a serious problem of soil phosphate depletion looming in the midwestern United States because of our finicky practice of draining sewage into streams which in turn deliver phosphate residues to the Gulf of Mexico (5).

The classic study employing adult man as his own model of chronic phosphorus deficiency was carried out by Lotz and Bartter in 1968 (6). In their normal adult subjects, phosphorus depletion was induced by feeding a phosphorus deficient diet. In addition, their studies suggested that if phosphate depletion were to become frankly symptomatic with anorexia, weakness, debility, and bone pain, one had to reduce serum phosphorus concentration below 1.0 mg/dL. This could be accomplished only by simultaneously administering phosphate binding antacids. This seemingly small point, namely, the addition of phosphate binding antacids to a phosphorus deficient diet to reduce serum phosphorus to a low value, is critically important in any model regardless of species. Otherwise, it appears that serum phosphorus concentration will remain sufficiently high to forestall acute cellular injury. Independently of chronic alcoholism, renal tubular defects, vitamin D deficiency or alimentation after severe weight loss, symptomatic phosphorus deficiency in man as a sporadic illness has occurred only in patients with a low phosphorus intake who also ingest phosphate-binding antacids.

If one administers a phosphorus deficient diet without phosphate-binding antacids to experimental animals, debility is not nearly so severe. The very first symptomatic response will be anorexia. For unknown reasons, physiological responses become activated that attempt to maintain a relatively normal cellular composition of ions and minerals. Thus, as phosphorus deficiency begins, urinary phosphorus excretion declines rapidly, and there follows an increased excretion of calcium, magnesium and potassium into the urine. All of the calcium and much of the magnesium excreted into the urine while feeding a phosphorus deficient diet derives from the skeleton. However, muscle will give up phosphorus, apparently to supply this vital element to critical organs such as the heart and brain which do not readily become phosphorus deficient (7). The loss of phosphorus from skeletal muscle is associated with a loss of the other major intracellular minerals and ions, namely magnesium and potassium, although to a lesser extent (8). Thereby, the internal milieu remains nearly normal. A lucid review expounding on the relationship between the relative constancy of intracellular ratios of nitrogen, magnesium, potassium and phosphorus in a number of different cell systems throughout the animal kingdom, including bacteria, was published by Wacker in 1968 (9). The spontaneous readjustment of cellular composition to correct selective deficiencies of any one of the 3 major ions with respect to nitrogen is apparently a fundamental property of life-regulatory systems in all species examined to date. In simple terms, one can summarize the foregoing statements as follows: if a healthy animal is deprived of phosphorus, the animal will reduce its food consumption, the cellular mass of skeletal muscle will shrink, phosphorus will leave the cell making itself available to maintain adequate levels in vital organs. In the process of dissolving lean mass, mostly skeletal muscle, the redundant quantities of potassium and magnesium leave the cell and are excreted into the urine. In a sense, the muscle cell displays compositional autoregulation.

I would now like to consider an additional important question. What is the effect of administering a phosphorus deficient diet with a phosphate binding antacid while simultaneously force-feeding the animals to circumvent the usual under-nutrition and weight loss?

As discussed in the preceding paragraphs, if a dog is fed a phosphorus deficient diet containing fewer calories than are needed to maintain body weight, skeletal muscle phosphorus content will usually remain normal (10). Figure 1 illustrates this fact. In this study, dogs were fed a phosphorus deficient diet and their caloric intake was about one-half normal. The tissue was measured again after the animals had lost 30 per cent of their initial body weight. Serum phosphorus concentration fell slightly. Muscle phosphorus content essentially remained normal. If on the other hand, the animal is fed the same phosphorus deficient diet and gavage fed its recommended daily

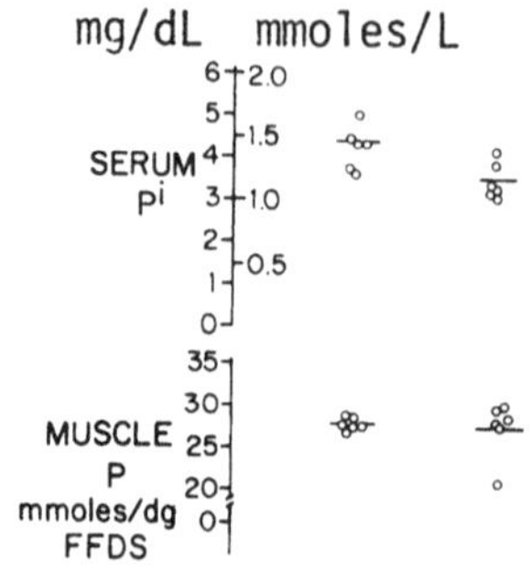

Figure 1

intake so as to avoid under-nutrition, alterations of skeletal muscle composition are much more pronounced. Figure 2 illustrates serial findings in muscle phosphorus content and serum phosphorus concentration in dogs gavage fed a phosphorus-deficient but otherwise normal diet for 28 days. Muscle phosphorus fell from 28.5 to 23.5 mmoles/100 gm fat-free dry tissue. Serum phosphorus concentration fell from 4.2 to 2.0 mg/100 ml. Apparently, the avoidance of malnutrition reduces the rate of atrophy of skeletal muscle cells, the tissue becomes deficient in phosphorus and after several weeks, evidence of cellular injury is evident. Evidence of tissue injury consists of an elevated sodium, elevated chloride and depressed potassium

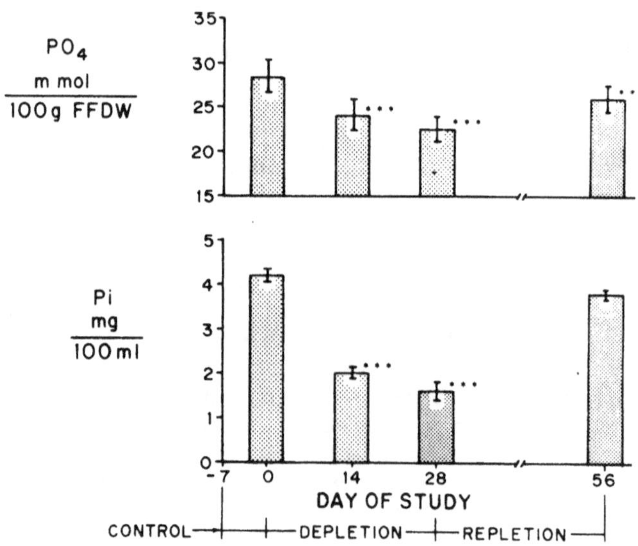

Figure 2

contents, and a depression of measured membrane potential. Each of these abnormalities becomes normal after restoring phosphorus to the diet.

The table shows data on phosphorus deficient rats (11). Skeletal muscle water content, sodium content and potassium content remain normal despite a fall of muscle phosphorus from 29.9 to 26.2 mmoles. Membrane potentials, not shown in this slide, do not fall in the rat with comparable phosphorus deficiency (12).

As is evident from other studies, dogs respond to chronic, severe phosphorus deficiency almost exactly as humans. They develop central nervous system dysfunction, rhabdomyolysis, myocardial insufficiency and probably impaired function of leukocytes and platelets. On the other hand, chronically phosphorus depleted rats show growth impairment, mobilization of skeletal calcium and magnesium, and under special circumstances, metabolic acidosis. However, they do not show evidence of acute tissue destruction like dogs. Rats have exceptionally tough skeletal muscle. For example, potassium deficiency can readily cause rhabdomyolysis in man or dog, but not the rat. In fact, potassium deficient, hypokalemic rats rarely if ever become paralyzed.

Based upon these species differences, it seems that the rat is an excellent model to study bone disease and acid base disorders but if the goal is to produce acute tissue destruction with phosphorus deficiency and hypophosphatemia, the dog is the preferable model.

The next issue I would like to address concerning models of

Table 1

MUSCLE COMPOSITION IN RATS FED A PHOSPHORUS DEFICIENT DIET
(Kreusser, PO_4 Conf. IV)

	H_2O % wet weight	Na	K	Pi
		mmol/g/ww		
PD (n = 12)	75.7 ± 0.59	21.9 ± 2.15	124 ± 7.17	26.2 ± 3.28
CONTROL (n = 12)	76.2 ± 0.56	21.8 ± 4.47	124 ± 3.0	29.9 ± 2.55
P	N.S	N.S	N.S	< 0.02

phosphorus deficiency is the so-called "pair-fed" control. To elucidate the characteristics of any nutritional disorder, we must compare the effects of our interventions to control animals. In my view, the ideal control is a normal animal. Many of the studies conducted on rats during the past two decades have simply offered a phosphorus deficient diet, realizing that both their food intake and weight gain will be less than rats allowed an ad lib normal diet. In such studies, the weight gain and food intake of the experimental rat is measured daily and the food intake of the control animal is restricted to the same quantity consumed by the rat receiving the phosphorus deficient diet. The control animal is thus "pair-fed". Unfortunately, the comparison is between two groups of abnormal animals. The first is phosphorus restricted, the second is undernourished. An assumption is made that undernutrition has no effects in a "normal" animal. Although serious effects probably do not occur in short term experiments, that long term undernutrition interferes with cellular ion transport is well known. Similarly, if one employs "pair-fed" animals in studies using weanling rats, the effects of undernutrition would likely appear much sooner. Using "pair-fed" controls is perhaps acceptable if one avoids designating the control animal as "normal". Although interpretation of data might become more difficult, it would seem better from my point of view that if pair-fed animals are to be utilized as controls, one should also compare a group of normal animals allowed to eat normal quantities of food to avoid misinterpretation of the effects of undernutrition.

I would now like to discuss hypophosphatemia itself. One should clearly differentiate the entities of phosphorus deficiency and hypophosphatemia. Clearly, phosphorus deficiency does not necessarily cause hypophosphatemia and conversely, hypophosphatemia does not necessarily indicate phosphorus deficiency (13).

Severe hypophosphatemia is arbitrarily defined as an inorganic phosphorus concentration in serum of 1.0 mg/100 ml or less. In fact, the most pronounced effects of hypophosphatemia in patients and dogs are seen when serum phosphorus has fallen to 0.5 mg/100 ml or less. In many rat studies, "severe" hypophosphatemia often means a level of 2.5 mg/deciliter or so, which may not be sufficiently low to cause problems.

Another tentative point is this. Based upon limited observations on patients and dogs, I have not seen convincing evidence that acute hypophosphatemia - of itself - has any harmful effect unless there is pre-existing cellular injury. The primary example is hypophosphatemia produced by respiratory alkalosis. This notion obviously needs substantiation.

One more important issue concerns the mechanism whereby hypophosphatemia is produced in the experimental animal. In one published study (14) examining distribution of phosphorus among various body tissues, hypophosphatemia was induced by injecting large quantities of glucose sufficient to evaluate blood glucose concentrations up to 1500 mg/100 ml (15). Although this method clearly produces hypophosphatemia, the associated massive osmotic gradients created across cellular membranes would almost certainly induce sufficient movement of electrolytes by solvent drag so that any data emanating from such a study could not be interpreted. How should one produce hypophosphatemia? Unfortunately, there is no good answer to this question. The method described earlier, namely, feeding a phosphorus deficient diet mixed with phosphate binding antacids and assuring a normal caloric intake is certainly one method. In some of our own studies, we have also induced hypophosphatemia very quickly in partially starved dogs by feeding a phosphorus deficient but otherwise normal diet containing sufficient glucose to provide 140 calories/kg/day (10). Unfortunately, this method does not circumvent the subtle cellular derangements induced by partial starvation *per se*. When it is desirable to produce acute severe hypophosphatemia to elicit cellular destruction, such methods appear to be useful. However, when one desires to study the effects of hypophosphatemia and phosphorus deficiency *per se*, the best method would seem to be dietary deprivation, antacids, and study at the most appropriate time. Finally, in my view, the dog is the ideal experimental animal to study the effects of phosphorus deficiency on tissue composition. Although this animal is unquestionably more expensive than laboratory rats, dogs can serve their own controls. In addition, one does not need to use "pair-fed" controls and the animal can be easily gavage fed if necessary. Rats commonly develop aspiration pneumonia when pair-fed. Based upon a good number of studies, the dog apparently responds to hypophosphatemia and phosphorus deficiency in a manner virtually identical to that of man.

1. Theiler, A. and Green H.H.: Aphosphorosis in ruminants. Nutr. Abs. and Rev. 1:359-385, (1932).
2. DuToit, P.J. and Bisschop, T.H.R.: The breeding of cattle on phosphorus-deficient veld. In: "15th Rept Direct Vet Services and Animal Lnd Union of South Africa." pp. 1050-1166, (1929).
3. Aubel, C.E.: The effects of low-phosphorus rations on growing pigs. Journal Agricultural Research 52(2):149-158, (1936).
4. Gilbert, F.A.: Mineral Nutrition and the Balance of Life. Univ. of Oklahoma Press, Oklahoma. (1957).
5. Phosphate - A Case Study of a Valuable Depleting Mineral in America. U.S. General Accounting Office - Quoted in Science, 209:372-376, (1980).

6. Lotz, M, Zisman, E., and Bartter, F.C.: Evidence for a phosphorus-depletion syndrome in man. NEJM 278(8):409-415, (1968).
7. Knochel, J.P., Haller, R., Ferguson, E.: Selective phosphorus deficiency in the hyperalimented hypophosphatemic dog and phosphorylation potentials in the muscle cell. In: "Phosphate and Other Minerals." pp. 323-334, (1979).
8. Fuller, T.J., Carter, N.W., Barcenas, C., and Knochel, J.P.: Reversible changes of the muscle cell in experimental phosphorus deficiency. JCI 57:1019-1024, (1976).
9. Wacker, W.E.C. and Williams, R.J.P.: Magnesium/calcium balances and steady states of biological systems. J Theoret Biol 20:65-78, (1968).
10. Knochel, J.P., Barcenas, C., Cotton, J.R., Fuller, T.J., Haller, R., and Carter, N.W.: Hypophosphatemia and rhabdomyolysis. JCI 62:1240-1246, (1978).
11. Kreusser, W., Ritz, E., Boland, R., and Brachmann, J.: Function of the sarcoplasmic reticulum (SR) in hypophosphatemic myopathy. In: "Phosphate and Other Minerals." pp. 313-321, (1979).
12. Kretz, J., Sommer, G., Boland, R., Kreusser, W., Hasselbach, W., and Ritz, E.: Lack of involvement of sarcoplasmic reticulum in myopathy and acute phosphorus depletion. Klin Wochenschr 58:833-837, (1980).
13. Knochel, J.P.: The pathophysiology and clinical characteristics of severe hypophosphatemia. Arch Int Med 137:203-220, (1977).
14. Derr, R. and Zieve, L.: Intracellular distribution of phosphate in the underfed rat developing weakness and coma folowing total parenteal nutrition. J Lab Clin Med:1398-1403, (1978).
15. Derr, R.F. and Zieve, L.: Weakness, neuropathy, and coma following total parenteral nutrition in underfed or starved rats: relationship to blood hyperosmolarity and brain water loss. J Lab Clin Med:521-528, (1978).

EFFECTS OF PHOSPHATE DEPLETION ON THE MYOCARDIUM

Nachman Brautbar, Ryszard Baczynski,
Christopher Carpenter, Shaul G. Massry

USC School of Medicine, Department of Medicine
2025 Zonal Avenue, Los Angeles, California. USA

Indirect evidence suggests that cardiac function may be affected by phosphate depletion (PD). Coburn and Massry (1) found that glomerular filtration rate is reduced during phosphate depletion and it returned to normal with phosphate repletion. They suggested that this phenomenon may be related to alteration in cardiac function. O'Connor, Wheeler and Bethune (2) evaluated the effect of PD on cardiac function in seven patients. They found that stroke work was reduced but returned to normal after phosphate administration. Cardiac output, as well as left ventricular stroke volume, were decreased and correlated with the rise in pulmonary artery wedge pressures. The authors showed that with the correction of the hypophosphatemia, left ventricular stroke volume improved and pulmonary artery wedge pressure decreased. Their studies were the first direct demonstration that phosphate depletion may affect cardiac function in man.

Fuller et al (3) studied cardiac function in dogs before and during PD. Stroke volume, maximum ascending aortic blood flow and maximum left ventricular time rate of change of pressure decreased significantly; all these changes disappeared upon phosphate repletion. The effects of pure phosphate depletion on cardiac function in patients have been described recently (4). Three patients who were ingesting excessive amounts of phosphate binding antacids, presented with cardiomyopathy and congestive heart failure. All had profound hypophosphatemia. Upon restoration of serum phosphorus to normal, the physical, radiologic and echocardiographic findings of congestive failure disappeared.

These studies from both patients and animals suggested impaired myocardial contractility as a result of PD. The process of myocardial contractility is energy dependent and requires energy production by mitochondrial oxidative phosphorylation, energy transfer from the outer membrane of the mitochondria via the creatine phosphate shuttle, and energy utilization by the myofibrils.

In an effort to evaluate the mechanisms responsible for the impaired myocardial function in PD, we examined myocardial energetics in 150-200 g Sprague-Dawley rats after 4, 8 and 12 weeks of selective phosphorus depletion produced by dietary phosphorus restriction. The animals were fed rat chow containing 0.025% phosphorus. Another group of weight and age matched, pair-fed rats received diet containing 0.35% phosphorus and served as control. The content of inorganic phosphorus, adenine nucleotides and creatine phosphate were measured in the myocardial tissue utilizing the Bessman automatic phosphate analyzer which is, in principle, high pressure liquid chromatography on an anion exchange column for separation of phosphorylated intermediates, and final ashing and colorimetric determinations upon completion of the separation (6). Mitochondrial functions were examined utilizing mitochondria isolated by a method described by Yang et al (7). The effect of PD on the activity of mitochondrial and myofibrilar creatine phosphokinase isoenzymes and on the ability to phosphorylate creatine at state 4 mitochondrial respiration were examined, utilizing a modification of the method described by Oscai et al (9). Cardiac myofibrils were isolated and purified according to the method of Solaro et al (10).

The concentration of serum inorganic phosphorus in PD rats was significantly ($p<0.01$) different than normal animals in 4 weeks (8.5 ± 0.1 vs 4.8 ± 0.5 mg/dl) and 12 weeks of PD (7.6 ± 0.3 vs 3.6 ± 0.1 mg/100 ml). The effect of PD on the intracellular concentration of inorganic phosphorus, adenine nucleotides and creatine phosphate of myocardium are presented in Figure 1, 2 and 3. A significant ($p<0.01$) reduction in the myocardial concentration of inorganic phosphorus was evident after 4 weeks of PD and remained low, thereafter. There was a significant and direct correlation between the concentration of inorganic phosphorus in the myocardium and serum inorganic phosphorus. The myocardial concentrations of ATP and ADP in PD rats were significantly ($p<0.01$) lower than those in control animals only after 12 weeks of PD. There was no correlation between the concentrations of these nucleotides and the serum levels of inorganic phosphorus or the cellular concentration of inorganic phosphorus. Phosphorylation potential was significantly increased at 4 weeks of PD and remained elevated throughout the study.

The myocardial concentration of creatine phosphate displayed a decrease after 4 weeks of PD but the decrements were statistically significant ($p<0.01$) after 8 and 12 weeks of PD. There were significant ($p<0.01$) and direct correlations between the myocardial

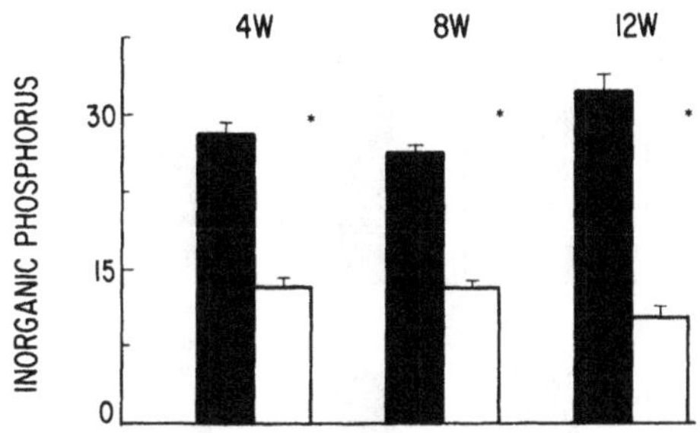

Figure 1. Myocardial inorganic phosphorus µmoles/gram protein. Controls (closed bars), PD (open bars), during 4, 8 and 12 weeks. The bars represent the mean data and the bracket SE of 12-14 rats *p<0.01).

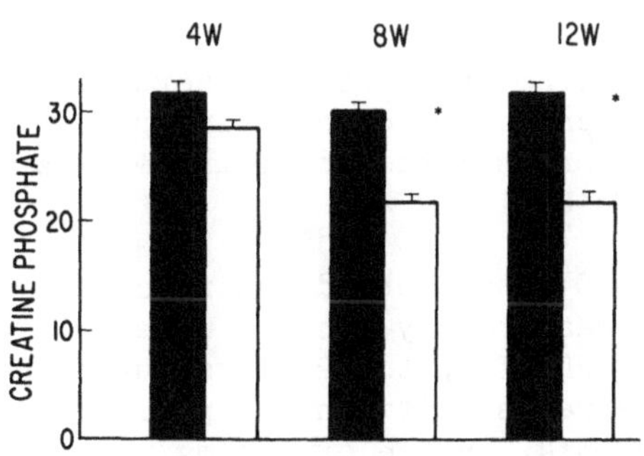

Figure 2. Myocardial creatine phosphate concentration µmoles/gram protein. Controls (closed bars), PD (open bars), during 4, 8 and 12 weeks. The bars represent the mean data and the bracket SE of 12 14 rats *(p<0.01).

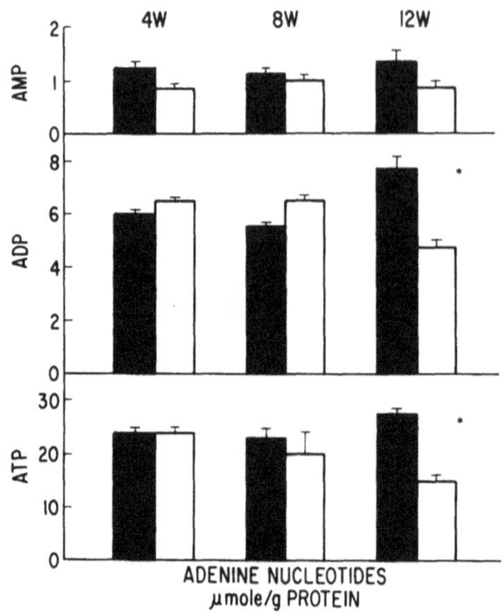

Figure 3. Myocardial concentration of adenine nucleotides. Controls (closed bars), PD (open bars), during 4, 8 and 12 weeks. The bars represent the mean data, and the bracket SE of 12-14 rats *($p<0.01$).

concentration of creatine phosphate and serum levels of inorganic phosphorus. The concentration of creatine phosphate was directly correlated with the concentration of intracellular inorganic phosphorus ($r=0.72$, $p<0.01$).

The effects of PD on mitochondrial functions are given in Figure 4, 5 and 6. Respiratory control rate (RC) and ADP:O ratio were not affected by PD of up to 12 weeks duration. Uptake of oxygen per unit time was significantly ($p<0.05$) reduced both after 8 weeks (94.0±10 vs 65±4.0 nmole oxygen/mg/protein/min) and 12 weeks (114±9.2 vs 82.0±8.0 nmole oxygen/mg/protein/min) of PD.

The activity of mitochondrial creatine phosphokinase isoenzymes was signficantly reduced after 4 weeks of PD (1.7±0.12 vs 0.50±0.10 IU/mg protein) and fell further after 12 weeks of PD. The addition of creatine to state 4 respiring mitochondria significantly enhanced oxygen consumption in mitochondria from control but not from PD animals as expressed by the ratio of oxygen consumption with and without creatine (Figure 6).

TABLE 1

EFFECTS OF PHOSPHATE DEPLETION ON THE ACTIVITY OF CREATINE PHOSPHOKINASE (IU/mg protein) HEART MYOFIBRILS

Control	PD 4 weeks	PD 8 weeks	PD 12 weeks
1.77±0.23	0.53±0.04	0.56±0.06	0.62±0.03
P value	<0.01	<0.01	<0.01

PD = Phosphate depletion
Data are mean±SE of 4 experiments

The effects of PD on the activity of creatine phosphokinase of heart myofibrils are shown in Table 1. There was a significant and marked decline in the activity of the enzyme which became apparent within 4 weeks of PD and remained reduced throughout the study.

These data show marked alterations in myocardial energetics at all steps of cellular energy metabolism, including energy production, transport and utilization.

Mitochondrial energy production was reduced as shown by reduced oxygen consumption at 8 weeks of PD. The observation that ATP levels were not reduced at the same time is compatible with reduced mitochondrial energy transport and utilization by the myofibrils. ATP levels fell at 12 weeks of phosphate depletion, as a result of greater reduction of mitochondrial energy production than the fall in energy utilization.

The energy generated by oxidative phosphorylation by the mitochondria in the form of ATP (11) is transferred via the synthesis of creatine phosphate at the mitochondrial membrane by creatine phosphokinase (11,12,13). The creatine phosphate then reaches the contractile myofibril and donates its phosphate to ADP producing ATP which is used in the contraction of the myofibrils (11). This process has been called the creatine phosphate energy shuttle. The demonstration in our study that creatine phophate of the rat myocardium is reduced during PD indicates that the transfer of energy from the mitochondria to the contractile apparatus (the creatine phosphate energy shuttle) is impaired.

The reduction in the myocardial cellular concentration of creatine phosphate could be the result of a) reduced ATP production

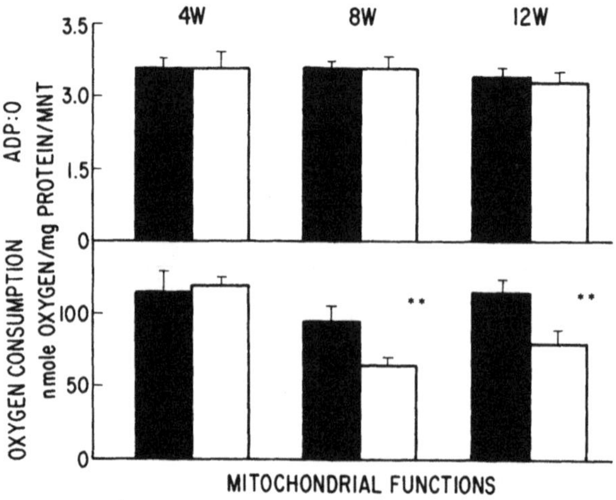

Figure 4. Mitochondrial functions from control (closed bars), and PD (open bars) rats. The bars represent the mean data and the bracket SE of 12-14 rats **(p<0.05).

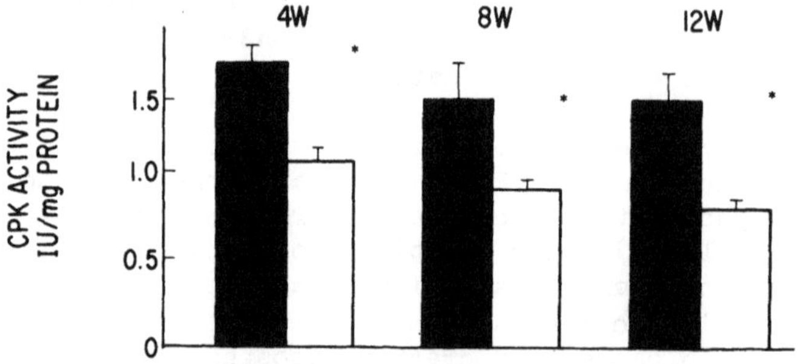

Figure 5. Mitochondrial creatine phosphokinase (CPK) activity in control (closed bars), and PD (open bars) rats. The bars represent the mean data and the brackets SE of 8-10 rats *(p<0.01).

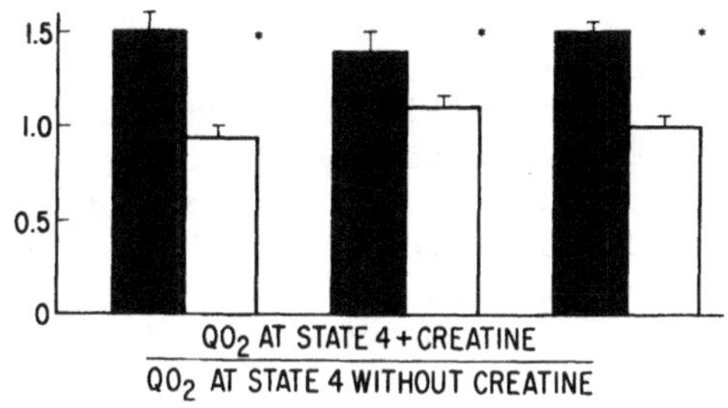

Figure 6. The ratio of maximal oxygen consumption (QO_2)of heart mitochondria at state 4 respiration with creatine/without creatine. Controls (closed bars), PD (open bars). The bars represent mean data, the brackets SE of 8-10 rats *($p<0.01$).

via the mitochondria, b) impaired creatine phosphorylation via the creatine phosphokinase system and c) tissue losses of creatine or decreased synthesis of creatine. The observation that creatine phosphate levels were reduced at 8 weeks of PD while ATP levels were still normal is against inadequate mitochondrial ATP supply for creatine phosphorylation. The reduced activity of the mitochondrial creatine phosphokinase isoenzyme occurred at 4 weeks of PD and preceded the fall in cellular creatine phosphate concentration. Since this enzyme is responsible for creatine phosphorylation, it is plausible to suggest that the reduced activity of the enzyme impaired mitochondrial energy transfer from ATP, and reduced creatine phosphorylation. Indeed, the observation of reduced maximal oxygen consumption at state 4 respiration of mitochondria from PD rats after the addition of creatine, is compatible with this notion. Finally, the possibility that cellular creatine stores were depleted secondary to tissue losses or reduced synthesis should be mentioned. Tissue creatine levels were reduced in the PD rats, and it is possible that this reduction in creatine levels is contributing to the reduced cellular creatine phosphate levels. The reduction in the activity of the creatine phosphokinase isoenzymes may play a critical role in the cardiomyopathy of phosphate depletion. These enzymes are involved in the regulation of mitochondrial (13) ATP production, energy transfer (13,14) and ATP utilization by the myofibrils (13,14).

Dietary phosphate restriction also caused a marked reduction in the concentration of inorganic phosphorus of the myocardium and this is, at least partly, due to the marked fall in the concentration of inorganic phosphorus in serum; indeed, there was a direct and significant correlation between these two parameters. The reduced cellular concentration of inorganic phosphorus occurred at early PD (4 weeks), preceded the fall in creatine phosphate and adenine nucleotides, and was accompanied by a fall in creatine phosphokinase isoenzyme activities at the mitochondrial and myofibrilar level.

This series of events suggests that the first abnormality to occur in phosphate depletion is reduced intracellular phosphorus stores. This, in turn, may impair creatine phosphokinase activity either secondary to reduced enzyme synthesis or impaired enzyme activation via phosphorylation. The reduced activity at both mitochondrial and mitofibrilar enzyme levels may further impair mitochondrial energy production, transport and utilization and, in turn, reduced myocardial contractility and bring about cardiomyopathy.

REFERENCES

1. J.W. Coburn, and S.G. Massry, Changes in serum and urinary calcium during phosphate depletion: Studies on mechanisms, J. Clin. Invest. 49:1073 (1970).

2. L.R. O'Connor, W.S. Wheeler and J.E. Bethune, Effect of hypophosphatemia on myocardial performance in men, New Engl. J. Med. 294:901 (1977).

3. T.J. Fuller, W.W. Nichols, B.J. Brenner and J.C. Peterson, Reversible depression in myocardial performance in dogs with experimental phosphorus deficiency, J. Clin. Invest. 62:1194 (1978).

4. J.R. Darsee and D.O. Nutter, Reversible severe congestive cardiomyopathy in three cases of hypophosphatemia, Ann. Int. Med. 89:867 (1978).

5. O.H. Lowry and J.B. Passanneau, A flexible system for enzymatic analysis, Academic Press, New York, p 123 (1972).

6. S.P. Bessman, P.J. Geiger, T. Sung-Cho-Lu and E.R.B. McCabe, Separation and automated analysis of phosphorylated metabolic intermediates. Analytical Biochemistry 59:533 (1974).

7. W.C.T. Yang, P.J. Geiger and S.P. Bessman, Formation of creatine phosphate from creatine and ^{32}P-labeled ATP by isolated rabbit heart mitochondria. Biochem. Biophys. Res. Com. 76:882 (1977).

8. B. Chance and G.R. Williams, Respiratory enzymes in oxidative phosphorylation. I. Kinestics of oxygen utilization, J. Biol. Chem. 217:383 (1955).

9. C.B. Oscai and J.O. Holloszy, Biochemical adaptation in muscle: II. Response of mitochondrial adenosinetriphosphatase, creatine phosphokinase and adenylate kinase activities in skeletal muscle to exercise, J. Biol. Chem 246:6968 (1971).

10. R.J. Solaro, D.C. Pang and F.N. Briggs, The purification of cardiac myofibrils with triton X-100, Biochem. Biophys. Acta. 245:259 (1971).

11. S.P. Bessman and P.J. Geiger, Transport of energy in muscle: The phosphorylcreatine shuttle, Science 211:448 (1981).

12. V.A. Saks, V.V. Kupriyanov and G. Elizarova, Studies of energy transport in heart cells, J. Biol. Chem. 255:755 (1980).

13. M.W. Seraydian and L. Artaza, Regulation of energy metabolism by creatine in cardiac and skeletal muscle cells in culture, J. Mole. Cell. Cardiol. 8:669 (1976).

14. B.J. Walker, Creatine biosynthesis, regulation and function, In Advances in Enzynology, Ed. A. Meisner, J. Wiley & Sons, New York, V50, p 177 (1979).

HYPOPHOSPHATEMIA AND OSTEOBLAST FUNCTION IN HUMAN BONE DISEASE

A.M. Parfitt and A.R. Villanueva

Bone and Mineral Research Laboratory
Henry Ford Hospital
Detroit, MI

There is experimental evidence from both in vitro and in vivo studies for three main effects of hypophosphatemia and phosphate depletion on bone. These are - an increase in osteoclastic resorption,[1,3] a decrease in the rate of collagen synthesis by osteoblasts,[3,4] and defective bone mineralization.[3,5] Studies in the intact rat using tetracycline labeling were reviewed by Ivey and colleagues at a previous Phosphate Workshop.[6] This paper summarizes the relationship between osteoblast function studied by double tetracycline labeling[7] and plasma inorganic phosphate (P) in various human metabolic bone diseases associated with chronic hypophosphatemia.

PATIENTS AND METHODS

The patient groups included 29 with surgically proven primary hyperparathyroidism, 18 with secondary hyperparathyroidism due to vitamin D deficiency, either nutritional or due to intestinal malabsorption, 9 with mild D deficiency osteomalacia with preservation of some double labeled surfaces, 19 with severe D deficiency osteomalacia without double labeled surfaces, 7 with osteomalacia due to primary renal hypophosphatemia (3 with juvenile onset and 4 with adult onset) and 5 with primary renal hypophosphatemia without osteomalacia. Mean values for age, and for plasma calcium (Ca), P and Ca x P are given in Table 1.

Definitions, units, and normal values for five indices of individual osteoblast function[8] are given in Table 2. Because of the difficulty in obtaining bone biopsies from healthy subjects in the United States, these values are based on embedded blocks from 16 healthy Danish subjects, provided by Dr. Flemming Melsen,

Table 1. Details of normal subjects and patients studied

	Normal Subjects	Primary HPT	Secondary HPT	OM (DL+)	OM (DL-)	Hypophosphatemia (OM-)	Hypophosphatemia (OM+)
n	16[1]/21[2]	29	18	9	19	5	7
Age (y) Mean	36.8±14.4	56.3±12.2	60.7±8.4	53.1±12.8	56.7±13.3	56.0±20.7	42.3±23.8
Range	23-76	33-76	43-77	40-73	32-76	31-83	20-77
Ca (mg/dl)	9.63±0.37	11.36±0.65	9.00±0.67	8.36±0.18	8.11±0.87	9.61±0.34	9.50±0.36
(%N)	100	118	93	87	84	100	99
P (mg/dl)	3.46±0.42	2.58±0.44	3.43±0.62	2.57±0.51	2.22±0.24	2.22±0.24	2.01±0.44
(%N)	100	75	99	86	74	66	58
CaxP (mg^2/dl^2)	33.25±3.72	29.42±5.18	30.63±5.05	24.43±3.00	20.54±5.28	21.36±2.52	18.97±3.73
(%N)	100	89	92	73	62	64	57

Data given as mean ± SD. [1]Subjects who had bone biopsy, with age data. [2]Subjects from whom biochemical data were obtained. HPT - hyperparathyroidism; OM - osteomalacia; DL - double labelled surface.

Table 2. Indices of osteoblast function and normal values

Index	Units	Normal Values All[1]	Old[2]	Young[3]	Abbrev.
1. Mean apposition rate (Mean ILD/ILT)	μm/d	0.794±0.130	0.790	0.795	AR
2. Labeled osteoid (LS/OS)		0.759±0.139	0.737	0.766	LO_f
3. Mean formation velocity (1 x 2)	μm/d	0.607±0.153	0.578	0.617	FV
4. Mean osteoid seam width	μm	11.28±2.55	10.88	11.41	OSW
5. Mineralization lag time (4/3)	d	19.33±4.93	19.38	19.31	MLT

ILD - interlabel distance; ILT - interlabel time; LS - labeled surface; OS - osteoid surface. [1]16 subjects mean age 36.8 y. [2]4 subjects mean age 57.3 y. [3]12 subjects mean age 30.0 y. There are no significant differences between the old and young normals for any of the five indices.

from which new sections were cut, stained and examined by the same methods as used for the patients[9]. This is preferable to using published normal data from other laboratories[10] because of possible technical differences such as in microscope calibration. The criteria for osteomalacia were osteoid seam width >15 μm, mineralization lag time >100 days and osteoid volume >10% of total bone volume[7]. The fraction of labeled osteoid was based on both single and double labeled surfaces except in osteomalacia, where only double labeled surfaces were counted.

RESULTS AND DISCUSSION

Mean values for formation velocity and osteoid seam width for each patient group are given in Table 3; values for the other indices are omitted because they correlated either less well, or (in most patient groups) not at all with plasma Ca, P or Ca x P. Formation velocity, which is the mineral apposition rate averaged over the entire osteoid surface, is, except in osteomalacia, an index of the mean rate of matrix synthesis by individual osteoblasts. This is because all matrix formed is eventually mineralized, so that the average rates of matrix apposition and mineral apposition must be equal[8]. In osteomalacia much of the matrix remains permanently unmineralized in the absence of treatment, and the mean rate of matrix apposition is greater (but usually not much greater) than the mean rate of mineral apposition. Formation

Table 3. Mean values (±SD) for formation velocity (FV) and osteoid seam width (OSW) in the patient groups from Table 1.

	FV		OSW	
	μm/d	%N	μm	%N
Primary HPT	0.318±0.122	52.4	11.90±4.17	105.5
Secondary HPT	0.445±0.145	73.3	12.87±2.60	114.1
OM (DL+)	0.102±0.054	16.9	18.90±3.62	167.5
OM (DL-)	0	0	34.02±13.03	301.6
Hypophosphatemia:				
(OM+)	0.032±0.042	5.3	34.16±19.89	302.8
(OM-)	0.083±0.091	13.7	8.94±2.49	75.1

velocity was significantly reduced in each patient group, an effect unlikely to be due to higher mean age than in the control subjects (Table 2).

In primary hyperparathyroidism there is significant depression of individual osteoblast function; this contrasts with the significant increase in total bone formation rate (not shown) that results from the increased activation of bone remodeling units and consequent increase in osteoblast birth rate and number[7,8]. Formation velocity did not correlate significantly with plasma Ca, P or Ca x P. Vernejoul and colleagues have recently found a significant inverse correlation between formation velocity and PTH in primary hyperparathyroidism[11].

In the patients with secondary hyperparathyroidism due to early vitamin D deficiency, the changes in osteoblast function were in the same direction as, but of smaller magnitude than, in primary hyperparathyroidism. In this group, unexpectedly, the mean plasma P was normal (Table 1). This may reflect the absence of hypercalcemia, which has an effect to reduce phosphate reabsorption which is independent of PTH[12]. As in primary hyperparathyroidism, no index of osteoblast function correlated with plasma P but there was a significant inverse correlation between osteoid seam width and plasma calcium ($r = 0.57$, $P < 0.02$). In the patients with osteomalacia and preservation of some double tetracycline labeling, there was a significant positive correlation between formation velocity and plasma P (Figure 1a) and a slightly stronger correlation with plasma Ca x P ($r = 0.73$, $P < 0.025$). If the patients with secondary hyperparathyroidism were included, the strength of both correlations was weakened, ($r = 0.48$ and 0.54 respectively) but the significance was strengthened ($P < 0.02$ and < 0.005 respectively) because of the increased n. It is not clear whether hypo-

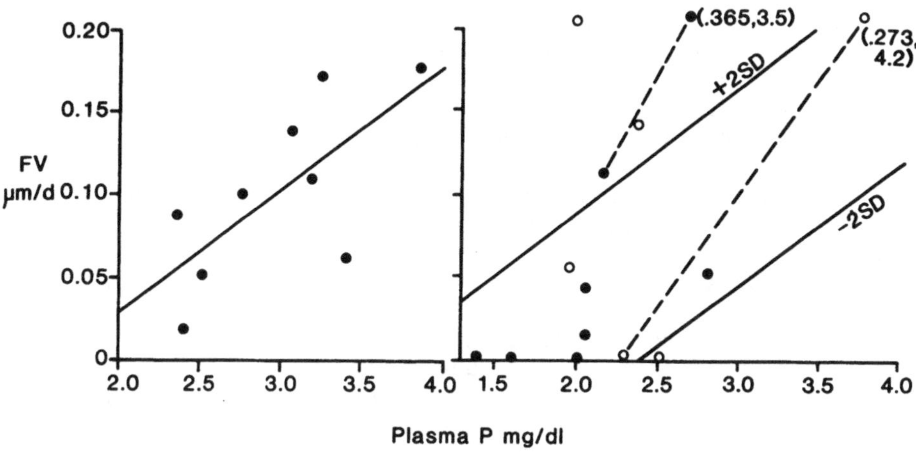

Fig. 1. The relationship between formation velocity (FV) and plasma P. On left (1a), scatter plot and regression line for 9 patients with mild vitamin D deficiency osteomalacia with preservation of some double tetracycline labeling. The regression equation is: FV = .075P - 0.12 (r = 0.71, P <0.05). The lower limit for FV in normal subjects is 0.3 µm/d, so that 5 of the 9 patients had significant depression of FV despite normal plasma P (<3.0 mg/dl). On right (1b), data from 12 patients with primary hypophosphatemia shown in relation to the confidence limits (±2SD) of the regression shown in Fig. 1a. For 6 of 7 patients with hypophosphatemic osteomalacia (closed circles) and for 3 of 5 patients with hypophosphatemic non-osteomalacia (open circles) the points lie within or very close to the confidence limits. The dotted lines join measurements made before and after supplemental phosphate administration to one patient of each group; the lines are of the correct slope and the coordinates of the post-treatment points are shown in parentheses.

phosphatemia is directly depressing osteoblast function or is simply a marker of increased PTH secretion or of some other consequence of D deficiency[13].

In primary hypophosphatemia and osteomalacia, osteoid seam width was increased to the same extent as in severe vitamin D deficiency (Table 3). Formation velocity was markedly reduced, and hypophosphatemia was more severe in this than in any other group. There was no significant correlation between these variables, but 6 of 7 points were within the confidence limits for the regression found in mild D deficiency osteomalacia (Figure 1b). Another group of patients with primary hypophosphatemia had very similar plasma Ca and P levels but markedly different bone histology. This group was clinically heterogenous, and hypophosphatemia came to light on investigation of vague rheumatic and/or skeletal pain; in one case the hypophosphatemia followed renal transplantation[14] but in the others no etiologic factor could be uncovered. There was no correlation of FV with plasma P, but 3 of 5 individual points fell within or close to the confidence limits of the regression found in mild osteomalacia (Figure 1b). In one patient with each type of primary hypophosphatemia, supplemental phosphate was followed by a rise in plasma P and a significant improvement in osteoblast function to normal or close to normal (Figure 1b).

There are several limitations to the interpretation of these data. First, no distinction has been made between hypophosphatemia and phosphate depletion, because of the frequent impossibility of deciding whether there is an intracellular as well as an extracellular phosphate deficit. Second, plasma P was in most patients measured on only a few occasions and in the fasting state, so that no account is taken of circadian or longer term fluctuation in plasma P, or of the duration for which hypophosphatemia had existed. Finally, it is not yet possible in clinical studies to distinguish between direct and indirect effects of hypophosphatemia on bone. Nevertheless, although hypophosphatemia is neither a necessary nor a sufficient condition for either impaired matrix synthesis by osteoblasts or for impaired bone mineralization, it is probably one of the factors that may influence both of these processes.

CONCLUSIONS

1. In primary hyperparathyroidism, hypophosphatemia is associated with reduced formation velocity (an index of matrix synthesis by individual osteoblasts) despite an increase in bone formation rate, but the former abnormalities were not correlated.

2. In secondary hyperparathyroidism due to vitamin D deficiency, osteoid seam width was correlated inversely with plasma calcium.

3. In mild osteomalacia due to vitamin D deficiency, formation velocity was correlated with plasma phosphate.

4. In primary renal hypophosphatemia with osteomalacia, the relationship between formation velocity and plasma phosphate was similar to that in vitamin D deficiency.

5. A clinically heterogenous group of patients had primary renal hypophosphatemia and impaired matrix synthesis by osteoblasts, but without osteomalacia, and with some evidence for a causal relationship.

6. The presence or absence of increased osteoid seam width in

hypophosphatemic patients is not fully explained by differences in plasma Ca and P levels.

REFERENCES

1. L. G. Raisz and I. Niemann, Effect of phosphate, calcium and magnesium on bone resorption and hormonal responses in tissue culture. Endocrinology 85:446 (1969).
2. P. Cuisineir-Gleizes, M. Thomassett, Sainteny-Debove, et al, Phosphorus deficiency, parathyroid hormone and bone resorption in the growing rat. Calcif Tiss Res 20:235 (1976).
3. D. Baylink, J. Wergedal, and M. Stauffer, Formation, mineralization, and resorption of bone in hypophosphatemic rats. J Clin Invest 50:2519 (1971).
4. L. G. Raisz, J. W. Dietrich, and D. Maina, Effects of phosphate on bone formation and resorption in tissue culture. in: "Phosphate Metabolism, Kidney and Bone," L. Avioli, Ph. Bordier, H. Fleish, S. Massry, E. Slatopolsky, ed., Armour Montagu, Paris (1976).
5. L. R. I. Baker, P. Ackrill, W. R. Cattell, T. C. B. Stamp, and L. Watson, Iatrogenic osteomalacia and myopathy due to phosphate depletion, Br Med J 3:150 (1974).
6. J. L. Ivey, E. R. Morey, and D. J. Baylink, The effects of phosphate depletion on bone, Adv Exp Biol Med 103:373 (1978).
7. A. M. Parfitt, C. Mathews, D. Rao, B. Frame, M. Kleereloper, and A.R. Villanueva, Impaired osteoblast function in metabolic bone disease, in: "Osteoporosis: Recent Advances in Pathogenesis and Treatment." H. F. DeLuca, H. Frost, W. Jee, C. Johnston, and A. M. Parfitt, ed., University Park Press, Baltimore (1981).
8. A. M. Parfitt, The physiologic and clinical significance of bone histomorphometric data, in: "Bone Histomorphometry. Techniques and Interpretations, R. Recker, ed., C. R. C. Press (in press).
9. A. R. Villanueva, Part II. Basic preparation and staining of undecalcified bone, in: "Theory and Practice of Histotechnology," 2nd Edition, D. C. Sheehan, B. B. Hrapchak, C. V. Mosby, St. Louis (1980).
10. F. Melsen and L. Mosekilde, Tetracycline double-labeling of iliac trabecular bone in 41 normal adults, Calcif Tiss Res 26:99 (1978).
11. M. C. de Vernejoul, L. Cancela, J. Gueris, J. L. Gardin, J. Bielakoff, D. Kuntz, A. Ryckewaert, and L. Miravet, Correlation between bone disease and 1,25-dihydroxy vitamin D in primary hyperparathyroidism, Min and Electrolyte Metab 6:270 (1981).

12. A. M. Parfitt and M. Kleerekoper, The divalent ion homeostatic system: Physiology and metabolism of calcium, phosphorus magnesium and bone, in: "Clinical Disorders of Fluid and Electrolyte Metabolism." M. Maxwell, C. R. Kleeman, 3rd Edition (1980.

13. D. J. Baylink, E. R. Morey, J.L. Ivey, and M. E. Stauffer, Vitamin D and bone, in: "Molecular Biology and Clinical Nutrition, A. W. Norman, ed., Marcel Dekker, Inc., New York (1980).

14. M. Kleerekoper, R.S. Bernstein, C. Cruz, N.W. Levin and A. M. Parfitt, Parathyroid hormone resistance in renal allograft recipients, Min and Electrolyte Metab, 6:246 (1981).

HYPOPHOSPHATEMIA AND GLUCOSE INTOLERANCE

Donald Simonson and Ralph A. DeFronzo

Department of Medicine
Yale University School of Medicine
New Haven, Connecticut 06510

INTRODUCTION

Hypophosphatemia is frequently observed in a variety of disease states including ketoacidosis, chronic alcoholism, malabsorption, severe burns, hyperparathyroidism, renal tubular defects, and re-feeding after starvation (1, 2). Since phosphate is a ubiquitous anion involved in such diverse functions as maintaining the structural integrity of the cell membrane, regulating a variety of intracellular enzymes, energy storage in the form of ATP, and regulating tissue delivery of oxygen through 2,3-DPG levels (2), it is not surprising that the clinical syndromes associated with phosphate depletion are equally diverse. Pathophysiologic disturbances associated with hypophosphatemia include hemolytic anemia, rhabdomyolysis, myopathy, impaired cardiac output, CNS abnormalities (encephalopathy, seizures), abnormal liver function tests, and platelet and leukocyte dysfunction (1, 2).

Phosphate depletion is especially common in the poorly controlled diabetic patient. Although the plasma phosphate concentration may be normal or only slightly reduced at the time of admission, total body phosphate stores are usually markedly reduced (2, 3). The negative phosphate balance is the result of several factors. Metabolic acidemia increases urinary phosphate excretion (4) and intracellular phosphate stores may remain depleted for up to 7-10 days following resolution of the acidemia (2). Furthermore, acidemia accelerates intracellular catabolism, thus facilitating the release of phosphate from tissues into the plasma (2). The osmotic diuresis which accompanies poorly controlled diabetes also contributes to the excessive urinary phosphate loss by inhibiting phosphate reabsorption by the proximal tubule (1, 2). Finally, insulin deficiency per se may be associated with impaired tubular reabsorption of phosphate and thus further exacerbate the phosphaturia (5, 6). With the institution of insulin therapy, the phosphaturia is rapidly reversed (7) but the hypophosphatemia may be worsened by the accompanying shift of phosphate into cells.

Despite the frequent presence of hypophosphatemia in the poorly controlled diabetic, its contribution to the impairment in glucose metabolism has not been clearly defined. Friedlander and Rosenthal were the first to suggest that hypophosphatemia per se may contribute to the impaired glucose tolerance. They demonstrated that intravenous administration of phosphate alone produced a decline in the plasma glucose concentration in the severe diabetic but had no effect on plasma glucose concentration in normal controls (8).

Recent studies examining glucose metabolism in patients with primary hyperparathyroidism have also provided evidence that hypophosphatemia may impair glucose utilization. Several groups have demonstrated that the plasma insulin response to both intravenous and oral glucose is significantly increased in patients with hyperparathyroidism and hypophosphatemia (9, 10). Since the plasma glucose response was similar in hyperparathyroid and control subjects, the hyperinsulinemia was construed to indicate the presence of insulin resistance. Since calcium infusion in the control subjects had no effect on the plasma glucose and insulin responses to oral and intravenous glucose, these authors concluded that the insulin resistance was secondary to the hypophosphatemia (9). However, one could argue that the calcium infusion and resultant hypercalcemia in the control subjects was not of sufficient duration to impair glucose metabolism. Alternatively, it is possible that the elevated levels of PTH per se were responsible for the insulin resistance in hyperparathyroid patients.

In an attempt to dissociate the effects of hypophosphatemia and elevated PTH levels on glucose metabolism, Harter et al examined the effects of chronic dietary induced hypophosphatemia on glucose tolerance and insulin secretion in dogs (11). After two months on a low phosphate diet, mean serum phosphorous levels declined from 4.1 to 1.1 mg/dl while the serum calcium concentration remained unchanged and serum PTH fell to undetectable levels. The hypophosphatemia was associated with a significant impairment in the intravenous glucose tolerance test (IVGTT) despite an augmented plasma insulin response (Figure 1). When calcium and/or PTH was administered to hypophosphatemic or control animals, no change in glucose tolerance or insulin release was observed. These results indicate that chronic phosphate depletion and hypophosphatemia are associated with impaired responsiveness to insulin.

QUANTITATION OF INSULIN SECRETION AND INSULIN RESISTANCE IN HYPOPHOSPHATEMIC MAN

Introduction

While the previously mentioned studies suggest that hypophosphatemia may impair glucose tolerance by diminishing tissue responsiveness to insulin, there are several methodologic problems which preclude an accurate quantitation of the degree of insulin resistance. During oral glucose administration, variable gastrointestinal absorption of glucose produces a continuously changing glycemic stimulus to the pancreatic beta cell. Since the plasma glucose concentration is significantly different in control and experimental groups and is changing at different rates, it is difficult to interpret the increased insulin response observed in hypophosphatemic animals. Furthermore, oral glucose stimulates the release of a variety of gut mediated factors which may alter insulin secretion. At present, it is unknown whether the release of these insulinotrophic factors are similar in normal and hypophosphatemic subjects. Lastly, since the rate of disappearance of plasma glucose after the IVGTT is slower in the hypophosphatemic subjects, a more prolonged hyperglycemic stimulus will be presented to the β-cell and this would be expected to enhance insulin release. One study (11), which attempted to measure insulin resistance more directly using the intravenous insulin tolerance test, failed to demonstrate any differences in either the rate of decline or nadir in plasma glucose concentration following intravenous insulin in hypophosphatemic dogs. It should be noted, however, that the hypoglycemic response to a pharmacologic bolus of exogenous insulin can not be used to accurately assess sensitivity to insulin since hypoglycemia results in a complex neuro-endocrine response leading to the secretion of epinephrine, glucagon, growth hormone, and cortisol. All of these counterregulatory hormones are known to antagonize the action of insulin and differences in their secretion and metabolic effects in normal and hypophosphatemic subjects have not been characterized.

To circumvent the problems of variable gastrointestinal absorption of glucose, gut hormone release following glucose ingestion, and variations in the glycemic stimulus presented to the beta cell, we have recently studied insulin secretion and insulin responsiveness in hypophosphatemic subjects using the hyperglycemic and euglycemic insulin clamp techniques respectively (12).

Study Population

Six hypophosphatemic subjects were studied: three had hypophosphatemic rickets, two had a renal phosphate leak, and one had adult onset hypophosphatemic osteomalacia (13). The mean plasma phosphate concentration, 2.4±0.2 mg/dl (range = 1.6-2.8 mg/dl) and maximum tubular rate of phosphate reabsorption, 2.0±0.2 (range = 1.2-2.4) mg/dl per 100 ml GFR, were significantly decreased compared to controls (P<0.01). Plasma calcium (9.3±0.1 mg/dl) and PTH (71±4 μl-eq/ml) concentrations were normal. All patients were within 20% of ideal body weight (mean = 112±2%) and were taking no medications. The mean age of the group was 45±9 years. The fasting plasma glucose concentration was normal in all of the hypophosphatemic subjects (range = 90-102 mg%).

Methods

Hyperglycemic Clamp. The plasma glucose concentration is acutely raised and maintained at 125 mg/dl above the fasting level by a prime-variable infusion of intravenous glucose. Under these steady-state conditions of hyperglycemia, the infusion rate of glucose (corrected for urinary glucose losses) must equal the amount of glucose metabolized by all of the tissues of the body and therefore provides a measure of overall glucose tolerance. The plasma insulin responses to this square wave hyperglycemic stimulus is biphasic with an early burst of insulin within the first 10 minutes. This is followed by a gradually increasing phase of insulin secretion that lasts until the end of the study. The total amount of glucose metabolized (M) divided by the plasma insulin response (I) during the two hour study period provides a measure of the tissue responsiveness to insulin (M/I ratio). Since hyperglycemia per se is known to enhance insulin-mediated glucose uptake and since part of the secreted insulin represents proinsulin (which has immunologic but little biologic activity) each subject also received a euglycemic insulin clamp study to provide a purer measure of tissue responsiveness to insulin.

Euglycemic Insulin Clamp. A prime-continuous infusion of insulin is administered to acutely raise and maintain the plasma insulin concentration at approximately 100 μU/ml above the basal level. The plasma glucose concentration is held constant at the fasting level by adjustment of a variable glucose infusion. Under these conditions of euglycemic hyperinsulinemia, the total amount of glucose infused must equal the total amount of glucose taken up by the cells since we have previously shown that hepatic glucose production is almost completely suppressed under such hyperinsulinemic conditions (14). Therefore, the glucose infusion rate required to maintain euglycemia provides a measure of tissue responsiveness to the exogenously infused insulin.

Results

Hyperglycemic Clamp. The total amount of glucose metabolized by the hypophosphatemic patients, 4.9±0.3 mg/kg·min was reduced by 36% (P<0.001) compared to normal controls, 7.6±0.4 mg/kg·min (Figure 2). The early (44±4 vs. 48±4 μU/ml), late (64±10 vs. 65±8), and total (62±9 vs. 65±8) plasma insulin responses were similar in hypophosphatemic and control subjects respectively (Figure 2). Consequently, the M/I ratio, a measure of tissue sensitivity to endogenously secreted insulin, was significantly reduced in the hypophosphatemic subjects, 8.7±1.4 vs. 12.1±0.7 mg/kg·min per μU/ml, $P<0.001$ (Figure 2).

Insulin Clamp. The rate of glucose metabolism during the euglycemic insulin clamp was reduced by 43% in hypophosphatemic patients, 3.8±0.6 mg/kg·min compared to controls, 6.7±0.3 mg/kg·min, $P<0.001$ (Figure 3). Since the steady-state plasma insulin levels were similar in the two groups, the M/I ratio was decreased ($P<0.001$) in hypophosphatemic subjects (Figure 3), indicating tissue insensitivity to insulin. The decrease in insulin-mediated glucose metabolism during the euglycemic insulin clamp correlated closely ($r = 0.90$, $P<0.01$) with the decrease in M/I ratio measured during the hyperglycemic clamp study.

Insulin Secretion

In the presence of decreased tissue sensitivity to insulin, the normal beta cell response is an increase in insulin secretion (15, 16). Because of the higher plasma insulin levels, glucose tolerance remains normal. It is noteworthy, therefore, that despite the presence of insulin resistance in our hypophosphatemic patients, insulin secretion was not increased during the hyperglycemic clamp study. This is in contrast to the elevated plasma insulin response observed in chronically hypophosphatemic dogs described by Harter et al (11) and suggests that hypophosphatemia, at least in man, may inhibit pancreatic insulin secretion. This possibility has received support from recent observations by Campillo et al (17). Using the isolated perfused rat pancreas, these investigators demonstrated that progressively decreasing the phosphate concentration in the perfusate let to a progressive diminution of both basal and stimulated insulin secretion. These results suggest that hypophosphatemia may also have an inhibitory effect on the beta cell.

Mechanism of Insulin Resistance

Although it seems fairly well established that hypophosphatemia is associated with resistance to the action of insulin, the cellular mechanisms underlying this disturbance in glucose metabolism remain to be defined. It has long been known that there is a direct relationship between glucose and phosphate transport by cells. In 1924, both Harrop et al (18) and Briggs et al (19) demonstrated that insulin administration stimulated the uptake of phosphate and glucose into muscle cells in a parallel fashion in diabetic and normal subjects. A similar effect was subsequently observed in the isolated perfused dog hind limb by Pollack et al (20). More recently, Walaas et al (21), using the isolated rat diaphragm, have shown that insulin, even in the absence of glucose in the incubation medium, stimulates phosphate transport and its accumulation within the cell as ATP and GTP. This insulin-stimulated phosphate transport could be blocked by ouabain as well as by substitution of potassium chloride or choline chloride for sodium chloride in the medium. These results suggest the presence of a specific membrane transport mechanism for phosphate which is closely coupled to sodium transport (21).

Although the transport of phosphate across the cell membrane appears to be facilitated by the presence of insulin and/or glucose, there is a paucity of information concerning the effects of hypophosphatemia on insulin-mediated glucose metabolism at the cellular level. While insulin-stimulated glucose uptake can occur in the rat soleus muscle (22) and the rat diaphragm (23) in the absence of phosphate, the doses of insulin employed in the incubation medium were in the pharmacologic range. Furthermore, chronic hypophosphatemia may alter the intracellular environment in a manner which is not reproduced by simply incubating isolated muscle in a phosphate-free medium. Since the first step in the intracellular metabolism of glucose is the phosphorylation by hexokinase to glucose-6-phosphate, it is possible that chronic hypophosphatemia, by depleting intracellular phosphate stores, may lead to an inhibition of glucose-6-phosphate formation (24). This would increase the concentration of free glucose within the cell and secondarily decrease glucose entry.

In addition to its role in the intracellular metabolism of glucose, phosphate may also be instrumental in the transport of glucose across the cell membrane. Lefevre et al have shown that phospholipids in the cell membrane are crucial for transport of glucose (as well as mannose, ribose, xylose, galactose, and other simple sugars) into the cell (25). If chronic hypophosphatemia induced a change in the properties of these membrane phospholipids, then a defect in glucose transport may result. Such an alteration of these membrane structures could also affect the insulin receptor and decrease its affinity for insulin.

SUMMARY

Hypophosphatemia of various etiologies results in insulin resistance and glucose intolerance. Studies, both in vivo and in vitro, have demonstrated that phosphate plays an important role in insulin-mediated glucose metabolism. Although phosphate is an integral component of the glucose transport system (membrane phospholipids) and is required for the intracellular metabolism of glucose (glucose phosphorylation), potential defects in these metabolic processes at the cellular level have not been critically examined in chronic hypophosphatemic states.

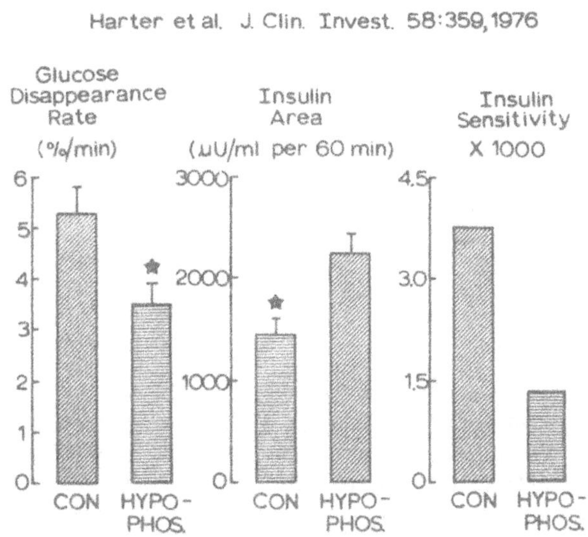

Figure 1. Glucose disappearance rate and insulin response (area under curve) in control (CON) and hypophosphatemic (HYPOPHOS) dogs following intravenous glucose administration. Insulin sensitivity was calculated by dividing the mean glucose disappearance rate by the mean insulin area and multiplying by 1000.

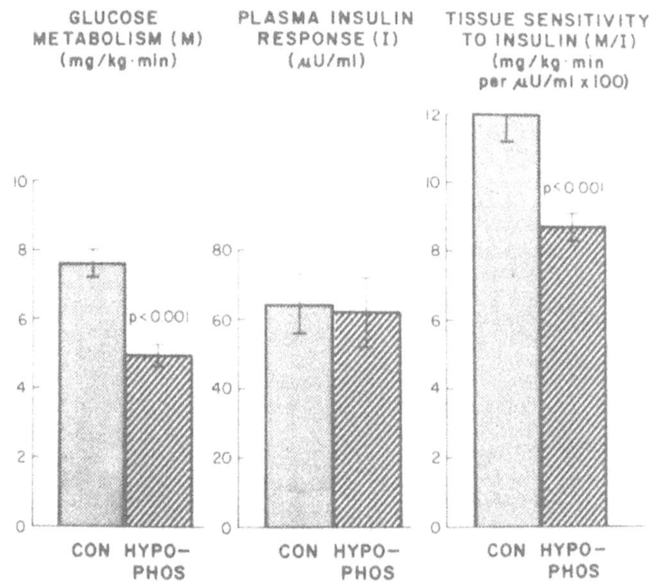

Figure 2. Glucose Metabolism, Plasma Insulin Response, and Calculated Tissue Sensitivity to Insulin during the Hyperglycemic-Clamp Study in Six Hypophosphatemic Subjects and 48 Control Subjects.

The plasma glucose concentration was acute raised and maintained at 125 mg per deciliter above the fasting level by a prime-variable infusion of glucose. Under these steady-state conditions of hyperglycemia, the glucose infusion rate must equal the amount of glucose taken up and metabolized by all the tissues of the body.

The rate of glucose metabolism (M) was reduced by 36 percent (P<0.001) in the hypophosphatemic group despite a plasma insulin response (I) that was similar in both groups. Consequently, the M/I ratio (a measure of tissue sensitivity to insulin) was significantly reduced (P<0.001) in the hypophosphatemic group.

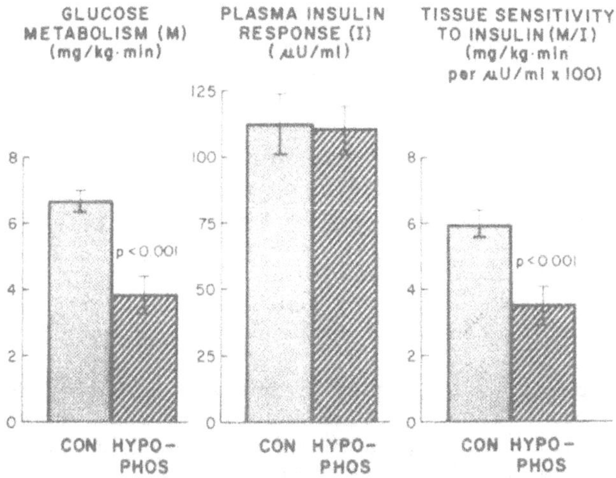

Figure 3. Glucose Metabolism, Plasma Insulin Response, and Calculated Tissue Sensitivity to Insulin during the Euglycemic Insulin-Clamp Study in Five Hypophosphatemic Subjects and 48 Control Subjects.

The plasma insulin concentration was acutely raised and maintained at a constant level about 100 μU per milliliter above the base line, and the plasma glucose concentration was maintained at the fasting level by a variable glucose infusion. Under these steady-state conditions of euglycemia, the glucose infusion rate must equal the rate of glucose uptake and metabolism by all the tissues of the body and thus provides a measure of tissue sensitivity to the infused insulin.

In hypophosphatemic subjects insulin-mediated glucose metabolism (M) was reduced by 43 percent ($P<0.001$) despite similar steady-state plasma insulin levels in both groups. Consequently, the M/I ratio (a measure of tissue sensitivity to insulin at euglycemic levels) was decreased ($P<0.001$) in the hypophosphatemic patients.

REFERENCES

1. J. P. Knochel, "Hypophosphatemia", Clin. Nephrology 7 (4): 131 (1977).

2. J. P. Knochel, "The pathophysiology and clinical characteristics of severe hypophosphatemia", Arch. Int. Med. 137: 203 (1977).

3. U. Keller and W. Berger, "Prevention of hypophosphatemia by phosphate infusion during treatment of diabetic ketoacidosis and hyperosmolar coma", Diabetes 29:87 (1980).

4. R. Mahnensmith, S. O. Thier, C. R. Cooke, A. Broadus, and R. A. DeFronzo, "Effect of acute metabolic acidemia on renal electrolyte transport in man", Metabolism 28:831 (1979).

5. R. A. DeFronzo, C. R. Cooke, R. Andres, G. R. Faloona, and P. J. Davis, "The effect of insulin on renal handling of sodium, potassium, calcium, and phosphate in man", J. Clin. Invest. 55:845 (1975).

6. R. A. DeFronzo, M. Goldberg, and Z. S. Agus, "The effects of glucose and insulin on renal electrolyte transport", J. Clin. Invest. 58:83 (1976).

7. D. W. Seldin and R. Tarail, "The metabolism of glucose and electrolytes in diabetic acidosis", J. Clin. Invest. 29: 552 (1950).

8. K. Friedlander, and W. G. Rosenthal, "Uber der Einflus des Phosphorsaureions auf den Blutund Harnzucker des normalen und des diabetischen Organismus", Arch. Exp. Path. Pharmakol 112:66 (1926).

9. H. Kim, R. K. Kalkhoff, N. V. Costrini, J. M. Cerletty, and M. Jacobson, "Plasma insulin disturbances in primary hyperparathyroidism", J. Clin. Invest. 50:2596 (1971).

10. K. Yasuda, Y. Hurukawa, M. Okuyama, M. Kikuchi and K. Yashinaga, "Glucose tolerance and insulin secretion in patients with parathyroid disorders", N. Eng. J. Med. 292:501 (1975).

11. H. R. Harter, J. V. Santiago, W. E. Rutherford, E. Slatopolsky, and S. Klahr, "The relative roles of calcium, phosphorous, and parathyroid hormone on glucose- and tolbutamide-mediated insulin release", J. Clin. Invest. 58:359 (1976).

12. R. A. DeFronzo, J. D. Tobin, and R. Andres, "Glucose clamp technique: a method for quantifying insulin secretion and resistance", Am. J. Physiol. 237:E214 (1979).

13. R. A. DeFronzo, and R. Lang, "Hypophosphatemia and glucose intolerance: evidence for tissue insensitivity to insulin", N. Engl. J. Med. 303:1259 (1980).

14. R. A. DeFronzo, "Glucose intolerance and aging. Evidence for tissue insensitivity to insulin", Diabetes 28:1095 (1979).

15. E. A. H. Sims, E. Danforth, E. S. Horton, G. A. Bray, J. A. Glennon, and L. B. Salans, "Endocrine and metabolic effects of experimental obesity in man", Rec. Prog. Horm. Res. 29:457 (1973).

16. O. G. Kolterman, J. Insel, M. Saekow, and J. M. Olefsky, "Mechanisms of insulin resistance in human obesity", J. Clin. Invest. 65:1272 (1980).

17. J. E. Campillo, J. I. Osuna, M. T. Pages, A. Blazquez, M. Castillo, and C. Osorio, "Effect of inorganic phosphate on basal and glucose-induced insulin release in vitro. Influence of magnesium concentration," Diabetologia 21:256 (1981).

18. G. A. Harrop, and E. M. Benedict, "The participation of inorganic substances in carbohydrate metabolism", J. Biol. Chem. 59:683 (1924).

19. A. P. Briggs, I. Koechig, E. A. Daisy, and C. J. Weber, "Some changes in the composition of blood due to the injection of insulin", J. Biol. Chem. 58:721 (1924).

20. H. Pollack, R. F. Millet, H. E. Essex, F. C. Mann, and J. L. Bollman, "Serum phosphate changes induced by injections of glucose into dogs under various conditions", Am. J. Physiol. 110:117 (1934).

21. O. Walaas, E. Walaas, and A. M. Wick, "The stimulatory effect by insulin on the incorporation of ^{32}P radioactive inorganic phosphate into intracellular inorganic phosphate, adenine nucleotides, and guanine nucleotides of the intact isolated rat diaphragm", Diabetologia 5:79 (1969).

22. I. H. Chaudry, and M. K. Gould, "Kinetics of glucose uptake in isolated soleus muscle", Biochem. Biophys. Acta 177:527 (1969).

23. P. J. Randle, and G. H. Smith, "Regulation of glucose uptake by muscle", Biochem. J. 70:501 (1958).

24. D. M. Kipnis, "Regulation of glucose uptake by muscle: Functional significance of permeability and phosphorylating activity", Ann. N. Y. Acad. Sci. 82:355 (1959).

25. P. G. LeFevre, K. I. Habich, H. S. Hess, and M. R. Hudson, "Phospholipid-sugar complexes in relation to cell membrane monosaccharide transport", Science 143:955 (1964).

ACUTE HYPOPHOSPHATEMIA DURING TOTAL PARENTERAL NUTRITION IN MAN: ITS EFFECTS ON MUSCLE CELL COMPOSITION

Alberto Montanari, Loris Borghi, Amedeo Curti, Mauro Canali, Mario Mergoni*, Paolo Zuccoli*, Almerico Novarini, Alberico Borghetti

Istituto di Semeiotica Medical e Cattedra di Anestesiologia e Rianimazione*, University of Parma, Italy

Acute hypophosphatemia (AHPP) may often develop in renutrition both chronic alcoholics and malnourished subjects and during recovery from diabetic ketoacidosis as well as in total parental nutrition (TPN), mainly in previously underfed patients (1,2).

A number of experimental evidences has shown a relationship between hypophosphatemia and/or phosphorus (P) depletion and muscle cell damage (3,4,5). On the other hand, the association of AHPP to either rhabdomyolysis (6,7) or alteration of muscle cell electrolyte composition (6) has been recognized in recovery from both diabetic ketoacidosis and alcoholism; this suggested that altered P homeostasis may play a role in muscle cell changes observed in these human clinical conditions (6). However, in alcoholism and ketoacidosis it may be difficult to distinguish the effects of AHPP on muscle from those possibly related to either other metabolic and nutritional disturbances, as hypomagnesemia, potassium depletion, acidosis or direct toxicity of ethanol "per se" (8).

In order to better point out the effects of AHPP on human muscle, our study was performed in a "pure" human model of AHPP, i.e. in TPN-fed, acutely hypophosphatemic subjects. Being TPN schedule complete and balanced (9) for all nutrients, electrolytes and minerals other than P, observed alterations of muscle cell composition can be reliably attributed to AHPP or P depletion rather than to other metabolic disturbances.

MATERIAL AND METHODS

H_2O, Cl, Na, K, Mg and total P were measured in muscle tissue obtained by needle biopsy (10) in healthy controls and 23 subjects with AHPP (serum Pi below 0.4 mM/l) which had appeared after 3-18 days of TPN treatment; TPN had been performed with 35-40 Kcal (50% dextrose) 1.5-2.0 mM Na, 1.2-1.8 mM K, 0.15-0.20 mM Ca, 0.16-0.20 mM Mg, no more than 0.08 mM P, 0.15-0.20 gr N (aminoacid solution) (amounts per Kg body weight per day). Ratios among the elements of TPN were similar to those known to have equilibrate effects on total body composition (9). Muscle biopsies were made into 12-24 hours after the recognition of AHPP. Subjects were divided into 2 groups: Group I: 11 subjects were malnourished and underweight; their deviation from ideal body weight, calculated on the basis of sex, age and height (11) was -16±8.7%. Clinical diagnosis was: gastrointestinal cancer (N=8), chronic alcoholism (N=2), protracted meningitidis (N=1). Group II: 12 previously well nourished (deviation from ideal body weight +5±4.5%), acutely ill patients were considered. Clinical diagnosis was: head injury (N=9), surgery for aortocoronary bypass (N=2) and for gastric perforation (N=1).

13 external balance studies for Na, K, Mg, P were performed in 12 subjects submitted to TPN and suffering from head injury. 9 out of 12 patients received muscle biopsy before and after a 5-11 day study period in which they were fed with a TPN formula identical to that reported above but with 10-15 mM P/day. 4 subjects of this group (AHPP-D) developed AHPP (serum Pi 0.2-0.4 mM/l) while the other 5 patients (AHPP-N) did not (serum Pi 0.9-1.5 mM/l). The last 4 subjects (AHPP-C) had a TPN-induced AHPP at the beginning of study period (serum Pi 0.2-0.4 mM/l) and P supplementation of 60-100 mM/day was given during 5-7 days, to correct AHPP up to serum Pi 1.1-1.3 mM/l at the time of second biopsy. Only 2 subjects from group AHPP-C were malnourished.

Each muscle sample, weighing 30-60 mg was freed from fat, connective and blood, then divided into 3 pieces which were dried and defatted with ether. In the first one both total muscle water (TW), by differential weighing after desiccation, and muscle Cl (Clm), by potentiometric titration after HNO_3-CH_3COOH extraction were measured. In the second one, digested with HNO_3-$HClO_4$ at 105°C, total muscle P (Pm) was determined by Chen's method (12). In the third fragment, extracted with HNO_3, K, Mg and Na (Km, Mgm, Nam) were measured by atomic absorption specgrophotometry (AAS). All muscle values were expressed as mM per Kg fat free dry solids (FFS). The partition into extra (ECW) and intracellular water (ICW) was estimated by the Cl method (13), according to Nernst equation and assuming a resting muscle membrane potential of -87.2 mV (14); ECW was calculated knowing Cle, Cli, Clm and TW (13). ICW was given by the difference between TW and ICW. Conventional balance techniques were employed; serum, urine and acid-digested stools were analyzed for Na, K and Mg by AAS and for P by Chen's method.

RESULTS

In our patients, fed by P-deficient TPN, AHPP had appeared into 3-8 days in Group I and into 7-18 days in Group II. At this time, serum Pi averaged 0.29 mM/l in both groups. Serum values did not show important extracellular disturbances; only acid-base parameters showed a moderate metabolic acidosis.

Table I summarizes muscle findings (mean±SEM) and P-values in all AHPP subjects in comparison with those obtained in healthy controls. Muscle K and Mg were significantly reduced, Cl and Na were increased in reference to FFS. TW was high because of a rise of ECW; ICW was unchanged. Intracellular Na and K concentration were respectively increased and reduced; intra/extracellular ratio for K, as well as Pm, were depressed. In Table II serum Pi, Pm, Nam, Km and Ki are compared between AHPP subjects with (Group I) and without malnutrition (Group II). Serum Pi values were similar in both groups; Pm was severely reduced in malnourished subjects of Group I, while it was only slightly depressed in Group II without malnutrition. Changes of Nam, Km and Ki, although highly significant versus controls in both groups were statistically more evident in subjects with malnutrition.

TABLE I

MUSCLE WATER ELECTROLYTES AND TOTAL P IN 23 SUBJECTS WITH TPN INDUCED AHPP COMPARED WITH HEALTHY CONTROLS (M±SEM *=.001; **=.005)

	AHPP	CONTROLS	(n=)	P
TW	3.68±.06	3.28±.04	(27)	*
ECW	1.03±.06	0.78±.05	(17)	**
ICW	2.65±.07	2.52±.06	(17)	NS
Clm	140±8	99±8	(17)	*
Nam	227±12	134±4	(27)	*
Km	379±10	458±5	(48)	*
Mgm	34±1	40±1	(38)	*
Pm	216±10	281±9	(17)	*
Nai	30±4	8±2	(17)	*
Ki	144±4	182±6	(17)	*
Ki/Ke	34±1	42±1	(17)	*

Data are expressed as mM (electrolytes and P) and Kg (water) per Kg FFS or Kg ICW

TABLE II

MUSCLE ELECTROLYTES IN 23 AHPP SUBJECTS WITH AND WITHOUT MALNUTRITION
(M ± S.E.M. * = .001; ** = .005; *** = .05 versus controls)

	Malnourished AHPP (n = 11)		P versus	Well-nourished AHPP (n = 12)	
Pis	.29 ± .03		NS	.29 ± .03	
Pm	177 ± 8	*	.001	252 ± 9	***
Nam	255 ± 18	*	.05	202 ± 13	*
Km	349 ± 12	*	.005	406 ± 14	*
Ki	134 ± 6	*	.025	153 ± 6	**

Balance studies. No significant alterations of extracellular electrolytes and acid base values were present at the beginning as well as at the end of study period except for a slight reduction of plasma bicarbonate (21.8 ± 1.0 mM/l). In figure 1 individual changes of serum Pi in each group of subjects submitted to balance studies are reported. Figure 2 represents mean values of external balances for K, Na, Mg and P in the groups of patients submitted to TPN. In AHPP-D Na balance was highly positive and K balance was severely negative. Significant gain of K was found in AHPP-C group. Changes of external balance of Mg were always marginal; P balance was slightly negative in both AHPP-D and N group while in AHPP-C significant retention of P was found due to 2 malnourished subjects with correction of initial low values of Pm to normal values.
Table III shows that TW and ECW increased in AHPP-D and decreased although at a lesser extent, in AHPP-C while no changes were found in AHPP-N. Individual data for muscle ECW in the groups are shown in

TABLE III

TW, ECW and ICW BEFORE AND AFTER BALANCE STUDY PERIOD DURING TPN
(* represents significant differences versus healthy controls)

	T.W.		E.C.W.		I.C.W	
	b	a	b	a	b	a
AHPP- D (n=4)	3.12±.03	3.65±.17*	0.75±.02	1.08±.06*	2.36±.04	2.56±.15
AHPP-N (n =5)	3.30±.07	3.20±.09	0.84±.08	0.72±.04	2.44±.12	2.47±.10
AHPP-C (n=4)	3.71±.18*	3.40±.10	1.10±.08*	0.93±.06	2.60±.14	2.47±.12

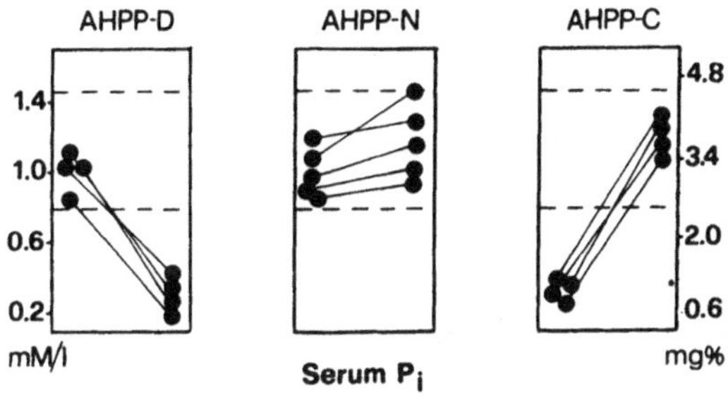

Figure 1. Changes of serum inorganic phosphorus (Pi) in 3 groups of subjects submitted to TPN: AHPP-D = patients who developed AHPP; AHPP-N = patients who did not develop AHPP; AHPP-C = correction of previously TPN-induced AHPP.

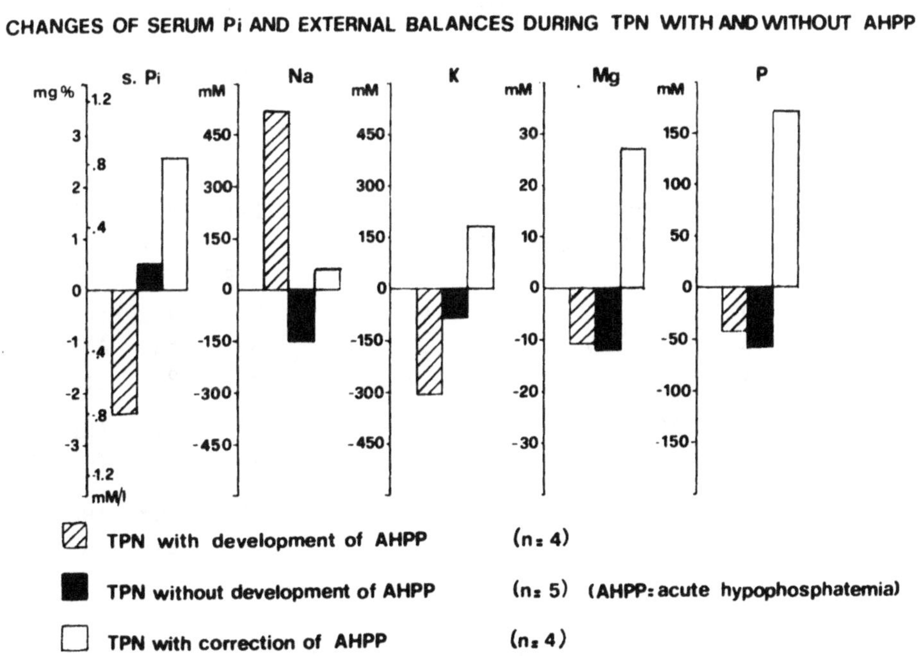

Figure 2. Mean values of external balances for Na, K, Mg and P in 3 groups of patients submitted to TPN (see figure 1).

figure 3. Table IV summarizes the variations of muscle electrolytes and total phosphorus in the same groups of subjects of table III; Clm and Nam increased and Km and Mgm decreased in patients who developed AHPP (AHPP-D). Similar alterations were found in AHPP-C group at the beginning of observation period and they were reversed by P supplementation for Nam, Km and Mgm while Clm was unchanged according to the only marginal changes of ECW we have reported above. All these values did not change significantly in subjects without AHPP (AHPP-N). Figures 4 and 5 enphasize the modifications of muscle Na and K during study period in the 3 groups of patients submitted to TPN.

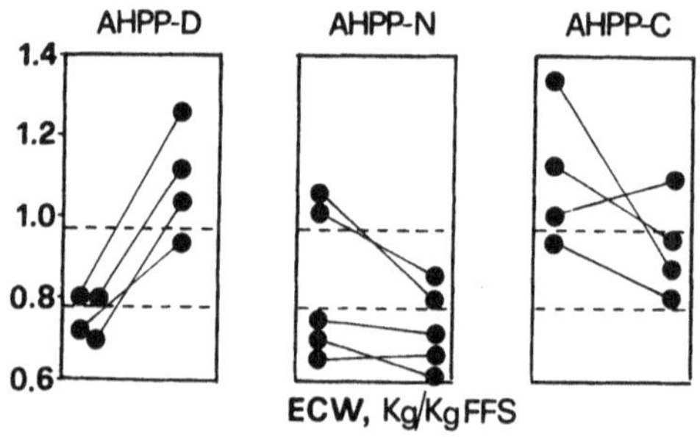

Fig. 3. Changes of ECW in patients submitted to TPN (see Fig. 1.)

TABLE IV

MUSCLE ELECTROLYTES AND TOTAL P BEFORE AND AFTER BALANCE STUDY PERIOD (SEE FIGURE 1 AND TABLE III FOR SYMBOLS)

Clm		Nam		Km		Mgm		Pm		
b	a	b	a	b	a	b	a	b	a	
109	154*	141	191*	465	357*	38	32*	284	256	AHPP-D
9	18	16	20	25	25	2	3	21	22	(n = 4)
123	117	139	126	442	424	39	38	307	284	AHPP-N
10	18	18	13	15	19	3	3	19	23	(n = 5)
143*	148*	213*	155	380*	433	32*	36	236*	240*	AHPP-C
18	15	15	10	25	12	2	2	36	21	(n = 4)

Table V represents the variations of muscle electrolytes expressed as concentration in ICW; also intra/extracellular ratio for K varied in opposite way in AHPP-D and AHPP-C groups, while it remained unchanged in AHPP-N one.

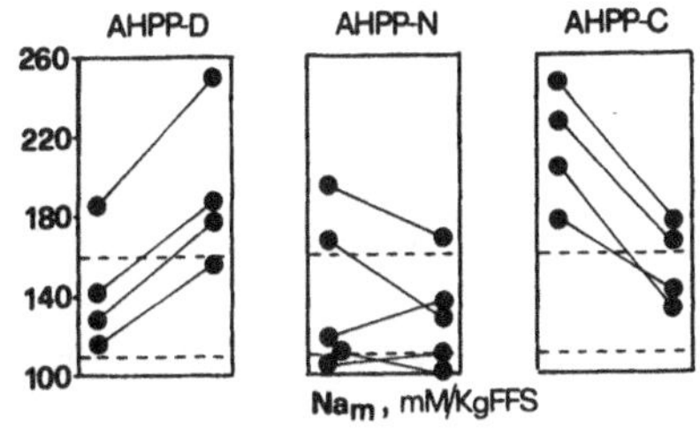

Figure 4. Changes of muscle Na in 3 groups of subjects submitted to TPN (see Figure 1).

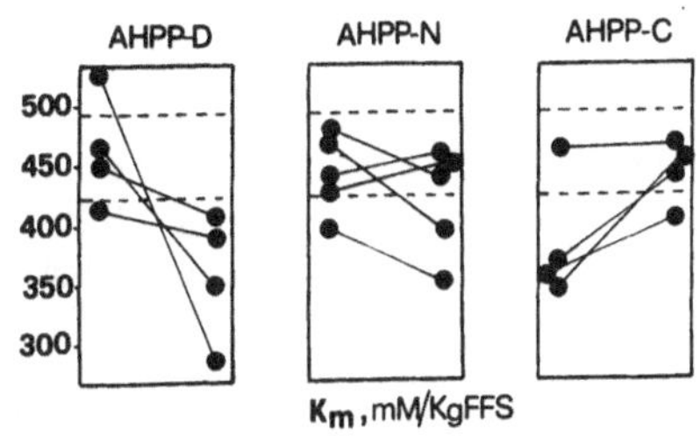

Figure 5. Changes of muscle K in 3 groups of subjects submitted to TPN (see Figure 1).

TABLE V

Na AND K CONCENTRATION IN MUSCLE ICW (mM/Kg ICW) AND Ki/Ke RATIO BEFORE AND AFTER BALANCE STUDY PERIOD DURING TPN

	Nai		Ki		Ki/Ke	
	b	a	b	a	b	a
AHPP-D (n = 4)	10±5	30±5	197±12	139±11 *	46±5	36±3 *
AHPP-N (n = 5)	4±2	6±3	182±14	168± 7	42±4	39±1
AHPP-C (n = 4)	20±11*	10±5	146±13*	176± 9	33±2*	40±2

DISCUSSION

The changes of muscle water and electrolyte composition we show in a human AHPP are quite similar to those found by others (4,5) in previously P depleted, partially starved dogs; in these animals, when intravenous hyperalimentation was undertaken, AHPP occurred associated with frank rhabdomyolysis, acute increase of muscle Na, Cl and TW and decline of K and P. All this picture was prevented or corrected by P supplementation. In fact, this latter experimental model seems to reproduce, at least in part, the mechanisms involved in clinical course of our previously underfed, acutely hypophosphatemic patients (Group I), even if clinical rhabdomyolysis was not seen. High muscle ECW, Cl and Na, low K and Mg in association with severely reduced Pm were prominent characteristics in our malnourished subjects, as well as in experimental dogs (4,5). However, in our patients severe muscle P depletion did not seem to be necessary to the development of muscle abnormalities in TPN induced AHPP; actually, we observed significant alterations of cell K, Mg and Na even in subjects without previous malnutrition and with normal or only slightly depressed Pm. This suggests that AHPP can alter cell electrolyte composition without true P depletion. Low Pm in malnourished subjects was associated to greater changes of cell composition; this may indicate that AHPP enhances previous alterations of cell composition due to either malnutrition, P depletion or toxic effects, as observed in experimental dogs (4,5) and humans with chronic alcoholism (6). Our balance studies confirm the role of acute fall of extracellular Pi in muscle cell derangement during TPN; actually, significant changes in muscle water and electrolytes were seen only when AHPP occurred during P-deficient TPN (AHPP-D), while subjects who did not develop AHPP (AHPP-N) had no significant alterations. Changes of muscle P were slight in AHPP-D and N groups; however, one cannot exclude that in malnourished subjects also muscle P depletion independently of AHPP contributes to muscle derangement according to the greater modifications seen in patients with low Pm. Also, the effects of P replacement in TPN-induced AHPP (AHPP-C) support a protective effect of adequate P intake against muscle cell changes in TPN.

The biochemical mechanism of cell alterations in AHPP and P depletion is unknown. Intracellular pattern observed in our AHPP subjects as well as in animal models of P depletion with or without AHPP (4,5) might be consistent with an altered ion transport across muscle cell plasma membrane; this could depend on either structural changes of membrane or reduced active Na efflux from (and K influx into) the cells by the Na/K pump, as previously supposed by others (2,3).

This interpretation can be supported by the finding of a reduced Ki/Ke ratio, which may suggest that muscle cell membrane is unable to ensure a normal intra/extracellular gradient for K; furthermore an impairment of Na/K pump was previously found by us in red cells of subjects with AHPP (15). However, the presence of such membrane defect also in a complex cellular model as muscle cell as well as its role in AHPP-associated muscle abnormalities must be further investigated.

In summary, our findings demonstrate that acute depletion of extracellular Pi per se has some clear effects on muscle cell compo- irrespectively to the presence or absence of severe muscle P depletion; thus, it is conceivable that in association to other toxic, metabolic or nutritional derangements hypophosphatemia contributes to muscle abnormalities found under different clinical conditions as alcoholism or diabetic ketoacidosis. Although some findings could suggest that a defect of transmembrane ion fluxes may play a role, the precise mechanism underlying these changes is not understood.

REFERENCES

1. KNOCHEL J.P.: The pathophysiology and clinical characteristics of severe hypophosphatemia . Arch.Int.Med.,137: 203-220 (1977)

2. PARFITT A.M., KLEEREKOPER M.: Clinical disorders of calcium, phosphorus and magnesium metabolism. In "Maxwell M.H., Kleeman C.R.: Clinical disorders of fluid and electrolyte metabolism" p. 947 (Mc Graw-Hill, New York, 1980).

3. FULLER T.J., CARTER N.W., BARCENAS C., KNOCHEL J.P.: Reversible changes of the muscle cell in experimental phosphorus deficiency. J.Clin. Invest. 57: 1019-1024 (1976).

4. KNOCHEL J.P., BARCENAS C., COTTON J.R., FULLER T.J., HALLER R., CARTER N.W.: Hypophosphatemia and rhabdomyolysis. J. Clin. Invest. 62: 1240-1246 (1978)

5. KNOCHEL J.P., HALLER R., FERGUSON E.: Selective phosphorus deficiency in the hyperalimented hypophosphatemic dog and phosphorilation potential in the muscle cell. In Massry S.G., Ritz E., Jahn H.: Advances in experimental medicine and biology vol. 128. Phosphate and mineral in healthy and disease, p. 323 (Plenum Press, New York, 1980).

6. ANDERSON R., HALLER R., ELMS J., CARTER N.W., KNOCHEL J.P.:Skeletal muscle phosphorus and magnesium deficiency in alcoholic

myopathy. Mineral Electr. Met. 4: 106-112 (1980).

7. KNIGHT A.H., WILLIAMS D.N., SPOONER R.J., GOLDBERG D.M.:Serum enzyme changes in diabetic ketoacidosis. Diabetes 23:126-131(1974)

8. BLACHLEY J.D.,FERGUSON E.R.,CARTER N.W.,KNOCHEL J.P.:Chronic alcohol ingestion induces phorphorus deficiency and my opathy in the dog. Trans.Am.Soc.Phys. 93:110-122 (1980)

9. RUDMAN D., MILLIKAN W.J.,RICHARDSON T.J.,BIXLER T.J.II,STACKHOUSE W.J.,McGARRITY W.C.: Elemental balances during intravenous hyperalimentation of underweight adult subjects.J.Clin.Invest.55:94-104 (1975)

10. BERGSTROM J.: Muscle electrolytes in man. Scand.J.Clin.Lab.Invest. 14:(suppl. 68), 7-117 (1962)

11. Metropolitan Life Insurance Statistical Bulletin,40,Nov-Dec.(1959)

12. CHEN P.S.Jr.,TORIBARA T.Y.Jr.,WARNER H.:Microdetermination of phosphorus. Anal.Chem. 28:1756-1758 (1956)

13. GRAHAM J.A., LAMB J.F., LINTON A.L.:Measurement of body water and intracellular electrolytes by means of muscle biopsy. Lancet ii: 1172-1176 (1967)

14. RIECKER G., BOLTE H.D., ROHL D.: Hypokaliamie und membran potential mikropunktionen einzelner muskelzellen beim menschen. Réanimation et organes artificiels. 1: 41-50 (1964).

15. MONTANARI A., BORGHI L., CANALI M., CURTI A., NOVARINI A., BORGHETTI A.: A sodium efflux defect from red blood cells in human severe hypophosphatemia. Min. Electr.Met. 2,106 A (1979).

PROXIMAL RENAL TUBULAR ACIDOSIS AND HYPOPHOSPHATEMIA INDUCED BY ARGININE

Daniel Batlle, Steven Hays, Richard Foley, Yun Chan,
Jose A.L. Arruda and Neil A. Kurtzman

Section of Nephrology
University of Illinois College of Medicine
Chicago, Illinois

INTRODUCTION

Arginine monohydrochloride is a cationic amino acid widely used to test pituitary function (1). In the recent past, its use for the treatment of severe metabolic alkalosis and hepatic encephalopathy was often recommended (2-4). Recognition of its potential for severe hyperkalemia (5,6) prompted the cautious use of this compound. Its use, however, is bound to continue in view of the widespread administration of amino acids in the course of hyperalimentation. This study was undertaken to systematically examine the effect of arginine, at a dose similar to that commonly used clinically, on urinary acidification and plasma electrolyte composition. Our results are in keeping with previous studies showing the development of metabolic acidosis and hyperkalemia during a brief infusion. They further demonstrate that arginine, like other cationic amino acids (7-9), markedly impairs proximal bicarbonate reabsorption. Of interest, a significant fall in plasma phosphate was uncovered by these studies. This could not be ascribed to renal phosphate wastage because phosphate excretion decreased markedly. Hence, arginine induces proximal renal tubular acidosis associated with hypophosphatemia without a renal phosphate leak.

METHODS

A total of thirty-one experiments were performed on fourteen female mongrel dogs, which weight ranged from 17 to 20 kg. The animals were anesthetized with sodium pentobarbital, 30 mg/kg, intravenously; light anesthesia, as judged by preservation of corneal reflexes, was maintained by subsequent small doses. A cuffed endotracheal tube was inserted and connected to a Bird respirator; plasma pCO_2 was maintained between 30 and 45 mmHg by appropriate manipulation of the respirator. A catheter was inserted in the femoral artery for blood sampling. A peripheral venous catheter was used to infuse 0.8% saline containing iothalamate-^{125}I (100 μCi/l) at a rate of 0.6 ml/min throughout the experiments as a marker of glomerular filtration rate (GFR). An equilibration period of at least 45 min was allowed before urine collections were started. Urine was collected via an indwelling Foley catheter.

The following set of experiments were performed:

Arginine infusion protocol

After completion of two clearance collections as described above, arginine monohydrochloride (3 mmol/kg body wt) was infused during 60 min. Six clearance collections of approximately 10 min duration were completed. Following completion of the above protocol, the dose of arginine monohydrochloride was increased to 6 mmol/kg body wt. This dose of arginine was infused during 60 min (i.e. second hour of arginine infusion). Six clearance collections were obtained. Following completion of the above, a 0.9M $NaHCO_3$ solution was infused at a rate of 2 ml/min during 60 min. During this period of time, arginine monohydrochloride infusion was sustained as in the second hour (i.e. 6 mmol/kg body wt.). Six clearance collections were obtained.

Ammonium chloride infusion protocol

Five dogs were prepared as described above and were infused with ammonium chloride in order to lower blood pH and plasma bicarbonate to a level similar to that observed in arginine monohydrochloride infused dogs (i.e. second hour of arginine infusion). Six clearance collections were obtained. This was followed by an infusion of 0.9M $NaHCO_3$ in a manner similar to that described in arginine-infused dogs. Six clearance collections were obtained.

Specimen collections, GFR, blood and urine electrolyte concentrations were determined as previously reported (10). Statistical analysis were performed using the student t test for paired and unpaired data when appropriate. Values are expressed as means ± SE.

RESULTS

Acid-base and urinary acidification data

During the last 30 min of the first hour of arginine chloride infusion, plasma bicarbonate fell slightly but not significantly (from 23.9 ± 0.8 to 22.9 ± 1.2 mEq/l). Blood pH also decreased slightly but not significantly (from 7.42 ± 0.01 to 7.39 ± 0.01). Blood pCO_2 fell from 40 ± 1.2 to 38 ± 1.5 mmHg, $p<0.05$. Plasma chloride increased significantly (from 115 ± 2.3 to 121 ± 2.0, $p<0.001$). The data obtained during the second hour of arginine infusion are presented in Table I. Observe that blood pH and blood bicarbonate fell markedly while plasma chloride increased significantly. The development of hyperchloremic metabolic acidosis was not associated with a significant fall in urine pH. Furthermore, fractional bicarbonate excretion increased from 4.5 ± 1.4 to 15 ± 5.6%, this increase did not achieve statistical significance. The finding of a high fractional bicarbonate excretion at normal and low plasma bicarbonate concentrations suggests the presence of a defect in proximal bicarbonate reabsorption (11,12).

The relationship of bicarbonate reabsorption (Tm/GFR) to plasma bicarbonate concentration during sodium bicarbonate infusion (i.e. during the third hour of arginine chloride infusion) is presented in the figure. It is clear from this figure that at low, normal, and high plasma bicarbonate concentrations, bicarbonate reabsorption was lower in arginine infused dogs than that of ammonium chloride treated controls. Prior to bicarbonate loading, blood pH and plasma bicarbonate were comparable in control dogs infused with ammonium chloride and arginine chloride infused dogs (Table II). Likewise, during sodium bicarbonate loading, the blood pH and plasma bicarbonate of ammonium chloride treated controls (7.51 ± 0.08 and 31.3 ± 0.8 mEq/l, respectively) were also not significantly different than those of arginine chloride infused dogs (7.47 ± 0.02 and 31.7 ± 2.7 mEq/l, respectively).

During sodium bicarbonate infusion, absolute bicarbonate excretion increased from 134 ± 50 to 571 ± 211 μEq/min. Urine pH and fractional bicarbonate excretion also increased further (Table I).

Plasma electrolyte and urinary electrolyte excretion

During the last 30 min of the first hour of arginine chloride infusion, plasma potassium increased from 3.3 ± 0.17 to 3.7 ± 0.2 mEq/l, $p<0.02$. No significant changes in plasma sodium, calcium, and plasma phosphate were observed.

Table III presents the data obtained during the second hour of arginine chloride infusion. Plasma potassium increased markedly and this increase was associated with a marked increase in fractional potassium excretion. Plasma phosphate decreased significantly. This decline in plasma phosphate occurred despite a fall in blood pH (Table I). Plasma calcium increased sligthly but not significantly. Both absolute and fractional phosphate excre-

TABLE I. Effect of arginine on urinary acidification

	Blood pH	Blood pCO_2 mmHg	Blood HCO_3 mEq/l	Plasma Cl mEq/l	Urine pH	Fractional HCO_3 Excretion (%)
BASELINE n=7	7.42 ±0.01	40 ±1.2	24 ±0.8	115 ±2.3	7.4 ±0.1	4.5 ±1.4
p<	0.001	NS	0.001	0.001	NS	NS
ARGININE (2nd hr)	7.31 ±0.01	37 ±1.2	17.7 ±0.5	140 ±1.9	7.2 ±0.07	15 ±5.6
p<	0.01	0.05	0.005	NS	0.05	0.02
ARGININE + $NaHCO_3$ (3rd hr)	7.47 ±0.02	46 ±2.3	31.7 ±2.7	143 ±7.5	7.53 ±0.08	42.5 ±9.3

TABLE II. Urinary acidification in dogs infused with arginine and NH_4Cl

	Blood pH	Blood pCO_2 mmHg	Blood HCO_3 mEq/l	Urine pH	HCO_3^- Tm/GFR
ARGININE (2nd hr)	7.31	37	17.7	7.2	15.1
n=7	±0.01	±1.2	±0.5	±0.07	±0.94
p<	NS	NS	NS	0.005	0.025
NH_4Cl	7.29	40	18.7	6.5	18.6
n=5	±0.08	±0.6	±0.7	±0.17	±0.79

TABLE III. Effect of arginine on plasma and urinary electrolyte excretion

	GFR	V	Plasma K	Plasma PO_4	Plasma Ca	Fractional Excretion			U_{Ca} x V	UPO_4 x V
						Na	K	PO_4		
	ml/min	ml/min	mEq/l	mmol/l	mEq/l		%		μEq/100ml	μmol/100ml
BASELINE	59	3.5	3.3	1.31	4.2	3.4	27	19	6.9	29
n=7	±3.3	±0.9	±0.2	±0.12	±0.1	±0.9	±4.3	±2.8	±1.9	±5.5
p<	0.01	0.01	0.01	0.05	NS	0.05	0.001	0.01	0.02	0.02
ARGININE	41	8.3	4.9	1.16	4.45	8.8	95	7.3	20.4	9.1
(2nd hr)	±3.0	±0.8	±0.3	±0.1	±0.1	±1.6	±11	±2.5	±3.6	±3.7
p<	0.02	0.05	NS	NS	NS	NS	0.05	NS	0.01	NS
ARGININE +	33.5	11	5.7	1.23	4.3	29	120	9.8	54	15
$NaHCO_3$ (3rd hr)	±4.1	±1.2	±0.4	±0.2	±0.1	±4.9	±6.9	±3.8	±2.3	±5.9

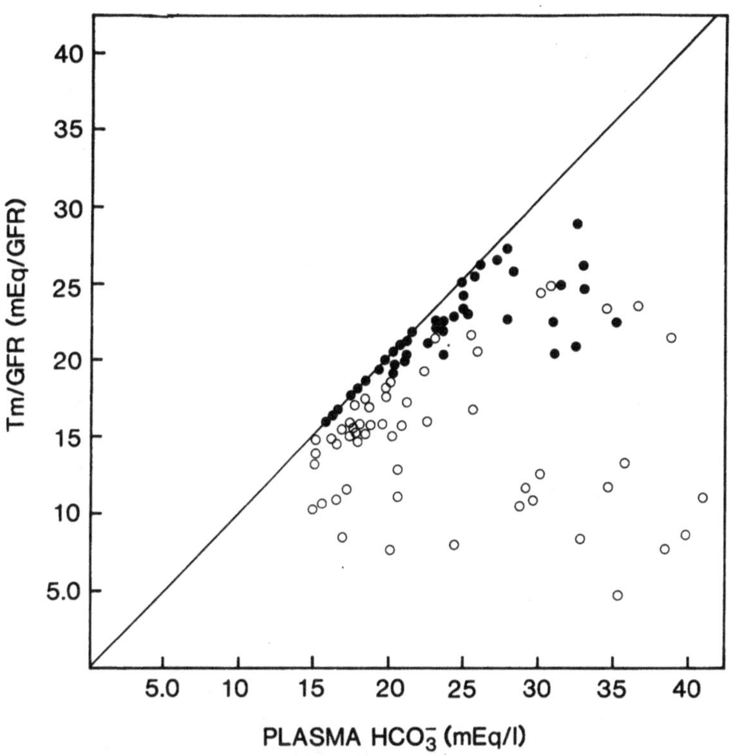

Fig. 1. Bicarbonate reabsorption (Tm/GFR) plotted against plasma bicarbonate concentration in arginine treated dogs (open circles) and ammonium chloride treated dogs (closed circles). Arginine treated animals exhibited a lower bicarbonate reabsorption at any plasma bicarbonate concentration than ammonium chloride treated control animals.

tion fell significantly. Hence, the decline in plasma phosphate did not result from increased phosphate excretion. In fact, during the last 20 min of arginine chloride infusion, urinary phosphate concentration was virtually undetectable (i.e. less than 0.1 mEq/l).

Glomerular filtration rate decreased significantly during arginine chloride infusion whereas urinary flow and fractional sodium excretion increased markedly. Absolute Ca excretion corrected per GFR also increased significantly.

Renal handling of electrolytes was also examined during sodium bicarbonate loading (Table III). Plasma potassium increased further (although not significantly) in arginine treated dogs despite superimposed infusion of sodium bicarbonate and an increase in blood pH. This was associated with a further increase in fractional potassium excretion. In contrast, sodium bicarbonate administration to control dogs infused with ammonium chloride lowered plasma potassium (from 4.6 ± 0.3 to 2.8 ± 0.1 mEq/l, $p<0.02$). In this group, sodium bicarbonate infusion also increased fractional phosphate excretion (from 2.5 ± 1.0 to 31 ± 9.9%, $p<0.05$). In arginine chloride infused dogs, sodium bicarbonate infusion did not exert a significant phosphaturic effect (Table II). Plasma phosphate did not change significantly but GFR further declined. Hence, filtered load of phosphate declined as well. Fractional sodium excretion increased further during sodium bicarboate loading. Calcium excretion increased markedly as well.

DISCUSSION

This study shows that an infusion of arginine monohydrochloride causes a profound impairment in overall bicarbonate reabsorption. The marked bicarbonaturic effect of arginine (i.e. fractional bicarbonate excretion around 15% at low plasma bicarbonate concentration) clearly indicates a defect in proximal bicarbonate reabsorption (11,12). Our data does not exclude an effect of arginine on distal bicarbonate reabsorption. A defect in the distal nephron, however, can not account for the large fractional bicarbonate excretion observed in this study in view of the limited capacity of this nephron segment for bicarbonate transport (11,12). The pattern of bicarbonate reabsorption disclosed in arginine-infused dogs (figure) is that seen in subjects with proximal bicarbonate wastage.

Arginine and other cationic amino acids can cause metabolic acidosis by generating HCl (13). The total dose of arginine infused during the first two hours (i.e. 180 mmols) of our protocol could generate 180 mEq of HCl after metabolism. This amount of arginine could fully account for the observed fall in plasma bicarbonate (i.e. approximately 7 mEq/l) only if it were metabolized rapidly (i.e. in less than two hours). Because such a rapid metabolism is unlikely, it follows that arginine induces metabolic acidosis at least in part by causing renal losses of bicarbonate (i.e. by causing proximal renal tubular acidosis).

A significant increase in plasma potassium was observed in arginine-infused dogs in agreement with previous observations (5,6,14). This effect was clearly independent of the fall in blood pH because plasma potassium continued to rise despite the administration of sodium bicarbonate. The increase in plasma potassium observed during arginine infusions has been ascribed to the translocation of potassium from cells to the extracellular compartment (15). Our data are consistent with this view and are further supported by the fact that potassium excretion increased markedly despite a significant fall in GFR.

It is of interest that plasma phosphate fell significantly during arginine chloride infusion (Table III). Bicarbonate wastage is often associated with depressed phosphate reabsorption. However, in this study, phosphate excretion decreased markedly. This was observed despite the development of acidosis, a potential phosphaturic factor. Furthermore, bicarbonate infusion failed to increase phosphate excretion. Therefore, arginine infusion caused hypophosphatemia unassociated with phosphate wastage. Whether arginine enhances tubular phosphate reabsorption or not, it is not clarified by this study, because the decrease in phosphate excretion occurred in the face of a fall in GFR and plasma phosphate concentration; thus the filtered load of phosphate fell markedly. The most likely explanation for the fall in plasma phosphate is that of translocation of phosphate from the extracellular space into the cellular space.

Hypophosphatemia is a common complication of hyperalimentation (16). This is often ascribed to the use of phosphate-poor parenteral preparations (17). It is possible, however, that the use of cationic amino acids such as arginine in hyperalimentation is a main determinant of the development of hypophosphatemia. This issue clearly requires investigation. Likewise, proximal bicarbonate wastage may contribute to the hyperchloremic metabolic acidosis developing during hyperalimentation using cationic amino acids. Plasma phosphate and blood pH as well as plasma potassium should be monitored during the use of arginine to test pituitary function or to treat hepatic encephalopathy.

REFERENCES

1. Merimee TJ, Rabinowitz D, Riggs L, Burgess JA, Rimoin DL, McKusick VA: Plasma growth hormone after arginine infusion. N Engl J Med 276:434-439, 1967.

2. Gennari FJ: Differential diagnosis and treatment of metabolic alkalosis, in Acid-Base and Electrolyte Balance, edited by Schwartz AB, Lyons H. New York, Grune and Stratton, 1977, p. 74.

3. Wolfe SJ, Fast BB, Stormont JM, Davidson CS: Treatment of hepatic coma: Use of certain Kreb's urea cycle intermediates (L-arginine, DL-ornithine). J Lab Clin Med 51:627-689, 1958.

4. Reynolds TB, Redeker AG, Davis P: A controlled study of the effects of L-arginine on hepatic encephalopathy. Am J Med 25:359-367, 1958.

5. Hertz P, Richardson JA: Arginine-induced hyperkalemia in renal failure patients. Arch Intern Med 130:778-780, 1972.

6. Bushinsky DA, Gennari J: Life-threatening hyperkalemia induced by arginine. Ann Intern Med 89:632-634, 1978.

7. Wallin JD, Brennar JP, Long DL, Aronoff SL, Rector FC, Jr, Seldin DW: Effect of increased distal bicarbonate delivery on free water reabsorption in the dog. Am J Physiol 224:209-218, 1973.

8. Gougoux A, Lemieux G, Vinay P: Bicarbonaturic effect of lysine in the dog. Kidney Internat 14:215-227, 1978.

9. Chan YL, Kurtzman NA: Effect of lysine on bicarbonate and fluid absorption in the rat proximal tubule. Am J Physiol (In press).

10. Kurtzman NA: Regulation of renal bicarbonate reabsorption by extracellular volume. J Clin Invest 49:586-595, 1970.

11. Batlle D, Arruda JAL: The renal tubular acidosis syndromes. Min elect Metab 5:83-99, 1981.

12. Sabastian A, McSherry E, Morris RC, Jr: Metabolic acidosis with special reference to the renal acidosis, in The Kidney, edited by Brenner B and Rector FC, Jr, Sauders, Philadelphia, 1976, p. 615.

13. Relman AS, Shelbourne PF, Talman A: Profound acidosis resulting from excessive ammonium chloride in previously healthy subjects. N Engl J Med 264:848, 1961.

14. Dickerman HW, Walker WG: Effect of cationic amino acid infusion on potassium metabolism in vivo. Am J Phsyiol 206:403-408, 1964.

15. Levinsky NG, Tyson I, Miller RB, Relman AS: The relation between amino acids and potassium in isolated rat muscle. J Clin Invest 41:480-487, 1962.

16. Sheldon GF, Grzyb S: Phosphate depletion and repletion: Relation to parenteral nutrition and oxygen transport. Ann Surg 182:683, 1975.

17. Travis SJ, Sugerman HJ, Rubery RL, Durick SJ, Delivoria-Papadopoulus M, Millor LD, Oski F: Alterations of red-cell glycolytic intermediates and oxygen transport as a consequence of hypophosphatemia in patients receiving hyperalimentation. N Engl J Med 285:763, 1971.

CARDIAC FUNCTION AND METABOLISM IN PHOSPHOROUS DEPLETED DOGS - EFFECTS OF HORMONAL STIMULATION

W.Kreusser, H.Vetter, H.Mittmann, U.Brückner, H.Hörl, E.Bäuerlein, D.Klormann, E.Ritz

Departments Internal Medicine, Experimental Surgery, Univ. of Heidelberg/Würzburg, and Max-Planck-Institut, Heidelberg, FRG

INTRODUCTION

Phosphorous depletion has recently been recognized as a cause of myocardial dysfunction in humans (1) and animals (2). O'Connor et al. (1) observed low stroke volume in acutely hypophosphatemic alcoholic patients. This abnormality returned to normal upon administration of phosphorous despite no change or even reduction of preload. Furthermore, in chronically phosphorous depleted patients, Darsee and Nutter (3) described a form of hypophosphatemic cardiomyopathy reversible upon phosphorous repletion. Finally, Fuller et al. (2) could reproduce the deleterious effect of phosphorous depletion on cardiac function in dogs with selective hypophosphatemia induced by dietary phosphorous depletion. The authors found a reversible depression of myocardial performance, i.e. of stroke volume, peak blood flow velocity and acceleration. These previous investigations were restricted to basal hemodynamic conditions and no information is available on the cardiac response to catecholamines. Furthermore, cardiac metabolism in phosphorous depletion has not been studied so far. Finally, changes of myocardial nucleotide content or calcium transport characteristics were discussed as possible mechanisms for depressed myocardial function (2). However, no experimentel evidence for such changes has been presented. The present study addresses these problems.

METHODS

12 female foxhounds (14.0 ± 0.67 kg) were examined during a control phase (CO), after 30 days of dietary phosphorous deprivation (PD), and (in 6 dogs) after 21 days of phosphorous repletion (PR). The dogs were anaesthesized with pentobarbital, intubated and artificially ventilated with a O_2/N_2O mixture (1:3). Basal hemodynamics as well as the response to norepinephrine (0.9 µg/kg/min.) and orciprenaline (0.5 µg/kg/min.) were measured.

Hemodynamic measurements: A Swan-Ganz catheter was inserted via the right jugular vein into the pulmonary artery for measurements of PAP (Statham transducer) and cardiac output (thermodilution), a Goodale-Lubin catheter to obtain coronary venous blood; a multipurpose catheter into the femoral artery for measurement of AOP; a catheter tip manometer (Miller) into the femoral artery for measurement of EDP and LVP. V_{pm} was calculated from the V_{CE} curve as described by Sonnenblick (4).

Blood chemistry: Phosphorous was measured after Fiske and Subarow (5); glucose with Technicon Autoanalyser; FFA after Novák (6); cAMP with a radioimmunoassay according to Steiner (7) and lactate or pyruvate enzymatically (8).
Sarcoplasmic reticulum (SR): SR from left ventricular myocardium was prepared according to Suko and Hasselbach (9). The initial rate of uptake and concentrating ability were measured. ATP and energy-rich nucleotides were measured as previously described (10) in quick frozen tissue specimens. Mitochondrial oxidation in heart mitochondria was studied (11).

RESULTS AND DISCUSSION

Table 1 gives biochemical data for control, P_i depletion and P_i repletion periods. PD was confirmed by low serum P_i, low skeletal muscle P_i content (PD 17.2 ± 0.70 pmol/g ww; PR 21.4 ± 0.54; r=6; $p < 0.01$) and hypercalcemia.
Lactate concentrations were significantly increased in the PD period in parallel with pyruvate and there was no difference of L/P-ratio in the CO and PD period. Higher arterial lactate concentrations would be consistant with increased anaerobiosis, but altered hepatic extraction of lactate cannot be excluded.
Under basal conditions, as shown in table 2, animals had resting tachycardia during their PD period. EDP

Table 1. Blood chemistry during control, phosphate depletion and repletion periods. Values are given as $\bar{x} \pm$ SEM.
*denotes significant difference between control and depletion period ($p < 0.01$)
§ denotes significant difference between depletion and repletion period ($p < 0.01$)

	Control period (n=12)	Depletion period (n=12)	Repletion period (n=6)
P_i (mmol/l)	2.35 ± 0.07	1.12 ± 0.03*	2.17 ± 0.08§
Ca (mmol/l)	2.37 ± 0.04	2.67 ± 0.07*	2.22 ± 0.02$
Mg (mmol/l)	0.80 ± 0.04	0.75 ± 0.02	0.74 ± 0.02
Creatinine (umol/l)	61.1 ± 2.65	55.8 ± 5.31	42.5 ± 0.88§
Urea (mmol/l)	5.90 ± 0.50	5.43 ± 0.60	4.53 ± 0.43
Glucose (µmol/l)	5833 ± 306	5583 ± 119	5761 ± 231
Lactate (µmol/l)	602 ± 42.8	945 ± 41.0*	871 ± 84.5
Free fatty acids (µmol/l)	-	424 ± 49.7	364 ± 34.7
CPK (U/l)	48.6 ± 3.1	48.8 ± 4.4	39.8 ± 4.5
Serum protein (g/l)	45.9 ± 1.30	43.3 ± 1.50	47.4 ± 1.30

Table 2. Hemodynamics under basal conditions and under infusion of noradrenaline (NA) and orciprenaline (ORC) in P_i-depleted dogs. Values are given as $\bar{x} \pm$ SEM. * significant difference between P_i depletion ($p<0.01$) Wilcoxon's test for paired differences for 12 animals. §significant difference between P_i depletion and P_i repletion ($p < 0.01$) Wilcoxon's test for paired differences for 6 animals.

	CONTROL PERIOD (n=12)			P_i DEPLETION (n=12)			P_i REPLETION (n=6)		
	Basal	NA	ORC	Basal	NA	ORC	Basal	NA	ORC
HR (min^{-1})	87.8 ± 6.50	89.4 ± 4.20	183 ± 7.60	113 ± 7.90*	89.3 ± 5.50	185 ± 7.10	98.7 ± 5.50§	80.7 ± 3.40	186± 13.2
EDP (mm Hg)	8.00 ± 0.80	14.4 ± 1.00	4.00± 0.70	7.00± 0.70	13.3 ± 1.00	5.50± 0.90	7.40 ± 1.00	11.5 ± 1.10	3.00± 0.70
LVP (mm Hg)	93.5 ± 2.70	141 ± 6.96	101 ± 1.91	99.7± 2.70	148 ± 4.93	113± 5.81	94.2 ± 3.07	136 ± 7.30	106± 2.59
CI (l/min./kg)	0.15 ± 0.01	0.18 ± 0.02	0.28± 0.02	0.16± 0.01	0.20 ± 0.01	0.30± 0.02	0.11 ± 0.01	0.14 ± 0.01	0.27± 0.04
dp/dt_{max} (mm Hg/sec.)	1814 ± 131	4332 ± 260	4445± 192	1982± 127	3705 ± 217*	3909± 260*	1508 ± 68	3275 ± 399	3500± 173
V_{PM} (circ./sec.)	2.90 ± 0.14	3.60 ± 0.14	3.76± 0.17	2.08± 0.18*	2.50 ± 0.20*	2.52± 0.24*	2.86 ± 0.10§	3.17 ± 0.06§	3.72± 0.18§

as an index of left ventricular function and compliance was unchanged under basal conditions. CI, SVI, LVP and dp/dt_{max} were unchanged. In contrast, V_{PM}, an index of myocardial contractile force, was significantly decreased and such decrease was reversed by P_i repletion.

Under infusion of noradrenaline (0.9 µg/kg/min.), LVP rose in the CO period as well as in the PD period. Similarly, dp/dt_{max} rose in the CO period (+ 109%), but to a significantly ($p < 0.01$) lesser extent in the PD period (+ 70.6%). V_{PM} increased markedly in the CO period and significantly less ($p < 0.01$) in the PD period.

During infusion of orciprenaline (0.5 µg/kg/min.), there were similar changes of HR and EDP in the CO and PD periods and virtually no change of LVP. There was a significant rise of dp/dt_{max} in the CO period and to a significant lesser extent in the PD period ($p < 0.01$). Similarly, V_{PM} increased significantly above basal values in the CO period and to a significant lesser extent ($p < 0.01$) in the PD period.

The present study clearly documents impaired myocardial contractile force and impaired inotropic response of the heart to catecholamines in dogs with phosphorous depletion. There was no evidence of overt cardiac insufficiency, since PAP and EDP remained in the normal range and rose to the same extent under infusion of pressor agents in PD and CO animals. However, latent cardiac insufficiency and increased sympathetic drive is suggested by the findings of resting tachycardia and increased arterial cyclic AMP concentration. Basal cAMP concentration was slightly higher in PD (CO: 15.6 ± 1.62 nmol/l; PD: 18.9 ± 1.88). The increment of arterial cAMP with infusion of noradrenaline was greater in the PD period (38.0 ± 5.63) than in the CO period (23.1 ± 0.62). Similar findings were obtained with orciprenaline. This finding suggests, that diminished contractile response to catecholamines involves steps distal to beta-sensitive adenylate cyclase in phosphorous depletion.

Fuller et al. (2) previously hypothesized that impaired calcium transport in the sarcoplasmic reticulum may be responsible for impaired myocardial function. In our study, there was no significant difference of the initial rate of uptake of Ca (PD 0.04 ± 0.005 µmol Ca/mg protein/min.; PR 0.052 ± 0.005) or concentrating ability (PD 0.240 ± 0.003 µmol Ca/mg protein; PR 0.241 ± 0.001). The finding of unchanged subcellular myocardial calcium transport, at least in vitro, is in agreement with our previous results in skeletel muscle

Table 3. Tissue electrolyte and nucleotide levels. ATP: adenosine triphosphate. ADP: adenosine diphosphate; AMP: adenosine monophosphate. Energy charge: ATP + 1/2 ADP/ATP+ADP+AMP. CP: creatine phosphate * denotes significant difference ($p < 0.01$) between phosphate depletion (PD) and repletion (PR) period. Values are given as $\bar{x} \pm$ SEM.

	HEART		SKELETAL MUSCLE	
	PD (n=6)	PR (n=6)	PD (n=6)	PR (n=6)
P_i (μmol/gww)	8.64 ± 0.35*	11.4 ± 0.38	23.39 ± 0.95*	29.10 ± 0.74
Mg (μmol/gww)	102.5 ± 3.48*	114.8 ± 2.61	90.3 ± 1.44*	110.4 ± 1.52
ATP (μmol/gww)	5.30 ± 0.22*	6.13 ± 0.20	4.31 ± 0.20*	5.66 ± 0.24
ADP (μmol/gww)	0.87 ± 0.109	0.90 ± 0.04	0.65 ± 0.03	0.75 ± 0.03
AMP (μmol/gww)	0.24 ± 0.01	0.29 ± 0.04	0.10 ± 0.03	0.12 ± 0.01
CP (μmol/gww)	1.90 ± 0.12*	2.39 ± 0.12	3.81 ± 0.29*	4.88 ± 0.15
Energy charge	0.89 ± 0.01	0.90 ± 0.01	0.92 ± 0.01	0.92 ± 0.01

of PD rats (12).

Finally, the concentration of high energy nucleotides were significantly diminished in PD, as shown in table 3. This finding is complemented by the observation of disturbed mitochondrial respiratory control ratio in hearts of PD rats (CO 5.65 $\pm$0.25 ; PD 4.30 $\pm$ 0.31 ; n=5, $p<0.05$) with no change of ADP/)-ratio (CO 2.50 $\pm$ 0.17; PD 2.30 $\pm$ 0.07). (glutamate/malate as substr).

In summary, the present studies demonstrate that phosphorous depletion impairs myocardial contractile force in the basal state and the inotropic response of the heart to catecholamines (catecholamine resistance). There was no evidence of disturbed subcellular transport, but evidence was obtained for abnormal high energy nucleotide levels and mitochondrial oxidation. These defects were completely reversible with phosphorous repletion.

REFERENCES

1. O'Connor, L.R., Wheeler, W.S., Bethune, J.E. (1977), Effect of hypophosphatemia on myocardial performance in man, N.Engl.J.Med., 297: 901
2. Fuller, T.J., Nichols, W.W., Brenner, B.J., Peterson, J.C. (1978), Reversible depression in myocardial performance in dogs with experimental phosphorous deficiency, J.Clin.Invest., 62: 1194
3. Darsee, J.R., Nutter, D. (1978), Reversible severe congestive cardiomyopathy in three cases of hypophosphatemia, Ann.Int.Med. 89: 867
4. Sonnenblick, E.H., Parmeley, W.W., Koschel, C.W. (1969), The contractile state of the heart expressed by force-velocity relations, Am.J.Cardiol. 23: 488
5. Fiske, C.H., Subbarow, Y. (1925), The colorimetric determination of phosphorous, J.Biol.Chem. 66: 375
6. Novâk, M. (1965), Colorimetric ultramicro method for the determination of free fatty acids, J.Lipid. Res., 6: 431
7. Steiner, A.L., Parker, C.W., Kipnis, D.M. (1972), Radioimmunoassay for cyclic nucleotides, J.Biol. Chem., 247: 1106
8. Bergmeyer, H.U. (1974), Methode der enzymatischen Analyse; 3rd. Ed. Acetoacetate p. 1887-1890; ß-hydroxybuturate, p. 1883-1886: Oxyglutarate p. 1624-1627; Citrate p. 1607-1611; Lactate p. 1510-1514; Pyruvate p. 1491-1496, Verlag Chemie, Weinheim

9. Suko, J., Hasselbach, W. (1976), Characterization of cardiac sarcoplasmic reticulum ATP-ADP phosphate exchange and phosphorylation of the calcium transport adenosine triphosphatase, Eur.J.Biochem. 64: 123-130
10. Kreusser, W.J., Kurokawa, K., Aznar, E., Massry, S.G. (1978), Phosphate depletion. Effect of renal inorganic phosphorous and adenine nucleotides, urinary phosphate and calcium, and calcium balance, Min.Electr. Metab. 5: 30-42
11. Methods in Enzymology, Vol. 10, p. 46-47 (1976)
12. Kreusser, W., Ritz, E., Boland, R., Brachmann, J. (1980), Function of the sarcoplasmic reticulum (SR) in hypophosphatemic myopathy, in: Phosphate and Minerals in Health and Disease, S.G. Massry, E. Ritz, H. John, ed., Plenum Press Corp.

CIRCULATORY RESPONSE TO PRESSOR AGENTS IN PHOSPHOROUS DEPLETION

W. Kreusser, H. Scholz, W. Rascher, A. Schömig, R. Dietz, D. Klormann, E. Ritz

Departments of Internal Medicine and Pharmacology, University of Heidelberg (FRG)

INTRODUCTION

Impaired function of myocardial muscle is a known feature of phosphorous depletion (PD) in man (1,2) and in experimental animals (3). Congestive heart failure has been described in patients, who were chronically phosphorous depleted secondary to ingestion of phosphorous binding agents (2). Furthermore, abnormalities of skeletal muscle function are common in PD (4). However, no information is available on smooth muscle function in PD. Specifically, control of blood pressure and the peripheral response to pressor agents has not been studied.

Some evidence points to abnormal sympathetic function in PD. First, our previous studies (5) showed a low myocardial glycogen content that was normalized by administration of beta-blockers. Second, abnormal cardiac response to catecholamines in PD is described by us in this issue.

In the present study, the function of vascular smooth muscle and its response to catecholamines were examined.

METHODS

12 female <u>foxhounds</u> (14.0 $\pm$ 0.67 kg) were studied after 2 weeks of adaptation on control diet (CO) and then switched to low P_i diet (0.03% P_i). During anaesthesia with sodium pentobarbital (Nembutal^R), measurement of AOP with Statham transducer was performed

in the resting state and after infusion of angiotensin II (Hypertensin[R]) at 0.1 µg/kg/min. Hemodynamic measurements were started when blood pressure had reached steady state.

In male Sprague Dawley rats phosphate depletion was induced by dietary phosphorous restriction for 6 weeks. Control animals were pairweighed to the PD group (6).

Reactivity of vascular smooth muscle to noradrenaline was measured in rats prepared for hind limb perfusion according to the method of Folkow et al. (7). Since flow was kept constant (10 ml/min./100 g tissue), changes in perfusion pressure, as measured via T-tube, directly reflect changes in vascular resistance (8). Cumulative dose response curves to NA were established by perfusion with concentrations of NA varying from 10^{-8} to 10^{-4} mol/l perfusate.

For determinations of plasma noradrenaline (NA), blood was obtained from a catheter inserted into the jugular vein (0.5 ml) the day before the experiment, in the awake rat. The concentration of noradrenaline was determined radioenzymatically (9).

The activities of neuronal and extraneuronal uptake for noradrenaline were determined in the isolated perfused rat heart preparation after Langendorff (perfusion with oxygenated modified Thyrode solution containing tritiated with NA (10^{-7} mol/l). The concentration of radioactive noradrenaline was measured in both perfusate and effluent following the separation procedure described by Graefe (10). The rates of uptake were calculated from the arterio-venous difference under steady state conditions before and after blockade of the neuronal uptake with cocain (3×10^{-5} mol/l) and after additional blockade of the extraneuronal uptake with corticosterone (10^{-4} mol/l).

RESULTS AND DISCUSSION

Blood pressure response to angiotensin in PD dogs (fig. 1).

In phosphate depleted dogs, serum P_i fell from 2.35 $\pm$ 0.07 mmol/l (CO) to 1.12 $\pm$ 0.03 (PD) and rose again during phosphate repletion (PR up to 2.17 $\pm$ 0.08). AOP during the different experimental period is shown in fig. 1. Under basal conditions there was no difference in AOP between CO, PD and PR period. During infusion of angiotensin II (0.1 µg/kg/min.) AOP rose significantly in the CO, PD and PR period. However, the increment of AOP was significantly ($p < 0.01$) smaller

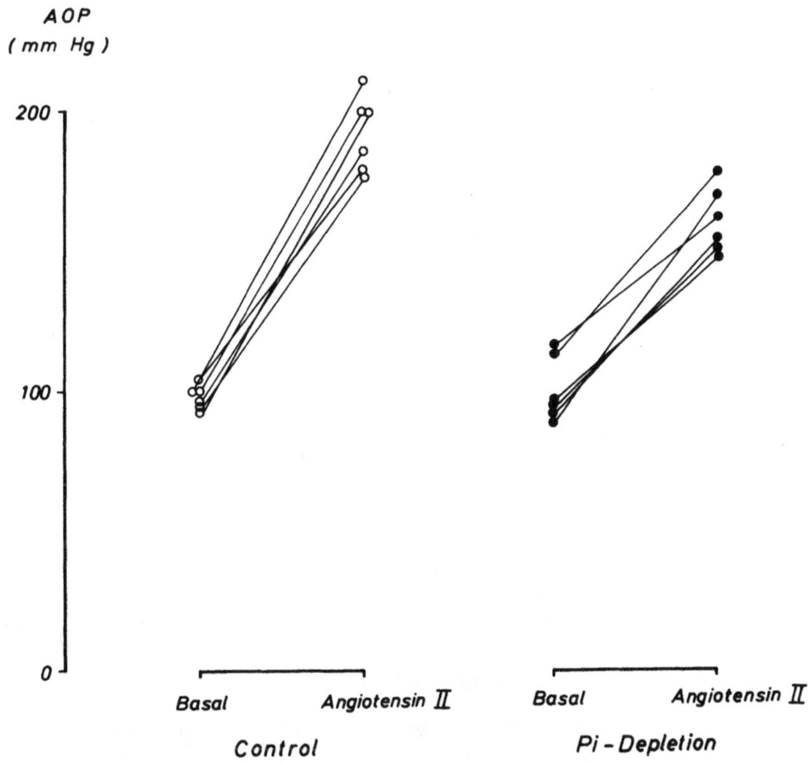

Fig. 1. Effect of P_i depletion on AOP (aortic pressure, mm Hg.) under basal conditions and after stimulation with angiotensin (0.1 µg/kg/min.)

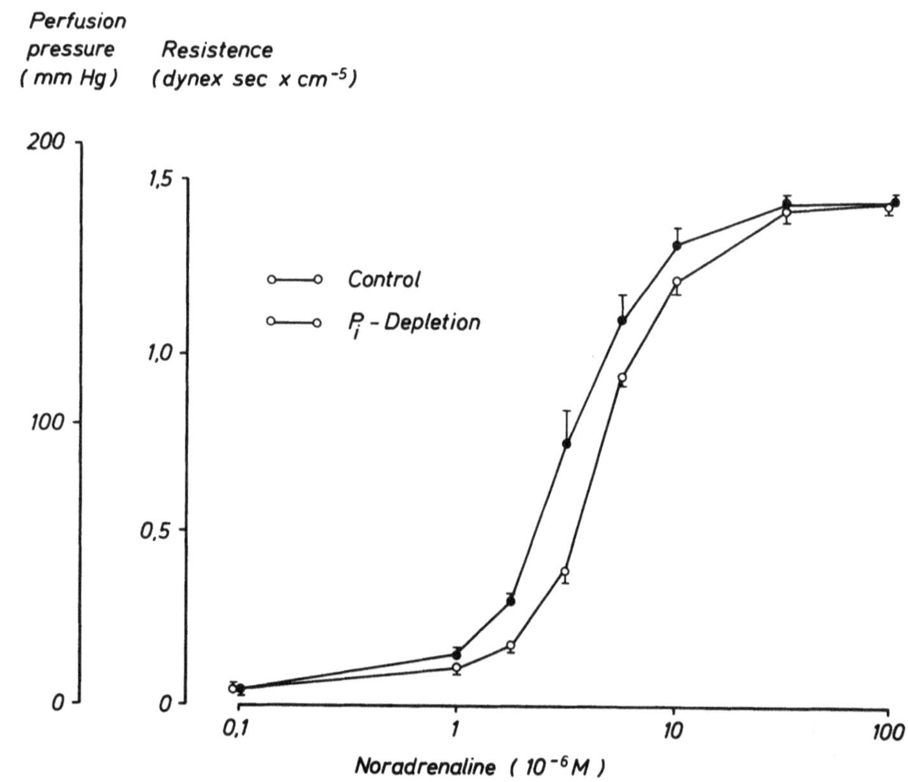

Fig. 2. Dose response curve to noradrenaline in the isolated perfused hind limb preparation of CO and PD animals (n=7). Response (ordinate) is given as the increase in vascular resistance which was calculated as the ratio of recorded increase in perfusion pressure and perfusate flow which was kept constant. Responses are given as mean ± SEM.

in PD animals (CO: + 88 ± 5.98 mm Hg; PD: + 68.2 ± 3.6 mm Hg) and such abnormal rise of AOP was normalized by P_i repletion. The failure of angiotensin II to raise arterial pressure to the same level during PD as in the CO phase (or PR phase) points to angiotensin-resistance of arterioles. To further elucidate the mechanism of such resistance, the following studies were performed.

Vascular reactivity to noradrenaline in PD rats (fig. 2).

Serum P_i was decreased significantly after 6 weeks of P_i depletion (CO 3.24 ± 0.11 mmol/l; PD 0.86 ± 0.09; n=9; $p < 0.001$). The dose response relationship between noradrenaline and vascular resistance in the isolated perfused hind limb of PD rats is given in fig. 2. Resistance was not different in CO and PD animals at maximal dilatation (no NA) and maximal contraction (10^{-4} mol NA/l). The dose response curve of the PD animals was shifted to the right, i.e. PD animals showed diminished responsiveness to submaximal doses of NA (2.5-5.75 x 10^{-6} mol NA/l). In the experiments shown in fig. 2, the ED_{50} was 3.31 ± 0.24 x 10^{-6} mol/l in CO animals and 4.37 ± 0.14 in PD animals (n=7) ($p < 0.01$).

In conclusion, the present study clearly demonstrates an abnormal pressor response (angiotensin II resistance) to angiotensin II of phosphate depleted dogs. The failure of angiotensin II to raise arterial pressure to the same level during phosphorous depletion as in the control phase points to abnormal function of resistance vessels. Further evidence for abnormal function of vascular smooth muscle is provided by the finding of diminished generation of vascular resistance in response to subnormal concentrations of noradrenaline in the isolated perfused hind limb of PD rats. Altered responsiveness to NA is not due to changes in vessel geometry, since no difference between CO and PD was observed at maximal vasodilatation and maximal vasoconstriction. It is of note that altered responsiveness to NA was also observed in heart (Kreusser et al., this issue) and hepatocytes (Hörl et al., this issue) of PD animals. Whether impaired vascular response to NA reflects abnormal function of the contractile apparatus, or other abnormalities (e.g. altered alpha/beta-receptor ratio, down-regulation of NA receptors, abnormal vascular prostaglandin metabolism etc.)remains to be established.

Plasma noradrenaline and uptake for noradrenaline in rats

The plasma noradrenaline concentration was significantly ($p < 0.01$) increased in PD animals (CO: 86 ± 4.69 pg/ml; PD: 221 ± 46.4). Similarly, after 45 min. of exposure to cold significantly higher plasma noradrenaline concentration was found in PD animals (CO: 162 ± 8.04 pg/ml; PD: 362 ± 85.2, n=6, $p < 0.01$).

Neuronal uptake for noradrenaline, i.e. the difference before and after blockade with cocaine ($3x10^{-5}$ mol/l) was slightly, but not significantly diminished in PD animals (CO: 128 ± 5.37 pmol/min./heart; PD: 115 ± 4.22, n=8, n.s.). Similarly, extraneuronal uptake, i.e. the difference before and after blockade with cocaine and corticosterone ($100x10^{-6}$ mol/l) was not significantly diminished in PD (CO:133 ± 6.57 pmol/min./heart; PD: 119 ± 5.16, n=7, n.s.).

Elevated circulating NA levels presumably point to increased sympathetic drive. Altered metabolism of NA is unlikely in view of unchanged neuronal and extraneuronal uptake of NA. Previous studies of our laboratory (5) provided evidence of increased sympathetic activity, i.e. a diminution of cardiac glycogen content which was normalized by beta-blockade. The cause of sympathetic overactivity may be either latent cardiac insufficiency (1-3) or diminished vascular responsiveness to NA or a combination of these factors. Finally, abnormal handling of NA by vascular tissue is unlikely in view of unchanged neuronal and extraneuronal uptake of NA by the heart, but formal exclusion of this possibility requires performance of the experiment with cocaine blockade.

This study shows that abnormal vascular function is another component of the known compromised cardiovascular performance in phosphorous depletion.

REFERENCES

1. O'Connor, L.R., Wheeler, W.S., Bethune, J.E. (1977), Effect of hypophosphatemia on myocardial performance in man, N.Engl.J.Med. 297: 901
2. Darsee, J.R., Nutter, D. (1978), Reversible severe congestive cardiomyopathy in three cases of hypophosphatemia, Ann.Int.Med. 89: 867
3. Fuller, T.J., Nichols, W.W., Brenner, B.J., Peterson, J.C. (1978), Reversible depression in myocardial performance in dogs with experimental phosphorous deficiency, J.Clin.Invest. 62: 1194

4. Kretz, J., Sommer, G., Boland, R., Kreusser, W., Hasselbach, W., Ritz, E. (1980), Lack of involvement of sarcoplasmic reticulum in myopathy of acute phosphorous depletion, Klin.Wschr. 58, 833-837
5. Hörl, W.H., Kreusser, W., Heidland, A., Ritz, E., Abnormalities of glycogen metabolism in cardiomyopathy of phosphorous depletion, in: "Phosphate and Minerals in Health and Disease", S.G. Massry, E. Ritz, H. Jahn, ed., Plenum Publishing Corp., New York and London (1980)
6. Kreusser, W., Kurokawa, K., Aznar, E., Massry, S.G. (1978), Phosphate depletion. Effect of renal inorganic phosphorous and adenine nucleotides, urinary phosphate and calcium, and calcium balance, Min. Electr. Metab. 5: 30
7. Folkow, B., Hallbäck, M., Lindgren, Y., Weiss, C. (1970), Background and increased flow resistance and vascular reactivity in spontaneously hypertensive rats, Acta Physiol. Scand. 80: 93
8. Schömig, A., Lüth, J.B., Dietz, R., Gross, F. (1976) Changes in vascular smooth muscle sensitivity to vasoconstrictor agents induced by corticosteroids, adrenalectomy and differing salt intake in rats, Clin.Sci.Mol.Med. 51: 61
9. Da Prada, M., Zürcher, G. (1976), Simultaneous radioenzymatic determination of plasma and tissue adrenaline, noradrenaline and dopamine within the femtomole range, Life Sciences 19: 1161
10. Graefe, K.H., Stefano, F.J.E., Langer, S.Z. (1973), Preferential metabolism of (-)-^{3}H-norepinephrine through the deaminated glycol in the rat vas deferens, Biochem. Pharmacol. 22: 1147

PHOSPHATE AND VANADATE REDUCE THE EFFICIENCY OF THE CHEMO-MECHANICAL ENERGY TRANSFORMATION IN CARDIAC MUSCLE

Joachim W. Herzig*, John W. Peterson**, Ross J. Solaro***, and Johann C. Rüegg ****

* Preclinical Research, Sandoz Ltd., CH-4002 Basle Switzerland

** Massachusetts General Hospital, Neurosurgical Service, Boston, MA 02114, USA

*** Department of Physiology, University of Cincinnati Cincinnati, OH 45267, USA

**** Department of Physiology II, University of Heidelberg, D-6900 Heidelberg, FRG (where the study was carried out)

SUMMARY

Trabecular preparations from the hog heart right ventricle were "skinned" by treatment with Lubrol WX and glycerol. Ca^{++} activated isometric contractions were gradedly relaxed by inorganic phosphate (P_i) in the millimolar range or vanadate (V_i) in the micromolar range while tension cost (ATP split/force generated) was increased by a factor of 1.75. From measurements of force, ATPase activity, immediate stiffness and stretch activation, evidence is provided that the mechanical deactivation and the increase in tension cost may result from an acceleration of the myosin cross-bridge cycle, due to a direct interference of P_i and V_i with the chemomechanical energy transformation at the contractile proteins. The possible significance of such a mechanism in cardiac failure or muscle fatigue is discussed.

INTRODUCTION

Inorganic phosphate (P_i) is one of the reaction products of adenosinetriphosphate (ATP) cleavage as it occurs in biological systems by the action of adenosinetriphosphatases (ATPases). With increasing energy demand, P_i may accumulate within the cell and is therefore proposed to be an important factor in muscle fatigue (Nassar-Gentina et al., 1976) or, at reduced energy supply, in ischaemia (Furchgott and Lee, 1961; Jacobus et al., 1977). Intracellular accumulation of inorganic phosphate may be one of the mechanisms causing cardiac failure, as Kübler and Katz (1977) reported cytosolic P_i concentrations of up to 48 mM in the ischaemic heart under conditions of early "pump" failure. With decreasing coronary flow, P_i liberation from the myocardial cell becomes impeded so that accumulation of inorganic phosphate may lead to a vicious circle. The nature and mechanism of the P_i induced loss of contractility are not yet completely understood. Kübler and Katz (1977) discuss an electro-mechanical uncoupling in terms of an enhancement of Ca^{++} sequestration, due to accumulation of cytosolic P_i. On the other hand, Rüegg et al. (1971) reported a deactivation of the contractile system of glycerol extracted insect flight muscle by P_i in the millimolar range, at constant, buffered Ca^{++} concentration. Similar results were obtained in glycerol extracted myocardial preparations (Herzig and Rüegg, 1977; Reiermann et al., 1977; Solaro et al., 1980a; Herzig et al., 1981a),demonstrating that, apart from a possible influence on Ca^{++} sequestration, a direct interaction of cytosolic P_i with the contractile proteins of the myocardial cell could be involved in P_i induced myocardial failure.

It is now widely accepted that force development results from the motion of myosin cross-bridges attaching to and detaching from the actin filaments, the force being generated in the attached state by stretching a linear elastic portion of the cross-bridge (Huxley and Simmons, 1971). It has been postulated that P_i interacts directly with the actomyosin ATPase cycle in terms of a product inhibition thereby possibly retarding the dissociation of P_i from the actomyosin-ADP-P_i complex (White, 1973; Taylor, 1979). In view of this, vanadate (V_i) may be a phosphate analogue as it forms a stable myosin-ADP-V_i complex, thereby inhibiting the myosin ATPase (Goodno, 1979). Furthermore, Solaro et al. (1980b) showed that vanadate inhibits myocardial myofibrillar ATPase with a K_i of about 50 μM without affecting Ca^{++} binding. Similar results, but at about 10x higher [V_i],were reported for chemically skinned vascular smooth muscle (Peterson, 1980). Despite this action, vanadate is known to have positive inotropic effects on the intact heart (Hackbarth et al., 1978).

In view of this background, we investigated the effects of P_i and V_i on the mechanics and the ATPase activity of the functionally isolated contractile structures of mammalian heart muscle, with special consideration of myocardial tension cost, defined as ATPase/force, and myosin cross-bridge kinetics.

METHODS

Thin (< 0.3 mm) strips were dissected from fresh hog right ventricular trabecula septomarginalis and immediately suspended in a Lubrol-glycerol extraction solution containing 50 % (vol/vol) glycerol, 0.5 % (wgt/vol) Lubrol WX, 10 mM NaN_3, 20 mM histidine, pH 7.3. In this solution, the preparations were shaken for two days at 4 °C and then transferred into 50 % (vol/vol) glycerol, 10 mM NaN_3, 20 mM histidine, pH 7.0 and stored at -18 °C for about one week before use.

The extracted preparations were mounted with a fast setting glue (cellulose nitrate dissolved in acetone) between a glass rod extending from a servo-feedback driven Ling Dynamics 101 vibrator performing rectangular length changes within 0.5 ms, and a carbon rod extending from an AME AE 801 force transducer (natural frequency 15 kHz).

After mounting, the preparations were relaxed in the relaxation solution. This consisted of 10 mM Mg ATP, 20 mM imidazole, 5 mM phosphoenolpyruvate (PEP), 20 U/ml pyruvate kinase (PK) (Sigma, type III), 5 mM NaN_3, 5 mM EGTA, pH 7.0 at 25 °C. KCl was added to adjust ionic strength to 0.15 M. pCa ($-\log[Ca^{++}]$) > 8. Graded sustained Ca^{++} activated contractions were elicited in the contraction solution which was identical to the relaxation solution with the exception of graded replacement of EGTA by Ca-EGTA thereby adjusting the pCa to values between 8 and 4.5 using the apparent association constants for the chelation of Ca^{++} and Mg^{++} calculated according to Portzehl et al. (1964). Experiments in presence of inorganic phosphate (P_i) or sodium vanadate (V_i, obtained from Fisher Chemicals) were performed in relaxation and contraction solutions in which KCl was reduced to keep ionic strength constant at 0.15 M. At pH 7.0, the predominant ionic species of vanadate is $H_2VO_4^-$ which we refer to as V_i.

During force measurements, the ATPase activity of the Lubrol-glycerol extracted preparations was determined in the well stirred incubation bath (1 ml) using an NADH coupled optical test for pyruvate which, by the action of the ATP reconstituting system, is formed in stoichiometric relation to the ATP split by the preparation, according to the following scheme:

$$ATP \longrightarrow ADP + P_i$$

$$ADP + PEP \xrightarrow[PK]{} ATP + pyruvate$$

For detection, pyruvate was then reduced to lactate by the lactate dehydrogenase (LDH) reaction:

$$\text{pyruvate + NADH} \xrightarrow[\text{LDH}]{} \text{lactate + NAD}$$

After 10 min of fibre incubation, a 0.8 ml sample of the bathing solution was mixed with 15 µl 13 mM β-NADH dissolved in 2 M Tris-HCl/400 mM $MgCl_2$, pH 8.6. Absorbance at 340 nm was determined before and after addition of 10 µl LDH (Sigma, type II). The absorbance - change was then related to ADP production using a calibration factor of 6 units ± 0.2 $A_{340\ nm}$/mM ADP, which was not affected by up to 1 mM V_i or 20 mM P_i. Non-incubated solution samples served for determination of background ADP and pyruvate. Typical absorbance differences above background were 0.15 - 0.20 (pCa 4.5, fibre dimensions ~0.2 x 5.0 mm). For normalization, the fibres were dissolved in boiling sodium dodecyl sulfate after each experiment, and subjected to total protein determination according to Lowry et al. (1951).

Immediate stiffness (S) as a measure for the number of myosin cross-bridges attached to actin at any one moment (Huxley and Simmons, 1971; Herzig, 1978) was determined from the extreme elastic force (ΔT) in response to a rectangular quick (0.5 ms) change in length (ΔL) according to:

$$S = \frac{\Delta T}{\Delta L}$$

The time constant τ of the delayed force development in response to quick stretch (stretch activation) was determined according to Kerzig and Herzig (1974) by extrapolation of the quasi exponential stretch activation transient. τ is defined as the time between the instant of stretch and the moment, at which the extrapolated transient reaches a value 1/e less than its maximum.

All experiments were carried out at a temperature of 25 ± 0.5 °C and a pH of 7.0.

RESULTS

Inhibition of Ca^{++} Activated Force by Phosphate and Vanadate

Incubation of the Lubrol-glycerol treated, functionally isolated contractile structures in Mg-ATP salt solutions containing different concentrations of free Ca^{++} ions resulted in graded isometric contractions. Relaxation was induced in the absence of Ca^{++} (pCa = $-\log[Ca^{++}] > 8$), maximal activation was reached at a pCa of 4.5 (~ 3 x 10^{-5} M Ca^{++}). At pCa 6.1, the force development was half maximal (Fig. 1). Addition of P_i or

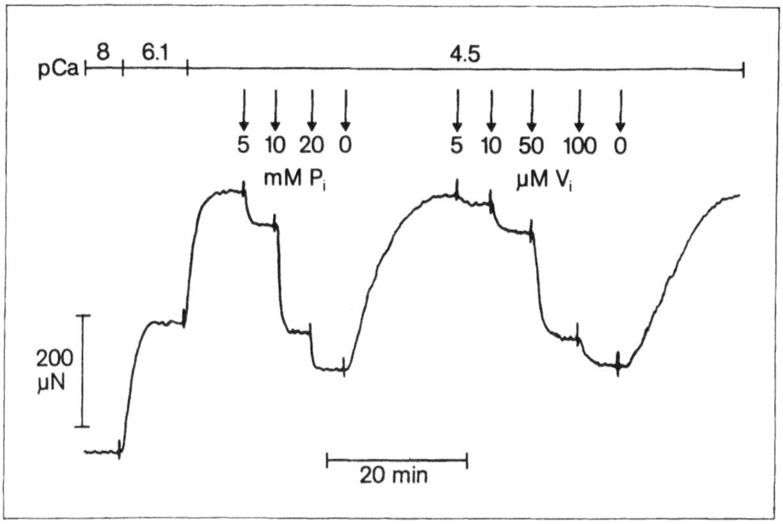

Fig. 1. Partial relaxation of Ca^{++} activated force by inorganic phosphate (P_i) or vanadate (V_i). Increasing the Ca^{++} concentration from pCa 8 over 6.1 to 4.5 induces graded isometric contractions which are reversibly partially relaxed by P_i in the millimolar range and V_i in the micromolar range. Note: addition of either 10 mM P_i or 50 µM V_i at pCa 4.5 leads to the same drop in force (by about 50 %) as a decrease in Ca^{++} concentration from pCa 4.5 to 6.1. Lubrol-glycerol extracted myocardial strip from the hog trabecula septomarginalis; 25 °C. For medium composition see Methods.

V_i in increasing concentrations of up to 20 mM or 100 µM led to graded relaxation of the maximally Ca^{++} activated preparations at a constant pCa of 4.5, buffered with 5 mM Ca-EGTA (Fig. 1). This relaxation was fully reversible by removal of P_i or V_i. Ionic strength was kept constant during the experiments (cf. Methods).

Influence of Phosphate and Vanadate on the Ca^{++} Activated ATPase of the Contractile Structures

During Ca^{++} activated isometric contractions, elicited at various pCa values and during relaxation, the ATPase activity of the functionally isolated contractile structures was measured in parallel to force. The suprabasal values of both parameters, exceeding the basal values in relaxation at pCa 8, were assumed to be due to Ca^{++} activation and are therefore referred to as "Ca^{++} activated ATPase" and "Ca^{++} activated force". Figure 2 shows

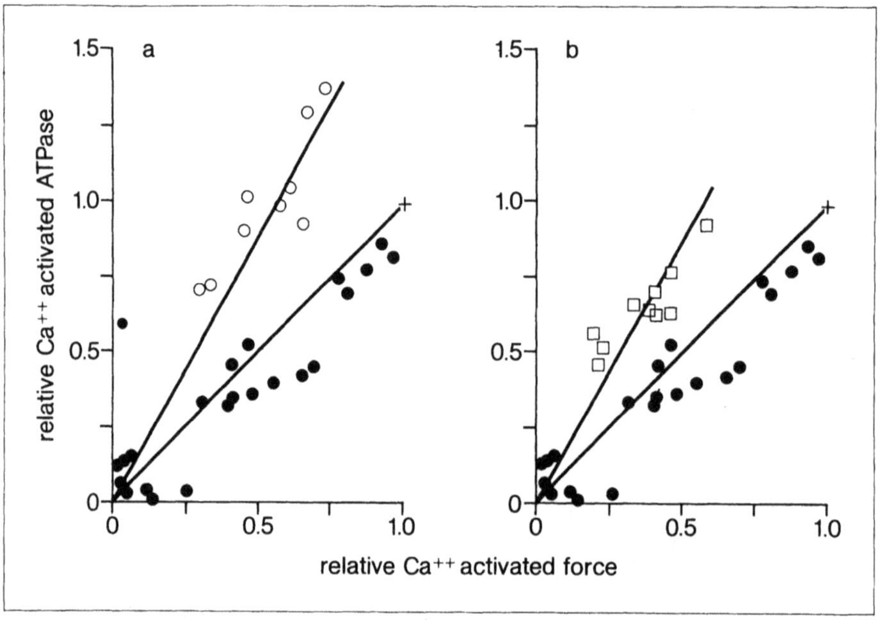

Fig. 2. Influence of P_i (a) or V_i (b) on the relationship between Ca^{++} activated force and Ca^{++} activated ATPase. a) and b): -●-control values obtained by variation of pCa in the absence of P_i or V_i (the corresponding line is the line of identity). a): -O- data obtained in various preparations at pCa 4.5 in presence of 20 mM P_i. b) -□- data obtained in various preparations at pCa 4.5 or 5 in presence of varying concentrations (20 - 50 µM) of V_i. Note: The tension cost (ATPase/force = slope of the diagram) increases in presence of P_i or V_i, rendering the chemo-mechanical energy transformation less economical. Lubrol-glycerol extracted strips from the hog trabecula septomarginalis; 25 °C. For medium composition see Methods.

that these two parameters are linearly correlated (cf. also Schädler, 1967). Typical values of ATPase activity were 30 - 40 nmolADP/mg protein per min in the fully Ca^{++} activated state and 6 - 8 nmolADP/mg protein per min in the relaxed state, induced by EGTA.

On addition of P_i or V_i in concentrations of up to 20 mM or 100 µM, Ca^{++} activated force was reduced in a concentration dependent manner at constant ionic strength and pCa (Fig. 1). P_i and V_i had negligible effects on the basal ATPase activity of the relaxed preparations at pCa >8. On the other hand, at any particular level of force development, P_i and V_i activated the ATPase above control values, obtained at the same force development achieved by varying pCa. At maximum Ca^{++} activation (pCa 4.5), addition of 20 µM V_i caused a 40 % decrease in force without a significant change in ATPase activity (Fig. 2b) while on addition of P_i, the ATPase activity even increased while force was reduced (Fig. 2a). This behaviour is reflected by an increase in the slope of the ATPase-force relation which, defined as ATPase/force, provides a relative measure of the tension cost of the contractile system. In figure 2, it is shown that both P_i and V_i increase the tension cost by a factor of 1.75 as compared to the control in absence of P_i or V_i.

Proportional Decrease of Force and Immediate Stiffness by Phosphate and Vanadate

To obtain further information about the chemo-mechanical energy coupling with P_i and V_i, immediate stiffness as a measure for the number of cross-bridges attached to actin at any one moment (Huxley and Simmons, 1971) was measured. At different states of partial relaxation by various concentrations of P_i and V_i at a constant pCa of 4.5 (cf. Fig. 1), quick rectangular length changes (rise time 0.5 ms) were applied to the contractile structures (cf. also Fig. 5). The extreme elastic force responses (T_1) reached during stretch and release, respectively, were plotted versus amplitude and direction of the length change applied (Fig. 3) in form of T_1-curves (cf. Huxley and Simmons, 1971). The points where the T_1-curves intersect the ordinate (force axis) represent the steady state forces (length change $\Delta L = 0$) of the contractile structures under conditions of complete Ca^{++} activation in absence or at partial relaxation induced by the presence of P_i (Fig. 3a) or V_i (Fig. 3b) at various concentrations. All T_1-curves may be described as straight lines deviating from the linear function in the range of release exceeding 1 % of the initial preparation length (L_i). With decreasing force, i.e. with increasing concentrations of P_i or V_i at a constant pCa of 4.5, the slopes of the T_1- curves ($\Delta T/\Delta L$ = immediate stiffness) decrease, indicating a decrease in the number of myosin cross-bridges attached to actin at any one moment. Extrapolation of the linear portions of all

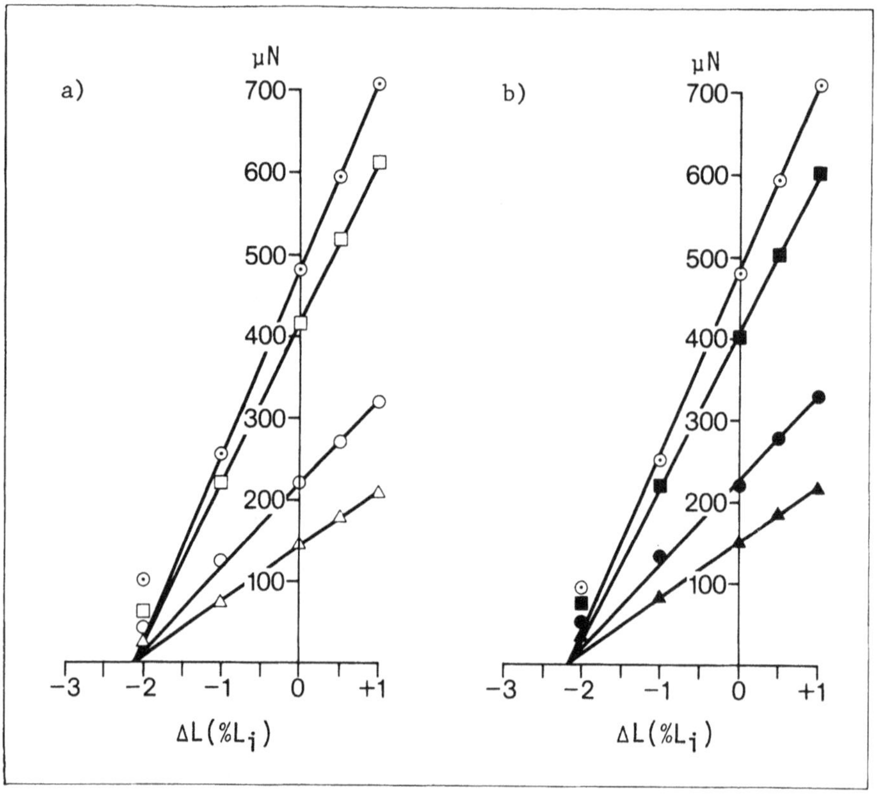

Fig. 3. Force-extension diagrams (T_1-curves) obtained in the absence or presence of P_i (a) or V_i (b). The immediate elastic response (μN) to stretch (+ΔL) or release (-ΔL) is plotted versus the length change (cf. Fig. 5). All data are obtained at pCa 4.5.

a) ⊙ without P_i, □ 5 mM P_i,
○ 10 mM P_i, △ 20 mM P_i.

b) ⊙ without V_i, ■ 10 μM V_i,
● 50 μM V_i, ▲100 μM V_i.

Note that all T_1-curves are straight lines deviating from the linear function in the range of large releases (> 1 %) and extrapolate to a common abscissa intercept at a release of 2.2 % of the initial length (L_i). Lubrol-glycerol extracted strip from the hog trabecula septomarginalis; 25 °C. For medium composition see Methods.

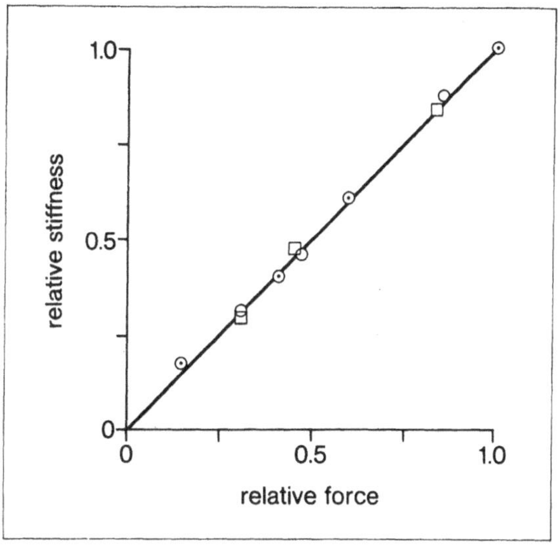

Fig. 4. Relationship between force and immediate stiffness as obtained from experiments as shown in figure 3 . Note that immediate stiffness, the slope of the T_1-curve, is altered in proportion to force, irrespective whether force is changed by alterations in Ca^{++} concentration - ⊙ - or by addition of P_i (- o -) or V_i (- □ -) at constant Ca^{++} concentration (pCa 4.5). Lubrol-glycerol extracted strips from the hog trabecula septomarginalis; 25 °C. For medium composition see Methods.

T_1-curves, in absence or presence of P_i or V_i, leads to a common abscissa intercept at a release of 2.2 % L_i. Plotting the slopes of the T_1-curves as a measure for immediate stiffness versus the corresponding isometric forces (ordinate intercepts) results in a straight line, i.e. stiffness and isometric force are linearly correlated, irrespective of whether force is altered by variation of pCa or by addition of P_i or V_i at constant pCa (Fig. 4).

Influences of Phosphate and Vanadate on the Kinetics of Stretch Activation

The finding of increasing ATPase activity at decreasing force and stiffness (increase in tension cost) suggests that P_i and V_i affect the kinetics of the myosin cross-bridges. Therefore, stretch activation transients were measured. According to Thorson and White (1969), the time constant τ of the delayed, quasi exponential tension rise following quick stretch (Fig. 5) provides a measure of the rate of cross-bridge detachment. τ is defined as the time which passes between the instant of stretch and the moment at which the exponentially extrapolated tension rise reaches a value 1/e less than its maximum (cf. Methods).

Figure 5 shows stretch activation transients, obtained at pCa 6.1 (half maximal Ca^{++} activation)and 4.5 (complete Ca^{++} activation) in absence and presence of P_i and V_i. It is shown that addition of 10 mM P_i or 50 µM V_i at a constant pCa of 4.5 (Fig. 5 C,D) reduces the steady state force (T_o) before stretch to approximately the value reached in the absence of P_i or V_i by reducing the Ca^{++} concentration to pCa 6.1 (Fig. 5B). Quick, rectangular stretch (rise time 0.5 ms) leads, after the initial "viscoelastic" peak (T_1), to a delayed, quasi exponential force development (stretch activation). It is clearly shown that in presence of 10 mM P_i (Fig. 5C) stretch activation is considerably faster than at pCa 4.5 or 6.1 in absence of P_i (Fig. 5A,B). τ values were 180 ms at pCa 4.5 with 10 mM P_i and 400/580 ms at pCa 4.5/6.1 without P_i. Also 50 µM V_i accelerates stretch activation (τ = 370 ms) as compared to the controls but the effect is much less pronounced than with P_i. Washout of P_i or V_i (Fig. 5E) restores steady state force and stretch activation to the values before administration of the minerals (compare Fig.5 E with A).

DISCUSSION

Our data obtained from measurements of force, ATPase activity, stiffness and stretch activation raise evidence that inorganic phosphate (P_i) and vanadate (V_i) interfere with the chemo-mechanical energy transformation at the myosin cross-bridges of the myocardial cell.

With variation of force (Fig. 1) induced either by changes in Ca^{++} concentration or by addition of P_i or V_i, the Ca^{++} activated ATPase activity in both cases is altered in proportion to force (Fig. 2). However, the tension cost, defined as the ratio ATPase/ force, is higher with P_i or V_i than in the absence of these minerals, i.e. P_i and V_i render the chemo-mechanical energy transformation less economical. Such a decrease in economy of force production could be brought about by two different mechanisms:

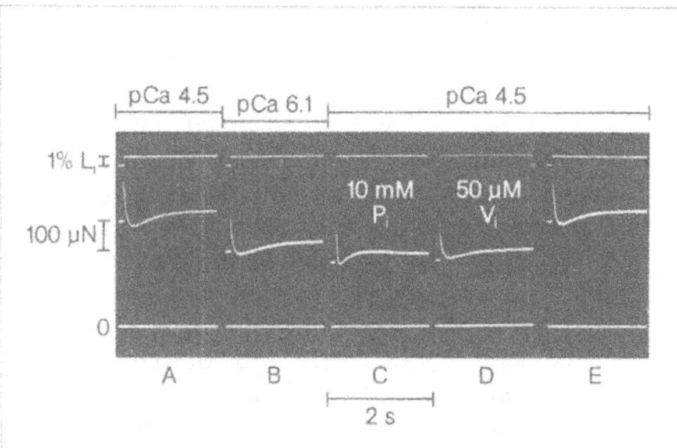

Fig. 5. Influence of Ca^{++}, P_i and V_i on the time course of force transients in response to quick stretch. pCa, $[P_i]$ and $[V_i]$ as given in the graph. Upper trace: time course of rapid stretch (rise time 0.5 ms). Middle trace: time course of force (force before stretch = T_o, extreme force reached during stretch = T_1, cf. figure 3). Lower trace = zero force. Note that 1) T_o is reduced by decreasing Ca^{++} concentration or by addition of P_i or V_i. 2) The time course of the quasi exponential rise in force (stretch activation) following the initial viscoelastic peak is accelerated by increasing Ca^{++} concentration or by addition of P_i or, less markedly, by addition of V_i. Lubrol-glycerol extracted strips from the hog trabecula septomarginalis; 25 °C. For medium composition see Methods.

1) The force produced by an individual cross-bridge (and therefore by a given amount of ATP split) could be reduced. According to Huxley and Simmons (1971) the force generating step of the cross-bridge cycle is the angular motion of the attached cross-bridge on the actin filament, thereby lengthening a series elastic bridge component (SEC) (cf. also Herzig et al., 1981b) the potential energy of which then contributes to force. The abscissa intercepts of the extrapolated T_1-curves (Fig. 3) are assumed to provide a measure for the amplitude of lengthening of the SEC in an individual cross-bridge and therefore a relative measure for the mechanical potential energy stored in it. As shown in figure 3, the abscissa intercepts obtained in absence and presence of P_i or V_i are identical. This rules out the possibility that P_i or V_i diminish the angular cross-bridge motion. This is also clearly demonstrated in figure 4 which shows that, irrespective of the absence or presence of P_i or V_i, a constant linear relationship is maintained between force and immediate stiffness which, according to Huxley and Simmons (1971), provides a measure for the number of cross-bridges attached to actin at any one moment. This suggests that the force produced by the individual cross-bridge is a constant.

2) The duration of the force generating step of the cross-bridge cycle could be diminished by P_i or V_i. This would reduce the probability of simultaneous force production by a certain number of cross-bridges at a given instant. This mechanism would imply an increase in the probability of cross-bridge detachment from the force generating state and would therefore shorten the cross-bridge cycle and increase the rate of ATP splitting by a single cross-bridge. This would then, consequently, lead to an increase in the ratio ATP split per force generated, i.e. to an increase in tension cost as it was observed in the present study (cf. Fig. 2).According to Thorson and White (1969), the rate of cross-bridge detachment is reflected by the reciprocal value of the time constant τ of the delayed tension development during stretch activation. Figure 5 shows that stretch activation is markedly accelerated by P_i and, less pronounced, by V_i indicating an increase in the rate of cross-bridge detachment.

It may be asserted that the P_i or V_i induced decrease in Ca^{++} activated force may be due to Ca^{++} complexation. There are two arguments against this assertion: a) The Ca^{++} concentration was buffered with EGTA so that changes in the free Ca^{++} concentration would be compensated. b) With decreasing Ca^{++} concentration, the time constant τ of stretch activation would increase (compare Fig. 5A with B) instead of decrease as it is the case with P_i or V_i (cf. Herzig and Herzig, 1974; Herzig and Rüegg, 1977).

It is concluded from our evidence that P_i and V_i interact with the contractile system of Lubrol-glycerol treated cardiac muscle, directly, rendering the chemo-mechanical energy transformation less economical. Our data suggest that this increase in tension cost results from a P_i or V_i induced acceleration of cross-bridge kinetics, possibly due to an increase in the rate of cross-bridge detachment. Such a mechanism is proposed to be involved in muscle fatigue or in energetic cardiac failure, i.e. in conditions when inorganic phosphate accumulates in the cytosol. As the phosphorylation degree of the contractile proteins plays an important role in the regulation of contractility and Ca^{++} responsiveness (Ray and England, 1976; McClellan and Winegrad, 1978; Herzig and Rüegg, 1980) it is tempting to suggest that the observed mechanical deactivation and the increase in tension cost may be due to interference of P_i of V_i with e.g. myosin light chain phosphatase which is known to be inhibited by inorganic phosphate.

ACKNOWLEDGEMENT

The authors thank Mrs D. Eubler for expert technical assistance. This study was supported by the Deutsche Forschungsgemeinschaft (SFB 90) and by the U.S.P.H.S. (grant R 01 HL 22231).

REFERENCES

Furchgott, R.F., and Lee, K.S., 1961, High energy phosphates and the force of contraction of cardiac muscle., Circ. Res., 24:416.

Goodno, C.C., 1979, Inhibition of the myosin ATPase by vanadate ion, Proc. Nat. Acad. Sci., 76:2620.

Hackbarth, I., Schmitz, W., Scholz, H., Erdmann, E. Krawietz, W., and Philipp, G., 1978, Positive inotropism of vanadate in cat papillary muscle, Nature, 275:67.

Herzig, J.W., 1978, A cross-bridge model for inotropism as revealed by stiffness measurements in cardiac muscle, Basic Res. Cardiol., 73:273.

Herzig, J.W., and Herzig, U.B., 1974, Effect of Ca-ions on contraction speed and force generation in glycerinated heart muscle, Symp. Biol. Hung., 17:85.

Herzig, J.W., Peterson, J.W., Rüegg, J.C., and Solaro, R.J., 1981a, Vanadate and phosphate ions reduce tension and increase cross-bridge kinetics in chemically skinned heart muscle, Biochem. Biophys. Acta, 672:191.

Herzig, J.W., and Rüegg, J.C., 1977, Myocardial cross-bridge activity and its regulation by Ca^{++}, phosphate and stretch, in: "Myocardial Failure", G. Riecker, A. Weber, J. Goodwin, eds., Springer, Berlin-Heidelberg-New York.

Herzig, J.W., and Rüegg, J.C., 1980, Investigations on glycerinated cardiac muscle fibres in relation to the problem of regulation of cardiac contractility - effects of Ca^{++} and c-AMP, Basic Res. Cardiol., 75:26.

Herzig, J.W., Yamamoto, T., and Rüegg, J.C., 1981b, Dependence of force and immediate stiffness on sarcomere length and Ca^{++} activation in frog skinned muscle fibres, Pflüger's Arch. Eur. J. Physiol., 389:97.

Huxley, A.F., and Simmons, R.M., 1971, Proposed mechanism of force generation in striated muscle, Nature, 233:533.

Jacobus, W.E., Taylor, G.J., Hollis, D.P., and Nunnally, R.L., 1977, Phosphorus nuclear magnetic resonance of perfused working rat hearts, Nature, 265:756.

Kübler, W., and Katz, A.M., 1977, Mechanism of early "pump" failure of the ischemic heart: possible role of adenosine triphosphate depletion and inorganic phosphate accumulation, Amer. J. Cardiol., 40:467.

Lowry, O.H., Rosebrough, N.D., Farr, A.C., and Randall, R.J., 1951, Protein measurements with the Folinphenol reagent, J. Biol. Chem., 193:265.

McClellan, G.B., and Winegrad, S., 1978, The regulation of the calcium sensitivity of the contractile system in mammalian cardiac muscle, J. Gen. Physiol., 72:737.

Nassar-Gentina, V., Passonneau, J.V., Vergara, J.L., and Rapoport, S.I., 1976, Relation of fatigue state in frog single muscle fibres to concentrations of glycogen, phosphocreatine (PCr) and ATP, Biophys. J., 16:206.

Peterson, J.W., 1980, Vanadate ion inhibits actomyosin interaction in chemically skinned vascular smooth muscle, Biochem. Biophys. Res. Com., 95:1846.

Portzehl, H., Caldwell, P.C., and Rüegg, J.C., 1964, The dependence of contraction and relaxation of muscle fibres from the crab maia squinado on the internal concentration of free calcium ions, Biochim. Biophys. Acta, 79:581.

Ray, K.P., and England, P., 1976, Phosphorylation of the inhibitory subunit of troponin and its effect on the calcium dependence of cardiac myofibril adenosine triphosphatase, FEBS Lett., 70:11.

Reiermann, H.J. Herzig, J.W., and Rüegg, J.C., 1977, Ca^{++} activation of ATPase activity, ATP-P_i exchange, and tension in briefly glycerinated heart muscle, Basic Res. Cardiol., 72:133.

Rüegg, J.C., Schädler, M., Steiger, G.J., and Müller, G., 1971, Effects of inorganic phosphate on the contractile mechanism, Pflüger's Arch. Eur. J. Physiol., 325:359.

Schädler, M.H., 1967, Proportionale Aktivierung von ATPase-Aktivität und Kontraktionsspannung durch Calciumionen in isolierten contractilen Strukturen verschiedener Muskelarten, Pflüger's Arch. Eur. J. Physiol., 296:70.

Solaro, R.J., Holroyde, M.J., Herzig, J.W., and Peterson, J., 1980a, Cardiac relaxation and myofibrillar interactions with phosphate and vanadate, Eur. Heart. J., 1 (Suppl. A):21.

Solaro, R.J., Holroyde, M.J., Matlib, A., Wang, T., Grupp, I., Grupp, G., and Schwartz, A., 1980b, Effects of vanadate on biochemical and contractile properties of rabbit hearts, J. Cardiovasc. Pharmacol., 2:445.

Taylor, E.W., 1979, Mechanism of actomyosin ATPase and the problem of muscle contraction, CRC Critical Rev. Biochem., 6:103.

Thorson, J., and White, D.C.S., 1969, Distributed representations for actin-myosin interaction in the oscillatory contraction of muscle, Biophys. J., 9:360.

White, D.C.S., 1973, Links between mechanical and biochemical kinetics of muscle, Cold Spring Harb. Symp. quant. Biol, 37:201.

EFFECTS OF HYPOPHOSPHATEMIA ON PULMONARY MUSCLE PERFORMANCE

Roque F. Planas, Reuben H. McBrayer and Peter A. Koen

Departments of Internal Medicine and Physiology
Eastern Virginia Medical School
Norfolk, Virginia

INTRODUCTION

Hypophosphatemia is a disorder often characterized by muscle weakness (1). In studies of cardiac performance in hypophosphatemic patients, O'Connor (2) found that muscle contractility could be increased by phosphate repletion. Similar results were obtained by Fuller (3) in dogs fed a phosphorus deficient diet. Studies in adult patients (4,5,6) have shown that pulmonary muscle weakness may also be associated with hypophosphatemia, although the decrease in muscle force has not been measured. We therefore investigated the effects of a dietary - induced phosphorus depletion on pulmonary muscle force in dogs.

Phosphate depletion may have separate effects depending on the rate of energy utilization by pulmonary muscle. The effect of hypophosphatemia on pulmonary force was thus evaluated in two separate experimental protocols. The static changes in pulmonary force were evaluated at the beginning and end of a 10 week period of phosphorus depletion in the first experimental protocol. Dynamic changes in pulmonary muscle force were evaluated in a second series of experiments by measuring the change in force following a series of fatiguing stimulations in both phosphate depleted and control animals.

METHODS

Static Changes in Pulmonary Muscle Force

Maximum mouth pressure (Pm) was measured in four male mongrel dogs weighing 18 ± 0.1 Kg (mean ± SE) in this portion of the protocol. On the day of the study the dogs were intubated with a side port of the endotracheal tube connected to a pressure transducer. Contraction of the diaphragm was achieved by inserting a stimulating electrode through a catheterized femoral vein. The electrode was positioned near the external border of the inferior vena cava above the right diaphragm. This permitted phrenic nerve stimulation since the nerve lies within the fascia of the inferior vena cava. The endotracheal tube was then occluded while measuring Pm during one-to-two seconds of tetanic phrenic nerve stimulation (120 hz, 0.2 ms duration). Phosphorus depletion was then induced by feeding the animals 350 grams per day of a low phosphate diet as described by Coburn and Massry (7) and by the administration of 60 ml/day of aluminum carbonate gel over a ten week period. On chemical analysis each 350 grams of the diet contained 91 mg of elemental phosphorus. Measurements of Pm and serum phosphorus were determined prior to placing the animals on the low phosphate diet and at the end of the depletion period.

Dynamic Changes in Pulmonary Muscle Force

The effect of hypophosphatemia on diaphragmatic fatigue was evaluated in three dogs (21 ± 2 kg) fed a normal diet and in six dogs (22 ± 2 kg) fed the same phosphorus deficient diet. The phosphorus depleted animals were studied once their plasma phosphorus was approximately 1 mg%. The dogs were intubated on the day of the study with a side port of the endotracheal tube connected to a pressure transducer for Pm measurement. Transdiaphragmatic pressure (Pdi), which is defined as the difference between gastric and esophageal pressures (Pgas - Ppl) was also measured. Both Pgas and Ppl were measured by two thin latex balloons attached to polyethylene catheters, which in turn were connected to pressure transducers. The esophageal balloon, which was used as an index of pleural pressure (8), was placed in the lower esophagus. The gastric balloon was placed in the stomach and was used as an index of abdominal pressure according to the method of Agostoni and Rahn (9).

Diaphragmatic fatigue was accomplished by repeatedly stimulating the diaphragm at two frequencies of stimulation (20 and 120 hz, 0.2 ms duration) using the transvenous electrode technique discussed in the last section. Fatigue has been previously quantified in the diaphragm (10,11) by measuring the force that the muscle generates at different frequencies of stimulation. The fatiguing sequence of stimulation consisted of 4 seconds of

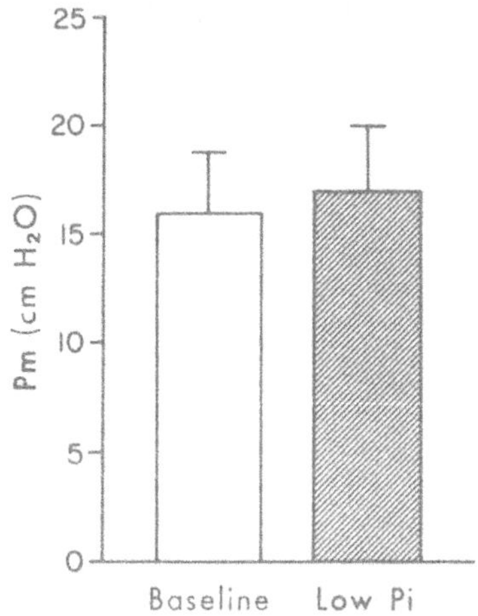

Figure 1. Change in mouth pressure (Pm) following 10 weeks of phosphorus depletion. Values are means ± 1 SE.

tetanus at 20 hz, 4 seconds of rest, 4 seconds of tetanus at 120 hz and 4 seconds of rest. This stimulation pattern was repeated over a 15 minute period with the airway left unoccluded. Both Pm and Pdi were measured before and after the fatiguing sequence at the two stimulation frequencies. Arterial blood samples were drawn both before and after the fatigue period and analyzed for PaO_2, $PaCO_2$ and pH.

RESULTS

Static Changes in Pulmonary Muscle Force

After administration of the low phosphate diet and aluminum carbonate gel, the serum phosphorus fell significantly ($p < 0.01$) from 4.4 ± 0.4 mg% at the beginning of the study to 1.5 ± 0.3 mg% at the end of the ten week period of depletion. There was, however, no significant change ($p > 0.50$) in Pm between baseline and week 10 of depletion (figure 1).

Dynamic Changes in Pulmonary Muscle Force

There was a significant difference ($p < 0.001$) in serum phosphorus between the control (5.7 ± 0.3 mg%) and phosphorus depleted group (1.1 ± 0.2 mg%) in this experimental protocol. The changes in Pm and Pdi at both stimulation frequencies are shown in figure 2 with each animal's pre-fatigue measurement used as baseline. The

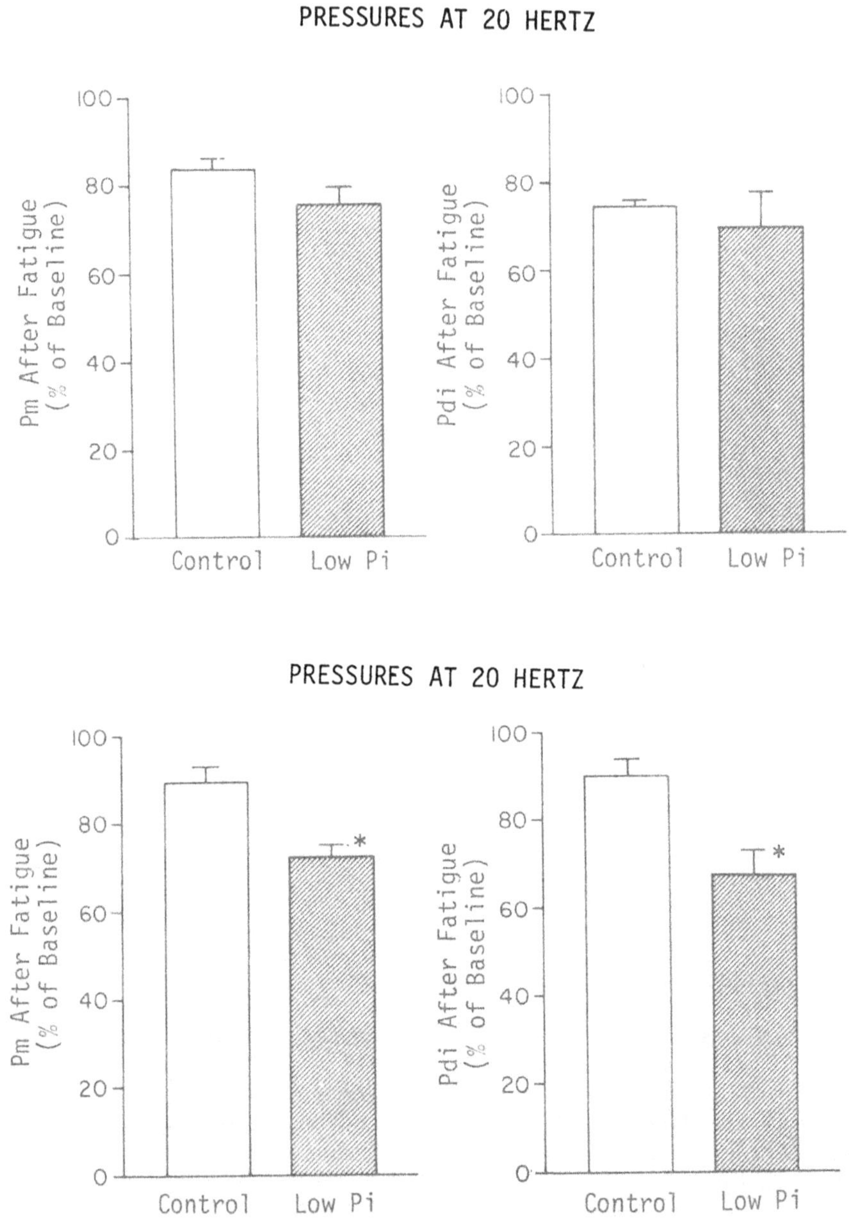

Figure 2. Change in mouth (Pm) and transdiaphragmatic (Pdi) pressure following a fatiguing series of stimulations. The top panel shows Pm and Pdi measured at a stimulation frequency of 20 hz. The bottom panel shows Pm and Pdi measured at a stimulation frequency of 120 hz. Values are means $\pm$ 1 SE. *Difference from control group of animals significant at $p < 0.05$.

The phosphorus deficient group fatigued significantly ($p < 0.05$) more than the control at the 120 hz stimulation frequency. There was no difference ($p > 0.10$) between the control and depleted group at the 20 hz stimulation frequency. There was no significant change ($p > 0.10$) in blood gases drawn before (pH = 7.38 $\pm$ 0.02, $PaCO_2$ = 30 $\pm$ 1 PaO_2 = 93 $\pm$ 5) and immediately after the fatiguing stimulation. (pH = 7.37 $\pm$ 0.01, $PaCO_2$ = 28 $\pm$ 1, PaO_2 = 97 $\pm$ 5).

DISCUSSION

Our results show that static changes in diaphragm strength as reflected by Pm do not change during a ten week period of phosphorus depletion. Hypophosphatemia, however, does cause a significant decrease in the high frequency force characteristics of the diaphragm after it is subjected to a series of fatiguing stimulations.

The lack of change in Pm during the ten week period of depletion initially appeared to be in conflict with the literature. Previous work by Fuller (3) in dogs during a five week period of phosphorus depletion has shown depressed myocardial function as evidenced by decreased stroke volume and peak blood flow velocity. Pulmonary failure has also been associated with hypophosphatemia in several studies (4,5,6). However, the apparent differences may be due to the more rapid utilization of energy supplies by the heart when compared to the diaphragm. Recently, Hörl et al (12) found reduced glycogen content in the cardiac muscle of phosphorus deficient rats when compared to normal phosphorus controls. The activity of enzymes involved in glycogen metabolism were also altered in the cardiac muscle of phosphorus deficient animals. Similar differences in skeletal muscle glycogen and enzyme activity between control and phosphorus deficient animals did not occur. Thus, the effects of hypophosphatemia on pulmonary muscle forces may only become apparent when the muscle is exercised. Presumably, the loss in force that occurred during the dynamic experiments was due to the more rapid depletion of energy supplies as a result of the fatiguing series of stimulations.

The importance of energy supplies during a similar series of fatiguing stimulations has been investigated by others. Edwards (13) found decreased adenosine triphosphate (ATP) and phosphorylcreatine (PC) in the quadriceps muscle in human subjects following a series of repeated contractions. Recent work by Rochester (14) in dogs found that increased contractile effort depletes ATP and PC more rapidly in the stimulated hemidiaphragm when compared to the contralateral unstimulated hemidiaphragrm. Therefore, the increased loss in force in the hypophosphatemic animals probably occurs in the presence of depleted energy stores. As a result pulmonary muscle weakness associated with hypophosphatemia (3,4,5) may then only occur when there is an increase in the work of breathing as might be associated with thoracic or pulmonary disease.

Theoretically, the loss in force evidenced in the hypophosphatemic animals following a fatiguing series of stimulations may occur at any site from the point of nerve stimulation down to the contractile elements of the muscle. Edwards et al (13) have postulated that high frequency fatigue results from a neuromuscular block or reduced excitability of the muscle fiber membrane. While at low frequencies the impairment involves the excitation-contraction coupling mechanism. High frequency fatigue may be related to a decreased sodium gradient across the sarcolemmal membrane. Recent work by Bigland-Ritchie, Jones and Woods (15) during a series of repeated high frequency stimulations of the human abductor policies muscle found evidence of slowed conduction velocity along the muscle membrane. A companion study by Jones, Bigland-Ritchie and Edwards (16) in isolated soleus muscle from rats found that the loss in force following repeated high frequency stimulation could be altered by changing the sodium concentration in the bathing solution. Based on these results they attributed high frequency fatigue to the inability of the sodium pump to maintain the normal sodium gradients. Changes in the intracellular concentrations of sodium could thus reduce the excitability of the muscle membrane. Fuller et al (17) have demonstrated an increased (hypopolarized) resting transmembrane potential in hypophosphatemic dogs. They felt that these changes could be due to either an abnormality of the sodium pump or an abnormality in the permeability of the sarcolemmal membrane. Thus, increased high frequency fatigue probably occurs in hypophosphatemic animals due to the higher intracellular sodium concentration which in turn reduces the probability of action potential propagation along the muscle fiber to a greater degree than in control animals.

ACKNOWLEDGEMENTS

The writers wish to thank Dr. James P. Baker for his guidance and continued support.

SUPPORT

Supported in part by NIH Biomedical Research Support Grant No. 2507 RR 0577.

REFERENCES

1. J. P. Knochel, The Pathophysiology and Clinical Characteristics of Severe Hypophosphatemia, Arch. Intern. Med., 137:203-220 (1977).
2. L. R. O'Connor, W. S. Wheeler, and J. E. Bethune, Effect of Hypophosphatemia on Myocardial Performance in Man, N. Engl. J. Med., 297:901-903 (1977).
3. T. J. Fuller, W. W. Nichols, B. J. Brenner and J. C. Peterson, Reversible Depression in Myocardial Performance in Dogs with Experimental Phosphorus Deficiency, J. Clin. Invest., 62:1194-1200 (1978)
4. J. H. Newman, T. A. Neff, and P. Ziporin, Acute Respiratory Failure Associated with Hypophosphatemia, N. Engl. J. Med., 296:1101-1103 (1973).
5. A. J. Furlan, M. Hanson, and A. Cooperman, Acute Areflexic Paralysis, Arch. Neurol. 32:706-707 (1975).
6. J. R. Darsee, and D. O. Nutter, Reversible Severe Congestive Cardiomyopathy in Three Cases of Hypophosphatemia, Ann. Intern. Med., 89:867-870 (1978).
7. J. W. Coburn, and S. G. Massry, Changes in Serum and Urinary Calcium During Phosphate Depletion: Studies on Mechanisms, J. Clin. Invest., 49:1073-1087 (1970).
8. J. Milic-Emili, J. Mead, J. M. Turner, and E. M. Glauser, Improved Technique for Estimating Pleural Pressure from Esophageal Balloons, J. Appl. Physiol., 19:207-211 (1964).
9. E. Agostoni, and Rahn, Abdominal and Thoracic Pressures at Different Lung Volumes, J. Appl. Physiol., 15:1087-1092 (1960).
10. M. Aubier, G. Farkas, A. DeTroyer, R. Mozes, and C. Roussos, Detection of Diaphragmatic Fatigue in Man by Phrenic Stimulation, J. Appl. Physiol., 50:538-544 (1981).
11. J. Moxham, A. J. R. Morris, S. G. Spiro. R. H. T. Edwards, and M. Green, Contractile Properties and Fatigue of the Diaphragm in Man, Thorax 36:164-168 (1981).
12. W. H. Horl, W. Kreusser, A. Heidland, and E. Ritz, Abnormalities of Glycogen Metabolism in Cardiomyopathy of Phosphorus Depletion, in: S. G. Massry, E. Ritz, and H. Jahn, eds., New York: Plenum Press, 128:343-350 (1980).
13. R. H. T. Edwards, D. K. Hill, D. A. Jones, and P. A. Marton, Fatigue of Long Duration in Human Skeletal Muscle After Exercise, J. Physiol, (Lond), 272:769-778 (1977).
14. D. R. Rochester, N. S. Arora, S. K. Goldberg, J. McCormak, and D. Moore, Diaphragm Energy Metabolism in Acute Respiratory Failure (abstract), Physiologist, 22:107 (1979).
15. B. Bigland-Ritchie, D. A. Jones, and J. J. Woods, Excitation Frequency and Muscle Fatigue: Electrical Responses

During Human Voluntary and Stimulated Contractions, Exper. Neur., 64:414-427 (1979)

16. D. A. Jones, B. Bigland-Ritchie, and R. T. Edwards, Excitation Frequency and Muscle Fatigue: Mechanical Responses During Voluntary and Stimulated Contractions, Exper. Neur., 64:401-413 (1979).
17. T. J. Fuller, N. W. Carter, C. Barcenas, and J. P. Knochel, Reversible Changes in the Muscle Cell in Experimental Phosphorus Deficiency, J. Clin. Invest., 57:1019-1024 (1976)

EXPERIMENTAL ALCOHOLISM INDUCES PHOSPHORUS AND MAGNESIUM DEFICIENCY IN SKELETAL MUSCLE

Evan R. Ferguson, Jon D. Blachley and James P. Knochel

VAMC and Southwestern Medical School
4500 South Lancaster Road
Dallas, Texas 75216

INTRODUCTION

Structural, electrochemical and biochemical derangements of skeletal muscle are exceptionally common findings in patients with severe, chronic alcoholism. Collectively, these abnormalities represent alcoholic myopathy. Studies conducted in our laboratories during the past eight years on patients and experimental animals suggest that skeletal muscle is consistently damaged by chronic exposure to ethanol[1-4]. In brief, prominent findings include a substantial depression of muscle cell phosphorus and magnesium content, while calcium is markedly elevated. As occurs in any injured cell, contents of sodium and chloride are elevated, while potassium tends to be reduced. These changes in muscle cell composition may occur either with or without elevated serum levels of creatine phosphokinase (CPK) activity.

Recently, we have developed a model of chronic alcoholism in the dog which successfully avoids the common problem of malnutrition[1,5]. Utilizing this model, we have shown derangements of canine skeletal muscle ionic composition after 8 weeks of alcohol ingestion which duplicate the changes seen in skeletal muscle of severe, alcoholic patients. In addition, we have demonstrated that these derangements of skeletal muscle ionic composition were accompanied by increases in active sodium transport of skeletal muscle microsomal preparations[1,5].

In the studies reported herein we were interested in ascertaining the effects of more prolonged ethanol consumption on skeletal muscle ionic composition and active sodium transport activity. In particular, we were interested in determining the temporal patterns of skeletal muscle electrolyte and divalent ion compositional changes induced by ethanol in the absence of malnutrition. Since internal sodium and potassium concentrations are regulated by the membrane-bound Na,K-ATPase, the enzymatic equivalent of the sodium pump[6], we were also interested in determining the temporal relationships between skeletal muscle electrolyte concentrations and active sodium transport. Finally, since active sodium transport requires the expenditure of metabolic energy, we were interested in ascertaining if changes in active sodium transport were supported by changes in skeletal muscle respiration.

METHODS

Eleven healthy dogs (20-30 Kg) were selected for study based on their willingness to consume a nutritious, synthetic diet mixed with ethanol. Only dogs that totally consumed the twice daily portions throughout the twelve days were selected for study. Following the selection process, the dogs were returned to diet plus water for a six week control period. Thereupon the experimental period began with the dogs consuming 3.2 gm ethanol/Kg body weight mixed with diet twice daily.

On the day preceding the period of ethanol administration and again at 1, 2, 3, 4 and 7 months the dogs were anesthetized with sodium thiopental, intubated, and the resting transmembrane electrical potential difference of skeletal muscle cells (Em) was determined _in situ_ using Ling-Gerard type electrodes on the gracilis muscle by techniques previously described[7]. 12-20 individual fiber potentials were obtained for each animal and the average calculated for each measurement. Following the measurement of the membrane potential, muscle samples were obtained from the contralateral gracilis muscle for electrolyte and mineral content, Na,K-ATPase activity, and muscle cell respiration.

Muscle wet, dry and fat-free dry weights and contents of sodium, potassium, chloride, magnesium, calcium and phosphorus were determined as previously described[8,9]. Total water content of muscle samples was determined gravimetrically on samples after vacuum drying at 80°C. Using the chloride distribution which in turn is calculated from the membrane potential (Em) and extracellular chloride content, the intracellular concentrations of sodium, potassium, and chloride were calculated using previously described equations[7].

Skeletal muscle microsomal fractions were prepared essentially as described by Asano et al[10] except the second homogenization step was eliminated. The ATPase assay conditions were as previously described except the reaction was carried out in 1.0 ml and terminated by the addition of 0.2 ml of iced 30% TCA[10]. The orthophosphate content of the supernatent was determined by the method of Fiske and Subbarow[11] and the protein content by the method of Lowry et al[12]. Na,K-ATPase activity was computed as the difference between total activity (without ouabain) and Mg^{++}-ATPase (with ouabain).

Skeletal muscle oxygen consumption was determined on triplicate samples of gracilis muscle using Clark Oxygen Electrodes. Parallel sets of samples were preincubated for 10 min at 37°C in oxygenated Na^+-Ringers solution and transferred for an additional 10 minutes in either Na^+-Ringers or K^+ free Ringers plus 1 mM ouabain[10]. The samples were then transferred to Clark Oxygen Electrode chambers and oxygen consumption measured in the presence and absence of ouabain. Following the measurement of oxygen consumption, the samples were blotted with filter paper and dry weight determined after heating to 80°C for 16-20 hours. Na^+-dependent respiration or $Q_{O_2}(t)$ was computed as the difference between total respiration (Q_{O_2}) determined in the absence of ouabain and sodium-independent respiration (Q_{O_2}') measured in K^+ free solution containing ouabain. Results were expressed as µl oxygen consumed/mg dry weight/hr.

Statistical analyses were performed using Analysis of Variance and Dunnett's test for statistical significance between multiple experimental groups and a single control. A p value <0.05 was considered statistically significant.

RESULTS

The average weight gained by these animals was 2.0 Kg after 7 months of ethanol administration. Throughout the 7 months of the ethanol administration the animals became visibly intoxicated twice daily. Following ingestion of the ethanol diet, peak concentrations of blood alcohol levels were seen at 2-3 hours and generally ranged from 150 to 350 mg/dL. In addition, throughout these studies no significant changes were observed in the plasma concentrations of electrolytes, divalent ions, or in venous pH, pCO_2, pO_2, or bicarbonate concentrations.

Skeletal muscle divalent ion content of alcoholic dogs is shown in figure 1. After one month of ethanol intake, skeletal muscle phosphorus content declined to 24.1 mmoles/100 gm FFDS (fat-free dry solids) and showed a further decline to 21.3 mmoles after 2 months. From 2-4 months, phosphorus content remained depressed and increased slightly at 7 months. Muscle magnesium content also declined from 9.3 to 8.0 mEq/100 gm FFDS during the first month of alcohol intake. Magnesium content remained depressed throughout the study ranging from 7.7 to 8.4 mEq/100 gm

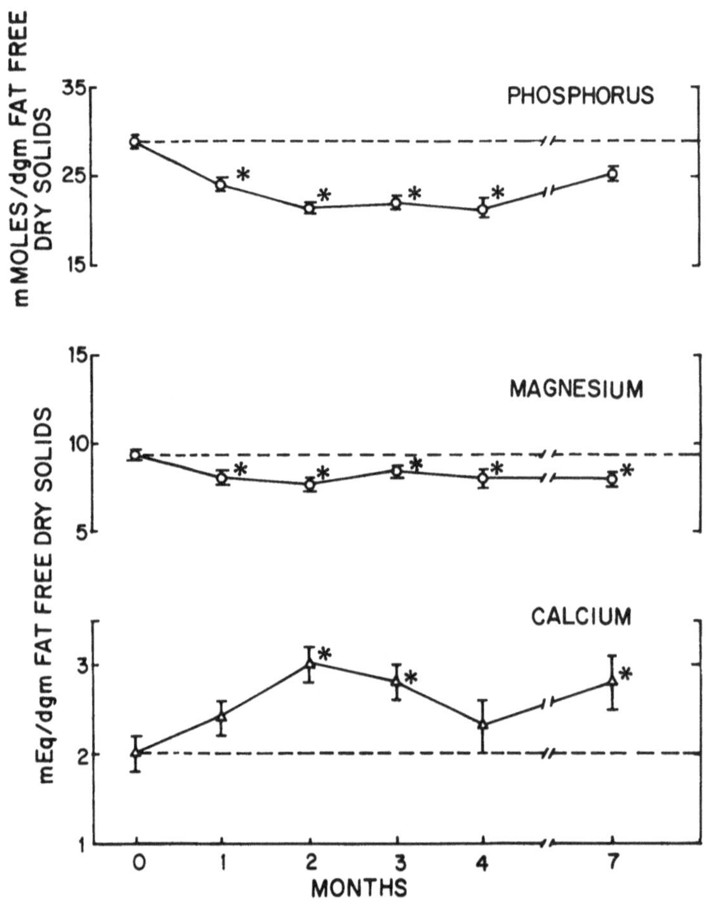

Fig. 1. Temporal patterns of divalent ion composition in alcoholic skeletal muscle. The first symbol and dashed line represent the control value. Each point is the mean $\pm$ S.E.M. of 11 determinations. * Significantly different ($p \leq 0.05$) from control value.

FFDS. Muscle calcium content was elevated from 1-7 months of alcohol intake but was significantly increased only at 2, 3, and 7 months.

The results of skeletal muscle electrolyte contents are seen in figure 2. Muscle cell sodium content rose significantly to 23.4 mEq/100 gm FFDS after one month of ethanol administration and reached a peak of 27.4 mEq/100 gm FFDS after 2 months. Thereafter, muscle sodium content declined slightly at 3 months and returned to normal after 4 months of alcohol intake. Chloride content mirrored

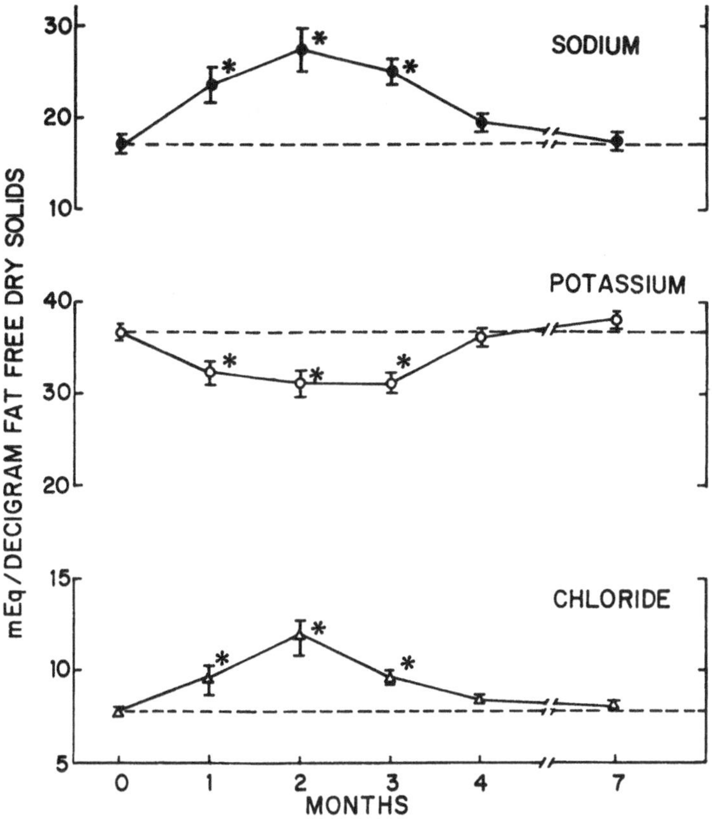

Fig. 2. Temporal patterns of electrolyte content changes in alcoholic skeletal muscle. The first symbol and dashed line represent the control value. Each point is the mean ± S.E.M. of 11 determinations. * Significantly different ($p \leq 0.05$) from control value.

that of sodium by increasing to a peak of 11.8 mEq/100 gm FFDS then declined, reaching normal limits at 4 months. Skeletal muscle potassium content reciprocated with that of sodium and chloride by declining to 32.3 mEq/100 gm FFDS after one month and to 31.1 mEq after 2 and 3 months of ethanol ingestion. After 4 months potassium content was within normal limits.

Since the data in figure 2 were expressed per 100 gm fat free dry weight, we were interested in determining if these changes reflected actual changes in intracellular ionic concentrations or reflected changes in both intracellular ions and water content. Total water content was determined gravimetrically and the partioning of water into intracellular and intracellular compartments determined from the chloride distribution[7]. Throughout the seven month experimental period there were no significant changes in total water, per cent water or in intracellular water. Using the calculated water partitions we then derived the intracellular concentrations of sodium, potassium and chloride expressed as mEq/liter cell water. As seen in figure 3, intracellular sodium rose to a maximum value of 55.8 mEq/liter cell water at 3 months

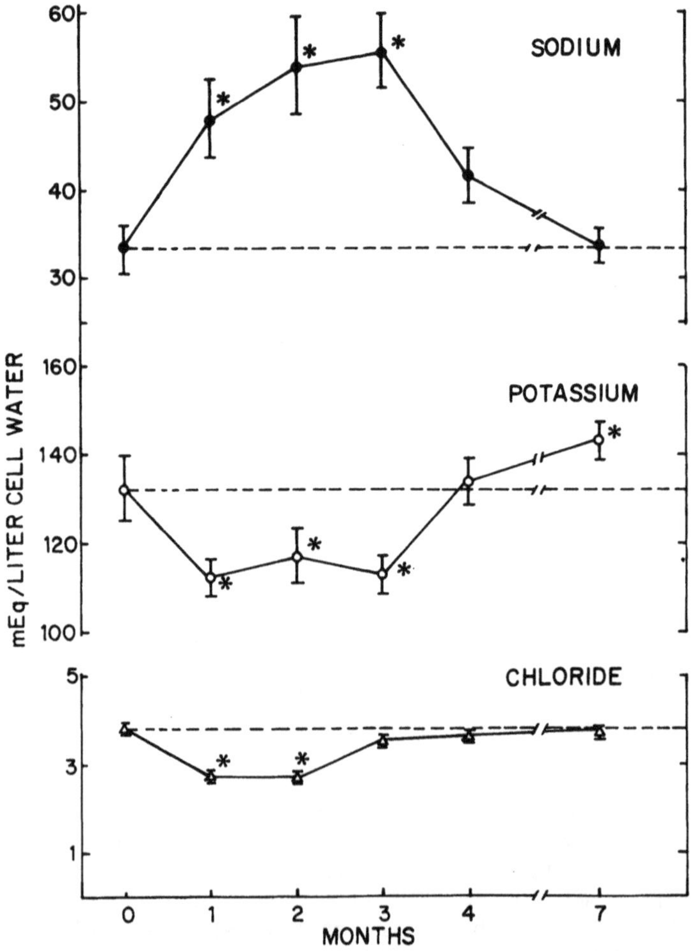

Fig. 3. Changes in electrolyte concentrations in alcoholic skeletal muscle. The first symbol and dashed line represents the control value. For method of calculation of the concentrations, see text. Each value is the mean ± S.E.M. of 11 determinations. * Significantly different ($\overline{p} \leq 0.05$) from the control value.

but returned to normal at 4 months. Intracellular potassium declined to 112.6 mEq/liter cell water after one month of alcohol intake, remained depressed at 2 and 3 months and returned to normal at 4 months. Intracellular chloride was depressed after 1 and 2 months of alcohol administration as expected since the transmembrane potential was hyperpolarized at this time (see figure 4) and intracellular chloride was derived from the Nernst potential assuming passive distribution of chloride. Of importance, the direction and magnitude of the changes seen in intracellular sodium and potassium in figure 3 duplicate the results of these ions expressed on a dry weight basis in figure 2.

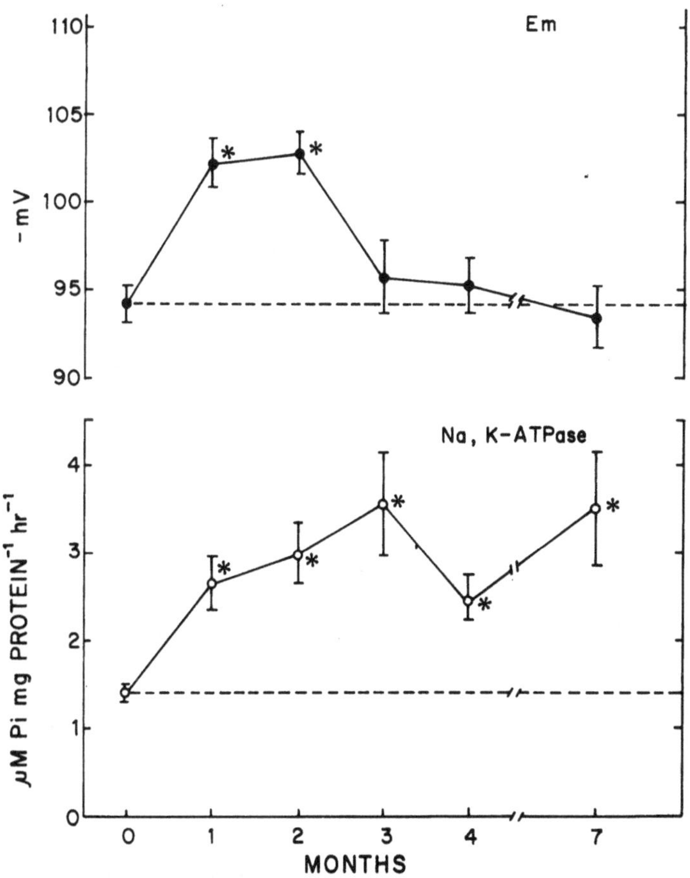

Fig. 4. Changes in skeletal muscle transmembrane potential (Em) and Na,K-ATPase activity during chronic alcoholism. The first symbol and dashed line represents the control value. Each point is the mean ± S.E.M of 11 determinations. * Significantly different ($p \leq 0.05$) from control value.

The results of the measurements of the transmembrane potential difference (Em) and Na,K-ATPase activities are seen in figure 4. After 1 month of ethanol intake the transmembrane potential was increased (hyperpolorized) to -102.2 mV and remained at this value after 2 months. At 3 months the membrane potential returned to normal and remained normal for the remainder of the study. Ouabain-sensitive, Na,K-ATPase activity was significantly increased after 1 month of ethanol intake and remained significantly

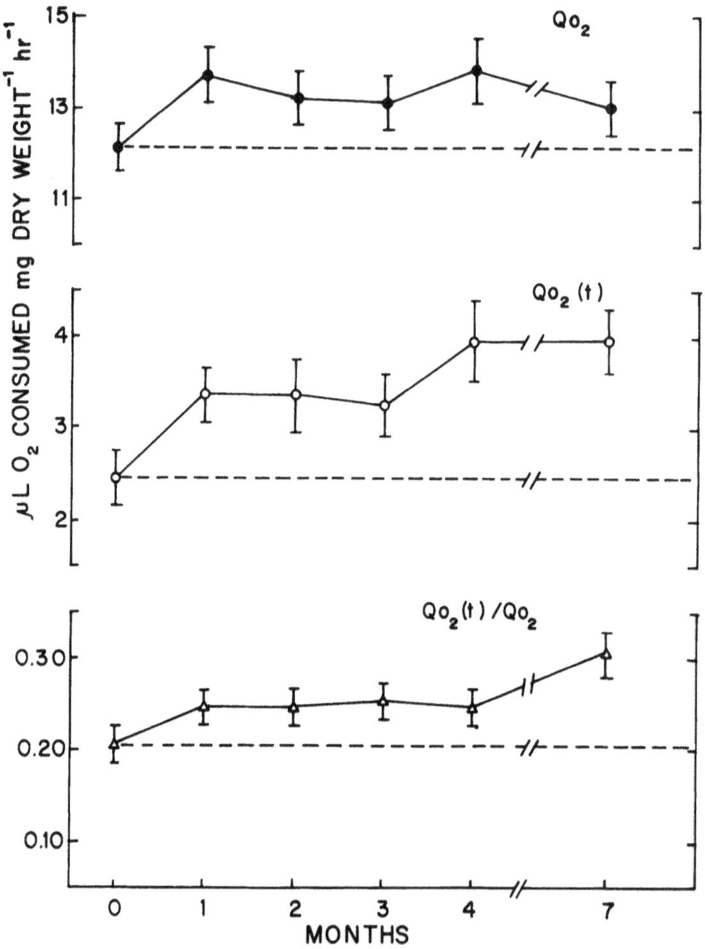

Fig. 5. Changes in skeletal muscle respiration [Q_{O2}], Na^+-dependent respiration [$Q_{O2}(t)$], and the percent of total respiration accounted for by active Na^+ transport [$Q_{O2}(t)/Q_{O2}$]. The first symbol and dashed line represents the control value. Each value is the mean ± S.E.M. of 30-36 determinations.

increased throughout the time period studied. After 7 months of alcohol administration, Na,K-ATPase activity was 250% that of the control value. Mg^{++}-ATPase activity (data not shown) was increased at 4 and 7 months.

Figure 5 shows the results of oxygen consumption measurements in alcoholic dog skeletal muscle. Total tissue respiration (Q_{O_2}) increased to 13.71 µl O_2 consumed/mg dry weight/hr at 1 month and remained elevated through 4 months of alcohol ingestion. Na^+-dependent respiration or $Q_{O_2}(t)$ also was increased to 3.35 µl O_2/mg dry weight/hr from 1-3 months, then further increased to 3.94 at 4 and 7 months. There were no significant changes in sodium-independent respiration or Q_{O_2}' (data not shown). The per cent of tissue respiration supporting active sodium transport or $Q_{O_2}(t)/Q_{O_2}$ increased by 5% from 1-4 months and showed a secondary rise to 30% of total respiration after 7 months.

DISCUSSION

These studies extend our previously reported observations made after 2 months of ethanol intake on skeletal muscle ionic composition and transport activity. As in the earlier studies, a demonstrable subclinical myopathy is evident after two months of alcohol ingestion i.e. muscle cell sodium, chloride, and calcium are elevated while potassium, magnesium, and phosphorus are depressed. Yet despite these changes, no clinical evidence of myopathy is evident. In addition, the magnitude and direction of the changes seen here at 2 months and in our earlier studies parallel those seen in patients with alcoholic myopathy[1,3,4]. These results indicate that ethanol (or a metabolite) may induce discernable effects on skeletal muscle despite a nutritious diet.

The alteration of divalent ion composition is difficult to explain since little experimental evidence has accumulated to assess the effects of ethanol on divalent ion composition. Severe alcoholic patients show derangements of muscle cell divalent ion composition similar to those observed here[4]. In addition, ethanol has been shown to induce magnesium losses in the urine and sequestration of calcium in muscle of alcoholic patients[13,14]. The latter effect is believed to be due to depression of calcium transport in the sarcoplasmic reticulum which may impair the supply of calcium to contractile elements[15]. Although we have demonstrated increases in muscle calcium content, to date we have not examined the possible underlying causes of calcium accumulation in alcoholic skeletal muscle. The depression of muscle magnesium and phosphorus occurs in spite of normal plasma levels of these ions. Similar observations have been made in alcoholic patients where plasma ion concentrations have been shown to be poor indicators of changes in muscle cell composition[3]. Since there were no apparent extrarenal losses and in the absence of balance studies, we assume that the cellular losses of magnesium and phosphorus were counterbalanced by urinary losses to result in no net changes in plasma concentrations.

In sharp contrast to the divalent ion derangements of alcoholic skeletal muscle are the results of the electrolyte compositional studies. Cellular sodium, potassium, and chloride show significant changes during the first three months of alcohol administration but return to normal after four months. We believe the early increase in both intracellular sodium concentration and Na,K-ATPase activity indicates that ethanol (or a metabolite) increases cellular permeability to sodium. The subsequent rise in intracellular sodium would thus stimulate increased Na,K-ATPase activity as has been implicated in other physiologic states[16,17]. In addition, the maintenance of apparently normal electrolyte concentrations with elevated Na,K-ATPase activity and sodium-dependent respiration indicates that increased sodium transport activity rectifies the derangements of electrolyte composition induced by ethanol. Whether the increased Na,K-ATPase activity results from a change in the kinetic parameters of the enzyme or an increased number of sodium transport units has not been assessed in alcoholic skeletal muscle. Studies by Edelman and his colleagues[10,18] and by Lin and Akera[19] in liver, kidney, and muscle indicate that thyroid hormone stimulated increases in Na,K-ATPase activity result from increased numbers of sodium transport units and not a change in the kinetic properties of the enzyme. Similar mechanisms may be operative in canine skeletal muscle under the influence of increased intracellular sodium concentrations resulting from ethanol administration.

The rectification of electrolyte concentrations with continued alterations in divalent ion composition indicates that separate mechanisms may be regulating electrolyte and divalent ion composition in alcoholic skeletal muscle. Indeed, to our knowledge, these results are the first to demonstrate normal electrolyte composition with alterations in skeletal muscle phosphorus, magnesium and calcium. This situation is in sharp contrast to that seen in severe alcoholics and probably results from the fact that most alcoholics studied to date have nutritional and/or intercurrent illnesses which may profoundly affect skeletal muscle. Thus, the subclinical myopathy seen in these studies may be observed only in the early stages of alcoholism where skeletal muscle may still adapt to electrolyte (but not divalent ion) derangements. The imposition of metabolic stress, nutritional deficiencies, etc. may then perturb skeletal muscle ionic composition to the state normally seen in severe alcoholics.

The membrane potential of alcoholic skeletal muscle was hyperpolarized at 1 and 2 months of alcohol intake. This hyperpolarization may result from increased Na,K-ATPase activity and increased electrogenic sodium pump activity in response to increased intracellular sodium concentrations. The return of the membrane potential (and electrogenic pump activity) to normal at 3 months may result from increased numbers of sodium transport units. Thus, in the early stages of skeletal muscle electrolyte derangements the muscle cell attempts to decrease intracellular sodium by changing the coupling ratio and activity of the sodium pump thereby increasing the electrogenic contribution to the transmembrane potential. With continued ethanol exposure, skeletal muscle may adapt either by increasing the number of sodium transport units to extrude more sodium and/or changing the membrane composition to decrease sodium permeability. Although either mechanism will result in decreased intracellular sodium, the sustained increase in Na,K-ATPase activity and sodium-dependent respiration indicates that the first alternative may be more likely. If this is indeed the case, then with increased numbers of sodium transport units available, the coupling ratio (and the electrogenic contribution thereof) would return to normal.

ACKNOWLEDGMENTS

We gratefully acknowledge the technical assistance provided by James T. Long, Marty Calabra, and Deloia Morris. We also thank Ms. Susan Kennedy for assistance in preparation of the manuscript.

REFERENCES

1. E.R. Ferguson, N.W. Carter, R. Haller, and J.P. Knochel, Chronic experimental alcoholism reproduces derangements of clinical alcoholic myopathy, Clin. Res. 27:794A (1980).
2. E.R. Ferguson, J.D. Blachley, and J.P. Knochel, Changes in rat skeletal muscle ionic composition and transport activity induced by chronic ethanol administration. Clin. Res. 28:843A (1980).
3. J.P. Knochel, G.L. Bilbrey, T.J. Fuller, and N.W. Carter, The muscle cell in chronic alcoholism: The possible role of phosphate depletion in alcoholic myopathy. Ann. New York Acad. Sci. 252:274-280 (1975).
4. R. Anderson, M. Cohen, R. Haller J. Elms, N.W. Carter, and J.P. Knochel, Skeletal muscle phosphorus and magnesium deficiency in alcoholic myopathy. Min. Electrol. Metab. 4:106:112 (1980).

5. E.R. Ferguson, N.W. Carter, R. Haller, and J.P. Knochel, Effects of chronic ethanol administration on skeletal muscle ionic composition and transport activity. Fed. Proc. 39:744 (1980).
6. J.C. Skou, Enzymatic basis for active transport of Na^+ and K^+ across cell membranes. Physiol. Rev. 45:596-617 (1965).
7. J.N. Cunningham, N.W. Carter, F.C. Rector, Jr., and D.W. Seldin, Resting transmembrane potential difference of skeletal muscle in normal subjects and severely ill patients. J. Clin. Invest. 50:49-59 (1971).
8. T.J. Fuller, N.W. Carter, C. Barcenas, and J.P. Knochel, Reversible changes of the muscle cell in experimental phosphorus deficiency. J. Clin. Invest. 57:1019-1024 (1976).
9. G.L. Bilbrey, N.W. Carter, M.G. White, J.F. Schilling, and J.P. Knochel, Potassium deficiency in chronic renal failure, Kid. Intl. 4:423-430 (1973).
10. Y. Asano, U.A. Liberman, and I.S. Edelman, Relationships between Na^+ dependent respiration and Na^+ + K^+ - adenosine triphosphatase activity in rat skeletal muscle. J. Clin. Invest. 51:368-379 (1976).
11. C.R. Fiske, and Y. Subbarow, The colorinetric determination of phosphorus. J. Biol. Chem. 66:375-400 (1925).
12. O.H. Lowry, N.J. Rosenbrough, A.L. Farr, and R.J. Randall, Protein measurement with the Folin phenol reagent. J. Biol. Chem. 193:265-275 (1951).
13. J.M. Kalbfleisch, R.D. Linderman, H.E. Ginn, and W.O. Smith, Effects of ethanol administration on urinary excretion of magnesium and other electrolytes in alcoholic and normal subjects. J. Clin. Invest. 42:1471-1475 (1963).
14. E. Rubin, Alcoholic myopathy in heart and skeletal muscle. N. Engl. J. Med. 301:28-33 (1979).
15. E. Rubin, A.M. Katz, and C.S. Lieber, Muscle damage produced by chronic alcohol consumption. Am. J. Pathol. 83:499-525 (1976).
16. T.B. Bolton, Effects of electrogenic sodium pumping in the membrane potential of longitudinal smooth muscle from terminal ileium of guinea pig. J. Physiol. 228:693-712 (1973).
17. R. Casteels, G. Droogmans, and H. Hendrickx, Active ion transport and resting potential in smooth muscle cells. Phil. Trans. R. Soc. Lond. B. 265:47-56 (1973).
18. C.H. Lo, and I.S. Edelman, Effect of triiodothyromine on the synthesis and degradation of renal cortical (Na^+ + K^+) - adenosine triphosphatase. J. Biol. Chem. 251:7834-7840 (1976).
19. M.H. Lin, and T. Akera, Increased (Na^+, K^+)-ATPase concentrations in various tissues of rats caused by thyroid hormone treatment. J. Biol. Chem. 253:723-726 (1978).

DEFECTIVE HORMONAL STIMULATION OF ISOLATED HEPATOCYTES IN PHOSPHOROUS DEPLETED RATS

Walter H. Hörl, Wilhelm Kreusser, August Heidland, Jan Stepinski, Eberhard Ritz

Depts. Internal Medicine, Univ. Würzburg and Heidelberg (FRG)

INTRODUCTION

In the past, some clinical evidence has been presented of disturbed liver function in patients with phosphorous depletion (PD) and hypophosphatemia. Frank and Kern (1) reported deterioration of hepatic function in a cirrhotic patient coincident with the development of hypophosphatemia. Furthermore, Rajan et al. (2) emphasized that hypophosphatemic patients with cirrhosis tend to undergo greater hepatic decompensation than do patients with normal blood phosphorous.
Finally, Klock et al. (3) found a defective hyperglycemic response to glucagon in alcoholic patients with hypophosphatemia. This abnormality was completely normalized after restoration of normal serum phosphorous levels.
In the present study, gluconeogenesis of isolated hepatocytes of PD rats was studied under basal conditions and after hormonal stimulation with glucagon and epinephrine.

METHODS

Male 130 g Sprague Dawley rats were phosphorous depleted by feeding with 0.03 % P_i (Altromin Comp., Lage, Lippe). Control animals (CO) were pairweighed with PD animals and received Altromin diet C 1000 which was identical with respect to all constituents with the exception of P_i (Ca 0.4 %, P_i 0.4 %). The animals were kept for 4 weeks. After a 24 h starvation period (to

Table 1

Serum phosphorous and glucose (mg/dl) in PD animals

	Phosphorous		Glucose
	overnight fasting (day 27)	24 h fasting (day 30)	24 h fasting (day 30)
PD (n=8)	2.79 ± 0.18	3.08 ± 0.14	172 ± 6.5
CO (n=8)	8.79 ± 0.16	9.55 ± 0.31	99.4 ± 6.5

$\bar{x}$ ± SEM, differences PD vs. CO, $p < 0.01$

deplete the liver of glycogen), hepatocytes were isolated after collagenase digestion according to Berry and Friend (4). Isolated hepatocytes were incubated for 30 min. in (P_i free) Krebs bicarbonate buffer (37°C; 95 % O_2, 5 % CO_2 atmosphere, pH 7.4) using 10 mmol/l pyruvate as substrate. After 30 min., glucose and lactate were measured enzymatically. The cells were counted with phase contrast microscopy, cell vitality was evaluated with the trypan blue exclusion method (maximally 50 % of cells took up trypan blue) and protein was measured according to Lowry et al. (5).

RESULTS AND DISCUSSION

An advanced degree of PD in the experimental animals is documented by severe fasting hypophosphatemia (table 1). Serum glucose in PD animals was significantly higher after an overnight fasting. The two groups may not be comparable, however, since CO animals tend to ingest food immediately whereas PD animals tend to consume food throughout the day; consequently, the true fasting period may have been longer in CO animals. Alternatively, hyperglycemia in PD animals may be an evidence of increased sympathetic drive or adrenaline excess which is known to exist in PD (6,7). Insulin resistance, as demonstrated by De Fronzo (8) in PD, may also play a role in the genesis of fasting hyperglycemia.

Glucose production from pyruvate by isolated hepatocytes of PD rats was markedly diminished (table 2). Under basal conditions, glucose production was 47.7 % higher in CO than in PD. Glucagon caused a highly significant increase of glucose production (+ 39.6 %; $p < 0.01$, Wilcoxon test for paired differences) in CO, whereas no significant change was observed in PD animals. A similar highly significant increase of glucose production was seen in CO with epinephrine (+ 22.9 %; $p<0.05$) whereas in PD a slight but not significant increase was observed. Both glucagon and epinephrine are known to stimulate hepatic cAMP production and activate phosphoenol-pyruvate kinase (9). Since measurements of cAMP were not performed in the study, it is unknown whether the defect is due to reduced hormone binding to the receptor, diminished cAMP production or inhibition of steps beyond cAMP generation. It is suggestive, that diminished hepatocellular ATP content, as demonstrated by us previously (10), would limit the rate of gluconeogenesis. Non-specific damage to hepatocytes of PD ani-

Table 2

Glucose production by isolated hepatocytes of PD rats

	Glucose production (nmol/mg protein/30 min)			
	basal	glucagon (28 nM)	epinephrine (10 µM)	PTH (1 U/ml)
PD (n=6)	195 ± 27	206 ± 24	223 ± 25	203 ± 23
CO (n=6)	$288 \pm 53^{+}$	$402 \pm 69^{+}$	$354 \pm 58^{+}$	282 ± 49

$\bar{x} \pm$ SEM, $^{+}$ denotes significant difference between PD and CO ($p < 0.05$)

mals, either intrinsic or subsequent to preparation with collagenase, is not definitely excluded but unlikely in view of unchanged cell vitality, as evaluated with the trypan blue exclusion method.

With the above preparation, no significant effect of PTH on glucose production was observed, although this has been demonstrated previously by Moxley et al. (11).

The above findings may have important clinical implication. Impaired gluconeogenesis may be considered as an index of hepatocellular dysfunction in PD. This may explain why hypophosphatemic patients with cirrhosis tend to undergo severe deterioration of liver function. Although in vivo, additional factors such as tissue hypoxia resulting from diminished erythrocyte 2,3-DPG levels (12), circulatory failure (7) with reduced liver perfusion or other factors cannot be excluded, the present finding points to some intrinsic abnormalities of hepatocytes.

Furthermore, diminished hepatic gluconeogenesis, in parallel with diminished renal gluconeogenesis as demonstrated by us previously (13), may lead to abnormal fasting blood glucose levels. Although this was not observed in the present experiment, hepatic and renal gluconeogenesis may become inadequate in prolonged fasting so that hypoglycemia would eventually ensue.

REFERENCES

1. Frank, B.W., Kern, F.Jr., 1962, Serum inorganic phosphorus during hepatic coma, Arch. Int. Med., 110: 101.
2. Rajan, K.S., Levinson, R., Leevy, C.M., 1973, Hepatic anoxia secondary to hypophosphatemia, Clin. Res., 21: 521.
3. Klock, J.C., Williams, H.E., Mentzer, W.C., 1974, Hemolytic anemia and somatic cell dysfunction in severe hypophosphatemia, Arch. Int. Med., 134:360.
4. Berry, M.N., Friend, D.S., 1969, High yield preparation of isolated rat liver parenchymal cells, J. Cell. Biol., 43:506.
5. Lowry, O.H., Rosebrough, N.J., Farr, A.L., Randall, R.J., 1951, Protein measurements with the folin phenol reagent, J. Biol. Chem., 193:265.

6. Hörl, W.H., Kreusser, W., Heidland, A., Ritz, E., 1980, Abnormalities of glycogen metabolism in cardiomyopathy of phosphorous depletion, Adv. Exper. Biol. Med., 128:343.
7. Kreusser, W., Vetter, H.,et al., in this issue.
8. De Fronzo, R.A., Lang, R., 1980, Hypophosphatemia and glucose intolerance: Evidence for tissue insensitivity to insulin, N. Engl. J. Med., 303:1259.
9. Johnson, M.E.M., Das, N.M., Butcher, F.R., Fain, J.N., 1972, The regulation of gluconeogenesis in isolated rat liver cells by glucagon, insulin, dibutyryl cyclic adenosine monophosphate, and fatty acids, J. Biol. Chem., 247:3229.
10. Kurokawa, K., Kreusser, W., Massry, S.G., 1978, Phosphate depletion and adenine nucleotide metabolism in kidney and liver, Adv. Exper. Biol. Med., 103:327.
11. Moxley, M.A., Bell, N.H., Wagle, S.R., Allen, D.O., Ashmore, J., 1974, Parathyroid hormone stimulation of glucose and urea production in isolated liver cells, Am. J. Physiol., 227:1058.
12. Travis, S.F., Sugerman, H.J., Tuberg, R.L., Dudrick, S.J., Delivoria-Papadopoulos, M., Miller, L.D., Oski, F.A., 1971, Alterations of red-cell glycolytic intermediates and oxygen transport as a consequence of hypophosphatemia in patients receiving intravenous hyperalimentation, N. Engl. J. Med., 285:763.
13. Kreusser, W.J., Descoeudres, C., Oda, Y., Massry, S.G., Kurokawa, K., 1980, Effect of phosphate depletion on renal gluconeogenesis, Mineral Electrolyte Metab., 3:312.

SHOULD HYPOPHOSPHATEMIA BE TREATED?

Charles R. Kleeman
Factor Family Foundation Professor of Nephrology, Medicine and Director, Center for Health Enhancement, Education and Research

University of California, Los Angeles
Division of Nephrology
School of Medicine
Los Angeles, California 90024

The answer to the question is yes. Phosphate treatment is necessary when hypophosphatemia is part of a true phosphate depletion syndrome (PDS). However, hypophosphatemia, even as low as 1.0-2.0 mg/dl in adults or 2.0-3.0 mg/dl in preadolescent children, does not necessarily mean or cause PDS. There are many examples in adult and child medicine of chronic hypophosphatemia caused by a high renal clearance of phosphorus (P) (low TmP/GFR) i.e. liberal amounts of P in the urine with low serum P. These do not develop a PDS unless there is superimposed a true lack of available P for the metabolic and growth needs of the patient. In the latter setting P excretion decreases markedly or disappears completely from the urine. This intense tubular reabsorption of P is an invariable feature of true phosphate depletion.

Long before phosphate depletion and PDS were described in the human medical literature the veterinarians where well aware of the problem in cattle or live stock grazing on P deficient pastures.

We quote from the in depth analysis of "Aphosphorosis in Ruminants" by Theiler and Green, 1932,[1] "Deficiency of phosphorus in the soil gives rise to a pasture limited in quantity by lack of essential plant food but still more limited in quality by a phosphorus content below minimal physiological requirements of the grazing animal (in relation to its caloric requirements or bulk intake).

Cattle subsisting on this vegetation develop, aside from other manifestations of malnutrition, a specific form of craving for phosphorus-rich material such as bones.

The search for bones leads to the ingestion of skeletal debris or carcase material which normal cattle naturally shun. To some extent the peaceful herbivore turns carnivore, even to the extent of crunching an occasional living tortoise between blood-stained jaws. On sparsely inhabited pastoral areas carcase debris is common enough--animals dying from any cause whatever, including game, hares, birds, lizards--and cattle find little difficulty in at least partially gratifying their unnatural craving even when there is not enough skeletal debris to cure it."

The essence of the pathogenesis of the problem is italicized in the first sentence of the quote from Theiler and Green. We may observe the PDS on an acute, subacute or chronic basis in many well known situations (Table 1). In all of these there is a persistent lack of a sufficient quantity of P to fulfill the immediate metabolic requirements of the animal i.e. an imbalance between availability and need. A vivid example of this imbalance is observed in the breastfed premature infant [2]. A 595 grm infant of 26 weeks gestation began feeding with breast milk expressed by her mother at 12 days of age and by one month all her nutrition was provided by human milk. Such a premature infant is born before the period of rapid intrauterine skeletal growth that normally occurs in the last trimester of pregnancy. The phosphorus content of human milk may be insufficient for the extremely rapid bone and soft tissue growth and bone mineralization which occurs exutero. This child at 5 months developed a most florid case of osteomalacia with multiple spontaneous fractures, ricketic changes at the epiphysis of the long bones, diffuse bone demineralization and failure to thrive. This syndrome was associated with frank hypercalcemia, 11.2-11.4 mg/dl, profound hypophosphatemia, 1.6-1.8 mg/dl, urine P of less than 0.4 mg/dl and TRP of greater than 99.9 percent, hypercalciuria of 15-20 mg/kg per day (normal 5-8), hydroxy proline excretion of 247 umols per day (normal 8 to 62), and circulating PTH was 53 uEq per ml (normal less than 90) with a 1,25 dihydroxy Vit D level of 200 pg/ml (normal 20-50). By supplementing the human milk with 20-25 mg/per kg per day of elemental phosphorus, the entire clinical biochemical and osseous syndrome responded rapidly and by 3 months the radiographs showed no evidence of rickets.

Starvation or semistarvation does not cause a PDS despite a zero or near zero Pintake. In fact Copp and Suiker [3] many years ago clearly demonstrated that in the phosphate depleted para-

TABLE 1

MAJOR CAUSES OF PHOSPHATE DEPLETION SYNDROME

I. Lack of phosphorus intake and/or absorption despite ingestion or administration of other nutrients.

   A. Chronic excessive intake of P binding antacids

   B. Chronic alcoholism

   C. Chronic mal absorption syndromes.

   D. Parenteral hyperalimentation with P deficient fluids.

   E. Chronic renal failure patients ingesting low P diets with or without antacids, and patients on chronic hemo or peritoneal dialysis with P free dialysate. Latter situation is, of course, withdrawing P from the body.

II. Any of these situations listed under I plus a rapid anabolic state (including growth) or a rapid formation of new protoplasma, i.e., the recovery phase of any severe catabolic state.

III. Any of the states listed under I and II plus chronic renal phosphate "leak" e.g. Hyperparathyroidism, chronic metabolic acidosis, chronic glucocorticoid administration, chronic renal tubular syndromes with inappropriately high clearance of phosphorus, vitamin D depletion.

thyroidectomized rat the characteristic hypercalcemia and hypophosphatemia reverted to the hypocalcemia and hyperphosphatemia of the hypoparathyroid state during 24-48 hours of fasting i.e. the phosphorus made available from lean tissue breakdown was adequate, in this period of time, to reverse the biochemical picture of P depletion.

The biochemical consequences (depletion of intracellular high energy phosphates) and their clinical manifestations of severe P depletion probably do not occur in humans unless the concentration of phosphorus in the plasma falls below 1.5 mg/dl in adults and 2.5 mg/dl in children. Knochel[3,4] has emphasized that these changes in phosphorus metabolism are more apt to produce overt PDS when they occur in an individual who is already sick from some form of acute or chronic dibilitating illness i.e. they start off with "sick cells" upon which P depletion is superimposed. This is consistent with our own personal experience and observations.

When under these circumstances the patient develops one or more of the varied clinical syndromes ascribed to phosphorus depletion (Table 2) oral or parenteral administration is necessary. This categorical statement is based on the innumerable clinical studies in the literature in which one or more of these abnormalities (Table 2) is reversed or totally corrected only by phosphorus replacement and correction of the profound hypophosphatemia[4-15]. It is true that many of these patients have associated electrolyte, acid-base and nutritional abnormalities which are often simultaneously corrected, and that very few controlled studies with and without P administration are available. However, in most of the reported experimental (16) and clinical studies[3-14] the probability is so strong that the phosphorus administration is primarily responsible for correction of the specific disorder (Table 2) that I believe we can accept the basic correctness of this conclusion.

In most of the reported cases the disorder or serious dysfunction caused by the PDS is such that we are not justified in withholding P replacement. However, randomized prospective studies with and without (phosphorus therapy) are still necessary. It may be possible to carry these out in those patients with phosphorus depletion whose specific symptomatalogy is minimal. Recently a study along these lines was carried out during the treatment of patients with diabetic ketoacidosis and non ketotic hyperosmolar coma (17). Keller and Berger randomly assigned a total of 40 cases to either standardized conventional treatment, alone, or combined with phosphate infusions from the beginning of therapy. The patients were appropriately matched for age, sex, and clinical characteristics. As usual the initial concentration of inorganic phosphate in the serum was normal or

TABLE 2

CLINICAL MANIFESTATIONS OF PHOSPHATE DEPLETION SYNDROME

1. Central and peripheral nervous system dysfunction with irritability, confusion, stupor to coma, focal neurologic abnormalities, abnormal EEG, EMG and impaired nerve conduction.

2. Muscle dysfunction and rhabdomyolysis with abnormal levels of CPK.

3. Red blood cell, leucocyte and platelet dysfunction with hemolytic anemia increased susceptibility to infection and bleeding tendency.

4. Myocardial dysfunction with forward and backward heart failure.

5. Pulmonary hypoventilation.

6. Impaired renal tubular function and reduced renal blood flow and glomerular filtration.

7. Loss of bone mass and osteomalacia.

8. Functional hypoparathyroidism.

9. Hypervitaminosis D due to excess synthesis of 1,25 $(OH)_2D_3$.

elevated in almost every patient. In these receiving phosphorus it fell to a low of 2.8-3 mg/dl by 8 hours while in the control group a low of 1.8 mg/dl was attained. These values persisted over the next 24-48 hours and the patients were followed very closely for at least 96 hours. Ad libidum food was permitted in both groups after the second day of treatment. The conclusion of this study was that a favorable effect of phosphate therapy on the clinical course of diabetic ketoacidosis or hyperosmolar coma could not be demonstrated. We are all aware of the fact that profound hypophosphatemia almost always develops during recovery from these conditions and the vast majority of clinical centers have not given (during the past 4-5 decades) parenteral P replacement. The most likely explanation for the failure to see a PDS in this setting is the fact that the oral intake of P containing nutrients is begun early in the course of treatment, usually by the end of the first 24 hours.

Parenteral P administration to the patient with a PDS should be done cautiously. These individuals have a state of physiologic hypoparathyroidism and, independent of the latter, their renal tubules continue to avidly reabsorb almost all the filtered phosphorus despite the development of hyperphosphatemia. The longer the duration of the P depletion, prior to its correction, the more persistent (many hours) are these physiologic dysfunctions. Therefore the absence of a normal increase in P excretion signifies that the kidney cannot play its essential role of preventing an abnormal rise of serum phosphate concentration. When the latter occurs it immediately causes a decrease in calcium ion concentration, at times to profound hypocalcemic levels. Thus in a matter of hours we may transform a phosphate depletion state into a phosphate "excess" one, much like the fasted P depleted hypoparathyroid rats of Copp and Suiker [3]. We would recommend that elemental P not be parenterally administered at a rate greater than 1 gram per 24 hours and that serum P and the rate of rise in urinary P be followed closely.

In conclusion, as stressed by the livestock veterinarians many decades ago "aphosphorosis" is a reality and it deserves prompt therapy [1]. We await more controlled clinical investigative studies to hopefully add increasing substances to our conclusion.

REFERENCES

1. A. Theiler, and H.H. Green, Aphosphorosis in ruminants. Nutr. Absts. and Rev. 1:359, (1932).
2. J.C. Rowe, D.H. Wood, D.W. Rowe and L.G. Raisz, Hypophosphatemic rickets in a premature infant fed breast milk. N.E.J.M. 300:293, (1979).
3. H. Copp and A.P. Suiker, Study of calcium kenetics in calcium and phosphorus deficient rats with the aid of radio calcium, in: Radio Isotope and Bone, P. Lacroix and A.M. Budy, eds., Blackwell Scientific Publications, Oxford, (1962).
4. J.P. Knochel, G.L. Bilhrey, T.J. Fuller, The muscle cell in chronic alcoholism. The possible role of phosphate depletion in alcoholic myopathy. Ann. N.Y. Acad. of Sc. 252:274, (1975).
5. J.P. Knochel, Hypophosphatemia in the alcoholic., editorial. Arch. Int. Med. 140:613, (1980).
6. Y. Yawata, Hebbel et al. Blood cell abnormalities complicating the hypophosphatemia of hyperalimentation: erythrocyte and platelet ATP deficiency associated with hemolytic anemia and bleeding in hyperalimented dogs. J. L and Clin Med. 84:643, (1975).
7. M.J. Sarg and C.S. Pitchumoni, Hypophosphatemic hemolytic syndrome of alcoholics a common city hospital problem. Amer. J. Med. Sc. 276:231, (1978).
8. G.E. Dent and C.S. Winter. Osteomalacia due to phosphate depletion from excessive aluminum hydroxide ingestion. B.M.J. 1:551, (1974).
9. J.H. Newman, T.A. Neff, P. Ziporin. Acute respiratory failure associated with hypophosphatemia. N.E.J.M. 296:1101, (1977).
10. P.R. Craddock, Y. Yawata et al. Acquired phagocyte dysfunction. A complication of the hypophosphatemia of parenteral hyperalimentation. N.E.J.M. 290:140B, (1974).
11. S.E. Silvis and P.D. Paragas, Jr. Parathesias, weakness, seizures, and hypophosphatemia in patients receiving hyperalimentation. Gastroent. 62:513, (1972).
12. P.A. Boelens, et al. Hypophosphatemia with muscle weakness due to antacids and hemodialysis. Am. J. Dis. Child. 120:350, (1970).

13. J.R. Darsee and D.O. Nutter. Reversible severe congestive cardiomyopathy in three cases of hypophosphatemia. Ann. Int. Med 86:867, (1978).
14. M. Lotz, R. Ney and F.C. Bartter. Osteomalacia and dibility resulting from phosphorus depletion. Trans of The Assoc. of Amer. Phys. 77:281, (1964).
15. D.B.N. Lee and C.R. Kleeman Phosphorus depletion in man. Clinical Digest McGaw Laboratories 5: No. 3, (1975).
16. N. Brautbar, D.B.N. Lee and C.R. Kleeman, In Print, Divalent ions calcium, phosphorus and magnesium, and Vitamin D. In Contemporary Metabolism Vol. 2 Ed. N. Frienkel Plenum Publ Corp., N.Y.
17. U. Keller and W. Berger. Prevention of hypophosphatemia by phosphate infusion during treatment of diabetic ketoacidosis and hyperosmolar coma. Diabetis 29:87, (1980).

TOPICS ON VITAMIN D METABOLISM

DEVELOPMENT AND APPLICATION OF AN

EXCHANGE ASSAY FOR 1,25-DIHYDROXYVITAMIN D_3

Anthony W. Norman, Marian R. Walters[§], Willi Hunziker[#] and Arie Bar[+]

Department of Biochemistry
University of California
Riverside, California

INTRODUCTION

1,25-Dihydroxyvitamin D_3 (1,25$(OH)_2D_3$), an active metabolite of the secosteroid vitamin D, is now generally considered to be a steroid hormone by classical criteria (1). Our recent data indicate that unoccupied 1,25$(OH)_2D_3$ receptors are present in crude chromatin fractions under low salt conditions in vitro (2,3). Consequently, quantitation of unoccupied receptor levels in the chick intestinal mucosa is best achieved by assay of the crude chromatin fraction (4). Due to the slow dissociation rate of 1,25$(OH)_2D_3$ from its receptor (2), only endogenously unoccupied 1,25$(OH)_2D_3$ receptors are detected by this method (incubation with [^{3}H]1,25$(OH)_2D_3$ at 4°C for 4 h).

The assay of endogenously occupied sites in addition to the unoccupied receptors has proven very useful in other steroid hormone systems (5-8). These assays require exchange of the endogenous ligand against ^{3}H-ligand in crude nuclear preparations in vitro. Since unoccupied 1,25$(OH)_2D_3$ receptors of the

[§]Present address: Department of Physiology, Tulane University School of Medicine, New Orleans
[#]Present address: Dept. of Pharmacology, School of Veterinary Medicine, University of Bern, Switzerland
[+]Institute of Animal Sciences, Volcani Center, Bet Dagan, Israel

chick intestinal mucosa are also associated with the nuclear/chromatin fraction (2), differentiation between and quantitative measurement of the unoccupied and occupied receptors is more complicated. We have recently described a method for differential detection and quantitative measurement of either in vivo occupied or unoccupied $1,25(OH)_2D_3$ receptors (9). In addition, described herein is the application of the $1,25(OH)_2D_3$ exchange assay to a study of certain aspects of the physiology of the vitamin D endocrine system including dietary phosphate depletion.

DEVELOPMENT OF $1,25(OH)_2D_3$ "EXCHANGE" ASSAY

The principles of a steroid "exchange" assay are summarized below in Table 1.

Our new $1,25(OH)_2D_3$ exchange assay method (9) provides differential measurement of either in vivo occupied or unoccupied receptors for 1,25-dihydroxyvitamin D_3 ($1,25(OH)_2D_3$) in the chick intestinal mucosa. The unoccupied receptors are quantitated in the chromatin fraction by incubation with $[^3H]1,25(OH)_2D_3$ at 4°C for 4 h without interference from the occupied sites. Fully occupied receptors can be measured at 37°C for 30 min with greater than 90% recovery. However, a mixture of occupied and unoccupied receptors cannot be directly quantitated at 37°C because of the high degradation rate of the unoccupied receptors at elevated temperatures (up to 50% degradation) which results in a falsely low total receptor estimate. Importantly, preincubation

Table 1. Principles of a Steroid-Receptor "Exchange Assay"

Steps	Assay Carried Out	Parameters Quantitated
(1)	$Rc + RcS + S^* \xrightarrow{4^\circ} RcS + RcS^*$	Unoccupied Sites
(2)	$Rc + RcS + S^* \xrightarrow{37^\circ} RcS^* + RcS^*$	Total Sites
(3)	Occupied Sites = [(2) - (1)]	
	or	
(4a)	$Rc + RcS + TPCK \xrightarrow{4^\circ} Rc\text{-blocked} + RcS$	Blocking of Unoccupied Sites
(4b)	$RcS + S^* \xrightarrow{37^\circ} RcS^*$	Occupied Sites

Here Rc represents the unoccupied receptor; RcS represents receptor occupied with nonradioactive ligand S, and S* = radioactive ligand.

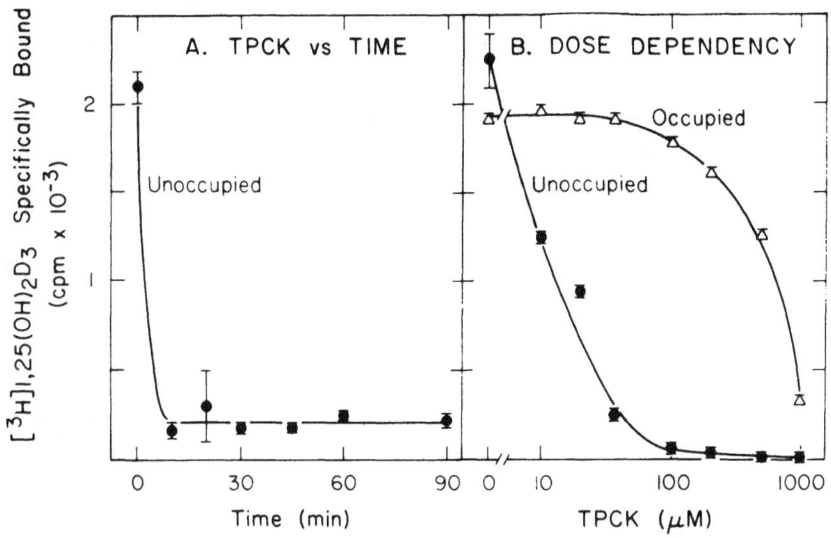

Fig. 1. Time (A) and dose dependency (B) of TPCK effects on $1,25(OH)_2D_3$ receptors. A, TED-chromatin from vitamin D_3-deficient chicks was preincubated with 50 M TPCK for the indicated times at 4°C before assay of $[^3H]1,25$-$(OH)_2D_3$ binding at 4°C for 4 h. B, TED-chromatin from vitamin D_3-deficient (●--●) or from $1,25(OH)_2D_3$-replete (△--△, 13 nmol of $1,25(OH)_2D_3$ 2 h prior to killing) chicks was preincubated with the indicated concentration of TPCK at 4°C for 30 min prior to assay with 8 nM $[^3H]$-$1,25(OH)_2D_3$ ± excess $1,25(OH)_2D_3$ at 4°C for 4 h (●--●) or at 37°C for 30 min (△--△). The values represent the means ± SEM of triplicate determinations.

at 4°C with L-1-tosylamide-2-phenylethyl chloromethyl ketone (TPCK, 100 μM) blocks the unoccupied $1,25(OH)_2D_3$ receptor sites allowing subsequent quantitation of exclusively occupied receptors by "exchange" incubation with $[^3H]1,25(OH)_2D_3$ at 37°C for 30 min (see figure 1).

With this exchange of $[^3H]1,25(OH)_2D_3$ in the presence of TPCK, there was no significant difference between total receptor levels in intestinal mucosa of chicks with fully occupied receptors (13 nmol $1,25(OH)_2D_3$ injected for 2 h) and the

Table 2. Concentrations of $1,25(OH)_2D_3$ in Intestinal Mucosa and Chromatin From Vitamin D-Replete Chicks as Measured by a Steroid Competition Assay, an Exchange Assay or After Continuous in vivo $[^3H]25(OH)D_3$ Labeling.*

Procedure	Steroid Competition Assay	Administration $[^3H]25(OH)D_3$ in vivo	Exchange Assay
Intestinal mucosa	1.44 ± 0.24	1.48 ± 0.20	1.42 ± 0.29
Intestinal chromatin	1.00 ± 0.25	1.34 ± 0.18	1.39 ± 0.35

*The results are expressed as a mean of 6 determinations ± SEM

receptor levels in chicks with only unoccupied receptors (8.01 ± 0.46 vs 7.82 ± 0.56 pmol/g tissue, respectively). We feel that this exchange assay allows quantitative measurement of occupied $1,25(OH)_2D_3$ receptors and/or unoccupied receptors in the chick intestinal mucosa.

Presented in Table 2 is a validation of the exchange assay measurement of $1,25(OH)_2D_3$ localized in the chick intestine. The amount of $[^3H]1,25(OH)_2D_3$ localized in the intestinal nucleus after in vivo administration of $[^3H]25(OH)D_3$ and the levels of nonradioactive $1,25(OH)_2D_3$ found in the intestinal nucleus as determined by the steroid competition assay (9) after organic solvent extraction were compared with the levels of occupied $1,25(OH)_2D_3$ receptors in the mucosal chromatin measured by the exchange assay (9). As shown in Table 2, no significant differences were detected in the duodenal or chromatin concentrations of $1,25(OH)_2D_3$ as determined by the specific activity of injected $[^3H]25\text{-}OH\text{-}D_3$ and $1,25(OH)_2D_3$ receptor occupancy measured by the exchange assay. These values were also similar to the levels of nonradioactive $1,25(OH)_2D_3$ determined by the competitive binding assay.

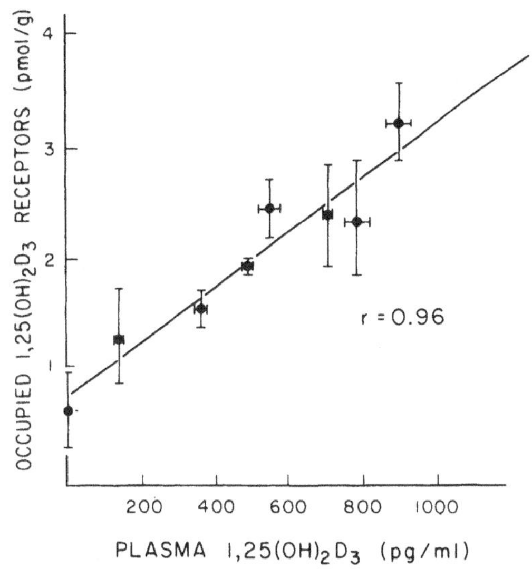

Figure 2. Correlation between serum $1,25(OH)_2D_3$ levels and levels of occupied chick intestinal $1,25(OH)_2D_3$ receptor after a subcutaneous dose of 1α-OH-D_3. Data points are the mean $\pm$ SEM on duplicate determinations on individual samples from 3 chicks.

Another form of validation of the $1,25(OH)_2D_3$ exchange assay which is particularly relevant to its application to the vitamin D endocrine system was an assessment of whether both unoccupied and occupied receptors $1,25(OH)_2D_3$ receptor levels were determined in the intestinal mucosa of $1,25(OH)_2D_3$-injected and noninjected vitamin D-deficient chicks. Importantly, there was no difference in the total receptor levels measured in the two groups of chicks (see Table 3). This result validates the receptor levels measured under nonexchange as well as under exchange conditions.

APPLICATION OF $1,25(OH)_2D_3$ "EXCHANGE" ASSAY

Figure 2 shows the close correlation existent 2 hr after an i.m. injection of 2-200 nmoles of $1\alpha(OH)D_3$ in the plasma level of $1,25(OH)_2D_3$ (measured by steroid competition assay) and the level of occupied intestinal receptor.

Table 3. Comparison of receptor levels in chromatin of the intestinal mucosa of vitamin D_3-deficient and of $1,25(OH)_2D_3$-replete chicks (mean $\pm$ SEM for 10 observations)

Chicks	Receptors		
	Unoccupied	Occupied	Total
		pmol/g	
Vitamin D_3-deficient	6.9 ± 0.5	0.9 ± 0.1	7.8 ± 0.6
$1,25(OH)_2D_3$-replete[a]	1.5 ± 0.2	6.5 ± 0.4	8.0 ± 0.6

[a]Injected with 19.5 nmol of $1,25(OH)_2D_3$ 2 h prior to killing.

Tissue responsiveness to estrogen or progesterone is regulated in part by a long-term increase (11) or decrease (12), respectively, in total receptor content following hormone administration. Thus we investigated whether vitamin D metabolites contribute to the regulation of intestinal $1,25(OH)_2D_3$ receptor levels. Since vitamin D deficient chicks were used, all changes in receptor levels can be attributed to the metabolite dosed and/or its *in vivo* derivatives. Daily treatment of chicks for 10 days with the indicated vitamin D metabolites resulted in different levels of occupied $1,25(OH)_2D_3$ receptors 24 h after the final injection (Fig. 3). In general, occupied receptor levels were higher in those animals treated with vitamin D derivatives which require one or more hydroxylations to generate a form with high affinity for $1,25(OH)_2D_3$ receptors. There was at least a 200-fold increase in the CaBP level with all the vitamin D forms; and there was a general correlation between the levels of CaBP and occupied receptor achieved with the metabolites. However, there was no effect of vitamin D treatment on the total tissue content of $1,25(OH)_2D_3$ receptors (Fig. 5). Similar data was obtained after daily treatment with these metabolites and 24, 48 and 72 h after a single injection of $1,25(OH)_2D_3$ or $24,25(OH)_2D_3$ (not shown). Thus these experiments suggest that the regulation of the total levels of the intestinal $1,25(OH)_2D_3$ receptor may not be directly related to the vitamin D status.

Intestinal responses to vitamin D and/or $1,25(OH)_2D_3$ appear to be decreased by glucocorticoids (12-14) and to be increased by progesterone (15) and estrogens (15). We therefore investigated whether these effects could be mediated through effects on the levels of intestinal $1,25(OH)_2D_3$ receptors. The effect of daily treatment with DES (5 mg), progesterone (1 mg)

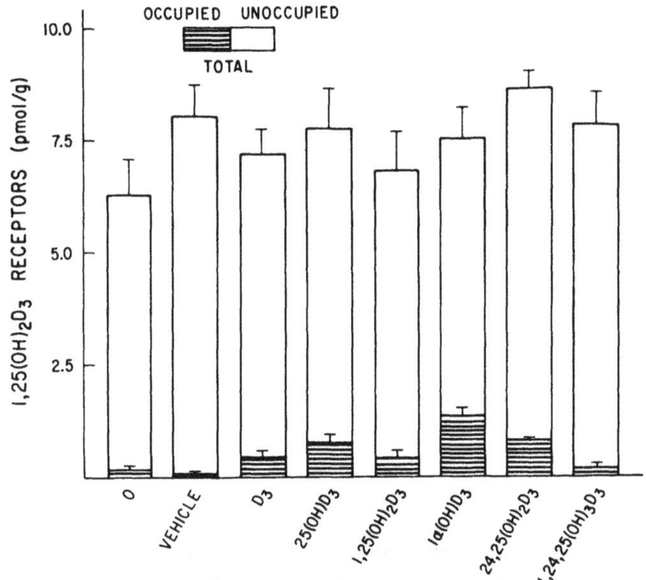

CaBP (μg/mg)	0.011 ±0.003	0.034 ±0.012	13.77 ±1.16	15.21 ±0.90	10.91 ±0.75	20.32 ±0.97	11.44 ±0.96	6.91 ±0.70

Fig. 3. Effect of vitamin D metabolites on $1,25(OH)_2D_3$ receptor levels in the intestinal mucosa. Rachitic chicks were treated i.m. daily for 10 days with 3.25 nmol of the indicated metabolites, and were sacrificed 24 h after the last injection. Data points represent the mean $\pm$ SEM of duplicate determinations in 8-10 chicks. The hatched bars represent occupied receptors, the open bars represent unoccupied receptors.

or cortisol (0.5 mg) was evaluated in chicks raised on a vitamin D-containing diet (Fig. 4). DES treatment resulted in increased $1,25(OH)_2D_3$ receptor occupancy, consistent with its reported effects on circulating $1,25(OH)_2D$ (16,17), as well as increased intestinal CaBP levels (15). However, there was no effect of any of these steroid hormones on the level of total $1,25(OH)_2D_3$ receptors in the intestinal mucosa (Fig. 4). Similar results were obtained after acute (24 h) and chronic (8 days) treatment

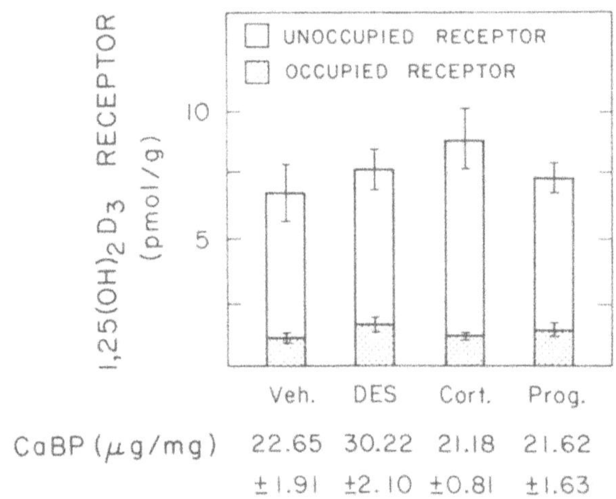

Fig. 4. Effect of estrogen, progesterone, and cortisol on $1,25(OH)_2D_3$ receptor levels in normal chicks. Chicks were raised from hatch on a vitamin D-containing diet. After three weeks they were injected i.m. daily for 8 days with vehicle (Neobee), 5 mg DES, 1 mg progesterone, or 0.5 mg cortisol and were sacrificed 24 h after the last injection. Data points represent the mean $\pm$ SEM of duplicate determinations in n = 6 individual chicks. Total bar heights represent total receptor levels, the hatched area represents occupied $1,25(OH)_2D_3$ receptors, and the open area represents the level of unoccupied receptors.

in vitamin D-deficient chicks (not shown). These results are consistent with our inability to detect estrogen receptors in the intestinal mucosa of vitamin D-deficient chicks (data not shown), despite the enhanced vitamin D-dependent CaBP production in the presence of DES (Fig. 4).

Under conditions of reduced dietary calcium or phosphorus, the activities of several aspects of the vitamin D endocrine system are stimulated (18-21). In order to determine whether

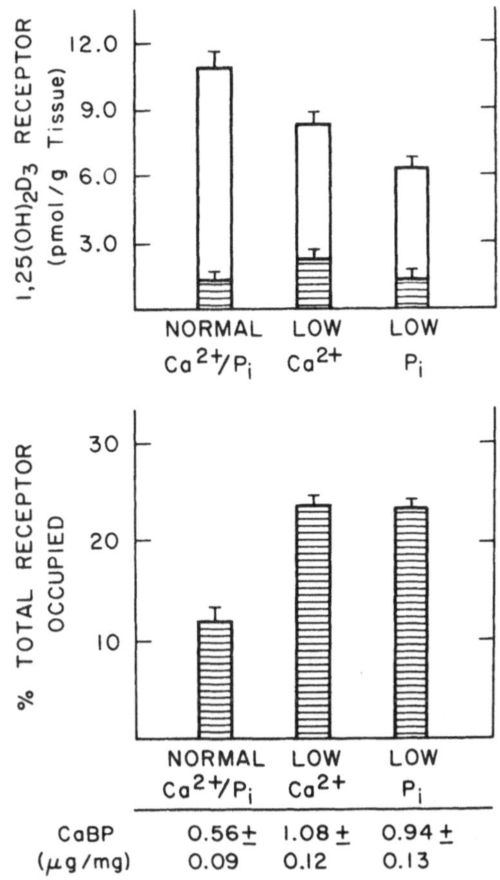

Fig. 5. Effect of Ca^{++} or phosphorus deficiency on 1,25-$(OH)_2D_3$ receptor levels in the intestinal mucosa of normal chicks. Chicks were raised on vitamin D-containing diets with normal levels of Ca^{++} (1.1%) and phosphorus (0.75%), low calcium (0.2% Ca^{++}, 0.75% phosphorus), low phosphorus (1.1% Ca^{++}, 0.25% phosphorus). Data points represent the mean ± SEM of n = 7-9 individual chicks. Upper panel presents level of occupied intestinal receptor, cross hatching represents occupied receptor, open bar represents unoccupied receptor, and total bar height represents the total receptor concentration. The bottom panel presents the percent occupied receptor.

these effects are mediated, in part, through regulation of intestinal $1,25(OH)_2D_3$ receptor levels, chicks were raised on vitamin D-containing diets with normal levels of Ca^{++} (1.1 %) and P (0.75%), low calcium (0.2% Ca^{++}, 0.75% P), or low phosphorus (1.1% Ca^{++}, 0.25% P). Receptor occupancy was increased in the mucosa of chicks fed the low Ca^{++} diet (Fig. 5), in agreement with reports of increased intestinal $1,25(OH)_2D_3$ content (18,19) and renal 25-hydroxyvitamin D-1α-hydroxylase stimulation (19) under these conditions. The total $1,25(OH)_2D_3$ receptor levels were lowered 25% ($P < 0.001$) by decreased dietary Ca^{++} and 46% ($p < 0.01$ vs. low Ca^{++} group) by reduced phosphorus (Fig. 5).

When the two variables of plasma concentration of $1,25(OH)_2$-D_3 and the concentration of occupied $1,25(OH)_2D_3$ receptors (Fig. 6A) were evaluated by linear regression analysis, a positive relationship was observed irrespective of whether the data from the low phosphate group were included or excluded. When individual values for plasma $1,25(OH)_2D_3$ concentration and the percent occupancy of $1,25(OH)_2D_3$ receptors in the duodenum (Fig. 6B) were evaluated by linear regression analysis, a positive relationship with a high r value (0.872 and 0.549) resulted when data for the low phosphorus group was included and omitted, respectively.

When plasma $1,25(OH)_2D_3$ concentration and the duodenal CaBP concentration were evaluated by linear regression analysis (Fig. 6C), a positive relationship was observed which was unchanged by including or excluding the data of the low P group. When the values for the plasma levels of $1,25(OH)_2D_3$ observed in control and calcium-deficient chicks and the total levels of intestinal $1,25(OH)_2D_3$ receptors were evaluated by linear regression analysis, a negative linear relationship was observed ($r = -0.683$, $y = 11.8-2.32\ X$; data not shown). When the values obtained from P-deficient chicks were included both the r value and the slope were changed ($r = -0.315$; $y = 9.7-1.8\ x$).

The linear regression relationship between occupied receptors and duodenal CaBP (Fig. 6) was unchanged in the presence and absence of the data from phosphorus-deficient chicks. Since the CaBP content of phosphorus-restricted birds was higher than in the controls, and the relationship to CaBP was unaffected by the values obtained from low phosphorus chicks, our methodology might be insufficient to determine relatively small changes in occupied receptors associated with large changes in CaBP levels. On the other hand, the concentration of total (occupied plus unoccupied) receptors was reduced by dietary calcium and, especially, by phosphorus restriction (Figure 5). As a consequence of this difference, the percent occupancy of intestinal $1,25(OH)_2D_3$ receptor in phosphorus-depleted chicks was as high as that in

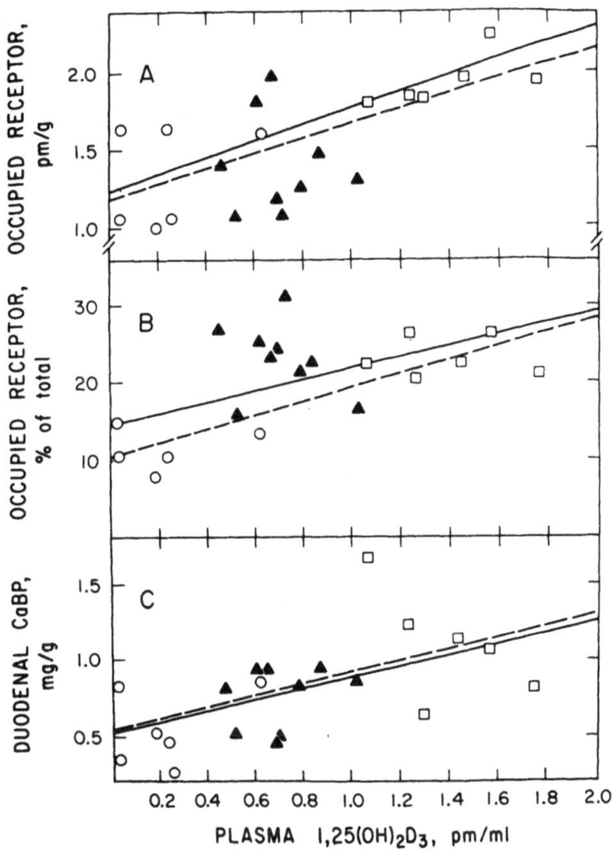

Fig. 6. Calculated linear regression relationships between plasma $1,25(OH)_2D_3$ concentration and occupied duodenal $1,25(OH)_2D_3$ receptor concentration both in pm/g (A), occupied receptor in percent total receptor (B) or duodenal CaBP in mg/g (C). Chicks were fed either a control diet containing normal Ca and normal P (o), or a low Ca or low P diet. Solid (I) and broken (II) lines represent the lines calculated including values from control (o), low calcium (□), low phosphorus (▲) groups, and from control (o) and low calcium (□), respectively.

The calculated lines and the r values are:

(A) I, y = 1.271 + 0.50 X, r = 0.799 (solid line);
II, y = 1.192 + 0.48 X, r = 0.610 (broken line).

(B) I, y = 10.43 + 9.04 X, r = 0.872;
II, y = 14.4 + 7.51 X, r = 0.549

(C) I, y = 0.509 + 0.381 X, r = 0.593;
II, y = 0.522 + 0.40 X, r = 0.522.

calcium-deficient chicks. These results may suggest a specific effect of phosphorus deficiency on either (a) the amount of receptor available or (b) that amount detected using our procedure. If the former is the case, then the high content of $1,25(OH)_2D_3$ previously observed in the intestinal mucosa of phosphorus-deficient birds (19) may have resulted from a higher portion of free $1,25(OH)_2D_3$ not bound to receptor proteins. Under these conditions, there might be an effect of this free $1,25(OH)_2D_3$ on the adaptive mechanism, suggesting the possibility of additional regulating factor(s) in this process. In the case of (b), a specific effect of phosphorus deficiency on either cell or nuclear membranes or cell biochemical properties, such as receptor stability, may be operative; this concept has been discussed previously (2). Experiments are currently underway to evaluate these possibilities.

The described method for differential measurement of unoccupied, occupied, and total receptor sites for $1,25(OH)_2D_3$ in the chick intestinal mucosa should be an important tool for future physiological studies in the vitamin D endocrine system. The procedure can be optimized for other target tissues and different species of animals including man. The small amounts of tissue required for the assay will be an asset in investigating disorders in the vitamin D system in humans.

ACKNOWLEDGEMENTS

This work was supported by USPHS Grant AM-09012-017 and USPHS Training Grant AM-07310.

REFERENCES

1. Norman, A.W., Vitamin D: The Calcium Homeostatic Steroid Hormone, Academic Press, New York, pp 490, (1979).

2. Walters, M.R., Hunziker, W. and Norman, A.W., Unoccupied 1,25 Dihydroxyvitamin D_3 receptors, J. Biol. Chem. 255:6799 (1980).

3. Walters, M.R., Hunziker, W. and Norman, A.W., Ubiquitous effects of the vitamin D endocrine system, Trends in Pharmacol. Sci. 2:42 (1981).

4. Walters, M.R., Hunziker, W. and Norman, A.W., Cytosol preparations are inadequate for quantitating unoccupied receptors for 1,25-dihydroxyvitamin-D_3, J. Receptor Res. 1(2):313 (1980).

5. Anderson, J.N., Clark, J.H., and Peck, E.J., Oestrogen and nuclear binding sites. Determination of specific sites by [^3H] oestradiol exchange, Biochem. J. 126:561 (1972).

6. Anderson, J.N., Peck, E.J. and Clark, J.H., Estrogen-induced uterine responses and growth: Relationship to receptor estrogen binding by uterine nuclei, Endocrinology 96:160 (1975).

7. Walters, M.R. and Clark, J.H., Cytosol and nuclear compartmentalization of progesterone receptors of the rat uterus, Endocrinology 103:601 (1978).

8. VuHai, M.T., Logeat, F. and Milgrom, E., Progesterone receptors in the rat uterus: Variation in cytosol and nuclei during the oestrous cycle and pregnancy, J. Endocrinology 76:43 (1978).

9. Hunziker, W., Walters, M.R. and Norman, A.W., 1,25-dihydroxyvitamin D_3 receptors, J. Biol. Chem. 255(20):9534 (1980).

10. Mourino, A., Lewicka-Piekut, S., Norman, A.W. and Okamura, W.H., Studies on vitamin D (calciferol) and its analogues. 20. Synthesis of 3-deoxy-3,3-dimethyl-1-hydroxyvitamin D_3 from vinylallene intermediates and related thermal and configurational studies, J. Organ. Chem. 45(20):4015 (1980).

11. Sarff, M. and Gorski, J., Control of estrogen binding protein concentration under basal conditions and after estrogen administration, Biochemistry 10:2557 (1971).

12. Kimberg, D.V., Baerg, R.D., Gershon, E., and Grandusius, R.T., Effect of cortisone treatment on the active transport of calcium by the small intestine, J. Clin. Invest. 50:1309 (1971).

13. Fehrer, J.J. and Wasserman, R.H., Intestinal calcium-binding protein and calcium absorption in cortisol-treated chicks: Effects of vitamin D_3 and 1,25-dihydroxyvitamin D_3, Endocrinology 104:547 (1979).

14. Spanos, E., Colston, K.W. and MacIntyre, I., Effect of glucocorticoids on vitamin D metabolism, FEBS Lett. 75:73 (1977).

15. Navickis, R.J., Dial, O.K., Katzenellenbogen, B.S. and Nalbandov, A.W., Effects of gonadal hormones on calcium binding protein in chick duodenum, Am. J. Physiol. 237:E409 (1979).

16. Kenny, A.D., Baksi, S.N. and Pang, P.K., Vitamin D metabolism: Physiological regulation in egg-laying Japanese quail, Am. J. Physiol. 230:1609 (1976).

17. Tanaka, Y., Castillo, L. and DeLuca, H.F., Control of renal vitamin D hydroxylases in birds by sex hormones (calcium/estrogen/testosterone/bone), Natl. Acad. Sci. USA 73:2701 (1976).

18. Edelstein, S., Harell, A., Bar, A. and Hurwitz, S., The functional metabolism of vitamin D in chicks fed low-calcium and low-phosphorus diets, Biochem. Biophys. Acta. 385:438 (1975).

EFFECTS OF SYSTEMIC pH ON CALCIUM REGULATING HORMONES AND BONE

John Cunningham and Louis V. Avioli

The Jewish Hospital and Washington University
School of Medicine
St. Louis, Missouri 63110 U.S.A.

Bone disease has long been recognized as a potential complication of chronic acidotic states[1]. By far the commonest of these is uremic acidosis, a situation in which deranged bone and mineral metabolism is invariably present. However, attempts to treat uremic bone disease by correction of an associated metabolic acidosis have been consistently unsuccessful[2], suggesting that factors other than systemic pH dominate the pathophysiology of this disease.

Chronic metabolic acidosis without uremia may result from renal tubular disorders or from surgical procedures which place a segment of bowel in continuity with the urinary tract. A proportion of these patients with hyperchloremic acidosis also develop bone disease, even when the glomerular filtration rate is normal or only minimally impaired[1,3]. In contrast to patients with uremic bone disease, in whom osteitis fibrosa and osteoclastosis is usually the predominant histological lesion seen, chronic hyperchloremic acidosis is attended by osteomalacia, histomorphometric evidence of parathyroid hormone excess being slight or absent. Furthermore, unlike uremic bone disease, osteomalacia complicating chronic hyperchloremic acidosis often responds well to correction of the acidosis by alkali therapy, whether or not vitamin D is given as well[4].

Of interest is that the development of rickets or osteomalacia appears not to depend on the presence of an intrinsic renal acidification defect causing bicarbonate depletion and acidosis. Thus, osteomalacia has been reported in patients with extrarenal bicarbonate depletion, for example following ureterosigmoidostomy, these subjects showing the same favorable response to alkali therapy, and vitamin D resistance, as is seen in the renal tubular acidoses[5,6].

The similarity of the skeletal lesions seen in chronic, non uremic, acidotic states to those of vitamin D deficiency, together with their favorable response to alkali therapy and poor response to even pharmacological doses of vitamin D, has raised the possibility of an acidosis-induced impairment of vitamin D bioactivation and/or resistance to the biological effects of the vitamin D metabolites.

It is now clearly established that normal vitamin D metabolism comprises sequential hydroxylation of the parent compound to 25-hydroxyvitamin D (25OHD) in the liver[7] and then to 1,25 dihydroxyvitamin D ($1,25OH_2D$) or 24,25 dihydroxyvitamin D ($24,25OH_2D$) in the kidney[8,9]. $1,25OH_2D$ serves as a calcemic hormone with potent effects on the gut and bone. Its biosynthesis is tightly modulated, parathyroid hormone (PTH), calcium and phosphate being the dominant controlling influences with a number of other factors including prolactin, growth hormone, insulin, estrogens, and possibly pH, also having demonstrable effects under certain circumstances[10,11,12]. Whether 25OHD and 24,25OHD serve as any more than precursor for $1,25OH_2D$ and inactive degradation product of 25OHD respectively remains controversial, although there is an increasing body of evidence suggesting unique effects of these metabolites on muscle[13], bone[14,15] and the developing fetus[16].

Many of the experimental models which have been devised to investigate the metabolism of vitamin D have yielded data which have been extrapolated successfully to human physiology and pathophysiology. Unfortunately this is not the case regarding acidosis and its effect (if any) on vitamin D metabolism, there being marked discrepancies between the information gained from experiments on laboratory animals and that from human studies.

In 1977, Sauveur et al[17] showed that a chronic metabolic acidosis, induced by ammonium chloride (NH_4Cl feeding) in vitamin D deficient chicks caused a 40% reduction of <u>in vitro</u> 1α-hydroxylase activity and that 24 hours after an intravenous injection of ^3H vitamin D_3, less ^3H $1,25(OH)_2D_3$ was recoverable from plasma, gut and bone in the acidotic animals than in controls. Acidosis did not affect plasma total calcium (ionized calcium was not measured), but raised plasma phosphate from 6.4 mg/dl to 9.5 mg/dl, leaving some doubt as to whether pH or phosphate was altering 1α-hydroxylation. Lee et al[18] studied the effect of an acute (3 day) NH_4Cl induced acidosis on the metabolism of intravenously injected ^3H $25OHD_3$ in vitamin D deficient rats and documented decreased circulating and intestinal accumulation of ^3H $1,25(OH)_2D_3$ in the acidotic animals, independent of changes in plasma calcium and phosphate. These data, although compatible with impairment of 1α-hydroxylation during acidosis, could also be explained, at least in part, by decreased tissue receptivity and/or increased degradation of preformed ^3H $1,25(OH)_2D_3$ in acidotic animals.

It should be remembered that in order to induce abundant and easily measured production of $1,25(OH)_2D$, the studies outlined above were all conducted on vitamin D and calcium depleted animals. Furthermore the apparent impairment of 1α-hydroxylation in these acidotic animals may not be specific, but merely part of a generalized depression of a variety of metabolic functions. In an attempt to resolve some of these questions, we have conducted studies using both vitamin D deficient and D replete animals to examine the interrelated effects of pH and vitamin D status. In vitro studies of chick renal 1α-hydroxylase activity during acute NH_4Cl induced acidosis produced changes similar to those seen in the more chronic studies of Sauveur et al[17], acidotic animals showing a 36% suppression of 1α-hydroxylase activity. However when the same experiments were performed on vitamin D replete animals raised on a nutritionally complete diet (0.9% calcium, 0.6% phosphorus), 24-hydroxylase activity was increased nearly fourfold by acidosis. These changes in enzyme activity were paralled by significant increments in plasma calcium and phosphate in the acidotic animals, either or both of which would be expected to decrease 1α-hydroxylase and increase 24-hydroxylase activity. When an increase in plasma calcium was induced in vitamin D replete animals by feeding a high calcium diet, the effect on 24-hydroxylase activity was similar to that of acidosis, despite no fall in pH and no rise in phosphate. These data indicate that effects of acidosis on the renal hydroxylases are demonstrable in the vitamin D replete state as well as in the vitamin D deficient state and that in the chick, they are accompanied by, and may be mediated by, changes in plasma calcium[19].

Preliminary studies in rats have produced similar results, with acidosis increasing plasma ionized calcium (though not total calcium or phosphate) and 24-hydroxylase activity and decreasing 1α-hydroxylase activity. In this model there is a temporal relationship between acidosis and the changes in the activity of the hydroxylases. Marked suppression of 1α-hydroxylase and augmentation of 24-hydroxylase were seen after 1 day of acidosis with loss of the 1α-hydroxylase effect by 6 days and of the 24-hydroxylase effect by 21 days, despite persisting acidemia and elevation of plasma ionized calcium. Thus, in the rat, some parameter of the acidotic state other than calcium, phosphate or pH appears to act early, but not late, in acidosis to alter the renal conversion of 25-hydroxyvitamin D.

Clearly the vitamin D resistance seen in acidosis need not necessarily be the result of impaired bioactivation of the parent compound but may instead reflect accelerated degradation of one or more of the dihydroxy metabolites, or decreased target organ receptivity to these metabolites. In this regard, Baran et al[20] have documented increased clearance of injected ^3H $1,25(OH)_2D_3$ from the circulation of acidotic chicks, though found no change in intestinal accumulation of this metabolite and Gafter et al[21] have shown that acute acidosis in rats does not impair the augmentation of intestinal calcium and phosphate absorption seen during their dietary deprivation.

Collectively, although the induction of acidosis is clearly associated with demonstrable alterations in vitamin D metabolism, the studies outlined above have failed to show a definite effect of pH per se on vitamin D metabolism at the level of the kidney, or on its action on the gut.

Data from human studies have generally been inconclusive. Brewer et al[22], using children with Fanconi's syndrome, administered ^3H 25OHD$_3$ and were unable to demonstrate the appearance of ^3H 1,25(OH)$_2$D$_3$ in plasma. However, they also failed to detect ^3H 24,25(OH)$_2$D$_3$ in 4 out of the 5 subjects, casting some doubt on their conclusion that 1,25(OH)$_2$D production may be decreased in Fanconi's syndrome. The induction of mild metabolic acidosis in man by high protein feeding or NH_4Cl loading has not been associated with measurable alterations of 1,25(OH)$_2$D production, although in some cases the techniques used may not have been sufficiently sensitive to detect small changes[23,24]. Another possible reason for the discrepancy between the human and animal studies may be the relatively more severe acidoses that have been induced in animals, although in this regard one of us (J.C.) has seen a patient with severe osteomalacia and metabolic acidosis in whom plasma levels of 25OHD and 1,25(OH)$_2$D were normal before and during successful treatment of the osteomalacia with alkali.

Data concerning the effects of acidosis on PTH are conflicting. Acid loading in normal man has been stated to increase[25], or to have no effect[23,24] on serum immunoreactive PTH. Irrespective of any tendency of acidosis to alter PTH secretion or metabolism, there exists the possibility of altered target organ responsiveness to PTH in acidotic states. Beck et al[26] examined the effect of acute acidosis on PTH mediated phosphaturia and cyclic AMP excretion in rats and found significant reductions in both during acidosis. Conversely, in humans, augmentation of PTH effects on the kidney have been reported during NH_4Cl loading[27]. Although not yet investigated, it is conceivable that PTH mediated stimulation of 1α-hydroxylase and suppression of 24-hydroxylase could be subject to these effects. At the level of bone the position seems clearer. In addition to the known direct action of acidosis to increase resorption, there is evidence that PTH-mediated bone resorption is augmented during acute acidosis in rats[28], and also that PTH-dependent cyclic AMP release by the isolated perfused canine tibia is increased in the presence of a simulated metabolic acidosis[29]. Therefore, the failure to demonstrate changes in PTH levels during acidosis may still be compatible with altered PTH action on the kidney and increased PTH action on the skeleton.

Interactions between acidosis and third major calcium regulating hormone, calcitonin, could be of considerable importance. However, Beck et al[28] have shown that the calcium lowering action of calcitonin, is unimpaired in acutely acidotic rats, suggesting that acidosis does not have any tendency to release resorptive forces from the normal controlling influence of calcitonin.

Common to all chronic metabolic acidoses is the major role played by bone in the defense of extracellular pH during the accumulation of non-volatile acids or the loss of base[30]. Acid administration results in rapid titration of extracellular bicarbonate which plateaus at a time when hydrogen ion balance is still positive. The apparent discrepancy can be accounted for by loss of bone carbonate and progressively greater negative calcium and phosphorus balances, finally reaching the point where bone mineral is the only significant contributor to the buffering of retained acid[31]. It is possible that these responses of the skeleton may in part be PTH dependent[32]. The potential for progressive calcium and phosphorus depletion is clear.

The foregoing discussion has attempted to relate some of the metabolic disturbances seen in acidotic animals to the clinical problem of osteomalacia with chronic acidosis. However, it is clear that at present, major discrepancies exist regarding the extrapolation of the experimental animal data to osteomalacia in humans. Despite the abundance of evidence indicating altered vitamin D metabolism and PTH action in appropriately acidotic models, there is at present no clear indication that acidosis induces a primary disturbance of calcium regulating hormones in man.

Addendum: Following completion of this report, it has come to our attention that in 1967 Verbanck and Kahn reported that NH_4Cl feeding resulted in a decrease in serum calcium in vitamin D-intoxicated hypercalcemic dogs (Actualites Nephrol. pp 241-248, 1967).

REFERENCES

1. F. Albright, C.H. Burnett, W. Parson, F.C. Reifenstein and A. Roos, Osteomalacia and late rickets: the various etiologies met in the United States with emphasis on that resulting from specific forms of renal acidosis, the therapeutic indication for each etiological subgroup and the relationship between osteomalacia and Milkman's syndrome, Medicine 25:399 (1946).
2. S.W. Stanbury and G.A. Lumb, Metabolic studies of renal osteodystrophy 1. Calcium, phosphorus and nitrogen metabolism in rickets, osteomalacia and hyperparathyroidism complicating chronic uremia and in the osteomalacia of the adult Fanconi syndrome, Medicine 41:1 (1962).
3. K.L. Pines and G.H. Mudge, Renal tubular acidosis with osteomalacia, Am. J. Med. 11:302 (1951).
4. P. Richards, M.J. Chamberlain and O.M. Wrong, Treatment of osteomalacia of renal tubular acidosis by sodium bicarbonate alone, Lancet 2:994 (1972).
5. P. Siklos, M. Davie, R.T. Jung and T.M. Chalmers, Osteomalacia in ureterosigmoidostomy: healing by correction of the acidosis, Brit. J. Urol. 52: 61 (1980).
6. W. Perry, L.N. Allen, T.C.B. Stamp, and P.G. Walker, Vitamin D resistance in osteomalacia after ureterosigmoidostomy, N. Engl. J. Med. 297:1110 (1977).
7. G. Ponchon and H.F. DeLuca, The role of the liver in the meta-

bolism of vitamin D, J. Clin. Invest. 48:1273 (1969).
8. D.R. Fraser and E. Kodicek, Unique biosynthesis by kidney of a biologically active vitamin D metabolite, Nature (London) 228:764 (1970).
9. M.F. Holick, H.K. Schnoes, H.F. DeLuca, R.W. Gray, I.T. Boyle, and T. Suda, Isolation and identification of 24,25-dihydroxycholecalciferol: a metabolite of vitamin D_3 made in the kidney, Biochemistry 11:4251 (1972).
10. M. Garabedian, M.F. Holick, H.F. DeLuca and I.T. Boyle, Control of 25-hydroxycholecalciferol metabolism by parathyroid glands, Proc. Nat. Acad. Sci. 69:1673 (1972).
11. M.R. Hughes, P.F. Brumbaugh, M.R. Haussler, J.E. Wergedal and D.J. Baylink, Regulation of serum 1α,25-dihydroxyvitamin D_3 by calcium and phosphate in the rat, Science 190:578 (1975).
12. Y. Tanaka and H.F. DeLuca, The control of 25-hydroxyvitamin D metabolism by inorganic phosphorus, Arch. Biochem. Biophys. 154:566 (1973).
13. S.J. Birge and J.G. Haddad, 25 hydroxycholecalciferol stimulation of muscle metabolism, J. Clin. Invest. 56:1100 (1975).
14. A. Arnoy, D. Goodwin, D. Noff and S. Edelstein, 24,25-dihydroxyvitamin D is a metabolite of vitamin D essential for bone formation, Nature 276:517 (1978).
15. P. Bordier, H. Rasmussen, P. Marie, L. Miravet, J. Gueris and A. Ryckwaert, Vitamin D metabolites and bone mineralization in man, J. Clin. Endocrinol. Metab. 46:284 (1978).
16. H.L. Henry and A.W. Norman, Vitamin D: Two dihydroxylated metabolites of vitamin D are required for normal chick hatchability, Science 201:835 (1978).
17. B. Sauveur, M. Garabedian, C. Fellot, P. Mongin and S. Balsan, The effect of induced metabolic acidosis on vitamin D_3 metabolism in rachitic chicks, Calcif. Tiss. Res. 23:121 (1977).
18. S.W. Lee, J. Russell and L.V. Avioli, 25-hydroxycholecalciferol to 1,25-dihydroxycholecalciferol: conversion impaired by systemic metabolic acidosis, Science 195:994 (1977).
19. J. Cunningham, D.D. Bikle, A. Fausto and L.V. Avioli, Effect of acidosis on chick renal 25-hydroxyvitamin D (25OHD) 1α and 24-hydroxylases, Calcif. Tiss. Int. 33:333A (1981).
20. D.T. Baran, S.W. Lee, O.D. Jo and L.V. Avioli, Acquired alterations in vitamin D metabolism in the acidotic state, Calcif. Tiss. Int. in press.
21. U. Gafter, J.A. Kraut, D.B.N. Lee, V. Silis, M.W. Walling, K. Kurokawa, M.R. Haussler and J.W. Coburn, Effect of metabolic acidosis on intestinal absorption of calcium and phosphorus, Am. J. Physiol. 239:G480 (1980).
22. E.D. Brewer, H.C. Tsai and R.C. Morris, Evidence for impairment of metabolism of 25-hydroxyvitamin D_3 ($25OHD_3$) in children with Fanconi's syndrome (FS), Clin. Res. 24:154A (1976).

23. H.P. Weber, R.W. Graw, J.H. Dominquez and J. Lemann, The lack of effect of chronic metabolic acidosis on 25-OH vitamin D metabolism and serum parathyroid hormone in humans, J. Clin. Endocrinol. Metab. 43:1047 (1976).
24. N.D. Adams, R.W. Gray and J. Lemann, The calciuria of increased fixed acid production in humans: evidence against a role for parathyroid hormone and $1,25(OH)_2$ vitamin D, Calcif. Tiss. Int. 28:233 (1979).
25. F.L. Coe, J.J. Firpo, D.L. Hollandsworth, L. Segil, J.M. Canterbury and E. Reiss, Effect of acute and chronic metabolic acidosis on serum immunoreactive parathyroid hormone in man, Kidney Int. 8:262 (1975).
26. N. Beck, H.P. Kim and K.S. Kim, Effect of metabolic acidosis on renal action of parathyroid hormone, Am. J. Physiol. 228:1483 (1975).
27. J.C.M. Chan and F.C. Bartter, Effect of metabolic acidosis and alkalosis on the renal response to parathyroid hormone infusion in normal man, Kidney Int. 14 Suppl:637 (1978).
28. N. Beck and S.K. Webster, Effects of acute metabolic acidosis on parathyroid hormone action and calcium mobilization, Am. J. Physiol. 230:127 (1976).
29. K.J. Martin, J.J. Freitag, E. Bellorin-Font, M.B. Conrades, S. Klahr and E. Slatopolsky, The effect of acute acidosis on the uptake of parathyroid hormone and the production of adenosine 3',5'-monophosphate by isolated perfused bone, Endocrinology 106:1607 (1980).
30. R.M. Blitz, E.D. Pellegrino and J.M. Letteri, Skeletal carbonates and acid base regulation, Min. Elec. Metab. 5:1 (1981).
31. J. Lemann, J.R. Litzow and E.J. Lennon, The effects of chronic acid loads in normal man: further evidence for the paticipation of bone mineral in the defense against chronic metabolic acidosis, J. Clin. Invest. 45:1608 (1966).
32. D.S. Fraley and S. Adler, An extrarenal role for parathyroid hormone in the disposal of acute acid loads in rats and dogs, J. Clin. Invest. 63:985 (1979).

INHERITED AND ACQUIRED DISORDERS OF VITAMIN D METABOLISM

John G. Haddad

Endocrine Section, Department of Internal Medicine
University of Pennsylvania School of Medicine
36th Street & Hamilton Walk
Philadelphia, PA 19104

Many human diseases have previously been characterized by their sensitivity or resistance to vitamin D, although direct information about mechanisms has been lacking. The development and application of radioisotopic materials and specific quantitative assays for vitamin D sterols have permitted direct analyses of vitamin D metabolism in patients affected by these diseases. Since there have been reviews of vitamin D metabolism in recent years (1-3), I shall confine this review to more recent studies of conditions which reflect inherited or birth-related, and acquired difficulties in vitamin D sterols' supply, metabolism and biological effects.

INHERITED OR BIRTH-RELATED DISORDERS

Since the discovery of vitamin D and its use as a dietary supplement during infancy and childhood, vitamin D deficiency rickets is seen less frequently and inherited rickets has received more attention. Prominent among these disorders are those associated with abnormalities in phosphorus translocation, with resulting phosphorus wasting and hypomineralization of bone. X-linked and sporadic autosomal hypophosphatemic syndromes are recognized. In addition, vitamin D-dependency is an autosomal recessive disorder in which effective production of 1,25-dihydroxyvitamin D is apparently impaired. Finally, true resistance to vitamin D is characterized in the reports of end organ hyposensitivity to 1,25-dihydroxyvitamin D and disorders of receptor content or binding characteristics in the tissues. Table I lists these disorders, and includes birth-related conditions of vitamin D status which derive from maternal factors and prematurity.

Table 1. Inherited Disorders of Vitamin D Metabolism

Condition	Transmission	Features
Vitamin D Deficiency	Maternal Vitamin D Deficiency and/or Prematurity	Hypomineralization, poor growth, secondary hyperparathyroidism
Vitamin D Dependent Rickets (Pseudovitamin D deficiency rickets)- Type I	Autosomal Recessive	Like D-deficiency 25OHD ↔ or ↑ 1,25 ↓ PTH ↑
End-organ Resistance to Vitamin D; Vitamin D Dependent Rickets - Type II	Autosomal Recessive	↑ 1,25, ↑ PTH ↓ Receptors Alopecia
Familial Hypophosphatemic Rickets	X-linked - usual Autosomal Dominant	PO_4 wasting PTH ↔ 1,25 ↔ or ↓
Pseudohypoparathyroidism	Sporadic ? Sex-linked dominant ?	↑ PTH ↓ Ca ↑ PO_4 ± Phenotype ↓ Renal response to PTH

Vitamin D-deficiency

Since intra-uterine life is devoid of effective solar irradiation, the fetus apparently depends entirely on placental transfer of vitamin D sterols to establish stores. It is not presently clear whether or not vitamin D metabolism *in utero* is essential to embryogenesis and fetal mineral homeostasis. Since calcium transfer is active from mother to fetus, fetal or cord parathyroid hormone (PTH) levels are low, as are plasma 1,25-dihydroxyvitamin D ($1,25-(OH)_2D$) concentrations, but calcitonin levels are elevated compared to those in adult blood[4,5]. Recently, the placenta has been shown to be capable of $1,25-(OH)_2D$ synthesis, but the importance of these hormones to the fetal skeleton is not understood. Since the maternal plasma binding protein for vitamin D (DBP) increases during pregnancy, the increased levels of $1,25-(OH)_2D$ in pregnancy reflect increased binding and stable "free" sterol concentrations[4]. Net fetal calcium gain increases only at the last few weeks of pregnancy, however.

Cord plasma, in several studies, contains amounts of 25-hydroxycalciferol (25-OHD) that are proportional to those in maternal plasma[6]. Earlier studies showed that vitamin D-deficient mothers gave birth to infants with neonatal rickets[7]. Clearly, maternal vitamin D status influences that of the newborn infant. With prematurity, there is evidence of fat and calcium malabsorption[8], poor vitamin D absorption and vitamin D 25-hydroxylation[9]. The incidence of D-deficiency in small prematures[10] demands an awareness of this possibility and its correction, since the myopathy further impairs compromised pulmonary function.

Vitamin D-Dependent Rickets - Type I

This condition closely simulates vitamin D-deficiency clinically and chemically, but is associated with a poor response to usual replacement doses of vitamin D[11]. Although plasma 25-OHD is normal and PTH levels are increased, plasma $1,25\text{-}(OH)_2D$ levels are inappropriately low[12]. Whereas massive doses of vitamin D can heal the rickets, small doses of $1,25\text{-}(OH)_2D$ are effective[13].

Available evidence suggests that the renal 25-OHD 1α-hydroxylase is defective in this autosomal recessive disorder, since $1,25\text{-}(OH)_2D$ levels are low when substrate (25-OHD) and stimulus (PTH) are plentiful. The assay of normal plasma 25-OHD levels in clinical vitamin D deficiency draws suspicion to this diagnosis.

Vitamin D-Dependent Rickets - Type II

Severe rickets, which is resistant to very high doses of vitamin D, and which also poorly responds to reasonable doses or endogenously high levels of $1,25\text{-}(OH)_2D$, has been noted by several workers[14,15,16,17]. In spite of adequate to high levels of bioactive sterols, intestinal absorption of calcium is poor and target-organ hyposensitivity or resistance was suspected. Recently, workers have succeeded in demonstrating nuclear uptake and cytosolic, high-affinity binding of $1,25\text{-}(OH)_2\{^3H\}D_3$ by normal fibroblasts in culture[18,19,20]. When fibroblasts from patients with this syndrome are tested, deficient binding of this sterol is apparent[20]. Since several steps are involved in the translocation and cellular expression of steroid hormones, a variety of defects seems possible in causing resistance to $1,25\text{-}(OH)_2D$ action. In some patients, total alopecia is seen. It is of interest that skin receptors for $1,25\text{-}(OH)_2D$ have been described, but a physiological role for this sterol in this tissue is not currently recognized. In two subjects, the plasma DBP levels were observed to be in the normal range[16].

Familial Hypophosphatemic Rickets

This disorder is certainly more familiar to most readers, since it has received more attention over a longer period. Best recognized in its x-linked form, sporadic cases of autosomal transmission are also recognized. The characteristic findings are hypophosphatemia and wastage of phosphorus into the urine. In contrast with the previously described disorders, myopathy, hypocalcemia, and secondary hyperparathyroidism are absent.

25-hydroxylation of vitamin D is recognized to be intact[21] and initial reports described normal plasma levels of 1,25-$(OH)_2D$[3]. Since then, however, others have found low-normal to sub-normal plasma levels of this sterol[12]. In contrast to the increased 1,25-$(OH)_2D$ concentrations seen in plasma from normal women during phosphorus depletion[22], these patients apparently do not respond to this stimulus.

Treatment with high dose vitamin D compounds alone has not improved the condition without endangering renal function through hypercalciuria and hypercalcemia. The addition of frequent, oral phosphate supplements has led to skeletal healing and improved growth[23]. Other compounds, such as DHT, 1$\alpha$$OHD_3$ and 1,25-$(OH)_2D_3$ have been used alone or with phosphate supplements[24,25] with some success. There is some evidence that 1,25-$(OH)_2D_3$ administration can cause improved renal tubular retention of phosphorus. Also, phosphate therapy alone can cause secondary hyperparathyroidism, which may be directly suppressed by sterol action on the parathyroids and/or by sterol stimulation of the variably depressed intestinal absorption of calcium. An acquired syndrome with similar features has been observed with certain types of connective tissue tumors[26].

Other Disorders

Neonatal dysfunctions in vitamin D metabolism can be traced to other disorders which compromise the production of effective vitamin D sterols. The presence of the hypoparathyroid state can be expected in the infant of the hypercalcemic mother, but this is a transient problem after delivery. In pseudohypoparathyroidism, however, the renal signal from PTH is not effective, and deficient 1,25-$(OH)_2D$ production is a problem. In addition, any urinary conduit abnormality _in utero_ which leads to renal damage can reduce the machinery for 1,25-$(OH)_2D$ synthesis. Since the renal 25-OHD-1α hydroxylase is a mitochondrial enzyme which requires substrate, NADPH, oxygen and favorable ionic milieu, it does not seem unreasonable that other inherited conditions of kidney function could be associated with impaired 1,25-$(OH)_2D$ synthesis.

Table 2. Acquired Disorders of Vitamin D Metabolism

SUPPLY AND ECONOMY

Deficiency
- Poor dietary content of anti-rachitic sterols
- Malabsorption of anti-rachitic sterols (gastro-intestinal surgery and diseases, hepato-biliary and pancreatic disorders, lipid-binding resins)
- Urinary wastage of anti-rachitic sterols (nephrotic syndrome); increased excretion of polar metabolites in G-I disorders
- Accelerated catabolism of anti-rachitic sterols (drug induction of microsomal P-450 enzymes)
- Poor cutaneous synthesis of vitamin D_3 (environment, clothing, customs, pigmentation, skin disorder)
- Maternal vitamin D-deficiency

Excess
- Pharamcologic doses of vitamin D, its metabolites and their analogs

METABOLISM

Deficiency
- Severe liver disease with impairment of 25-hydroxylation
- Severe renal disease with impairment of 1-hydroxylation
- Hypoparathyroid states with decreased 1-hydroxylation
- Non-parathyroid hypercalcemia with decreased 1-hydroxylation
- Oncogenic osteomalacia
- Marked hyperphosphatemic states
- Old age
- Accelerated catabolism of sterols (anti-convulsant drugs)

Excess
- Sarcoidosis and other granulomatous disorders
- Idiopathic hypercalciuria
- Hyperparathyroid states
- Response to hypocalcemic challenge

ACTION

Deficiency
- Diseases of target organs
- Glucocorticoid therapy
- Estrogen therapy
- ? increased DBP

Excess
- ? age (youth)
- ? decreased DBP

ACQUIRED DISORDERS OF VITAMIN D METABOLISM

A variety of conditions have been identified in which vitamin D supply, economy and/or efficient metabolism are threatened, resulting in a deficiency of vitamin D or its metabolites. Similarly, other conditions are recognized in which exaggerated supplies of vitamin D or augmented metabolism to its bioactive form results in excessive vitamin D effects. For the purpose of this brief review, let's consider these as examples of problems in the supply, economy, metabolism and action of these sterols.

Supply and Economy

Sources. Evidence has accumulated to indicate that cutaneous production of vitamin D is the major source of this sterol under normal conditions. Clearly, however, many factors (abundance of effective u-v rays, clothing, customs, dietary vitamin D, etc.) can influence the adequacy or dominance of this source, and lead to disease[27]. Since illness in general is frequently the cause of anorexia and limited mobility, vitamin D stores can be taxed during periods of poor intake and limited exposure to solar irradiation. Conversely, persons with heavy u-v light exposure are known to have high levels of plasma 25-OHD[28,29].

Deficiency Although "pure" vitamin D deficiency is still seen in some areas where effective cutaneous synthesis is precluded by clothing and weather and dietary supplements are insufficient[31], most cases now recognized in this country are attributable to other problems such as intestinal malabsorption and anti-convulsant therapy. Deficiency states are characterized by low plasma 25-OHD, an excellent index of vitamin D stores in most instances. Other polar metabolites are usually in low titer as well, but normal to high levels of plasma 1,25-$(OH)_2D$ have been observed[32]. This appears to be an appropriate response to the secondary hyperparathyroidism attending this state. However, recent analyses of the plasma sterol response to low dosage vitamin D replacement is of interest[33]. Following a modest increase in vitamin D and 25-OHD availability, plasma 1,25-$(OH)_2D$ levels increase dramatically and stay at high levels for months. These levels are certainly higher than those seen in some cases of early vitamin D deficiency, and one wonders if normal or slightly elevated 1,25-$(OH)_2D$ levels in plasma from D-deficient subjects are inappropriately low, reflecting the lack of sufficient substrate (25-OHD). It is not presently clear if PTH or other factors are responsible for the continued high plasma levels of 1,25-$(OH)_2D$ during the phases of the later healing of vitamin D deficiency. Certainly, the continued low plasma levels of 24,25 $(OH)_2D$ and 25,26-$(OH)_2D$ during this healing are not supportive of their having a role in the skeletal repair.

Intoxication In the past, chronic, high doses of vitamin D were required to bring about hypercalciuria and hypercalcemia. Subsequently, dihydrotachysterol, now known to have an A ring similar to that of 1,25-$(OH)_2D$, caused these changes more quickly at lower dosage. Bypassing 25-hydroxylation by administration of 25-OHD_3 is followed in hours by increased plasma 25-OHD[30]. Intoxication with vitamin D is associated with high plasma 25-OHD, but normal to low 1,25-$(OH)_2D$ levels[3]. 1αOHD administration results in its 25-hydroxylation to 1,25-$(OH)_2D$, and this sterol can abruptly cause an increase in serum calcium.

Hepatic and Intestinal Disorders Although low 25-OHD concentrations are observed in plasma from subjects with liver diseases[34], it is possible that this represents low dietary vitamin D and poor sunlight exposure in addition to deficient 25-OHD and plasma DBP production. Certainly, subjects with severe liver disease are capable of 25-hydroxylation if substrate is delivered intravenously[35]. In some instances, increased catabolism of sterols, bile flow and urinary excretion of polar materials are noted.

A variety of intestinal disorders and diseases of the pancreatic-biliary system imperil fat absorption. Dietary vitamin D is poorly absorbed, thus endangering those patients with marginal exposure to effective ultra-violet rays in the 280-310 nm range. The suggestion that an enterohepatic circulation for vitamin D sterols might further tax D-status is not supported by studies which indicate that most of the sterols are polar, biologically inactive compounds[37]. The need for a reliable parenteral preparation of vitamin D is underscored by the variation of vitamin D content in some oily depot products[38]. The bioavailability of oral and parenteral preparations [38] suggests that a parenteral preparation of 25-OHD_3 might be a useful addition to presently available preparations.

Other threats to supply The therapeutic application of resins designed to reduce lipid absorption can reduce absorption of vitamin D. In cases of severe proteinuria, both plasma DBP and bioactive sterols are lost into the urine[39], and deficiency disease can occur[40].

Metabolism

Parathyroid hormone and kidney. The original observations of the stimulative action of PTH on the 25-OHD-1λhydroxylase have been confirmed in human disease states. Primary and secondary hyperparathyroidism are associated with increased plasma 1,25-$(OH)_2D$ levels, if sufficient 25-OHD is available. Conversely, hypoparathyroid conditions are associated with low plasma concentrations of 1,25-$(OH)_2D$[3]. When PTH is administered to hypoparathyroid subjects, plasma 1,25-$(OH)_2D$ increases.

Interferences in the signal from PTH to the kidney, such as in pseudohypoparathyroidism, results in levels of $1,25\text{-}(OH)_2D$ that are inappropriately low for the increased levels of circulating PTH[41]. When the sterol synthetic mechanism is reduced by kidney disease, the $1,25\text{-}(OH)_2D$ responses to PTH are also less than expected[3].

Non-parathyroid, ionic effects Evidence has accumulated to suggest direct influences by calcium and phosphorus on the 1α hydroxylases. In the absence of PTH, low extracellular phosphate has been associated with increased plasma $1,25(OH)_2D$[22,42], and hypercalcemia has been observed to suppress plasma $1,25\text{-}(OH)_2D$ concentrations[43]. A previous review of the hydroxylation reaction has considered the possible mechanisms for these ionic effects[1]. Clinically, these ionic influences can be considered as a function of pathophysiologic events. However, under physiologic conditions, a positive correlation between PTH and $1,25\text{-}(OH)_2D$ is clear and useful.

Diseases attended by non-parathyroid hypercalcemia, such as hyperthyroidism[44] and cancer[45] are associated with low plasma concentrations of $1,25\text{-}(OH)_2D$. Similar effects are appreciated during immobilization and vitamin D intoxication. The latter condition appears to not be attributable to elevated $1,25\text{-}(OH)_2D$ production, a remarkable tribute to the regulation of this synthesis. In disorders characterized by a tendency to hypocalcemia and secondary hyperparathyroidism, such as might occur in osteoblastic malignancy, appropriate increases in plasma $1,25\text{-}(OH)_2D$ are expected.

Anti-convulsant therapy Patients receiving long-term treatment with drugs, such as diphenylhydantoin and barbituates, experience an exaggerated metabolism of many substances following stimulation of hepatic microsomal P-450 hydroxylase enzymes[3]. 25-OHD levels in plasma can be reduced[46], and strikingly frequent deficiency disease has been reported[47]. Prior to severe depletion, plasma $1,25\text{-}(OH)_2D$ levels may be normal or elevated, which is consistent with a secondary hyperparathyroidism.

Sarcoidosis In granulomatous diseases, hypercalcemia has been noted and previously thought to be due to an increased sensitivity to vitamin D. Non-toxic amounts of vitamin D are poorly tolerated in sarcoidosis and increased (inappropriate to low PTH levels) plasma levels of $1,25\text{-}(OH)_2D$ are seen[48]. Recently, an anephric patient with sarcoidosis has been described to have elevated $1,25\text{-}(OH)_2D$ and calcium in plasma[49]. The calcium and $1,25\text{-}(OH)_2D$ levels fall in response to corticosteroid therapy. Whether sarcoid tissue can produce a $1,25\text{-}(OH)_2D$-stimulating factor (also operative at non-renal sites) or produce the sterol is not presently known.

Idiopathic hypercalciuria Subjects with this disorder exhibit levels of plasma $1,25\text{-}(OH)_2D$ which are inappropriate to the prevailing (mostly normal) plasma PTH concentrations[50]. The mechanism of exaggerated 1,25-$(OH)_2D$ production is not known, but the sterol appears to be responsible for the hyperabsorption of calcium from the intestinal lumen in this condition.

Oncogenic osteomalacia In certain connective tissue tumors, phosphaturia and suppressed plasma 1,25-$(OH)_2D$ levels are associated with osteomalacia[26,51]. Removal of these neoplasms corrects the biochemical abnormalities and leads to skeletal healing, but the mechanism of these effects is not understood.

Other Whereas other factors have been proposed to directly influence the 1α-hydroxylase, such as cortisol, growth hormone, prolactin, sex steroids, insulin, and hydrogen ion, reports are controversial, and the possibility of indirect effects through PTH and change in ionic milieu should be considered. Finally, the renal mitochondrial hydroxylase is subject to several trophic and constitutive influences as have been studied in analogous adrenal systems[1].

In early phase renal failure due to rhabdomolysis, plasma 1,25-$(OH)_2D$ levels are low and not responsive to PTH increases. The hyperphosphatemia may be a factor here, but the nature of the inhibition is not known[52].

Actions

During glucocorticoid therapy, the intestinal response to 1,25-$(OH)_2D$ is blunted, since calcium malabsorption persists in spite of adequate sterol levels in plasma and tissue. There is some evidence that the 1α-hydroxylase activity falls off with aging, and that target tissue accumulation of 1,25-$(OH)_2D$ is also decreased[53,54].

The delivery of 1,25-$(OH)_2D$ to tissues is apparently conditioned by the plasma DBP concentration, as is recognized in other hormone-plasma binding protein systems[4]. Since estrogen increases plasma DBP levels[55] less "free" sterol may become available with increased binding protein. Conceivably, some clinical phenomena might be explained by such a mechanism, since estrogen therapy can ameliorate hyperparathyroidism[56] and antagonize effective vitamin D treatment of hypoparathyroid states.

SUMMARY

Sources continue to be an important concern in many areas of the world because of environment, nutrition practices, and customs. We should remember that aging and many illnesses can tend to reduce the opportunity for effective u-v light exposure and diminish adequate dietary vitamin D intake. Our very first source is *in utero*, and is crucial to the subsequent period of growth. Prematurity threatens our *in utero* sources, and rickets in surviving premature infants may reflect inadequate sources as well as faulty vitamin D metabolism, poor mineral intake and/or poor target tissue responses. Pharmacological amounts of vitamin D lead to large increases in blood 25-OHD and intoxication, but chronic and intense u-v light exposure appears to result in sub-toxic accumulations of vitamin D and 25-OHD.

The conservative aspects of vitamin D economy appear to carefully protect us against brief periods of poor sources. There is little esterification or oxidation of normal supplies of sterols, and steady-state maintenance of blood 25-OHD levels appears to require about 200 units or 3-4 μg of 25-OHD replacement daily under conditions of average utilization. With certain drugs, an exaggerated transformation of vitamin D to 25-OHD and other inactive products occurs, and 25-OHD and 1,25-$(OH)_2$D might also be catabolized and excreted more rapidly. With adequate sources of vitamin D, the waste pathways and the normal metabolic pathways can be served and disease prevented. With severe nephrotic states, sources can be strained due to heavy losses of DBP and sterols in urine. Normally, most of the bile's content of vitamin D material appears to be biologically inactive, and enteric reclamation of useful sterol appears to be quite small. Malabsorptive disorders, therefore, appear to interfere with dietary sources of the vitamin. The large, circulating vitamin D binding capacity favors sterol retention - and while this protects us against variations in sources, it appears to contribute to the protracted periods of vitamin D intoxication.

The known metabolic steps certainly point to liver and kidney diseases as conditions in which sufficient 25-OHD and 1,25-$(OH)_2$D production could be threatened. Apparently, very severe liver damage must be present before 25-OHD production is compromised in the presence of sufficient substrate. Loss of nephrons can be correlated to deficient 1,25-$(OH)_2$D synthesis. An important role for PTH stimulation of the 1-hydroxylase is established, and a negative feedback loop (direct or through calcium ion) seems likely. Other direct endocrine influences on the 1-hydroxylase appear to be less certain, permissive or non-regulatory, with controversial information available and secondary influences through PTH more likely. Unknown stimulators (sarcoidosis, idiopathic hypercalciuria) and inhibitors (tumor-related osteomalacia) await identification. Drugs, such as the diphosphonate, disodium etidronate, and certain cations inhibit the 1-hydroxylase.

Apparent resistance to 1,25-$(OH)_2$D has been reported in some patients. The biological action of vitamin D appears to involve high-affinity receptors for 1,25$(OH)_2$D in target tissues, and disorders of sterol access into or action at the cell can be anticipated. The natural antagonism of vitamin D action by glucocorticoids might provide a probe to elucidate the biochemical steps in vitamin D action. With improved appreciation of sterol action and better techniques, a new family of disorders might be uncovered which would allow us to better define vitamin D "sensitivity" and "resistance" at the target level.

Clearly, the potential exists for the existence of many inherited and acquired disorders which could compromise effective vitamin D action. I've touched on a few, but the list is certain to grow.

REFERENCES

1. D.R. Fraser, Regulation of the metabolism of vitamin D, Phys. Revs. 60:551 (1980).
2. H.F. DeLuca, and H. Schnoes, Metabolism and mechanics of action of vitamin D, Ann. Rev. Biochem. 929:631 (1977).
3. M. Haussler, and T. McCain, Basic and clinical concepts related to vitamin D metabolism and action, New Eng. J. Med. 297:974 and 1041 (1977).
4. R. Bouillon, F. Van Assche, H. Van Baelen, W. Heyns, and P. De Moor, Influence of the vitamin D binding protein on the serum concentration of 1,25-$(OH)_2$D, J. Clin. Invest. 67:589 (1981).
5. L.S. Hillman, S. Rojanasathit, E. Slatopolsky, and J. Haddad, Serial measurements of serum calcium, magnesium, parathyroid hormone, calcitonin and 25-OHD in premature and term infants during the first week of life, Ped. Res. 11:739 (1977).
6. L. Hillman, and J. Haddad, Perinatal vitamin D metabolism. I. 25-OHD in maternal and cord blood, J. Pediat. 84:742 (1974).
7. M. Moncrieff, and T. Fadahunsi, Congenital rickets due to maternal vitamin D deficiency, Arch. Dis. Child 49:810 (1974).
8. J.C.L. Shaw, Evidence for defective skeletal mineralization in low-birth weight infants: the absorption of calcium and fat, Pediat. 57:16 (1976).
9. L. Hillman, and J. Haddad, Perinatal vitamin D metabolism. II. Serial 25-OHD concentrations in sera of term and premature infants, J. Pediat. 86:928 (1975).
10. N. Hoff, J. Haddad, S. Teitelbaum, W. McAlister, and L. Hillman, Serum concentrations of 25-OHD in rickets of extremely premature infants, J. Pediat. 94:460 (1979).
11. D. Fraser, and C.R. Scriver, Familial forms of vitamin D-resistant rickets revisited: x-linked hypophosphatemia and autosomal recessive vitamin D dependency, Am. J. Clin. Nutr. 29: 1315 (1976).
12. C.R. Scriver, T.M. Reade, H.F. DeLuca, and A.J. Hamstra, Serum 1,25-$(OH)_2$D levels in normal subjects and in patients with hereditary rickets or bone disease, New Eng. J. Med. 229:976 (1978).

13. E. Devlin, F. Glorieux, P. Marie, and J. Pettifor, Vitamin D dependency; replacement therapy with calcitriol, J. Pediat. 99:26 (1981).
14. M. Brooks, N. Bell, L. Love, P. Stern, E. Orfei, S. Queener, A. Hamstra, and H. DeLuca, Vitamin D-dependent rickets type II. resistance of target organs to $1,25(OH)_2D_3$, New Eng. J. Med. 298:996 (1978).
15. S. Marx, A. Spiegel, E. Brown, D. Gardner, R. Sowns, M. Attie, A. Hamstra, and H. DeLuca, A familial syndrome of decrease in sensitivity to $1,25\text{-}(OH)_2D_3$, J. Clin. Endocrinol. Metab. 47: 1303 (1978).
16. J. Rosen, A. Fleischman, L. Finberg, A. Hamstra, and H. De Luca, Rickets with alopecia: an inborn error of vitamin D metabolism, J. Pediat. 94:729 (1979).
17. Y. Tsuchiya, N. Matsuo, H. Cho, M. Kumagai, A. Yasaka, T. Suda, H. Orimo, and M. Shiraki, An unusual form of vitamin D-dependent rickets in a child: alopecia and marked end-organ hyposensitivity to biologically active vitamin D, J. Clin. Endocrinol. Metab. 51:685 (1980).
18. C. Eil, and S. Marx, Nuclear uptake of $\{^3H\}1,25\text{-}(OH)_2D_3$ in dispersed fibroblasts cultwad from normal human skin, Proc. Natl. Acad. Sci. U.S.A. 78:2562 (1981).
19. D. Feldman, T. Chen, M. Huist, K. Colston, K. Karasek, and C. Cone, Demonstration of $1,25\text{-}(OH)_2D_3$ receptors in human skin biopsies, J. Clin. Endocrinol. Metab. 51:1463 (1980).
20. C. Eil, U. Liberman, J. Rosen, and S. Marx, A cellular defect in hereditary vitamin D-dependent rickets Type II: defective nuclear uptake of $1,25\text{-}(OH)_2D$ in cultured fibroblasts, New Eng. J. Med. 304:1588 (1981).
21. J. Haddad, K. Chyu, T. Hahn, and T.C.B. Stamp, Serum concentrations of 25-OHD in sex-linked hypophosphatemic vitamin D-resistant rickets, J. Lab. Clin. Med. 81:22 (1973).
22. J. Dominquez, R. Gray, and J. Lemann, Dietary phosphate deprivation in women and men: effects on mineral and acid balances PTH and the metabolism of 25-OHD, J. Clin. Endocrinol. Metab. 43:1056 (1976).
23. C. West, J. Blanton, F. Silverman, and N. Holland, Use of phosphate salts as an adjunct to vitamin D in the treatment of hypophosphatemic vitamin D refractory rickets, J. Pediat. 64:469 (1964).
24. G. Hirschman, H. DeLuca, and J. Chan, Hypophosphatemic vitamin D-resistant tickets: metabolic balance studies in a child receiving $1,25\text{-}(OH)_2D_3$, phosphate and ascorbic acid. Pediatrics 61:451 (1978).
25. H. Rasmussen, M. Pechet, C. Anast, A. Mazur, J. Gertner, and A. Broadus, Long-term treatment of familial hypophosphatemic rickets with oral phosphate and $1\alpha OHD_3$, J. of Pediat. 99:16 (1981).
26. M. Drezner, and M. Feinglos, Osteomalacia due to $1,25\text{-}(OH)_2D_3$ deficiency: association with a giant cell tumor of bone,

27. W.F. Loomis, Rickets, Sci. Amer. 223:77 (1970).
28. J. Haddad, and K. Chyu, Competitive protein-binding radioassay for 25-OHD$_3$, J. Clin. Endocrinol. Metab. 33:992 (1971).
29. T.C.B. Stamp, J. Haddad, and C. Twigg, Comparison of oral 25-OHD$_3$, vitamin D and ultraviolet light as determinants of circulating 25-OHD in man, Lancet 1:1341 (1977).
30. J. Haddad, and S. Rojanasathit, Acute administration of 25-OHD$_3$ in man, J. Clin. Endocrinol. Metab. 42:284 (1976).
31. G.A. Lamb, and S.W. Stanbury, Parathyroid function in human vitamin D deficiency and vitamin D deficiency in primary hyperparathyroidism, Am. J. Med. 56:833 (1974).
32. H. Rasmussen, R. Baron, A. Broadus, R. Defronzo, R. Lang, and R. Horst, 1,25-(OH)$_2$D$_3$ is not the only D metabolite involved in the pathogenesis of osteomalacia, Am. J. Med. 69:360 (1980).
33. S.E. Papaponlos, L. Fraber, T. Clemes, J. Gleed, and J.L. O'Riordan, Metabolites of vitamin D in human vitamin D deficiency: effect of vitamin D$_3$ or 1,25-(OH)$_2$D$_3$, Lancet 2: 612 (1980).
34. M. Imawari, Y. Akanuma, J. Itakura, Y. Muto, K. Kosaka, and D. Goodman, The effects of diseases of the liver on serum 25-OHD and on the serum binding protein for vitamin D and its metabolites, J. Lab. Clin. Med. 93:171 (1979).
35. E. Krawitt, M. Grundman, and E.B. Mawer, Absorption, hydroxylation, and excretion of vitamin D$_3$ in primary biliary cirrhosis, Lancet 2:1246 (1977).
36. L. Mosekilde, F. Melsen, I. Hessov, M. Christensen, B.J. Lund, B.I. Lund, and O.H. Sorensen, Low serum levels of 1,25-(OH)$_2$D and histomorphometric evidence of osteomalacia after jejunoileal bypass for obesity, Gut 21:624 (1980).
37. R. Kumar, The metabolism of 1,25-(OH)$_2$D, Endocrine Reviews 1: 258 (1980).
38. M. Whyte, J. Haddad, D. Walters, and T.C.B. Stamp, Vitamin D bioavailability: serum 25-OHD levels in man after oral, subcutaneous, intramuscular, and intravenous vitamin D administration. J. Clin. Endocrinol. Metab. 48:906 (1979).
39. J. Barragry, N. Carter, M. Beer, W. France, J. Auton, B. Boucher, and R. Cohen, Vitamin D metabolism in nephrotic syndrome, Lancet 2:629 (1977).
40. H. Malluche, D. Goldstein, and S. Massry, Osteomalacia and hyperparathyroid bone disease in patients with nephrotic syndrome, J. Clin. Invest. 63:494 (1979).
41. M. Drezner, F. Nelson, M. Haussler, H. McPherson, and H. Lebovitz, 1,25-(OH)$_2$D$_3$ deficiency: The probable cause of hypocalcemia and metabolic bone disease in pseudohypoparathyroidism, J. Clin. Endocrinol. Metab. 42:62 (1976).
42. Y. Tanaka, and H. DeLuca, The control of 25-OHD metabolism by inorganic phosphorus, Arch. Biochem. Biophys. 154:566 (1973).
43. K. Hove, R. Horst, and E. Littledike, PTH and plasma Ca: conflicting signals for regulation of plasma 1,25-(OH)$_2$D levels

in PTH-infused calves, Program of the 63rd Endocrine Society Meeting, pg. 122 (1981).
44. R. Bouillon, E. Muls, and P. DeMoor, Influence of thyroid function on the serum concentration of 1,25-$(OH)_2D_3$, J. Clin. Endocrinol. Metab. 51:793 (1980).
45. A. Stewart, R. Horst, L. Deftos, E. Cadman, R. Lang, and A. Broadus, Biochemical evaluation of patients with cancer-associated hypercalcemia, New Eng. J. Med. 303:1377 (1980).
46. T. Hahn, B. Hendin, C. Scharp, and J. Haddad, Effect of chronic anticonvulsant therapy on serum 25-OHD levels in adults, New Eng. J. Med. 287:900 (1972).
47. H. Sherk, M. Cruz, and J. Stambaugh, Vitamin D prophylaxis and the lowered incidence of fractures in anti-convulsant rickets and osteomalacia, Clin. Orthop. & Rel. Res. 129:251 (1977).
48. P. Stern, J. DeOlazabal, and N. Bell, Evidence for abnormal regulation of circulating 1,25-$(OH)_2D$ in patients with sarcoidosis and normal calcium metabolism, J. Clin. Invest. 66:852 (1980).
49. G. Barbour, J. Coburn, E. Slatopolsky, A. Norman, and R. Horst, Hypercalcemia in an anephric patient with sarcoidosis: evidence for extrarenal generation of 1,25-$(OH)_2D_1$, New Eng. J. Med. 305:440 (1981).
50. A. Caldas, R. Gray, and J. Lemann, The simultaneous measurement of vitamin D metabolites in plasma: studies in healthy adults and in patients with calcium nephrolithiasis, J. Lab. Clin. Med. 91:840 (1978).
51. Y. Fukumoto, S. Tarin, K. Tsukujama, K. Ichihara, K. Moriwaki, K. Nonaka, T. Mizushima, Y. Kobayashi, S. Dokoh, M. Fukumaga, and R. Marita, Tumor-induced vitamin D-resistant hypophosphatemic osteomalacia associated with proximal renal tubular dysfunction and 1,25-$(OH)_2D$ deficiency, J. Clin. Endocrinol. Metab. 49:873 (1979).
52. F. Llach, A. Felsenfeld, and M. Haussler, The pathophysiology of altered calcium metabolism in rhabdomyolysis-induced acute renal failure, New Eng. J. Med. 305:117 (1981).
53. R. Horst, H. DeLuca, and N. Jorgensen, The effect of age on calcium absorption and accumulation of 1,25-$(OH)_2D_3$ in intestinal mucosa of rats, Metab. Bone Dis. Relat. Res. 1:29 (1978).
54. H. Armbrecht, T. Zenser, and B. Davis, Effect of age on the conversion of 25-OHD_3 to 1,25-$(OH)_2D_3$ by kidney of rat, J. Clin. Invest. 66:1118 (1980).
55. J. Haddad, and J. Walgate, Radioimmunoassay of the binding protein for vitamin D and its metabolites in human serum. Concentrations in normal subjects and patients with disorders of mineral homeostasis, J. Clin. Invest. 58:1217 (1976).
56. J. Gallagher, and B.E.C. Nordin, Treatment with estrogens of primary hyperparathyroidism in postmenopausal women, Lancet, 1:503 (1972).

THE MOLECULAR NATURE OF 1,25-$(OH)_2$-D_3-INDUCED CALCIUM-BINDING PROTEIN BIOSYNTHESIS IN THE RAT

Felix Bronner and Michael Buckley

Department of Oral Biology
School of Dental Medicine
University of Connecticut Health Center
Farmington, Connecticut 06032

ABSTRACT

Exogenous 1,25-$(OH)_2$-D_3, administered to vitamin D-replete animals on a high calcium diet, induces biosynthesis of the duodenal, cytosolic calcium-binding protein (CaBP) in less than 2 h. This process can be blocked by simultaneously administered cycloheximide, but not by actinomycin D. In vitamin D-replete animals on a low Ca diet, on the other hand, 1,25-$(OH)_2$-D_3 administration leads to new CaBP synthesis only after about 7 h; this process can be blocked by actinomycin D. In vitamin D-deficient animals on a high calcium diet who have no CaBP, treatment with 1,25-$(OH)_2$-D_3 induces CaBP formation in $\simeq$ 8 h; this process is known to be blocked by actinomycin D. Thus in D-replete animals on a low calcium diet and in D-deficient animals, CaBP biosynthesis proceeds by a transcriptional route, whereas in D-replete animals on a high calcium diet the rapid response appears to be posttranscriptional. This finding points to the possibility of a more rapid regulatory action of vitamin D than previously reported and how vitamin D might function in the D-replete state.

INTRODUCTION

Duodenal calcium transport involves two processes, one that is saturable and vitamin D-dependent and a second non-saturable, diffusional-type process[1]. The former is regulatable inasmuch as it varies inversely with calcium intake[2], varies with age[3] and correlates directly with the duodenal content of the vitamin D-dependent, cytosolic calcium-binding protein (CaBP)[2]. CaBP content in turn varies inversely with calcium intake[4] and in the steady state is a direct reflection of the circulating level of 1α,25-dihydroxyvitamin D_3 (1,25-$(OH)_2$-D_3), biologically the most active metabolite of vitamin D_3[5,6]. While there thus now exists substantial evidence correlating the steady-state levels of CaBP with saturable calcium transport in the vitamin D-replete animal, studies comparing the time-course of appearance of CaBP and calcium transport in the vitamin D-deficient rat[7] or -deficient chick[8] have been able to dissociate the two events, with transport induction preceding CaBP. It therefore seemed of interest to see whether such dissociation can also be demonstrated in the vitamin D-replete state. As a first step to this end we have studied the appearance of CaBP in vitamin D-replete and -deficient animals following an intraperitoneal injection of 1,25-$(OH)_2$-D_3.

MATERIALS AND METHODS

Male Sprague-Dawley rats (ARS, Madison, WI) were used throughout. To make animals vitamin D-deficient, weanlings were placed on a high calcium (1.5% Ca), high phosphorus (1.5% P) semi-synthetic vitamin D-deficient diet (III-D, TD # 78250, Teklad Mills, Madison, WI) for 5-6 wks, when their plasma calcium level had dropped to below 7 mg/dl. Vitamin D-replete animals weighed 75-100g when purchased and were placed on either a high calcium, high phosphorus diet (III, TD # 78249) or a low calcium (0.06% Ca), low phosphorus (0.2% P) diet (I, TD # 78245) for 10 days or more. Both diets contained 2200 i.u. vitamin D_2/kg. On the day of the experiment, some animals from each diet group received 0.5 μg 1,25-$(OH)_2$-D_3 (obtained in crystalline form from Hoffman-LaRoche, Inc., Nutley, NJ) by intraperitoneal injection. The animals were killed at intervals following the injection, their duodena removed, rinsed and processed for CaBP analysis by an equilibrated column technique, as previously described[9]. Results are expressed either as nmol CaBP/g mucosa or as nmol Ca_{bound}/g mucosa. 1 nmol CaBP = 2 nmol Ca_{bound}. In some experiments, animals received by i.p. injection actinomycin D (50 μg) or cycloheximide (20 μg). These drugs were given to control animals and simultaneously to animals that were receiving 1,25-$(OH)_2$-D_3. In the experiments with inhibitors of protein synthesis, the animals treated with 1,25-$(OH)_2$-D_3 and/or inhibitors were killed ≃ 3 h after treatment in the case of diet III and ≃ 9 h after treatment in the case of diet I.

RESULTS

Fig 1 shows the time-course of CaBP response to exogenous 1,25-$(OH)_2$-D_3 in the three groups of animals studied. Vitamin D-deficient animals, whose pretreatment CaBP levels were undectable, showed no increase in CaBP until after 8 h; by 20 h after metabolite injection, CaBP levels had reached a maximum, where they remained for about 20 h more, when they began to decline[9]. The delay in response to the metabolite was similar to that reported by Thomasset et al.[7]

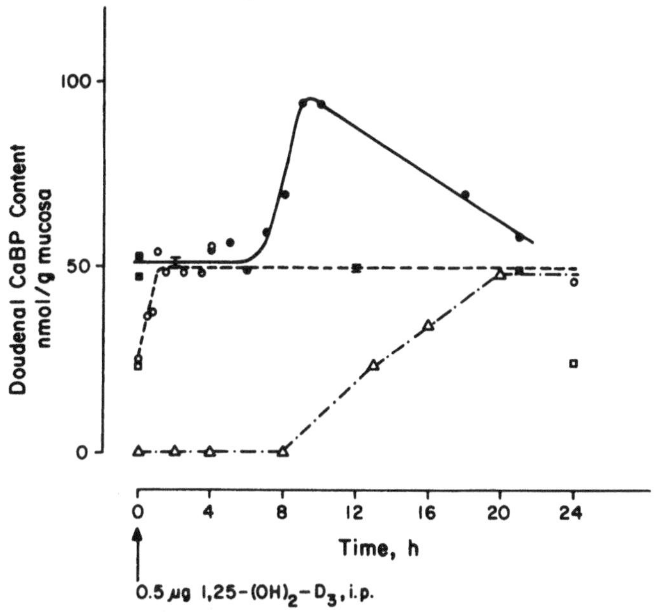

Fig. 1 The Effect of Exogenous 1,25-Dihydroxyvitamin D_3 on CaBP Levels in Rat Duodenum. The solid line and closed circles refer to CaBP levels in vitamin D-replete animals on the low calcium diet I treated with 1,25-(OH)$_2$-D$_3$. The dashed line and open circles refer to CaBP levels in vitamin D-replete treated animals on the high calcium diet III, and the dash-dot line and open triangles to CaBP levels in treated vitamin D-deficient animals on the high calcium, vitamin D-deficient diet III-D. The square symbols refer to CaBP levels in untreated vitamin D-replete controls; open squares: diet III; closed squares: diet I.

In the case of the vitamin D-replete animals, on the other hand, the time of response was either much earlier (<2 h) or at about the same time (7-8 h) as for the vitamin D-deficient animals, depending on whether the animals had been on a high- or a low-calcium diet. In both groups the rate at which CaBP rose in the intestine was much faster than in the case of the D-deficient animals. The D-replete animals differed also with respect to the rate of return to the preinjection level. In the case of the animals on the high calcium diet (III), Fig 1 shows that CaBP remained at the new level for about 24 h. Over the succeeding 24 h period the duodenal CaBP declined to the pre-injection level[9]. In the case of the animals on the low calcium diet (I), however, CaBP began declining very soon after it had reached its peak (Fig. 1). The rate of decline was much faster than had been found[9] for the animals on diet III.

To determine whether the same or different mechanisms were involved in these responses, two types of inhibitors of protein synthesis were utilized, actinomycin D which prevents transcription, and cycloheximide, which inhibits translation. Table 1 shows that in diet III animals, actinomycin did not inhibit the 1,25-$(OH)_2$-D_3-stimulated induction of CaBP, whereas cycloheximide did. In the diet I animals, on the other hand, actinomycin D administration inhibited the CaBP response to simultaneous 1,25-$(OH)_2$-D_3 treatment. These results suggest that the early CaBP response observed in diet III animals does not require transcription, whereas the delayed response in the diet I animals does.

Table 1. Effect of protein synthesis inhibitors on CaBP response.

	CaBP content, nmol Ca_{bound}/g mucosa	
	Diet III	Diet I
control	57	99
+1,25-$(OH)_2$-D_3 (0.5 μg)	118	186
+actinomycin D (50 μg)	55	113
+actinomycin D + 1,25-$(OH)_2$-D_3	112	123
+cycloheximide (20 μg)	68	not done
+cycloheximide + 1,25-$(OH)_2$-D_3	60	not done

Animals treated with 1,25-$(OH)_2$-D_3 and/or inhibitors were killed 3 h after treatment in the case of the diet III group and 9 h after treatment in the case of the diet I group. The dose administered per animal is indicated in parentheses.

DISCUSSION

The results reported above show that the lag between 1,25-$(OH)_2$-D_3 administration and CaBP response varies with calcium intake in vitamin D-replete animals, an early (<2 h) response occurring in animals on a high calcium diet, while in animals on a low calcium diet the response does not occur for about 7 h. Since the early response does not appear to depend on transcriptional events (Table 1), it seems reasonable to suppose that the administration of $1,25-(OH)_2-D_3$ leads to the expression of already formed messenger molecules. One might suppose that in the diet III animals there exists a pool of active and inactive messenger molecules and that their proportion in the steady state is determined by the luminal and ultimately cytosolic calcium level. Support for this notion comes from experiments that have shown that duodenal CaBP rises diurnally and inversely with the cytosolic calcium[4]. The latter in turn varies directly with food intake.

In animals on the low calcium diet, on the other hand, where CaBP levels are twice as high as in the animals on diet III (Fig. 1) and where no early response to $1,25-(OH)_2-D_3$ has been observed, most messenger molecules would appear to be fully expressed. Therefore treatment with quite high doses of the metabolite effected no early response and the response at 7 h may have been the result of added synthesis of mRNA for CaBP. This interpretation is consistent with the inhibitory effect of actinomycin D administered simultaneously with the vitamin D metabolite (Table 1). It is also consistent with the 7-8 h delay observed in vitamin D-deficient animals (Fig. 1), in whom actinomycin D has been reported to inhibit CaBP synthesis[10].

From a physiological viewpoint, it is interesting that rapid regulation can be effected under conditions that resemble normal nutrition, inasmuch as CaBP levels of rats on "typical" calcium diets (0.6% Ca, 0.6% P) are closer to those of animals on diet III than to animals on diet I (Freund and Bronner, unpublished observations). In animals whose CaBP levels are below maximum, one can imagine that a drop in luminal calcium can effect release of the calcium-related inhibition of translation so that CaBP levels go up rapidly. If saturable calcium transport also increases, a rapid transport response would result. Preliminary data, obtained with everted duodenal sacs from vitamin D-replete animals, have shown[11] that calcium transport increases following $1,25-(OH)_2-D_3$ injection in a manner similar to that displayed in Fig. 1.

ACKNOWLEDGMENT

Support by the National Institutes of Health, grants AM 26174 and AM 14261, the National Science Foundation, grant PCM 782366, and the University of Connecticut Research Foundation is gratefully acknowledged.

REFERENCES

1. F. Bronner, Intestinal calcium absorption and transport, in: "Membrane Transport of Calcium", E. Carafoli, ed., Academic Press, London (1982, in press).
2. D. Pansu, C. Bellaton and F. Bronner, The effect of calcium intake on the saturable and non-saturable components of duodenal calcium transport. Am. J. Physiol. 240: G32-G37 (1981).
3. F. Bronner, C. Bellaton and D. Pansu, Calcium absorption and calcium-binding protein (CaBP) in suckling rats. Fed. Proc. 40: 899 (abstract), (1981).
4. T. Freund and F. Bronner, Regulation of intestinal calcium-binding protein by calcium intake in the rat. Am. J. Physiol. 228: 861-869 (1975).
5. S. Edelstein, D. Noff, L. Sinai, A. Harell, J. B. Puschett, E. E. Golub and F. Bronner, Vitamin D metabolism and expression in rats fed on low-calcium and low-phosphorus diets. Biochem. J. 170: 227-233 (1978).
6. A. W. Norman, "Vitamin D. The Calcium Homeostatic Steroid Hormone", Academic Press, New York (1979).
7. M. Thomasset, P. Cuisinier-Gleizes and H. Mathieu, 1,25-dihydroxycholecalciferol: dynamics of the stimulation of duodenal calcium-binding protein, calcium-binding protein, calcium transport and bone calcium mobilization in vitamin D- and calcium-deficient rats. FEBS Letters 107: 91-94 (1979).
8. R. Spencer, M. Chapman, P. W. Wilson and D. E. M. Lawson, The relationship between vitamin D-stimulated calcium transport and intestinal calcium-binding protein in the chicken. Biochem. J. 170: 93-101 (1978).
9. M. Buckley and F. Bronner, Calcium-binding protein biosynthesis in the rat: regulation by calcium and 1,25-dihydroxyvitamin D_3, Arch. Biochem. Biophys. 202: 235-241 (1980).
10. D. D. Bikle, D. T. Zolock, R. L. Morissey and R. H. Herman, Independence of a 1,25-dihydroxyvitamin D_3-mediated calcium transport from de novo RNA and protein synthesis. J. Biol. Chem. 253: 484-488 (1978).
11. F. Bronner, J. Lipton, D. Pansu, M. Buckley, R. Singh and A. Miller III, Molecular and transport effects of 1,25-dihydroxyvitamin D_3 in rat duodenum, Fed. Proc. (1982, in press).

EFFECTS OF 1,25-DIHYDROXY VITAMIN D_3 IN PATIENTS WITH EARLY RENAL FAILURE

Mildred Lam and Francisco Llach

University of Oklahoma Health Sciences Center and
Veterans Administration Hospital
Oklahoma City, Oklahoma 73104

INTRODUCTION

Patients with chronic renal failure commonly develop secondary hyperparathyroidism as creatinine clearances decrease to less than 30 ml/min.[1] However, biochemical abnormalities have also been noted in patients with early renal failure (ERF), with higher creatinine clearances (30 to 90 ml/min). These abnormalities include hypocalcemia, hypophosphatemia, and elevated serum levels of parathyroid hormone (PTH).[2-4] Such abnormalities indicate that secondary hyperparathyroidism may be present even in the early stages of chronic renal failure.

Serum levels of 1,25-dihydroxy vitamin D_3 (1,25$(OH)_2D_3$) have been shown to be normal or decreased in early renal failure.[5,6] Administration of 1,25$(OH)_2D_3$ has been shown to have beneficial effects on patients with endstage renal disease and patients on chronic dialysis.[7-10] However, little data is available about the effects of 1,25$(OH)_2D_3$ on patients with ERF. Therefore, our study was designed to investigate the chronic effects of 1,25-$(OH)_2D_3$ on patients with creatinine clearances between 30 and 90 ml/min. This was accomplished by studying the following: 1) skeletal resistance to PTH, as evaluated by calcemic response to an infusion of parathyroid hormone extract; and 2) response to an oral phosphate load.

METHODS

The study group consisted of four male patients, ages 50 to 72, with stable creatinine clearances ranging from 40 to 80 ml/

min. The cause of chronic renal failure in all patients was tubulointerstitial disease; no patient had nephrotic-range proteinuria or evidence of associated systemic disease. The subjects remained on a regular diet and took no diuretics, antacids, or vitamin D preparations during the study. Other medications (such as digoxin and anithypertensive drugs) were continued. All studies were carried out on an inpatient metabolic ward. All subjects gave consent to a protocol approved by the Human Experimentation Committee.

Each subject had 2 baseline studies. The first was a parathyroid hormone extract (PTE) infusion test, in which bovine PTE (Eli Lilly; Indianapolis, Indiana) was given intravenously at a rate of 1 unit/kg/hr for 10 hours. Blood was obtained through an indwelling plastic intravenous catheter at baseline and at 2, 6, 10, and 12 hours after the beginning of the infusion. Serum calcium, phosphate, creatinine, and PTH were measured. A 24-hour urine for calcium, phosphate, and creatinine were collected prior to study in each patient. A fractional urine for calcium, phosphate, and creatinine was also collected from the beginning of PTE infusion until 24 hours later.

The second baseline study was an oral phosphate loading test, in which one gram of sodium potassium phosphate was administered as a single oral dose. Serum calcium, phosphate, creatinine, and PTH were measured at baseline and hourly for 6 hours after the oral phosphate load. Hourly urine collections for calcium, phosphate, and creatinine were also obtained at baseline and for 6 hours following the phosphate load.

Following completion of baseline studies, each subject was placed on $1,25(OH)_2D_3$, 0.25 mcg orally, twice a day. After six weeks of treatment with $1,25(OH)_2D_3$, the 24-hour urine collection, PTE infusion, and phosphate loading tests were repeated.

Calcium, phosphate, and creatinine were measured using a multichannel Technicon SMA 12-60 AutoAnalyzer. Renal phosphate threshold ($TmPO_4/GFR$) was determined using the nomogram of Walton and Bijvoet.[11] Serum PTH was measured by radioimmunoassay; the carboxy-terminal fragment was measured using antibody GP-5 (at a dilution of 1:100,000) and the amino-terminal fragment was measured using antibody R-4 (dilution 1:20,000). The GP-5 antiserum was developed by immunization of a guinea pig with purified bovine PTH: its major antigenic-recognition site is located in the amino acid sequence 35-84 of the PTH molecule. The R-4 antiserum was developed by immunization of a rabbit with a synthetic fragment of bovine PTH containing the amino acid sequence 1-34.[12]

Results were analyzed using standard statistical methods.

Statistical significance was determined using Student's t-test.

RESULTS

Baseline serum calcium increased from 9.1 ± 0.3 mg/dL (mean ± SEM) to 9.8 ± 0.2 mg/dL after six weeks of treatment with $1,25-(OH)_2D_3$ ($p<.05$) (Fig. 1). Baseline serum phosphate increased from 3.4 ± 0.2 to 3.8 ± 0.2 mg/dL ($p<.05$) (Fig. 2). Twenty-four-hour urinary calcium excretion increased from 38 ± 8 to 120 ± 28 mg ($p<.05$) (Fig. 3). PTH, C-terminal, did not change significantly: it was 0.61 ± 0.12 ng/ml (normal, <0.5 ng/ml) before treatment and 0.75 ± 0.26 ng/ml after $1,25(OH)_2D_3$. Likewise, N-terminal PTH was 0.28 ± 0.05 ng/ml (normal, <0.4 ng/ml) before and 0.36 ± 0.14 ng/ml after treatment.

Results of the PTE infusion before and after 6 weeks of $1,25-(OH)_2D_3$ are shown in Figures 4 and 5. Mean serum calcium was significantly higher after $1,25(OH)_2D_3$ at nearly every point during the study. Mean serum phosphate was also higher at all points after treatment, but the differences were not statistically significant.

Results of the oral phosphate loading test are shown in Figure 6. Mean serum phosphate was higher, although not significantly so, at every point during the test after 6 weeks of $1,25(OH)_2-D_3$. Six-hour urinary phosphate excretion did increase significantly after $1,25(OH)_2D_3$, from 265 ± 31 to 363 ± 15 mg ($p<.025$). Serum PTH, both C-terminal and N-terminal, increased in all patients during the phosphate loading test, but the amount of increase did not appear to be significantly affected by $1,25(OH)_2-D_3$. When results before and after $1,25(OH)_2D_3$ were compared, tubular reabsorption of phosphate and $TmPO_4$/GFR were not significantly different during the PTE and oral phosphate loading tests.

DISCUSSION

The present study suggests the presence of mild $1,25(OH)_2D_3$ deficiency in patients with ERF and provides evidence for the possible beneficial effects of this sterol in these patients.

Patients with chronic renal failure develop elevated serum levels of PTH when creatinine clearances decrease to less than 30 ml/min.[1] Hypocalcemia, hypophosphatemia, and elevated serum PTH have also been demonstrated in patients with mild renal failure, that is, creatinine clearances between 30 and 90 ml/min.[2-4] Thus, these biochemical abnormalities in patients with ERF indicate that secondary hyperparathyroidism may develop early in the course of chronic renal failure.

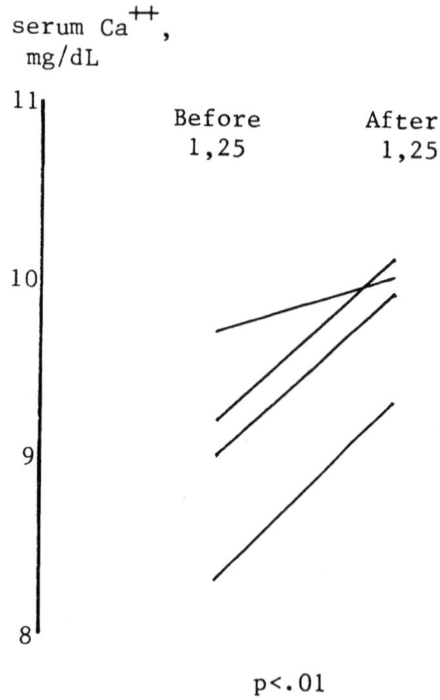

Figure 1. Baseline serum calcium before and after $1,25(OH)_2D_3$.

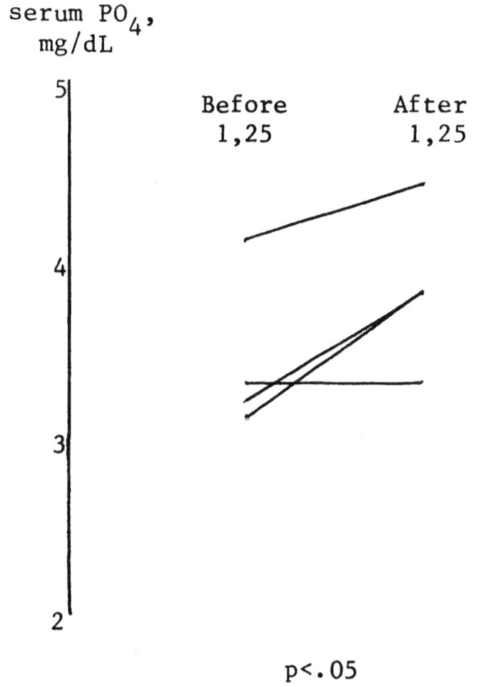

Figure 2. Baseline serum phosphate before and after $1,25(OH)_2D_3$.

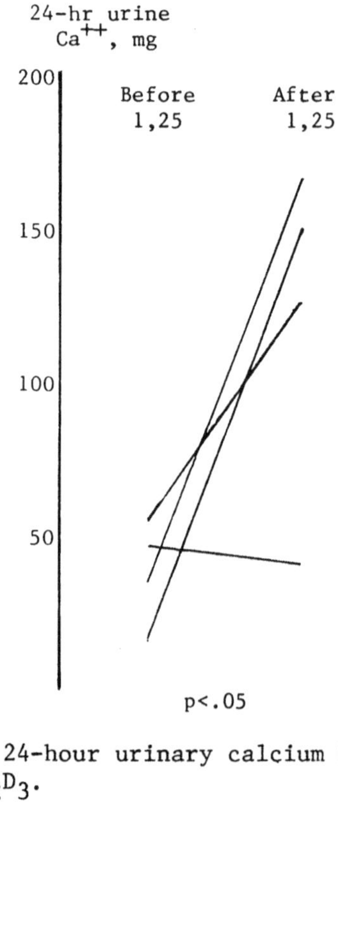

Figure 3. Baseline 24-hour urinary calcium before and after $1,25(OH)_2D_3$.

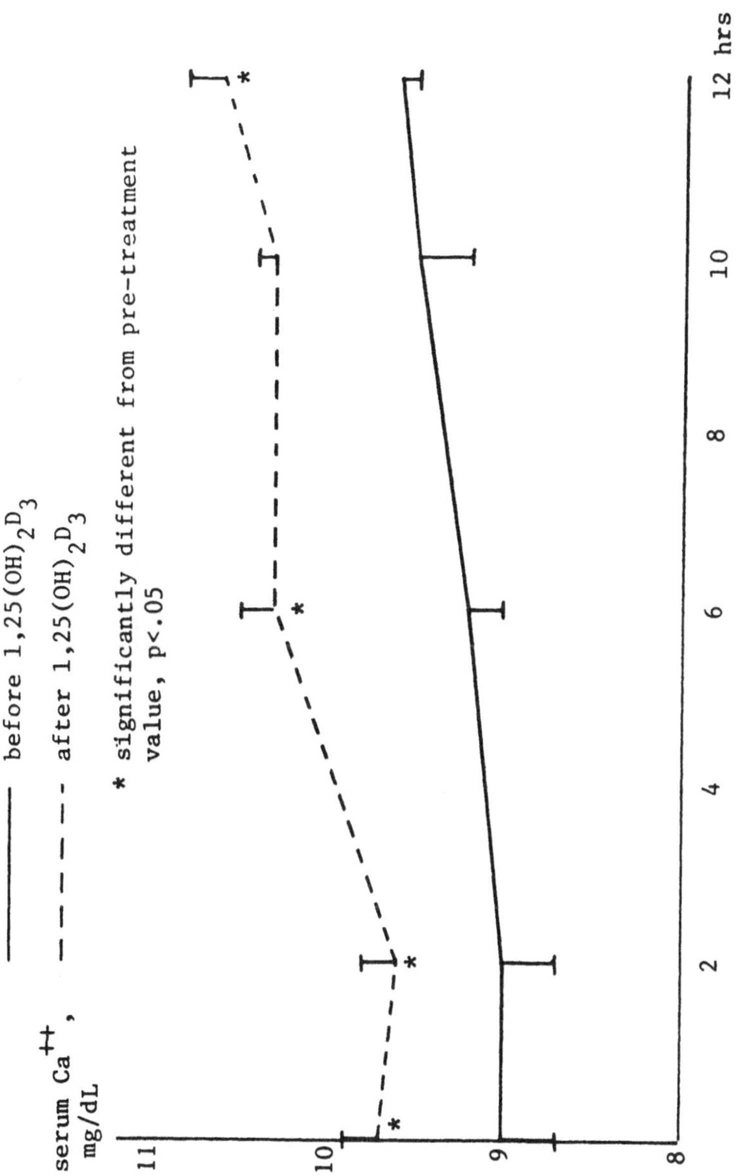

Figure 4. Mean serum calcium during and after PTE infusion, before and after $1,25(OH)_2D_3$.

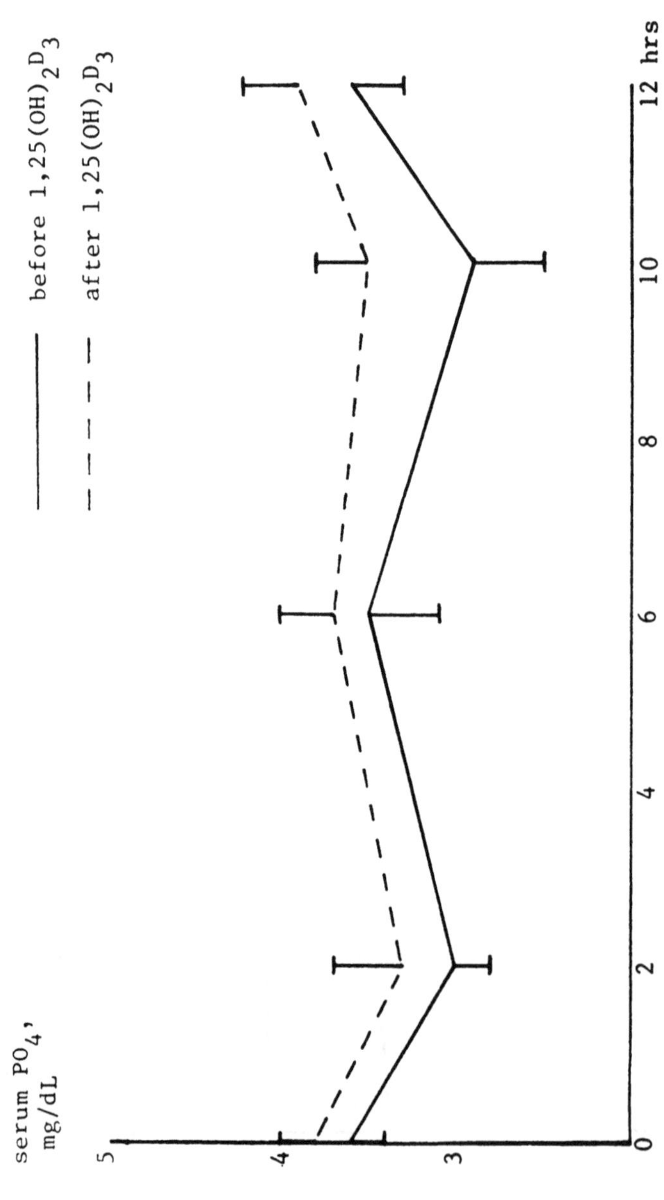

Figure 5. Mean serum phosphate during and after PTE infusion, before and after $1,25(OH)_2D_3$.

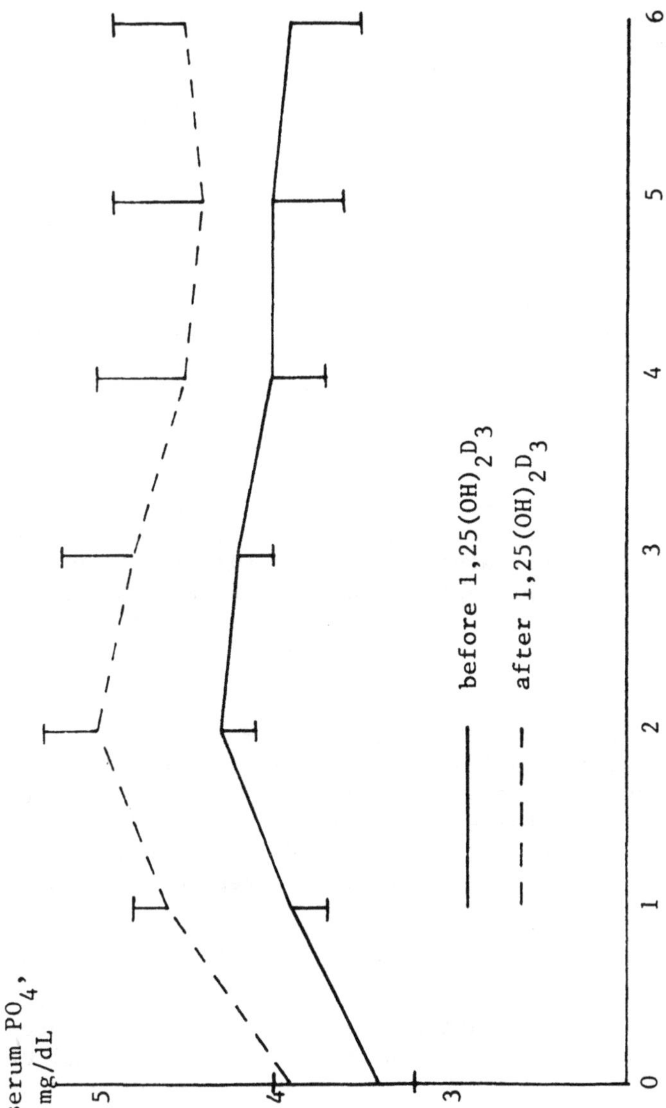

Figure 6. Mean serum phosphate following the oral phosphate load, before and after 1,25(OH)$_2$D$_3$.

There are several explanations for the pathogenesis of secondary hyperparathyroidism in ERF. The first of these is the phosphate retention hypothesis. Bricker et al postulate that, as chronic renal failure progresses, with each decrement in glomerular filtration rate a small increase in serum phosphate occurs.[13] This is accompanied by a reciprocal small decrease in serum ionized calcium, which in turn stimulates PTH secretion. The elevated PTH then results in phosphaturia, returning serum phosphate and thus serum calcium to normal levels, at the expense of an elevated serum PTH. However, this hypothesis does not explain the hypophosphatemia observed in subjects with ERF.

A second hypothesis, postulated by Llach et al, states that patients with ERF have skeletal resistance to the calcemic action of PTH, with decreased bone reabsorption in response to endogenous PTH, resulting in hypocalcemia, hypophosphatemia, and elevated serum PTH.[14] A third hypothesis states that decreased synthesis of $1,25(OH)_2D_3$ by the diseased kidney is responsible for the development of secondary hyperparathyroidism in ERF. Although Slatopolsky et al[15] have measured serum levels of $1,25(OH)_2D_3$ in patients with serum creatinines of 1.5 to 3.5 mg/dL and have found them to be within normal range, some investigators feel that such levels are inappropriately low for the decreased serum calcium levels and elevated PTH levels which are usually noted in these patients. More recently, decreased serum $1,25(OH)_2D_3$ levels have been demonstrated in patients with ERF.[6] Decreased levels of $1,25(OH)_2D_3$ probably induce hypocalcemia and hypophosphatemia both by impairing intestinal absorption of calcium and phosphate[16] and by contributing to the skeletal resistance of PTH.[17]

Administration of physiologic doses of $1,25(OH)_2D_3$ to patients with endstage renal disease on chronic dialysis has been shown to have multiple beneficial effects. These include decrease in musculoskeletal symptoms (e.g., pain and weakness), increase in serum calcium and phosphate, decrease in serum alkaline phosphatase and PTH, and improvement or arrest of deterioration in bone histologic characteristics.[7-10]

However, little data is available about the effects of $1,25(OH)_2D_3$ on patients with ERF. Llach et al showed that dietary phosphate restriction in patients with creatinine clearances between 46 and 70 ml/min resulted in increased intestinal calcium absorption, decreased serum PTH, increased calcemic response to PTH, and improved bone histology.[18] The investigators felt that $1,25(OH)_2D_3$ production in their patients was impaired by small intermittent elevations in serum phosphate which were eliminated by dietary phosphate restriction, and that the improvement in biochemical and histologic characteristics observed after phosphate restriction could be explained by an increase in $1,25(OH)_2D_3$ synthesis. The study thus provides indirect evidence for the role of decreased $1,25(OH)_2D_3$ synthesis in the genesis of secondary hyperparathyroidism in ERF.

More direct evidence for the effects of $1,25(OH)_2D_3$ deficiency in such patients was provided by a more recent study. Healy et al[19] studied 3 patients with ERF who were given $1,25(OH)_2D_3$, 0.5 mcg daily for 6 months, and demonstrated modest increases in serum total and ionized calcium and in urinary calcium excretion. Intestinal calcium absorption also increased, and bone histology demonstrated healing of osteomalacia and decrease in signs of hyperparathyroid bone disease.

The results of our study provide further evidence for the beneficial effects of chronic treatment with $1,25(OH)_2D_3$ on patients with ERF. Our patients demonstrated increases in baseline serum calcium and phosphate, as well as in urinary calcium excretion. The calcemic response to PTE improved following 6 weeks of $1,25(OH)_2D_3$, suggesting a decrease in skeletal resistance to PTH and/or an increase in intestinal absorption of calcium. The short course of $1,25(OH)_2D_3$ also affected the response to an oral phosphate load: the peak serum phosphate and 6-hour urinary phosphate excretion following the oral load increased, possibly reflecting improved intestinal phosphate absorption.

We did not demonstrate a significant decrease in serum PTH following treatment with $1,25(OH)_2D_3$. This could be either because the treatment period was too short to allow hypertrophied parathyroid glands to shrink in size, or most likely because not all of the patients selected for this study had clearly elevated baseline PTH levels. Further studies are currently being done in our laboratory on patients with ERF and elevated baseline PTH levels, to evaluate the effects of $1,25(OH)_2D_3$ on elevated serum PTH levels.

The question arises as to whether all of the results of this study could be explained simply by improved intestinal absorption of calcium and phosphate occurring as a physiologic response, rather than as an improvement in impaired absorption. Preliminary observations in our laboratory on two normal volunteers treated with $1,25(OH)_2D_3$ for 6 weeks indicate that subjects with normal renal function show no change in baseline serum calcium, phosphate, or PTH, nor in response to an oral phosphate load. Therefore, the changes seen in patients with ERF after treatment with $1,25(OH)_2D_3$ appear to reflect a decrease in skeletal resistance to PTH and/or improved intestinal absorption of calcium and phosphate. Our data support the role of $1,25(OH)_2D_3$ deficiency in the pathogenesis of early renal failure. Further clinical studies are needed to confirm the beneficial effects of 1,25-$(OH)_2D_3$ in patients with ERF, in particular the effects upon bone histology.

REFERENCES

1. Arnaud CD: Hyperparathyroidism and renal failure. Kidney Int 4:89-95, 1973.

2. Reiss E, Canterbury JM, Bilinsky RT: Measurement of serum parathyroid hormone in renal insufficiency. Trans Assn Am Phys 81:104-114, 1968.

3. Massry SG, Coburn JW, Lee DBN, Jowsey J, Kleeman CR: Skeletal resistance to parathyroid hormone in renal failure: studies in 105 human subjects. Ann Intern Med 78:357-364, 1973.

4. Coburn JW, Koppel MH, Brickman AS, Massry SG: Study of intestinal absorption of calcium in patients with chronic renal failure. Kidney Int 3:264-272, 1973.

5. Massry SG, Ritz E: The pathogenesis of secondary hyperparathyroidism of renal failure: Is there a controversy? Arch Intern Med 138:853-856, 1978.

6. Tessitore N, Lund BJ, Bonucci B, Sorenson E, Maschio OH: unpublished data.

7. Brickman AS, Coburn JW, Sherrard DJ, Wong EGC, Norman AW, Singer FR: Clinical effects of 1,25-dihydroxyvitamin D_3 in uremic patients with overt osteodystrophy. Contrib Nephrol 18:29-41, 1980.

8. Berl T, Berns AS, Huffer WE, Alfrey AC, Arnaud CD, Schrier RW: Controlled trial of the effects of 1,25-dihydroxycholecalciferol in patients treated with regular dialysis. Contrib Nephrol 18:72-81, 1980.

9. Goldstein DA, Malluche HH, Massry SG: Long-term effects of $1,25(OH)_2D_3$ on clinical and biochemical derangements of divalent ions in dialysis patients. Contrib Nephrol 18:42-54, 1980.

10. Sherrard DJ, Coburn JW, Brickman AS, Singer FR, Maloney N: Skeletal response to treatment with 1,25-dihydroxyvitamin D in renal failure. Contrib Nephrol 18:92-97, 1980.

11. Walton RJ, Bijvoet OL: Nomogram for derivation of renal threshold phosphate concentration. Lancet 2:309-310, 1975.

12. Mayer GP, Hurst JG, Barto JA, Keaton JA, Moore MP: Effect of epinephrine on parathyroid hormone secretion in calves. Endocrinology 104:1181-1187, 1979.

13. Bricker NS, Slatopolsky E, Reiss E, Avioli LV: Calcium, phosphorus, and bone in renal disease and transplantation. Arch Intern Med 123:543-553, 1969.

14. Llach F, Massry SG, Singer FR, Kurokawa K, Kaye JH, Coburn JW: Skeletal resistance to endogenous parathyroid hormone in patients with early renal failure: A possible cause for secondary hyperparathyroidism. J Clin Endocrinol Metab 41:339-345, 1975.

15. Slatopolsky E, Gray R, Adams ND, Lewis J, Hruska K, Martin K, Klahr S, DeLuca H, Lemann J: Low serum levels of 1,25-dihydroxycholecalciferol are not responsible for the development of secondary hyperparathyroidism in early renal failure (abstract). Kidney Int 14:733, 1978.

16. Tanaka Y, DeLuca HF, Omdahl J, Holick MF: Mechanism of action of 1,25-dihydroxycholecalciferol on intestinal calcium transport. Proc Natl Acad Sci USA 68:1286-1288, 1971.

17. Metz SA, Baylink DJ, Hughes MR, Haussler MR, Robertson RP: Osseous resistance to parathyroid hormone due to 1,25-dihydroxycholecalciferol deficiency. N Engl J Med 297:1084-1090, 1977.

18. Llach F, Massry SG, Koffler A, Malluche HH, Singer FR, Brickman AS, Kurokawa K: Secondary hyperparathyroidism in early renal failure: Role of phosphate retention (abstract). Kidney Int 12:459, 1977.

19. Healy MD, Malluche HH, Goldstein DA, Singer FR, Massry SG: Effects of longterm therapy with calcitriol in patients with moderate renal failure. Arch Intern Med 140:1030-1033, 1980.

INCREASED SERUM 1,25-$(OH)_2$-VITAMIN D CONCENTRATIONS FAIL TO AFFECT SERUM OR URINE PHOSPHATE IN HUMANS

J. Lemann, Jr., W.J. Maierhofer, N.D. Adams and R.W. Gray

Departments of Medicine and Biochemistry, Medical College of Wisconsin, Milwaukee, WI

Patients with recurrent calcium oxalate/apatite nephrolithiasis in association with hypercalciuria (idiopathic hypercalciuria) may exhibit low serum inorganic phosphate concentrations (1,2,3,4) in association with normal rates of urinary phosphate excretion implying the existence of impaired renal tubular phosphate reabsorption. In fact, such calcium stone formers exhibit impaired renal phosphate conservation in response to ingestion of a diet low in phosphate (5). They also exhibit higher than normal salivary phosphate concentrations (6) implying the presence of a more generalized abnormality of phosphate transport. Dietary phosphate deprivation in animals is accompanied by increased synthesis of the calcium mobilizing steroid 1,25-$(OH)_2$-vitamin D_3 by the kidney (7) and elevated serum levels of this hormone (8). Similarly renal synthesis of 1,25-$(OH)_2$-D is increased in hypercalciuric kidney stone formers (9) and high serum 1,25-$(OH)_2$-D concentrations among these patients may be inversely related to the degree of hypophosphatemia (4). Collectively, these observations are consistent with the view that an abnormality in phosphate metabolism underlies the enhancement of renal 1,25-D synthesis among some patients with idiopathic hypercalciuria; the defect in phosphate transport thus ultimately causing increased intestinal calcium absorption and hypercalciuria. On the other hand, although vitamin D or 1,25-$(OH)_2$-D administration to vitamin D deficient patients or animals augments intestinal phosphate absorption (10,11,12,13), the administration of physiologic doses of 1,25-$(OH)_2$-D_3 to thyroparathyroidectomized rats augments urinary phosphate excretion (14). The latter observation thus raises the possibility that the tendency for patients with idiopathic hypercalciuria to exhibit low serum phosphate concentrations might be a consequence of elevated serum 1,25-D concentrations to enhance renal phosphate excretion. To evaluate the possible effects of serum 1,25-D concentrations on phosphorus metabolism it thus becomes necessary to determine whether experimentally increased serum 1,25-$(OH)_2$-D concentrations affect serum phosphate levels and/or urinary phosphate excretion. The opportunity to obtain such data became available during the course of studies primarily designed to assess the effects of chronic oral 1,25-$(OH)_2D_3$ (calcitriol) administration on calcium metabolism in healthy men.

METHODS

We carried out 26 studies of 20 healthy men in the Medical College of Wisconsin Clinical Research Center with the consent of the subjects and the approval of the Medical College of Wisconsin Human Research Review Committee. Ten studies were performed while the subjects ate constant diets providing a normal calcium intake averaging 19.5±0.4 SD mmol Ca/day and 44.7±2.1 mmol PO_4/day. Sixteen studies were carried out while the subjects ate a low calcium diet providing an average of only 4.3±0.7 mmol Ca/day and 48.8±6.6 mmol PO_4/day. The subjects were studied first during a control period and then during an experimental period beginning at least four days after the initiation of continuing oral calcitriol administration every six hours. Among the subjects studied while eating the normal Ca diet two subjects received 0.25 μg, four subjects received 0.5 μg and four subjects received 0.75 μg calcitriol six hourly. Among the subjects eating a low Ca diet two subjects received 0.25 μg, six subjects received 0.5 μg and eight subjects received 0.75 μg calcitriol six hourly. All of the control and experimental observations of the subjects eating the normal calcium diet and six of the sixteen studies of the subjects eating the low calcium diet were during three or four day study periods. The remaining ten studies of subjects eating the low calcium diet involved complete metabolic balances during one or two six day control periods followed by one to three six day experimental periods beginning four days after the start of calcitriol administration.

Daily 24 hour urines were collected for the measurement of phosphate and creatinine. Serum 1,25-$(OH)_2$-D concentrations were measured on three to ten occasions during the control and during the experimental phases of the study of each subject. Fasting morning serum phosphate and creatinine concentrations were measured on two to six occasions of each study phase. In each subject a two hour fasting morning urine together with a serum specimen was obtained on two occasions in the control and in the calcitriol phases for the measurement of phosphate and creatinine and estimation of $TmPO_4$/GFR by the method of Bijvoet (15). Dietary and fecal phosphate were measured during the balance studies. Net intestinal phosphate absorption was calculated as dietary phosphate minus fecal phosphate while percent dietary phosphate absorption was calculated as net intestinal phosphate absorption divided by dietary phosphate intake times one hundred. The analytical methods employed have been reported (4,16).

Results are presented as mean ± standard deviation.

RESULTS

Effects of elevated serum 1,25-$(OH)_2$-D on intestinal phosphate absorption

Table I presents group mean values for daily calcitriol dose, serum 1,25-$(OH)_2$-D concentrations, dietary phosphate intake, net intestinal phosphate absorption and percent intestinal absorption of dietary phosphate during the control and experimental balances in ten of the subjects studied while eating the low Ca diet. Net intestinal PO_4 absorption increased slightly but significantly during calcitriol administration by an average of +3.9±3.3 mmol/day ($p<0.01$) or by +7±6% of daily phosphate intake ($p<0.01$). As shown in Figure 1, percent absorption of dietary PO_4 was positively correlated to serum 1,25-$(OH)_2$-D concentrations when the data for the control and experimental periods was considered together; $p<0.025$.

TABLE I - Effects of Calcitriol Administration on Serum 1,25-$(OH)_2$-D Concentrations and Net Intestinal Phosphate Absorption During Studies of 10 Subjects Eating Low Calcium Diets

	Control	Taking Calcitriol	Mean Change From Control	P
Calcitriol Dose* nmol/day	0	6.2±1.2	+6.2±1.2	<0.001
Serum 1,25-$(OH)_2$-D, pM	103±19	184±39	+81±31	<0.001
Diet PO_4	52.4±5.8	524±5.8	0	NS
Net Intestinal PO_4 Absorption, mmol/day	34.3±4.9	38.2±5.5	+3.9±3.3	<0.01
Percent Intestinal Absorption of Dietary PO_4	66±6	73±4	+7±6	<0.01

*Four subjects were given 4.8 nmol calcitriol/day while six were given 7.2 nmol calcitriol/day; Mean body weight for the 10 subjects averaged 71.5±8.8 kg and did not change during calcitriol administration.

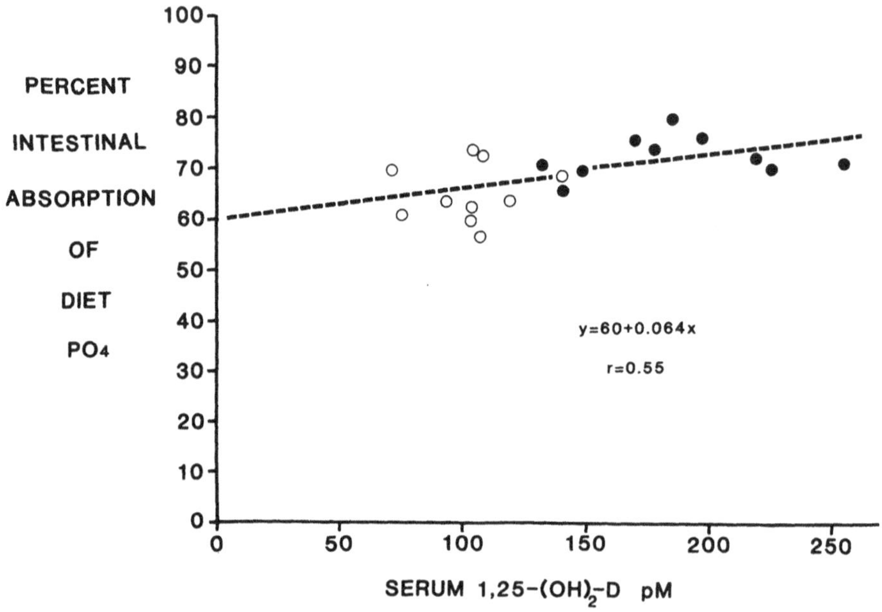

Figure 1 - Percent intestinal absorption of dietary PO_4 as a function of serum 1,25-$(OH)_2$-D concentration among subjects eating the low Ca diet during control (0) and during calcitriol administration (●).

<u>Effects of elevated serum 1,25-$(OH)_2$-D concentrations on serum and urinary phosphate</u>

Table II presents mean serum 1,25-$(OH)_2$-D concentrations, fasting serum phosphate concentrations, daily urinary phosphate excretion and fasting $TmPO_4$/GFR during control and during calcitriol administration for the ten studies of subjects who ate the normal Ca diet and, separately the 16 studies of subjects who ate the low Ca diet. As expected, serum 1,25-$(OH)_2$-D concentrations were about 25% higher during control when the subjects ate the low Ca diet as compared to the normal Ca diet; $p<0.025$ (16). However, the reduction in dietary Ca intake had no detectable effect on fasting serum phosphate, daily urinary phosphate excretion or $TmPO_4$/GFR. During the administration of calcitriol similar increments in and absolute levels of 1,25-$(OH)_2$-D concentrations were produced regardless of dietary Ca intake. The elevated serum 1,25-$(OH)_2$-D concentrations had no detectable effect on serum PO_4 or urinary PO_4 excretion in the studies of subjects eating a normal Ca diet. By contrast, mean fasting serum PO_4 concentrations and daily urinary PO_4 excretion rose slightly but very significantly when calcitriol was administered to subjects eating a low Ca diet. Despite these changes, mean fasting $TmPO_4$/GFR was not altered while the subjects ate the low Ca diet. As shown in Figure 2, fasting $TmPO_4/GFR$ did not vary as a function of prevailing serum 1,25-$(OH)_2$-D concentrations in these studies regardless of calcium intake.

Table II - The Effects of Elevated Serum 1,25-$(OH)_2$-D Concentrations on Serum and Urine Phosphate

	Normal Calcium Diet 10 Studies			
	Control	Taking 1,25-$(OH)_2$-D	Δ	P
Serum 1,25-$(OH)_2$-D, pM	84±23	172±38	+89±45	<0.001
Serum PO_4, mM	1.34±0.16	1.39±0.19	+0.05±0.09	NS
Urine PO_4, mmol/day	36.9±5.4	36.5±4.3	-0.4±3.8	NS
Fasting $TmPO_4/GFR$, mM	1.28±0.15	1.29±0.13	+0.01±0.10	NS
	Low Calcium Diet 16 Studies			
	Control	Taking 1,25-$(OH)_2$-D	Δ	P
Serum 1,25-$(OH)_2$-D, pM	106±20	183±40	+.77±29	<0.001
Serum PO_4, mM	1.32±0.15	1.41±0.16	+0.09±0.10	<0.005
Urine PO_4 mmol/day	34.0±3.6	39.3±5.4	+5.4±4.6	<0.001
Fasting $TmPO_4/GFR$, mM	1.41±0.20	1.39±0.16	-0.02±0.15	NS

As shown in Table III, we have compared fasting morning serum PO_4 levels in 26 men with recurrent nephrolithiasis, hypercalciuria and spontaneously elevated serum 1,25-$(OH)_2$-D concentrations to similar measurements in 15 healthy men without a personal or family history of stones. Both groups were studied as outpatients while they ate their usual diets. Serum PO_4 levels were significantly lower among the stone formers whose average serum 1,25-$(OH)_2$-D level was almost twice that of the healthy subjects. It should also be noted that serum PTH levels did not differ between the groups. The stone formers exhibited, as expected, hypercalciuria.

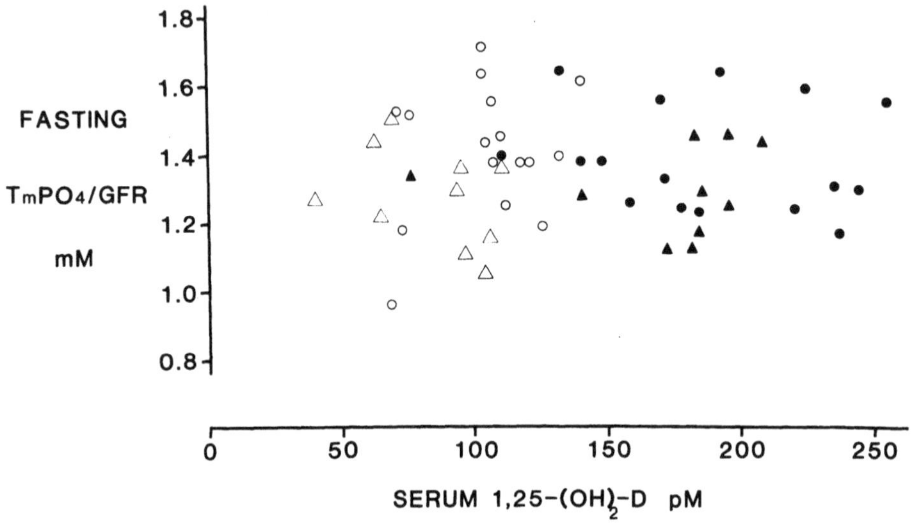

Figure 2 - Fasting $TmPO_4$/GFR as a function of serum 1,25-$(OH)_2$-D concentration during control (open symbols) and during calcitriol administration (closed symbols) while subjects ate normal Ca diets (triangles) or low Ca diets (circles).

Table III - Comparison of Ca Stone Formers Exhibiting Elevated Serum 1,25-$(OH)_2$-D Levels to Healthy Subjects

	15 Healthy Men	28 Men With Ca Nephrolithiasis and Elevated Serum 1,25-$(OH)_2$-D Concentrations	P
Serum 1,25-$(OH)_2$-D, pM	84±24	188±37	<0.001
Serum PO_4, mM	1.23±0.15	1.03±0.18	<0.005
Serum Ca, mM	2.46±0.10	2.47±0.12	NS
Serum PTH, μlEq/ml	5.4±2.6	6.0±2.1	NS
Urine Ca, mmol/day	4.7±1.3	8.7±2.7	<0.001

DISCUSSION

Previous observation of the relationship between intestinal absorption and serum 1,25-$(OH)_2$-D levels in our laboratory among healthy volunteers and patients with spontaneously varying serum 1,25-$(OH)_2$-D concentrations showed that net intestinal phosphate absorption was positively but not significantly dependent on serum levels of the hormone: percent absorption of dietary $PO_4 = 64 + 0.045 +$ serum 1,25-$(OH)_2$-D, pM; $r = 0.30$ (17). The present observations extend and confirm those results. Even though we have now observed a significant dependence of PO_4 absorption on serum 1,25-$(OH)_2$-D concentrations, it is evident that the bulk of intestinal PO_4 absorption must be independent of 1,25-$(OH)_2$-D.

The observation that experimental elevations of serum 1,25-$(OH)_2$-D concentrations as a result of chronic oral calcitriol administration are not associated with significant reductions in fasting serum PO_4 concentrations or fasting $TmPO_4$/GFR does not support the view that 1,25-$(OH)_2$-D inhibits tubular reabsorption of phosphate in humans. Instead, the observations are consistent with previous proposals that the low serum PO_4 concentrations observed among patients with hypercalciuric nephrolithiasis and spontaneously elevated 1,25-$(OH)_2$-D concentrations may contribute to the accelerated renal synthesis of 1,25-$(OH)_2$-D and thus the high serum levels of the hormone.

Supported in part by USPHS RR-00058, AM15089 and AM22014

REFERENCES

1. Henneman, P.H., Benedict, P.H., Forbes, A.P. and Dudley, H.R. 1958. Idiopathic hypercalciuria. N. Eng. J. Med. 259: 802.

2. Coe, F.L., Canterbury, J.M., Firpo, J.J. and Reiss, E. 1973 Evidence for secondary hyperparathyroidism in idiopathic hypercalciuria. J. Clin. Invest. 52: 134.

3. Shen, F.H., Baylink, D.J., Neilsen, R.L., Sherrard, D.J., Ivey, J.L. and Haussler, M.R. Further evidence supporting the phosphate leak hypothesis of idiopathic hypercalciuria. Proceedings of the Third International Workshop on Phosphate and other Minerals, Madrid, July, 1977. In Homeostasis of Phosphate and Other Minerals, S.G. Massry, E. Ritz and A. Rapado, Editors. Plenum Press, New York, 1978, 217.

4. Gray, R.W., Wilz, D.R., Caldas, A.E., and Lemann, J. Jr. 1977 The importance of phosphate in regulating plasma 1,25-$(OH)_2$-

vitamin D levels in humans: Studies in healthy subjects, in calcium-stone formers and in patients with primary hyperparathyroidism. J. Clin. Endocrinol. Metab. 45: 299.

5. Lemann, J. Jr., Gray, R.W., and Wilz, D.R. 1978. Evidence for a renal PO_4 leak in patients with calcium nephrolithiasis. Proceedings of the Third International Workshop on Phosphate and other minerals, Madrid, July, 1988. In Homeostasis of Phosphate and Other Minerals, S.G. Massry, E. Ritz and A. Rapado, Editors. Plenum Press, New York, 225.

6. Lemann, J. Jr., Gray, R.W., Wilz, D.R. and Adams, N.D. 1979. Is there a disorder of phosphate metabolism in idiopathic hypercalciuria? Proceedings of the 4th Workshop on Phosphate, Strasbourg, June, 1979. In Phosphate and Minerals in Health and Disease, S.G. Massry, E. Ritz, and H. Jahn, Editors. Plenum Press, New York, 1980, 427.

7. Gray, R.W., 1981. Dietary phosphate deprivation increases 1,25-$(OH)_2$-vitamin D_3 synthesis in rat kidney. Federation Proceedings: 40: 899.

8. Hughes, M.R., Haussler, M.R., Wergedal, J. and Baylink, D.J. 1975. Regulation of serum 1α,25-dihydroxy-vitamin D_3 by calcium and phosphate in the rat. Sci 190: 578.

9. Maierhofer, W.J., Gray, R.W., Adams, N.D., Smith, G.A. and Lemann, J. Jr. 1981. Synthesis and metabolic clearance of 1,25-dihydroxyvitamin D as determinants of serum concentrations: A comparison of two methods. J. Clin. Endo. Metab. 53: 472.

10. Harrison, H.E., Harrison, H.C. 1961. Intestinal transport of phosphate: Action of vitamin D, calcium and potassium. Am. J. Physiol. 201: 1007.

11. Chen, T.C., Castillo, L., Korycka-Dahl, M., et al. 1974. Role of vitamin D metabolites in phosphate transport of rat intestine. J. Nutr. 104: 1056.

12. Brickman, A.S., Hartenbower, D.L., Norman, A.W. and Coburn, J.W. 1977. Actions of 1α-hydroxyvitamin D_3 and 1,25-dihydroxyvitamin D_3 on mineral metabolism in man. J. Clin. Nutr. 30: 1064.

13. Perlik, M. and Wasserman, R.H. 1978. Effect of vitamin D on transepithelial phosphate transport in chick intestine. Am. J. Physiol. 234: E399.

14. Bonjour, J-P, Preston, C. and Flesch, H. 1977. Effect of 1,25-dihydroxyvitamin D_3 on the renal handling of Pi in thyroparathyroidectomized rats. J. Clin. Invest. 60: 1419.

15. Walton, R.J., Bijvoet, O.L.M. 1975. Nomogram for the derivation of renal threshold phosphate concentration. Lancet 2: 309.

16. Adams, N.D., Gray, R.W. and Lemann, J. Jr. 1979. The effects of oral $CaCO_3$ loading and of dietary calcium deprivation on plasma 1,25-$(OH)_2$-vitamin D concentrations in healthy adults. J. Clin. Endo. Metab. 48: 1008.

17. Wilz, D.R., Gray, R.W., Dominguez, J.H. and Lemann, J. Jr. 1979. Plasma 1,25-$(OH)_2$-vitamin D concentrations and net intestinal calcium, phosphate and magnesium absorption in humans. Am. J. Clin. Nutr. 32: 2052.

ADRENERGIC BLOCKADE MAY INHIBIT THE INCREASE IN PLASMA 1,25-$(OH)_2$-VITAMIN D DURING PHOSPHATE DEPRIVATION IN THE RAT

Richard W. Gray

Departments of Biochemistry and Medicine
Medical College of Wisconsin
Milwaukee, WI

Dietary phosphate deprivation in rats is accompanied by a 4 to 5 fold increase in the plasma concentration of 1,25-$(OH)_2$-Vitamin D. This increase in plasma levels has recently been shown to be the result of increased renal synthesis of the hormone (1), and is not mediated by PTH or gonadal hormones (2-4). Earlier work by Tanaka and DeLuca (5) had suggested that this response might be mediated by hypophosphatemia *per se*, but recent experiments in rats have shown that hypophysectomy completely abolishes the response despite a comparable degree of hypophosphatemia in the phosphate-deprived hypophysectomized (hypox) animals (4). In addition, hypox rats retain their ability to increase plasma 1,25-$(OH)_2$-D levels on a low Ca diet (4). Finally, replacement of phosphate-deprived hypox rats with either growth hormone or, independently, with thyroid hormone at least partially restores the ability of such animals to increase their plasma 1,25-$(OH)_2$-D levels on a low phosphorus diet (6). These results would suggest that the low-phosphate stimulus to renal 1,25-$(OH)_2$-D synthesis is, at least in part, hormonally mediated. The present studies were undertaken to determine whether various pharmacologic blocking agents could be used as probes to gain further insight into possible hormonal mechanisms which might mediate the increase in plasma 1,25-$(OH)_2$-D levels during dietary phosphate deprivation.

METHODS

Six-week old male Sprague-Dawley rats were maintained on a synthetic diet containing 0.56% phosphorus, 0.63% calcium and 3 IU of vitamin D_3 per g for 1 to 2 days after being received from the supplier. Bromocriptine, aminophylline, imidazole, and chlorpheniramine together with cimetidine were administered intraperi-

Table 1. Plasma PO_4 and 1,25-$(OH)_2$-D Concentrations during Dietary Phosphate Deprivation in Rats Treated with Various Pharmacological Agents

Drug	Dose	Plasma P mM	Plasma 1,25-$(OH)_2$-D pM
Control	No Rx	1.77±0.50 (10)	931±466 (11)
Bromocriptine	3 mg/kg	1.58±0.50 (4)	913±299 (4)
Aminophylline	100 mg/kg	1.53±0.13 (4)	761±213 (4)
Imidazole	100 mg/kg	1.49±0.08*(4)	937±322 (4)
Chlorpheniramine	5 mg/kg	1.49±0.16 (4)	1452±352 (4)
& Cimetidine	45 mg/kg		
Inodomethacin	5 mg/kg	1.64±0.26 (4)	1217±444 (4)
Reserpine	0.5 mg/kg	1.88±0.56 (8)	414±137†(8)

*$p<0.05$ vs. control
†$p<0.01$ vs. control

toneally in divided dosages twice daily for 1 day prior to and then during 4 days of dietary phosphate deprivation. Indomethacin was administered in corn oil via gavage on the same schedule. Reserpine and 6-hydroxydopamine were administered as a single intraperitoneal dose on the morning before the 4 days of dietary phosphate deprivation were begun. Phosphate deprivation was achieved using a synthetic diet providing only 0.02% phosphorus and 0.63% calcium. After 4 days of phosphate deprivation, the animals were weighed, anesthetized with ketamine or ether and exsanguinated from the abdominal aorta into heparinized syringes. Plasma 1,25-$(OH)_2$-D concentrations, Ca and PO_4 were measured as previously described (3,7). Results are presented as group mean ± S.D.

RESULTS

Table 1 shows the results of a screening assay in which several pharmacologic blocking agents were administered during 4 days of dietary phosphate deprivation. Bromocriptine was given to inhibit prolactin secretion (8). Aminophylline and imidazole were given to inhibit or stimulate breakdown of cyclic AMP, respectively (9,10). Chlorpheniramine and cimetidine were given together to block H_1 and H_2 receptors (11). Inodomethacin was given to inhibit prostoglandin synthesis and reserpine was given to induce adrenergic blockade (12). Of all of these drugs, only reserpine administration resulted in a significant decrease in plasma 1,25-$(OH)_2$-D levels in comparison to untreated rats after 4 days of dietary phosphate deprivation.

Since it appeared that adrenergic blockade may have some in-

Table 2. Comparison of Plasma 1,25-$(OH)_2$-D, Ca and PO_4 Levels during Control Condition and Phosphate Deprivation in Rats with or without 6-Hydroxydopamine Treatment

NORMAL DIET	1,25-$(OH)_2$-D pmol/l	Ca mM/l	P mM/l
No Treatment	228±76 (40)	2.52±0.2 (19)	2.67±0.26 (36)
6-Hydroxydopamine (150 mg/kg as a single dose)	132±32* (4)	2.69±0.1 (3)	2176±0.25 (3)
LOW P DIET			
No Treatment	931±466† (11)	3.03±0.26† (10)	1.77±0.5† (10)
6-Hydroxydopamine (150 mg/kg as a single dose)	371±98*† (5)	2.78±0.2 (4)	1.44±0.23† (4)

*$p<0.025$ vs. no treatment
†$p<0.005$ vs. normal diet

hibitory effect on the increase in plasma 1,25-$(OH)_2$-D levels in response to phosphate deprivation, this effect was further examined by administration of another adrenergic blocker, 6-hydroxydopamine, to animals eating a low phosphorus diet as well as to animals eating a diet providing normal quantities of phosphorus (Table 2). Among animals eating the normal phosphorus diet, the administration of 6-hydroxydopamine reduced plasma 1,25-$(OH)_2$-D concentrations to a mean level slightly but significantly below that of untreated control animals. Plasma calcium and phosphorus concentrations were unaffected by the drug. When 6-hydroxydopamine was administered during phosphate deprivation, plasma 1,25-$(OH)_2$-D levels rose but reached a mean level of only 371 ± 98 pM, significantly lower than the mean level of 931 ± 466 pM observed in untreated rats deprived of phosphate ($p<0.025$). Moreover, relative to animals eating the control normal P diet, plasma 1,25-$(OH)_2$-D rose only by an average of 2.8 fold during phosphate deprivation in the presence of the drug in comparison to an average of 4.1 fold in untreated animals. Finally, the mean plasma 1,25-$(OH)_2$-D level of 371 ± 98 pM observed when phosphate-deprived animals were given 6-hydroxydopamine was similar to the mean level of 414 ± 137 pM observed in phosphate-deprived animals given reserpine (Table 1).

DISCUSSION

Adrenergic blockade achieved by either reserpine or 6-hydroxydopamine was the only pharmacologic probe tested which produced a significant inhibition of the elevation of plasma 1,25-$(OH)_2$-D levels that normally occurs in response to phosphate deprivation in the rat. However, interpretation of this effect is difficult since 6-hydroxydopamine administration also resulted in lower plasma 1,25-$(OH)_2$-D levels in animals not deprived of phosphorus and did not completely abolish the rise in plasma 1,25-$(OH)_2$-D levels in response to phosphate deprivation. There are several possibilities which might account for these results. First, it is possible that both reserpine and 6-hydroxydopamine have a direct effect on the kidney to inhibit 1,25-$(OH)_2$-D synthesis independent of their adrenergic blocking effects. Second, it is possible that the doses of the drugs used as well as their method of administration may have resulted in incomplete adrenergic blockade which might explain the lack of complete inhibition of the increase in plasma 1,25-$(OH)_2$-D levels in response to phosphate deprivation. Finally, and speculatively, the effect of adrenergic blockade may be mediated by inhibition of growth hormone secretion, since adrenergic agonists stimulate growth hormone secretion and growth hormone very likely plays a permissive role in the response of renal 1,25-$(OH)_2$-D synthesis to phosphate deprivation (6,14). All of these possibilities can be tested experimentally, and such experiments are currently in progress.

The lack of an effect of the other pharmacological probes on the response of plasma 1,25-$(OH)_2$-D levels to phosphate deprivation also has some implications. The failure of bromocriptine to blunt the response would suggest that increased prolactin secretion in response to phosphate deprivation is not a mechanism which mediates the rise in plasma 1,25-$(OH)_2$-D during phosphate deprivation. This interpretation is consistant with unpublished observations in our laboratory that plasma prolactin levels do not rise in phosphate-deprived rats. The failure of either aminophylline or imidazole to inhibit the rise in plasma 1,25-$(OH)_2$-D levels during phosphate deprivation would suggest that changes in cyclic AMP levels do not significantly affect this response. Similarly, the failure of either the combination of chlorpheniramine and cimetidine or inodomethacin to block the rise in plasma 1,25-$(OH)_2$-D during phosphate deprivation would suggest that neither histamine nor prostaglandins are involved in the response.

Supported in part by USPHS RR00058 and AM22014.

REFERENCES

1. R. W. Gray, Dietary phosphate deprivation increases 1,25-$(OH)_2$-Vitamin D_3 synthesis in rat kidney, Fed. Proc. 40:899 (1981).

2. M. R. Hughes, M. R. Haussler, J. Wergedal and D. J. Baylink, Regulation of serum 1α,25-dihydroxyvitamin D_3 by calcium and phosphate in the rat, Science 190:578 (1975).
3. R. W. Gray, Effects of age and sex on the regulation of plasma 1,25-$(OH)_2$-D by phosphorus in the rat, Calcif. Tissue Int. (In press), (1981).
4. R. W. Gray, The control of plasma 1,25-$(OH)_2$-vitamin D concentrations by calcium and phosphorus in the rat: effects of hypophysectomy, Calcif. Tissue Int. (In press), (1981).
5. Y. Tanaka, H. F. DeLuca, The control of 25-hydroxyvitamin D metabolism by inorganic phosphorus, Arch. Biochem. Biophys. 154:566 (1973).
6. R. W. Gray, T. L. Garthwaite and L. S. Phillips, The increase in plasma 1,25-$(OH)_2$-vitamin D in response to dietary phosphate deprivation in the rat requires growth hormone or triiodothyronine, Calcif. Tissue Int. 33:334 (1981).
7. A. E. Caldas, R. W. Gray, and J. Lemann, Jr., The simultaneous measurement of vitamin D metabolites in plasma: Studies in healthy adults and in patients with calcium nephrolithiasis, J. Lab. Clin. Med. 91:840-849 (1978).
8. H. M. Lloyd, J. D. Meares and J. Jacobi, Effects of oestrogen and bromocryptine on in vivo secretion and mitosis in prolactin cells, Nature 255:497-498 (1975).
9. W. T. Beck, R. W. Bellantone and E. S. Canellakin, The in vivo stimulation of rat liver ornithine decarboxylase activity by dibutyryl cyclic adenosine 3'5'-monophosphate, theophylline, and dexamethazone, Biochem. Biophys. Res. Comm. 48:1649-1655 (1972).
10. P. Prig-Parelloda and J. M. Planas, Pharmacological properties of imidazole. II. Actions on the normal body temperature regulation in rats, Life Sci. 14:457-462 (1974).
11. C. J. Levy, M.E. Carroll, J. C. Smith and K. G. Hofer, Antihistamines block radiation-induced taste aversions, Science 186:1044-1045 (1974).
12. R. E. Zigmond, F. Schon and L. L. Iversen, Increased tyrosine hydroxylase activity in the locus coeruleus of rat brain stem after reserpine treatment and cold stress, Brain Research 70:547-552 (1974).
13. A. Kawa, T. Kamisaki, T. Ariyama, T. Kawabata, Y. Maeda, O. Okamoto and T. Kanehisa, The effects of intraperitoneal injection of 6-hydroxydopamine on the turnover and the levels of plasma corticosterone in rats, Clin. Exp. Pharmacol. Physiol. 6:123-128 (1979).
14. M. T. Bluet-Pajot, C. Schaub, F. Mounier, A. Segalen, J. Duhault and C. Kordon, Monoaminergic regulation of growth hormone in the rat, J. Endocrinol. 78:387-396 (1980).

TOPICS ON BONE METABOLISM

REGULATION OF OSTEOBLAST ACTIVITY AND THE OSTEOBLAST-OSTEOCYTE TRANSFORMATION

William A. Peck and Leonard Rifas

Department of Medicine, The Jewish Hospital of
St. Louis, Washington University School of Medicine
216 South Kingshighway, St. Louis, Missouri 63110

According to currently held concepts of bone formation (Table 1), osteoblasts develop from mitotically competent marrow stromal cells by a process of non-mitotic differentiation (modulation) (1,2). Osteoblasts are attracted to the bone surfaces, and are activated to elaborate lamellae of collagen-rich organic matrix (osteoid) which is subsequently mineralized. Inactive osteoblasts, having completed a cycle of bone formation, remain attached to bone, where they appear as flattened, biosynthetically dormant cells. A small proportion of osteoblasts are trapped in the newly secreted osteoid and are buried in successively formed layers of bone. These internalized cells, termed osteocytes, remain connected to each other and to surface osteoblasts by slender processes that traverse the microcanalicular system of bone (3), yielding an apparent syncytium that provides an enormous surface area for mineral exchange and a mechanism for conducting ions from bone to vascular channels. Indeed, the osteocyte network may mediate, at least in part, the role of the skeleton in maintaining mineral and acid-base homeostasis (Table 1).

Table 1. The Cellular Basis of Bone Formation

1. Expansion of the Marrow Mesenchymal (Stromal) Cell Pool by Mitosis.
2. Specialization of Preosteoblasts and Their Attraction to Bone Surfaces.
3. Activation of Mature Osteoblasts.
4. Synthesis and Mineralization of Osteoid.
5. Entrapment of Some Osteoblasts (Osteocyte Formation), Inactivation of Others.

Little is known about the regulation of osteoblast growth, differentiation, activation and deactivation, nor is there substantive information about their conversion to osteocytes. Circumstantial evidence has accumulated to suggest that local as well as systemic factors may be important in controlling these events. Bone formation is temporally and spatially linked to two intraskeletal phenomena: the formation of calcified cartilage template cores at the epiphyseal growth plate and the resorption of bone (Table 2). Factors released from resorbing bone and from cartilage templates, locally synthesized hormones, and other agents may serve to promote bone formation (Table 2).

Since our initial observation in 1977 of an autologous growth promoting substance released by calvaria cells in primary culture (4), a number of peptides have been obtained from bone, cartilage, isolated bone cells and chondrocytes that have the capacity to modify bone cell behavior (5-11). Well-characterized growth factors of non-skeletal origin, fibroblast growth factor (FGF), epidermal growth factor (EGF) and multiplication stimulating activity (MSA) have also been found to enhance bone cell and chondrocyte growth (12-17). The studies described herein demonstrate that isolated chondrocytes *in vitro* release a substance (or substances) that promotes the growth of chondrocytes and osteoblasts, but not of fibroblasts. We also report on the development of an *in vitro* system that may well permit the study of osteoblast specialization and transformation into osteocytes.

In order to examine the elaboration of growth factors by cartilage cells, we selectively cultured chondrocytes obtained from rat chondrocranium in a previously described chemically defined, protein-free incubation medium (18). In brief, the chondrocranial portions of the calvaria of 19-21 day old rat fetuses were excised and the chondrocytes dispersed by exposure to crude collagenase. Harvested, washed cells were cultured in 35 mm petri plates containing 1 ml of medium. The chondrocytes rapidly attached to the plastic support surface, spread, proliferated and aggregated to

Table 2. The Local Regulation of Bone Formation

1. Local Conditions that Promote Formation
   a. Bone Resorption (Membranous Osteogenesis)
   b. Cartilage Template Cores (Endochondral Osteogenesis)
2. Possible Mechanisms of Local Regulation
   a. Locally Elaborated Agents (e.g., Growth Factors, Catecholamines, Prostaglandins)
   b. Surface Charge Changes
   c. Chemotactic Factors
   d. Ions (e.g., Calcium)

form three-dimensional clusters or nodules that have been shown to contain cartilage matrix by multiple criteria (typical histochemical reactions and transmission electron-microscopic appearance, synthesis of type II collagen and cartilage proteoglycans) (19).

To explore the possibility that chondrocyte growth in serum and hormone-free medium was engendered by an autologous growth factor, we dialyzed and concentrated incubation medium which had been conditioned by exposure to the chondrocytes for 7 days and tested the effect of the concentrate on chondrocyte growth in mature (confluent) cultures. This crude material stimulated thymidine incorporation into DNA and cell proliferation, but only at high concentrations (100 to 500 μg/ml (4). By contrast, EGF and FGF were effective in this system at concentrations ranging from 10 to 100 ng/ml (9). We then embarked on a purification sequence, beginning with ion-exchange chromatography, an approach employed previously to purify MSA from the conditioned medium bathing Buffalo rat liver tumor cells in culture (20,21). This system yielded two peaks of activity, eluting at pH 9 and pH 11, respectively. Each peak contained material which promoted chondrocyte DNA synthesis and proliferation and which acted at a low concentration (1 μg/ml) (9). In order to test for target cell specificity, we employed skin cells (presumptive fibroblasts) derived from the same rat fetuses used for chondrocyte harvests by the same method and cultured under similar conditions. Neither the pH 9 nor the pH 11 fraction stimulated DNA synthesis in the skin cell system, whereas EGF was effective (9). To examine this specificity further, we examined the effects of pH 9 and pH 11 fractions on DNA synthesis in chondrocytes and skin cells in the presence of the growth inhibitor dexamethasone (Fig. 1). Dexamethasone decreased DNA synthesis in the chondrocyte and the skin cell cultures. Concomitant exposure to each fraction obscured the inhibitory effect of dexamethasone in the cartilage cell system, but not in the skin cells, pointing to the relative specificity of this material (Fig. 1).

In collaboration with Drs. Ernesto Canalis and Lawrence Raisz of the University of Connecticut, we tested the possibility that the pH 9 and pH 11 fractions might stimulate osteoblast as well as chondrocyte growth. Organ cultured calvaria, known to be rich in osteoblasts, were exposed to the pH 9 and pH 11 fractions and the incorporation of radioactively labeled thymidine into DNA as well as total DNA assessed. Both fractions promoted DNA synthesis in this system, suggesting that osteoblasts may be responsive to these substances (10).

Consequently, chondrocytes in primary culture elaborate a substance (or substances) which has the capacity to promote multiplication in chondrocytes, perhaps in osteoblasts, but not in a skin cell system. Although the substance chromatographically resembles the now purified MSA in that it lacks sulfation factor activity in vitro. Our working hypothesis is that this factor may be important in chondrocyte and osteoblast growth during embryogenesis and could be essential for the wave of osteoblast proliferation that follows cartilage maturation during endochondral bone growth.

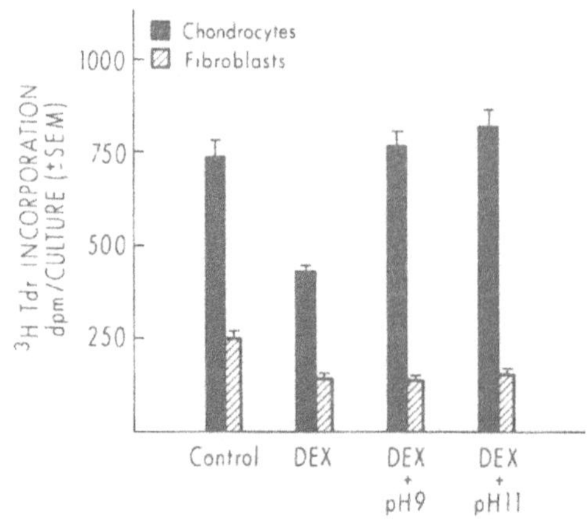

Fig. 1. Chondrocytes and fibroblasts isolated from rat chondrocranium and skin fragments, respectively, were grown to confluence in primary culture. The cells were then exposed to agents [dexamethasone (10^{-7} M), pH 9 (1 μg/ml) and pH 11 (1 μg/ml)] as indicated for 24 hours. ^{3}H thymidine was added 24 hours before termination. Data are presented as means and standard errors of four separate cultures.

Absence of appropriate in vitro model systems has impeded acquisition of knowledge about the transformation of osteoblasts to osteocytes. Existing cell and organ culture systems have not been found to support this degree of bone cell specialization. In ex-

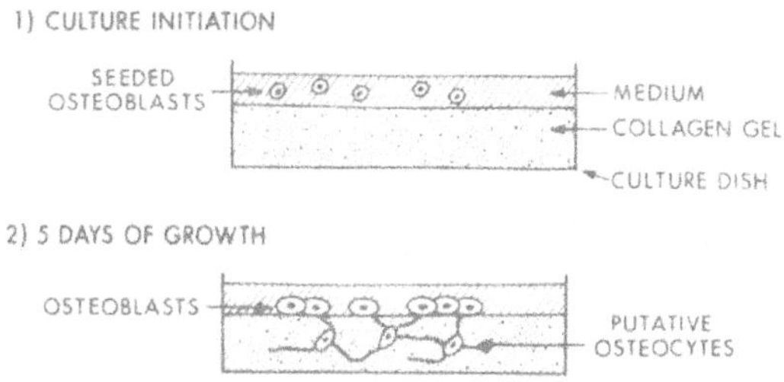

Figure 2. Osteoblast-Osteocyte Transformation; In Vitro Model

ploring new methods for studying this phenomenon, we selected a culture system that would present cultured osteoblasts with a "preformed" organic matrix for possible penetration and osteocytic transformation (Fig. 2). Collagen gels composed of highly purified rat tail tendon collagen were used to serve as a cell support on the bottoms of 35 mm culture vessels. Osteoblast-like cells, dispersed from cartilage-free segments of fetal rat calvaria, were added to the gels in the presence of the same serum-free incubation medium used previously in culturing chondrocytes (18). These cultures were incubated for up to 21 days, and the incubation medium was changed every third or fourth day.

Spherical, osteoblast-like cells, enriched in cytoplasmic alkaline phosphatase, attached to the surfaces of the gels within minutes. After 1-2 days, it was apparent that some but not all of the attached cells had penetrated the gels and had become stellate in shape. The cells entrapped in the gels retained copious cytoplasmic alkaline phosphatase activity and exhibited slender cytoplasmic extensions that appeared to interact with those of neighboring cells, forming a continuum. Electron microscopic examination disclosed that the cells located within the gels retained osteoblast features; abundant mitochondria and endoplasmic reticulum. Their extended cell processes contained clearly identifiable microfilament bundles as well as microtubular structures. Specialized junctions linked the cell bodies of osteoblasts on the surface of the gels. In general, these were tight junctions but gap junctions were noted on occasion. Similar junctions could be seen to

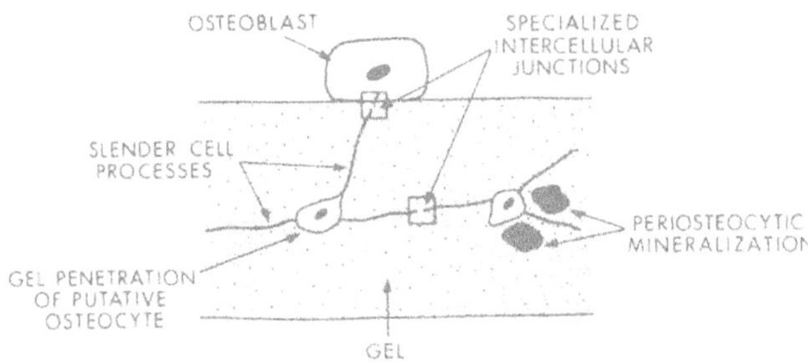

Figure 3. Features of the In Vitro Osteocyte Model

join the cell processes of the stellate cells within the gel, thus indicating the presence of a syncytium. After two weeks in culture, calcium deposits appeared in the gels adjacent to the cells.

These results suggest that the study of osteoblast behavior on collagen gels may provide a useful model for examining the events involved in skeletal mineralization and osteoblast-osteocyte transformation. Our observations indicate that certain osteoblasts penetrate the collagen gels upon which they are cultured yet retain histochemical evidence of their osteoblast heritage. The putative osteocytes have extended processes that interact with those of adjacent cells via specialized junctions and are associated with local mineralization (Fig. 3). It will be of interest to examine the effects of hormones and bone cell growth factors in this system.

Acknowledgement

The work described herein was supported by NIH Grant 5R01 AM19855.

References

1. Friedenstein, A.J., Precursor cells of mechanocytes, Internat. Revs. Cytol. 47: 327 (1976).
2. Ashton, B.A., Allen, T.D., Howlett, C.R., Eaglesom, C.C., Hattori, A., and Owen, M., Formation of bone and cartilage by marrow stroma cells in diffusion chambers in vivo, Clin. Orthop. Rel. Res. 151: 294 (1980).

3. Pritchard, J.J., in: "The Biochemistry and Physiology of Bone," G.H. Bourne, ed., Academic Press, New York (1956).
4. Peck, W.A., and Burks, J.K., Proliferation and specialization of bone cells cultured in serum-free medium, in "Proceedings, Workshop on Mechanisms of Hard Tissue Destruction," J. Horton, T. Tarpley, and W. Davis, eds., Calc. Tissue. Abstr., pp. 3-12 (1978).
5. Klagsbrun, M., Langer, R., Levenson, R., Smith, S., and Lillihei, C., The stimulation of DNA synthesis and cell division in chondrocytes and 3T3 cells by a growth factor isolated from cartilage, Exp. Cell Res. 105: 99 (1977).
6. Azizkhan, J.C., and Klagsbrun, M., Chondrocytes contain a growth factor that is localized in the nucleus and is associated with chromatin, Proc. Natl. Acad. Sci. USA 77: 2762 (1980).
7. Klagsbrun, M., and Smith, S., Purification of a cartilage-derived growth factor, J. Biol. Chem. 255: 10859 (1980).
8. Burks, J.K., and Peck, W.A., Growth and differentiation of isolated calvarium cells in a serum-free medium, Int. Rev. Cytol., Suppl. 10, 103-115 (1979).
9. Peck, W.A., Kohler, G., and Rifas, L., Bone cell function studied in vitro: the importance of local chemical signals, in "Proceedings, Tenth Steenbock Symposium (Osteoporosis: Recent Advances in Pathogenesis and Treatment), Madison, Wisconsin, June 8-12, 1980, pp. 275-282.
10. Canalis, E., Peck, W.A., and Raisz, L.G., An autologous growth factor which stimulates DNA and collagen synthesis in cultured fetal rat calvaria, Science 210: 1021 (1980).
11. Howard, G.A., Bottemiller, B.L., Turner, R.T., Rader, J.I., and Baylink, D.J., Parathyroid hormone stimulates bone formation and resorption in organ culture: evidence for a coupling mechanism, Proc. Natl. Acad. Sci. USA 78: 3204 (1981).
12. Canalis, E., and Raisz, L.G., Effect of fibroblast growth factor on cultured fetal rat calvaria, Metabolism, Clinical and Experimental 29: 108 (1980).
13. Canalis, E., and Raisz, L.G., Effect of epidermal growth factor on bone formation in vitro, Endocrinol. 104: 862 (1979).
14. Canalis, E., and Raisz, L.G., Effect of multiplication-stimulating activity on DNA and protein synthesis in cultured fetal rat calvaria, Calcif. Tiss. Internat. 29: 33 (1979).
15. Van Wyk, J.J., and Underwood, L.E., in "Biochemical Actions of Hormones," G. Litwack, ed., Academic Press, New York (1978).
16. Jones, K.L., and Addison, J., Pituitary fibroblast growth factor as a stimulator of growth in cultured rabbit articular chondrocytes, Endocrinol. 97: 359 (1975).
17. Gospodarowicz, D., and Mescher, A.L., A comparison of the responses of cultured myoblasts and chondrocytes to fibroblast and epidermal growth factors,J. Cellular Physiol. 93: 117 (1977).

18. Burks, J.K., and Peck, W.A., Bone cells: a serum-free medium supports proliferation in primary culture, Science 199: 542 (1978).
19. Rifas, L., Uitto, J., Memoli, V.A., Kuettner, K.E., Henry, R.W., and Peck, W.A., The selective emergence of differentiated chondrocytes during serum-free culture of cells derived from fetal rat calvaria, J. Cell. Biol., in press.
20. Dulak, N.C., and Temin, H.M., A partially purified polypeptide fraction from rat liver cell conditioned medium with multiplication-stimulating activity for embryo fibroblasts, J. Cell. Physiol. 81: 153 (1973).
21. Dulak, N.C., and Temin, H.M., Multiplication-stimulating activity for chicken embryo fibroblasts from rat liver cell conditioned medium: a family of small polypeptides, J. Cell. Physiol. 81: 161 (1973).

ROLE OF MONOCYTES IN BONE RESORPTION

Gregory R. Mundy

University of Texas Health Science Center
7703 Floyd Curl Drive
San Antonio, TX 78284

ROLE OF MONOCYTES IN THE PROCESS OF BONE RESORPTION

Bone remodeling occurs in Haversian systems and on endosteal bone surfaces throughout life. The classic or traditional concept of bone remodeling holds that the initial event in bone turnover is osteoclastic bone resorption. Osteoclastic bone resorption causes degradation of the bone matrix and release of bone mineral and the formation of resorption bays or Howship's lacunae. This phase of osteoclastic bone resorption is followed by a phase of bone formation by osteoblasts. The attraction of osteoblasts to the site of the resorption defect and the activation of the osteoblasts to lay down new bone leads to repair of the resorption bay. Although this coupling of bone formation to bone resorption occurs under physiological and most pathological circumstances, the mechanisms which are responsible for linking bone formation to bone resorption are unknown. Recently some workers have described a putative coupling factor found in bone which leads to increased bone formation (Howard et al., 1980). We have found a chemotactic factor released by resorbing bone which causes unidirectional migration of cells with the characteristics of osteoblasts (Mundy et al., 1980). These factors could explain the coupling or linkage which exists between bone resorption and bone formation.

The initial cause of osteoclast activation during physiological bone turnover is not understood. The mechanisms which have been postulated are: a) stress or trauma, as suggested by Frost (1964), b) local signals released by cells in the bone marrow microenvironment which activate osteoclasts, such as osteoclast activating factor or prostaglandins (Mundy and Yoneda, 1981), c) systemic hormones which increase osteoclastic bone resorption such as PTH or 1,25-

dihydroxyvitamin D, and d) changes in osteoblast activity due to alterations in shape as suggested by Boyde and co-workers (Jones et al., 1978), or release by osteoblasts of a factor which stimulates osteoclasts, as suggested recently by Martin and Rodan (1981).

Monocytes are frequently found at bone resorbing surfaces. Since they are normal constituents of the bone marrow cavity, they are present in the cell population which lies adjacent to bone resorbing surfaces during normal bone remodeling. They are also present in increased numbers in conditions which are associated with excessive bone resorption such as metastatic tumors, rheumatoid arthritis and periodontal disease. There is increasing evidence that these cells are not simply innocent bystanders, but rather are critically involved in the process of bone resorption. In this review, I will attempt to summarize the evidence which supports the concept that the monocyte is a key cell in the process of bone resorption.

POTENTIAL ROLE OF MONOCYTES IN BONE RESORPTION

There are a number of ways in which monocytes could influence bone resorption *in vivo*. For each of these there is experimental evidence from *in vitro* studies. However the *in vivo* evidence is still circumstantial since it is difficult to show that the function of an individual cell or cell population which has been demonstrated *in vitro* also occurs *in vitro*. It is always possible that other cells could be responsible for any activity or function that is observed in *in vivo* experiments. Nevertheless it seems likely that monocytes are important to the process of bone resorption. The ways in which monocytes could be involved in bone resorption are:

1. Monocytes may be precursors for osteoclasts. There is strong circumstantial evidence that a circulating mononuclear cell, probably a monocyte, is the precursor cell for the osteoclast. Walker showed in osteopetrotic mice that the defect could be cured by allowing normal circulating mononuclear cells access to the marrow compartment either by inoculation or by parabiosis (Walker, 1972; Walker, 1975a; Walker, 1975b). Ash et al., (1980a,b) showed that macrophages were responsible for the development of the marrow cavity in the osteopetrotic mice by using donor cells with characteristic large lysosomal markers. Others had shown that osteoclasts or their precursors are of hematogeneous origin, probably arising from circulating mononuclear cells, and are formed by fusion rather than nuclear division (Kahn and Simmons, 1975; Fischman and Hay, 1962; Jee and Nolan, 1963; Gothlin and Ericsson; 1973; Buring, 1975). It is possible that there is only a subset of circulating cells which are capable of forming osteoclasts. Monocytes which appear identical by morphologic criteria at the light microscopic level have been shown to have different functional capabilities (Roubin and Zolla-

Pazner, 1979; Ciancoli and Snyderman, 1981). To date, no one has been able to culture monocytes and observe them fuse to form osteoclasts in vitro, although it is possible for monocytes to form multi-nucleated cells in culture. Presumably the in vitro systems currently available lack the appropriate differentiating factors or helper cells which are necessary to accomplish this transformation.

2. Monocytes may directly resorb bone. Monocytes are capable of resorbing bone directly in vitro. This has been shown by Mundy et al. (1977) using fetal rat long bones previously devitalized to remove endogenous bone cells and by Kahn et al. (1978) who used peritoneal macrophages and bone chips. Neither of these groups has been able to show a hormonal response of the cells. Minkin et al. (1977) found a slight increase in cyclic AMP content in elicited peritoneal macrophages in response to parathyroid hormone.

3. Monocytes may assist osteoclasts in the process of bone resorption. Heersche has postulated that monocytes or mononucleated cells may play a helpful role with the osteoclasts during the process of bone resorption (Heersche, 1978). The osteoclast does not phagocytose the bone matrix. Heersche has suggested that the osteoclasts may be responsible primarily for releasing mineral from bone and that mononucleated cells, possibly macrophages, may be responsible for degrading further the proteinaceous bone matrix.

4. Monocytes are helper cells to the activated lymphocyte during the process of release of OAF. Recently we have found that prostaglandins are necessary for OAF production by activated lymphocytes (Yoneda and Mundy, 1979a,b). In the presence of indomethacin inhibitors, activated leukocytes consisting of lymphocytes and monocytes do not produce OAF. The cell source of origin of OAF is the lymphocyte and the cell source of the prostaglandins necessary for OAF release is the monocyte. Experiments in which monocytes are depleted from a leukocyte population by successive cycles of adherence to plastic surfaces cause decreased OAF production which can be restored by the addition of monocyte conditioned media, monocytes, or exogenous prostaglandins (Yoneda and Mundy, 1979b). This effect of prostaglandins to permit the lymphocyte to release OAF is mediated by cyclic AMP and can be replaced by agents which increase lymphocyte cyclic AMP content such as isoproterenol, dibutyryl cyclic AMP or isobutyl methyl xanthine (IBMX) (Yoneda and Mundy, 1981).

5. Monocytes may regulate adjacent osteoclastic activity by producing prostaglandins. Monocytes are capable of producing large amounts of prostaglandins in response to appropriate stimuli (Bray et al., 1974; Hines et al., 1977; Dominguez and Mundy, 1980). Prostaglandins are powerful bone resorbing factors. In experiments we have performed in which we have co-cultured peripheral blood monocytes with fetal rat long bones, we have found that the monocytes

stimulate bone resorption, that this bone resorption is mediated by prostaglandins and can be inhibited by adding indomethacin and other drugs which block prostaglandin synthesis to the cultures (Dominguez and Mundy, 1980). It is possible that this is a mechanism by which monocytes may control osteoclast activity at endosteal bone surfaces.

6. Monocytes produce a Mononuclear Cell Factor (MCF) or factors which cause synovial cells and gingival fibroblasts to release prostaglandins and collagenase (Dayer et al., 1976; 1977a,b). Release of this protein is stimulated by activated lymphocytes (Dayer et al., 1979), aggregated IgG and Fc fragments (Dayer et al., 1980a) and Types II and III collagen (Dayer et al., 1980b). This complicated cell-cell interaction between monocytes and synovial cells may cause osteoclastic bone resorption via prostaglandin production by synovial cells or collagen degradation due to collagenase release from these cells.

CHEMOTAXIS OF MONOCYTES BY FACTORS DERIVED FROM BASE

If monocytes are key cells in the process of bone resorption and bone remodeling, then one could postulate that there should be some mechanism of recruitment of circulating mononuclear cells to endosteal bone surfaces. Recently we and others have described factors which are produced by resorbed or remodeling bone which are chemotactic for monocytes (Mundy et al., 1978; Minkin et al., 1981). These bone derived factors cause the unidirectional migration of monocytes in Boyden chemotactic chambers *in vitro*. In these experiments, circulating mononuclear cells are incubated in the upper compartment of a Boyden chamber. In the lower compartment is placed media which has been harvested from resorbing bone cultures. When bones are stimulated to resorb, they release factors which cause unidirectional migration of monocytes. These chemotactic factors which are generated by resorbing bones appear independent of the mechanism of bone resorption. The more the bone is resorbed, the more chemotactic factor that is generated. The nature of this chemotactic factor is unknown, but it appears to be macromolecular. Similar chemotactic factors are generated from resorbing bone to cause chemotaxis of tumor cells (Orr et al., 1978; Orr et al., 1980).

Some products of the bone matrix may be chemotactic for monocytes. Collagen and fragments of collagen are chemotactic for monocytes (Postlewaite and Kang, 1976). The bone matrix is composed of more than 90% Type I collagen which is degraded and released as fragments during the process of bone resorption and bone remodeling. Another prominent protein component of bone is the vitamin K-dependent protein osteocalcin, which contains gamma-carboxy glutamic acid moities, and which is also chemotactic for monocytes. The relationship of these chemotactic factors to each other is not known at present.

Recently we have found another chemotactic factor for monocytes which could be important for recruiting these cells to bone resorbing surfaces during bone metastasis. Cultured tumor cells produce a soluble chemotactic factor for elicited mouse peritoneal macrophages and circulating human mononuclear cells. Monocytes make up an important component of the heterogeneous cell population which is present in tumors which metastasize to bone. The role they play in the destruction of bone which occurs adjacent to these tumor deposits is unknown, but for reasons already explained could be substantial. They may also play an important role in the host-immune response to the tumor. Clearly factors produced by tumor cells which influence monocyte migration and function could be very important in tumor cell biology.

In summary, there are many ways in which monocytes could be influential in controlling or regulating the process of bone resorption. How important each of these individual functions is, or how these functions interact and are regulated, is not known at the present time. More research will hopefully provide some answers to these questions. I believe that a clear understanding of the cell biology of the process of bone resorption is necessary to understand the pathophysiology of bone loss associated with a variety of diseases which cause bone loss, including common metabolic bone diseases such as osteoporosis, and to devise therapeutic programs to prevent or inhibit the changes in bone cell biology which occur with advancing age.

REFERENCES

Ash, P., Loutit, J.F., and Townsend, K.M.S., 1980a, Giant lysosomes, a cytoplasmic marker in osteoclasts of beige mice, J. Pathol., 130:237.

Ash, P., Loutit, J.F., and Townsend, K.M.S., 1980b, Osteoclasts are derived from haemopoietic stem cells, Nature, 283:669.

Bray, M.A., Gordon, D., and Morley, J., 1974, Proceedings: Role of prostaglandins in reactions of cellular immunity, Br. J. Pharmacol., 52:453P.

Buring, K., 1975, On the origin of cells in heterotopic bone formation, Clin. Orthopaed. Rel. Res., 110:293.

Ciancoli, G.J., and Snyderman, R., 1981, Monocytes responsiveness to chemotactic stimuli is a property of a subpopulation of cells that can respond to multiple chemoattractants, J. Clin. Invest., 67:60.

Dayer, J.M., Krane, S.M., Russell, R.G.G., and Robinson, D.R., 1976, Production of collagenase and prostaglandins by isolated adherent rheumatoid synovial cells, Proc. Natl. Acad. Sci. USA, 73:945.

Dayer, J.M., Robinson, D.R., and Krane, S.M., 1977a, Prostaglandin production by rheumatoid synovial cells has stopped stimula-

tion of myofactor from human mononuclear cell, J. Exp. Med., 145:1399.
Dayer, J.M., Russell, R.G.G., and Krane, S.M., 1977b, Collagenase production by rheumatoid synovial cells: Stimulation by a human lymphocyte factor, Science, 195:181.
Dayer, J.M., Breard, J., Chess, L., and Krane, S.M., 1979, Participation of monocyte-macrophages and lymphocytes in the production of a factor which stimulates collagenase and prostaglandin release by rheumatoid synovial cells, J. Clin. Invest., 64:1386.
Dayer, J.M., Passwell, J.H., Schneeberger, E.E., and Krane, S.M., 1980a, Interactions among rheumatoid synovial cells and monocyte-macrophages: Production of collagenase-stimulating factor by human monocytes exposed to conconavalin A or immunoglobulin Fc fragments, J. Immunol., 124:1712.
Dayer, J.M., Trentham, D.E., David, J.R., and Krane, S.M., 1980b, Collagens stimulate production of mononuclear cell factor (MCF) and prostaglandins (PGE_2) by blood mononuclear cells, Clin. Res., 28:551A.
Dominguez, J.H., and Mundy, G.R., 1980, Monocytes mediate osteoclastic bone resorption by prostaglandin production, Calcif. Tiss. Int., 31:29.
Fischman, D.A., and Hay, E.D., 1962, Origin of osteoclasts from mononuclear leukocytes in regenerating newt limbs, Anat. Rec., 143:329.
Frost, H.M., 1964, Dynamics of bone remodeling, in: "Bone Biodynamics," H.M. Frost, ed., Little Brown and Company, Boston.
Gothlin, G., and Ericsson, J.L.E., 1973, On the histogenesis of the cells in fracture callus. Electron microscopic autoradiographic observations in parabiotic rats and studies on labeled monocytes, Virchows Arch. B. (Cell Pathology), 12:318.
Heersche, J.N.M., 1978, Mechanisms of osteoclast bone resorption. A new hypothesis, Calcif. Tiss. Res., 26:81.
Hines, J.L., Bonney, R.J., Pelus, L., Dahlgren, M.E., Sadowski, S.T., Kuehl, F.A., and Davies, P., 1977, Macrophages synthesize and release prostaglandins in response to inflammatory stimuli, Nature, 269:149.
Howard, G.A., Bottemiller, B.L., and Baylink, D.J., 1980, Evidence for the coupling of bone formation to bone resorption in vitro, Metab. Bone Dis. Rel. Res., 2:131.
Jee, W.S.S., and Nolan, P.D., 1963, Origin of osteoclasts from the fusion of phagocytes, Nature, 200:225.
Jones, S.J., and Boyde, A., 1978, Scanning electron microscopy of bone cells in culture, in: "Endocrinology of Calcium Metabolism," D.H. Copp and R.V. Talmage, eds., Excerpta Medica, Amsterdam, pp. 97-104.
Kahn, A.J., and Simmons, D.J., 1975, Investigation of cell lineage in bone using a chimera of chick and quail embryonic tissue, Nature, 258:325.
Kahn, A.J., Stewart, C.C., and Teitelbaum, S.L., 1978, Contact-

mediated bone resorption by human monocytes in vitro, Science, 199:988.

Martin, T.J., and Rodan, G.A., 1981, Personal communication.

Minkin, C., Blackman, L., Newbrey, J., Prokress, S., Posek, R., and Walling, M., 1977, Effects of parathyroid hormone and calcitonin on adenylate cyclase in murine mononuclear phagocytes, Biochem. Biophys. Res. Commun., 76:875.

Minkin, C., Posek, R., and Newbrey, J., 1981, Mononuclear phagocytes and bone resorption: Identification and preliminary characterization of a bone derived macrophage chemotactic factor, Metab. Bone Dis. Rel. Res., 2:363.

Mundy, G.R., Altman, A.J., Gondek, M.D., and Bandelin, J.G., 1977, Direct resorption of bone by human monocytes, Science, 196: 1109.

Mundy, G.R., Varani, J., Orr, W., Gondek, M.D., and Ward, P.A., 1978, Resorbing bone is chemotactic for monocytes, Nature (London), 275:132.

Mundy, G.R., DeMartino, S., and Rowe, D.W., 1980, Collagen and collagen fragments are chemotactic for tumor cells, Clin. Res., 28:526A.

Mundy, G.R., and Yoneda, T., 1981, Release of the lymphokine osteoclast activating factor requires cyclic AMP accumulation, Calcif. Tiss. Int., in press.

Orr, W., Varani, J., and Ward, P.A., 1978, Characteristics of the chemotactic response of neoplastic cells to a factor derived from the fifth component of complement, Am. J. Pathol., 93: 405.

Orr, F.W., Varani, J., Gondek, M.D., Ward, P.A., and Mundy, G.R., 1980, Partial characterization of a bone derived chemotactic factor for tumor cells, Am. J. Pathol., 99:43.

Postlewaite, A.E., and Kang, A.H., 1976, Collagen - and collagen peptide-induced chemotaxis of human blood monocytes, J. Exp. Med., 143:1299.

Roubin, R., and Zolla-Pazner, S., 1979, Markers of macrophage heterogeneity. I. Studies of macrophages from various organs of normal mice, Eur. J. Immunol., 9:972.

Walker, D.G., 1972, Congenital osteopetrosis in mice cured by parabiotic union with normal siblings, Endocrinology, 91:916.

Walker, D.G., 1975a, Bone resorption restored in osteopetrotic mice by transplants of normal bone marrow and spleen cells, Science, 190:784.

Walker, D.G., 1975b, Spleen cells transient osteopetrosis in mice, Science, 190:786.

Yoneda, T., and Mundy, G.R., 1979a, Prostaglandins are necessary for osteoclast activating factor (OAF) production by activated peripheral blood leukocytes, J. Exp. Med., 149:279.

Yoneda, T., and Mundy, G.R., 1979b, Monocytes regulate osteoclast activating factor production by releasing prostaglandins, J. Exp. Med., 150:338.

Yoneda, T., and Mundy, G.R., 1981, Release of the lymphokine osteoclast activating factor requires cyclic AMP accumulation, Calcif. Tiss. Int., in press.

COUPLING FACTOR

David Baylink[1], John Farley[1], Guy Howard[2], Rolf Drivdahl[3], Ed Puzas[4], Takeshi Masuda[5], Joel Ivey[2], Helen Gruber[6]

[1]Pettis Memorial VA Hospital and Loma Linda University Loma Linda, CA
[2]American Lake VA Hospital, Tacoma WA and University of Washington, Seattle, WA
[3]Evergreen St. College, Olympia, WA
[4]Department of Orhtopedics, University of Rochester Rochester, NY
[5]Department of Orthopedics, Hokkaido University Hospital, Sapporo, Japan
[6]Division of Nephrology, University of Southern California, Los Angeles, CA

Several years ago we intiated studies to clarify the problem of osteoporosis. On the basis of historical prospective, we reasoned that a disease of an organ is always attributable to inadequate regulation. That regulatory dysfunction may, in turn, be due to an overwhelmed regulatory mechanism, or to a faulty regulatory mechanism. Thus, inasmuch as osteoporosis is a disease of too little bone, we sought to characterize the regulation of bone volume.

One of the first clues to understanding the regulation of bone volume was the demonstration by Harris and Heaney that bone formation and bone resorption are correlated (i.e., coupled) in humans (1). This coupling implies that as bone resorption goes up or down, for whatever reason, bone formation will change in a corresponding direction. Theoretically, the correlation could also apply when the initial change is in bone formation. We felt that understanding this relationship was essential to understanding bone volume regulation, and for this reason, we set out to develop a rat model of coupling in vivo. We knew that PTH stimulated bone resorption but also inhibited bone formation, at least acutely, Nonetheless, we used PTH to produce an increase in bone resorption; however, we studied the chronic rather than the acute affects of the hormone administration. Thus, rats treated with PTH, 60 units

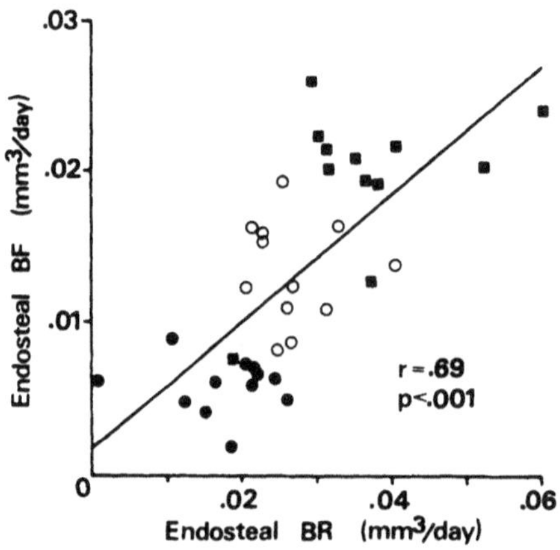

Fig. 1. Relationship between endosteal bone resorption and endosteal bone formation in data pooled from control rats and rats treated with two different doses of PTE (15 and 30 units/day) for 10 days. Each point is from an individual rat.

TABLE 1. Effects of PTE Treatment, 60 U/day for 10 Days on Serum Ca and Endosteal Bone Formation and Resorption

	Control	PTE-treated	P Value
Serum Ca, mg/dl	10.6 ±1.4[a]	10.8 ± 0.9	NS
Bone Resorption Rate, $mm^3/d \times 10^4$	175 ± 71	368 ± 109	<.001
Bone Formation Rate, $mm^3/d \times 10^4$	59 ± 18	198 ± 51	<.001

[a]Mean ± S.D.

per day for 10 days, exhibited the expected increase in bone resorption, and this, to our delight, was attended by a highly significant increase in bone formation (Table 1). Additionally, when different doses of PTH were administered to different groups of rats, the pooled data revealed a correlation between bone formation and bone resorption at the tibial endosteum (Fig. 1) (2). Thus, we had confirmed and extended the work of Harris and Heaney by showing that in a longitudinal study an increase in bone resorption was attended by an increase in bone formation.

The next step was to determine why and how the chronic administration of PTH, which was known to acutely inhibit bone formation, could stimulate bone formation. To determine whether this paradoxical increase in bone formation was peculiar to PTH, we tested another bone resorber, a high dose of vitamin D. We found that, like PTH, chronic administration of vitamin D increased bone resorption and that this increase in bone resorption was attended by an increase in bone formation (2). Thus, the increase in bone formation appeared to be a specific response to the increase in resorption, rather than to the nature of the bone resorber used.

This observation suggested that the coupled increase in bone formation was an intrinsic counterregulatory mechanism in bone. The fact that we could find no correlation between serum PTH, $1,25\text{-}(OH)_2D_3$, calcium, phosphorus, or magnesium and the coupled increase in bone formation argued against systemic regulation by these effectors (3). Additionally, the serum production of $^3H\text{-}24,25\text{-}(OH)_2D_3$ was not increased in our PTH-treated rats (4). This was considered pertinent because experimental evidence suggested that this metabolite of vitamin D could stimulate bone formation *in vitro* (5).

Together these data favored a local coupling mechanism that was inherent in bone rather than a sytemically mediated coupling mechanism. If this were true, we reasoned that it should be possible to demonstrate coupling *in vitro*. To test this possibility, it was necessary to develop an *in vitro* bone organ culture model in which both bone resorption and bone formation were occurring under basal conditions. We also wished to use tissue culture medium without serum to simplify data interpretation in terms of the causes of the changes in bone formation. These prerequisites were met by an embryonic chick long bone culture system employing eight-day-old chick long bones and BGJ_b (Fitton Jackson modified, GIBCO) medium without added protein (Fig. 2)(6). As can be seen in Figure 2, both bone formation and resorption were evident during a 12 day culture period under basal conditions. When PTH was added for the first 24 hours of the culture to induce bone resorption, there was a prolonged increase in bone resorption beginning a few hours after addition of the hormone and continuing until the end of the culture period. This increase in bone

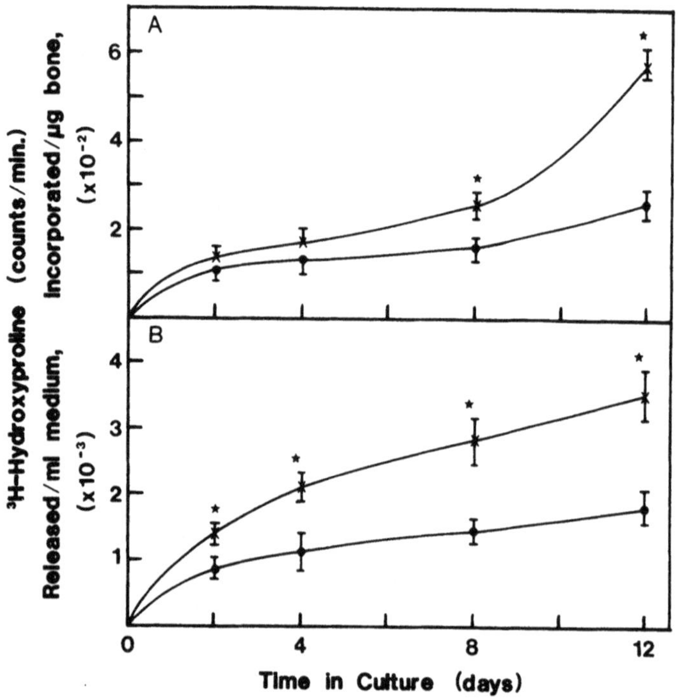

Fig. 2. In vitro bone metabolism over 12 days. The values obtained from the 8-day embryonic chick bones cultured in modified BGJ_b medium without added PTE (controls) are shown by the closed circles and the PTE-treated bones by the (x). The medium was changed each 2 days. PTE (10^{-12} M) was included in the test medium for the initial 24 hours of the experiment only. Each point represents the mean ± S.D.; N=6-8 bones; * = P <.001 by Student's t test. Panel A shows data for bone formation, and panel B shows data for bone resorption. ^{3}H-OH-pro released was summed per ml of medium over the days in culture for the data in panel B. The dry weights of the bone shafts at zero time were 100-200 µg, and increased to 600-700 µg by the end of the 12 day incubation.

TABLE 2. Effect of Dialyzed Conditioned Medium on Bone in Organ Culture[1]

	Tibial shaft	
	Dry wt, μg	^{3}H-OH-pro, cpm/ μg
Control medium	519 ± 74	126 ± 31
Conditioned medium, dialyzed		
Experiment 1	693 ± 66	193 ± 26
Experiment 2	742 ± 87	221 ± 56
Experiment 3	701 ± 91	182 ± 32

[1] ^{3}H-pro was added to the medium for the last 24 h of incubation.

resorption was attended by a similar prolonged increase in bone formation (Fig. 2). Not shown is the acute, significant inhibition of bone formation that occurred at approximately 16 hours, but dissipated after about 24 hours (6). As an alternative to our interpretation that these data represent coupling *in vivo*, one might argue that the removal of PTH after the first 24 hours exposure was ineffective, and that the bones were continuously exposed to PTH. Since the concentration of PTH used to stimulate bone resorption was only 10^{-12} M, a level too low to measure by radioimmunoassay, we cannot exclude the possibility of continuous exposure to PTH. However, the fact remains that PTH acutely (which presumably reflects its primary action) inhibits bone formation, a finding confirmed in this work (6).

We interpret these data to strongly suggest that coupling occurs *in vitro*. If so, one is forced to conclude that the coupling of bone formation to bone resorption is a mechanism which is intrinsic to bone. This coupling mechanism tends to oppose the resorptive effect of PTH and thus tends to conserve bone mass, and accordingly, we feel that coupling could be a control mechanism designed to regulate bone volume.

Having obtained this strong experimental evidence that coupling is an inherent activity of bone, our obvious next question was: How is this coupling mediated? One likely possibility was that the observed increase in bone resorption was releasing a coupling factor into bone water and thus perhaps into the medium. We tested this possibility, and the results (shown in Table 2) demonstrated that conditioned medium obtained from resorbing chick bone, when applied to fresh chick bone cultures at dilution of 1:20 (diluted with fresh BGJ_b medium), increased bone formation significantly.

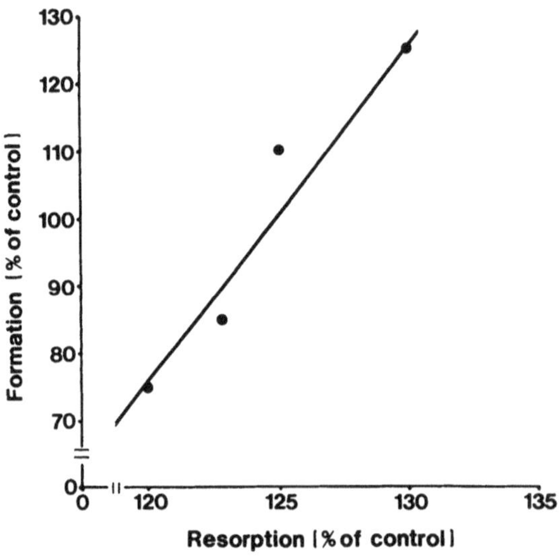

Fig 3. Relationship between bone formation and bone resorption. The data were obtained from the experiment shown in Fig 2. Included are only those points after the actue inhibition of formation. r=.96; P<.05; estimated by Student's t test.

Because these bones grew without added protein, one might argue that the protein concentration in the medium was increased by the process of cell death and/or resorption and that, instead of coupling, we had witnessed a nonspecific stimulation of bone formation caused by adding protein to this protein-free medium. This seems unlikely, because the protein concentration in our conditioned medium was only about 35 ng/ml, a concentration more suggestive of a specific growth stimulation(7).

The next question was: What is the source of this putative coupling factor? The answer to this question must satisfy the constraint that the amount of, or at least the response to, the putative coupling factor is proportional to the extent of bone resorption. Indeed, the proportionality between formation and resorption was evident not only in humans and in our rat and chick

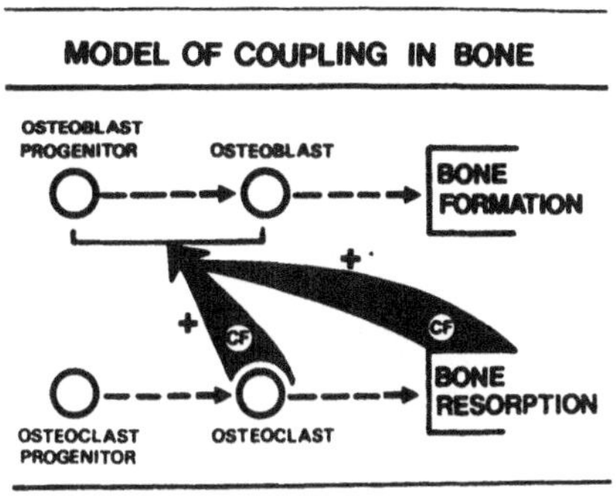

Fig 4. Theoretical model of coupling in bone. Two potential sources of coupling factor are illustrated (bone matrix and osteoclasts). See text for rationale.

models, but also in vitro in response to PTH treatment (Fig. 3.). A model illustrating two potential sources of the putative coupling factor is shown in Fig. 4. First, the osteoclast might produce coupling factor in proportion to its resorptive activity and thus satisfy the correlation between formation and resorption. Second, coupling factor might reside in bone and be released in proportion to the amount of bone resorbed. In the previous studies, we had developed a procedure to isolate osteoclasts (80% pure) which were viable in monolayer cultures for at least 7 days. Using such a preparation we examined osteoclast conditioned medium and aqueous extracts of osteoclasts and found no evidence of coupling factor activity as determined by the ^{3}H-TdR assay described below.

At this stage of our investigations, we realized that to purify and characterize our putative coupling factor in a reasonable length of time we would have to develop a bioassay for coupling factor activity which was much more rapid than the organ culture

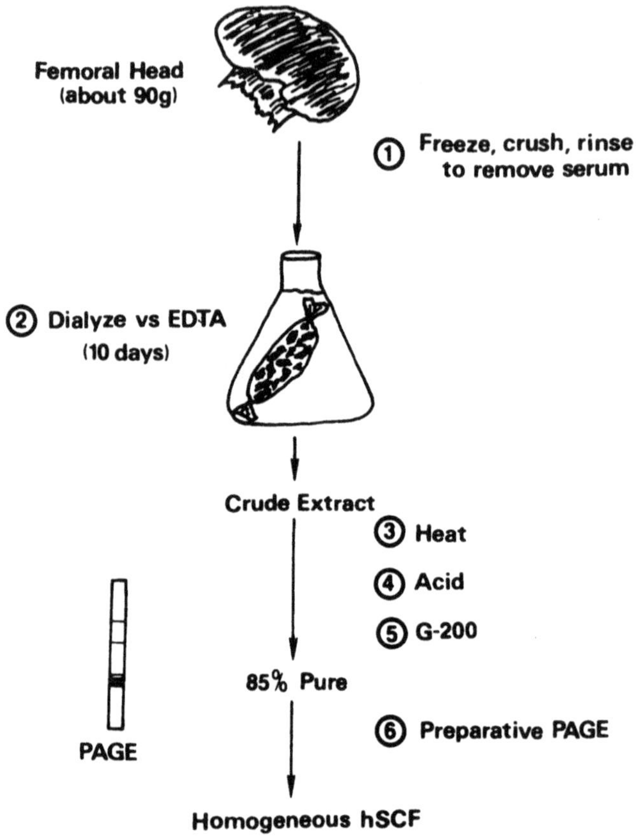

Fig 5. Purification schema of human skeletal coupling factor. See text for discussion.

assay. To solve this problem we developed an assay to measure the incorporation of tritiated thymidine (^{3}H-TdR) into isolated calvarial cells (8). This assay satisfied our requirement for speed and we have used it for the remainder of our work, periodically confirming the results obtained with the corresponding results from the organ culture assay. This thymidine incorporation assay was used in the experiments referenced above to evaluate whether osteoclasts might be the source of coupling factor. Despite our negative findings, we do not feel that these studies exclude the possibility that a growth factor is produced by osteoclasts. Our reasons for this latter position include the fact that our method for isolating osteoclasts only provides about 500,000 cells, and such a small number of cells might be insufficient to produce detectable amounts of growth factor.

Simultaneous studies examining the possibility that bone itself was the source of our putative coupling factor afforded positive results. Aqueous extracts of the shafts of embryonic chick bone tissue were found to contain a potent cell growth stimulator (9). These extracts also increased the growth of chick embryonic bone in vitro. Thus, the crude factor obtained from chick bone had effects identical to those of the factor in conditioned medium as tested by both assay systems. We have not yet, however, shown that the bone extract activity and the conditioned medium activity are the consequence of an identical factor.

Because no one would be surprised to find a growth factor in embryonic tissue (and this, of course, would include embryonic bone) and because we were primarily interested in skeletal coupling in adult humans,* our next undertaking was to determine if adult human bone contained a factor which was positive in our two assay systems. Crude extracts of human bone were prepared according to the schema shown in Fig. 5. Femoral heads obtained from patients operated on for osteoarthritis were washed to remove serum and cleaned of marrow tissue, and then frozen in liquid nitrogen and crushed into small particles to increase the surface area in an effort to increase the subsequent rate of extraction. After additional rinsing, the small bone particles were placed in a dialysis bag which had a 10,000 molecular weight cutoff. The dialysis bag was then suspended in a beaker containing a large volume of 10% EDTA. The extraction procedure was carried out at $4^{\circ}C$. After several days the retentate was dialyzed against phosphate buffer to remove the EDTA, and this preparation constituted our crude extract. Parenthetically, we should like to emphasize that because we use the ^3H-TdR incorporation assay to monitor purification, periodically throughout the purification procedure, we did cell counts to establish that the observed increase in thymidine incorporation was not the consequence of a change in thymidine pool size, or some other change which might result in a spurious conclusion regarding the cellular proliferation activity of this factor, Thus, various preparations of human skeletal coupling factor (hSCF) consistently increased cell number as well as the incorporation of ^3H-TdR into DNA.

The initial purification steps consisted of heat and acid precipitations, hSCF activity being resistant to both, and large amounts of nonspecific protein were removed from the crude extract by these maneuvers (10). Further purification was achieved by Sephadex G-200 column chromatography, followed by preparative polyacrylamide gel electrophoresis. The latter procedure provided gels containing one major band of protein which was hSCF and three minor bands which were evident when the gel was stained with coomassie blue. The major hSCF band was then excised from unstained gels to provide an apparently homogenous protein by the criteria of subsequent PAGE (overloaded to identify minor bands of impurities if present), isoelectric focusing and HPLC (10).

*Our interest in the more general topic of adult human coupling has only a peripheral bearing on these studies.

Subsequently, we determined some of the characteristics of this purified putative coupling factor (10). We found that putative coupling factor has a molecular weight of 83,000 (as determined by native polyacrylamide gel electrophoresis using gel concentrations ranging from 5% to 15%); that it is insensitive to heat

CELL SPECIFICITY OF hSCF

Cell Type	Effect on DNA Synthesis*	Sig.
Bone - calvarial	192 +/- 67%	p<.001
Bone - femoral	118 +/- 40%	p<.001
Cartilage - sternum	148 +/- 71%	p<.001
Skin	none	NS
Kidney	none	NS
Muscle	none	NS
Liver	none	NS

*Increase above control

Fig 6. Cell specificity of human skeletal coupling factor. Cells were prepared from 17 day embryonic chick tissue, plated at 250 cells/mm^2; cultured 48 hr in 1% FCS and then 24 hr in serum-free BGJ_b before addition of hSCR (6 μg/ml). All types of cells grew to comparable densities before addition of hSCR. ^{3}H-TdR incorporation into DNA was used to estimate effect on DNA synthesis. Values are given as mean increase (± S.D.) above control.

and extremes of pH; that it is inactivated by trypsin, but not by collagenase treatment and thus is a noncollagenous protein; and that it is not inactivated by reducing agents, at least not by 1% β-mercaptoethanol (10). A molecular weight of 83,000 is admittedly large for a growth factor, but as yet we have no evidence for smaller subunits under non-denaturing conditions.

An important aspect of the characterization of any growth factor is organ specificity. Our results on this issue are shown in Fig. 6. As can be seen, putative coupling factor acts exclusively on bone and cartilage cells. While our standard assay uses chick cells, we have examined the effects of human skeletal coupling factor on human bone cells and have found a stimulation of up to 1,000% in serum-free medium. Preliminary findings from our investigations into the source of this putative coupling factor indicate no such factor acting to increase thymidine incorporation in bone cells in extracts obtained from liver, kidney, or muscle tissue from the embryonic chick. The only other tissue that we have examined that appears to contain the factor which specifically stimulates bone and cartilage cell proliferation is cartilage, and this includes both sternal and articular cartilage.

I would now like to turn to the question of the physiological significance of this factor, and more specifically to the issue raised in the introduction, namely, whether this factor truly is involved in bone volume regulation. All of our evidence is consistent with this possibility, but we have no definitive proof that such a working hypothesis is indeed correct. Moreover, it would be difficult to prove this hypothesis since one cannot ablate the skeleton as one would do as a standard procedure to establish the function of a particular endocrine gland. On the other hand, there are several techniques which will allow us to approach this problem, and these are now being employed to further evaluate our hypothesis. Meanwhile, based on our evidence thus far we feel that our working hypothesis, that putative coupling factor acts on bone to promote cell self-renewal, is tenable and consistent with our data.

Turning back to the issue of osteoporosis and bone volume regulation, we have recently shown that when bone formation is plotted as a function of bone resorption in Paget's Disease, the slope is 1.06 (i.e., skeletal balance is unity regardless of the turnover rate)(11). In sharp contrast, the corresponding slope in postmenopausal osteoporosis is 0.46, with an intercept on the Y axis, such that patients with postmenopausal osteoporosis are in negative calcium balance for all turnover rates except those less than 200 mg/day. Moreover, the higher the turnover, the greater the negative calcium balance (11). Thus, there is perfect coupling in Paget's disease and poor coupling in postmenopausal osteoporosis.

Further evidence invoking a key role for poor coupling in postmenopausal osteoporosis is the finding that this disease is due to neither an increase in bone resorption above normal, nor to a decrease in bone formation below normal. Instead, bone formation and bone resorption are both within the normal range (12); they are abnormal in that they are not regulated to the extent that they are precisely equal as they are in normal young adults. Accordingly, further studies on the mechanism whereby coupling regulates bone volume may well help clarify the etiology of this important disease.

REFERENCES

1. W.H. Harris and R.P. Heany, Skeletal renewal and metabolic bone disease, New Engl. J. Med., 280:253 (1969).

2. D.J. Baylink and C.C. Liu, The regulation of endosteal bone volume, J. Periodontol., 50(4 spec. No.):43(1979).

3. D.J. Baylink, E.R. Morey, J.L. Ivey, and M.E. Stauffer, Vitamin D and bone, in: "Molecular Biology and Clinical Nutrition," A.W. Norman, ed., Marcel Dekker, Inc., New York (1980).

4. J.I. Rader, R.T. Turner, G.A. Howard, and D.J. Baylink, Effect of treatment with parathyroid extract on bone parameters and metabolism of ^{3}H-25-hydroxyvitamin D_3 in hypocalcemic thyroparathyroidectomized rats, Metab. Bone Dis. Rel. Res. 1:313 (1979).

5. A. Ornoy, D. Goodwin, D. Noff and S. Edelstein, 24,25-Dihydroxyvitamin D_3 is a metabolite of vitamin D_3 essential for bone formation, Nature 276:517 (1978).

6. G.A. Howard, B.L. Bottemiller, and D.J. Baylink, Evidence for the coupling of bone formation to bone resorption in vitro, Metab. Bone Dis. Rel. Res. 2:131 (1980).

7. G.A. Howard, B.L. Bottemiller, R.T. Turner, J.I. Rader, and D.J. Baylink, Parathyroid hormone stimulates bone formation and resorption in organ culture: Evidence for a coupling mechanism, Proc. Natl. Acad. Sci. USA 78(5):3204 (1981).

8. J.E. Puzas, R.H. Drivdahl, G.A. Howard, and D.J. Baylink, Endogenous inhibitor of bone cell proliferation, Proc. Soc. Exp. Biol. Med. 166:113 (1981).

9. R.H. Drivdahl, J.E. Puzas, G.A. Howard, and D.J. Baylink: Regulations of DNA synthesis in chick calvaria cells by factors from bone organ culture. Proc. Soc. Exp. Biol. Med., in press, (1981).

10. J.R. Farley and D.J. Baylink, Purification of a putative human skeletal coupling factor, in: "Transactions of the American Physicians," in press, (1981).

11. J.L. Ivey and D.J. Baylink, Postmenopausal osteoporosis: Proposed roles of defective coupling and estrogen deficiency, (editorial) Metab. Bone Dis. Rel. Res., 3:3 (1981).

12. H.E. Gruber, J.L. Ivey, C.H. Chestnut, and D.J. Baylink, unpublished.

GLUTAMINE: A NEW METABOLIC SUBSTRATE

R.M. Biltz, J.M. Letteri, E.D. Pellegrino, L. Pinkus

Department of Medicine, Nassau County Medical Center
East Meadow, New York, and The Catholic University of
America, Washington, D.C., and S.U.N.Y., Stony Brook, N.Y.

Glutamine serves important metabolic functions in a variety of tissues, but it has only recently been recognized as a new component of the metabolism of bone. Glutamine and glutamate are present as free amino acids in bone water at concentrations 2.5 and 40 times greater than their respective concentrations in plasma. The mediated transport of glutamine into calvaria occurs almost exclusively by Na^+-dependent system(s). Glutamine uptake is not inhibited by N-methyl-D-L-alanine or 2-(methylamino)-isobutyric acid which are inhibitors of the A system of transport.[2] Calvaria, when incubated *in vitro* degrade significant amounts of glutamine to ammonia, glutamate, other amino acids (alanine, aspartate, proline, ornithine) and CO_2. The purpose of this report is to further delineate several of these processes with a view to their possible physiological significances.

METHODS AND PROCEDURES

Calvaria were obtained from newborn rats and incubated at 37° in Erlenmeyer flasks (25 ml) containing 2 ml of basal salt solution (BSS) consisting of 125 mM NaCl, 0.75 mM NaH_2PO_4, 1.2 mM KH_2PO_4, 5.4 mM KCL, 0.81 mM $MgSO_4$, 1.5 mM $CaCl_2$ and 22 mM $NaHCO_3$, pH 7.4. The gas phase was 5% CO_2 - 95% O_2. A gyratory water shaker bath was employed at 90 oscillations per minute. Glucose, glutamine and other compounds were added as indicated.

Metabolic studies were terminated by the addition of trichloroacetic acid. Bone and precipitated protein were removed by centrifugation and the medium was subsequently analyzed for lactic acid with lactic dehydrogenase and for ammonia and glutamate with glutamic dehydrogenase.[3]

Incubations performed to measure amino acid formation from glutamine were terminated by freezing and thawing three times at -70°. The soluble amino acids released into the medium were lyophilized, redissolved in 0.2 ml of 5% sulfosalicylic acid and separated on a Beckman 119 C Amino Acid Analyzer with a lithium citrate buffer system.

Phosphate-Dependent Glutaminase (PDG) Activity

Calvaria when incubated in a bicarbonate-buffered physiologic salt solution at 37°, converts glutamine to ammonia and glutamate in nearly equimolar amounts, suggesting that hydrolysis of the glutamine amide group is the initial step in its metabolism (Figure 1). Glutamine uptake and activity of PDG is dependent on the concentration of glutamine in the medium (Figure 2) with an apparent $K_{\frac{1}{2}}$ of 1.0-1.5 mM. This is similar to the apparent K_m^{gln}

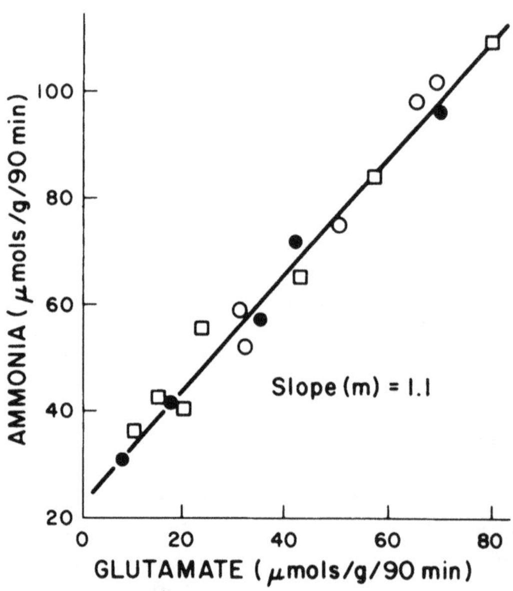

Figure 1. Stoichiometry of ammonia and glutamate formation in calvaria incubated in BSS at 37° with glutamine. Variations in pH (7.0-7.8), open squares; phosphate concentration (2.0-7.0 mM), open circles or glutamine concentration (0.5-10 mM), closed circles, although influencing the rate of the process, did not significantly affect the stoichiometry.

of 2.3 mM exhibited by PDG in bone homogenates.[1] The data indicate that soluble products of glutamine are in part released from the tissue. Ammonia production from calvaria increases containing up to 7.0 mM of inorganic phosphate. Phosphate activated PDG in homogenates with an apparent $K_{\frac{1}{2}}$ of 25 mM. Ammonia and glutamine formation increase about 5 fold between pH 7.0 and 7.8 and were, therefore, sensitive to changes in the extracellular pH. 6-Diazo-5-oxo-L-norleucine (DON) was a potent inhibitor of PDG in

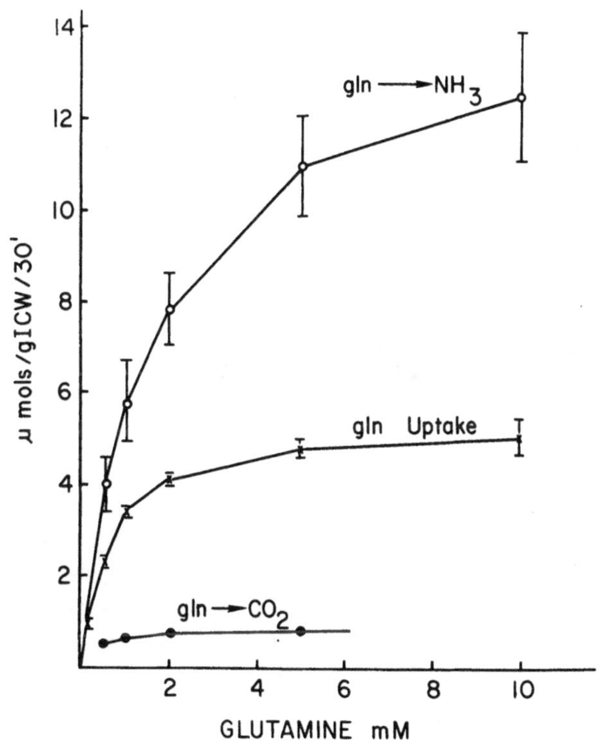

Figure 2. Dependence of Ammonia Production, $^{14}CO_2$ Production and Glutamine Uptake Upon Glutamine Concentration. Calvaria were incubated with 5.5 mM glucose plus the indicated concentration of [U-^{14}C] glutamine for a period of 30 minutes. Acid soluble products were extracted from the calvaria (glutamine uptake). Ammonia and $^{14}CO_2$ (trapped in hyamine) were measured in the medium.

homogenates and also severely imparied ammonia formation in intact calvaria. The rate of $^{14}CO_2$ formation from [U-^{14}C] glutamine was weak (Figure 2) indicating that relatively little of the glutamate formed was oxidized. DON treatment inhibited glutamine oxidation by >90%.

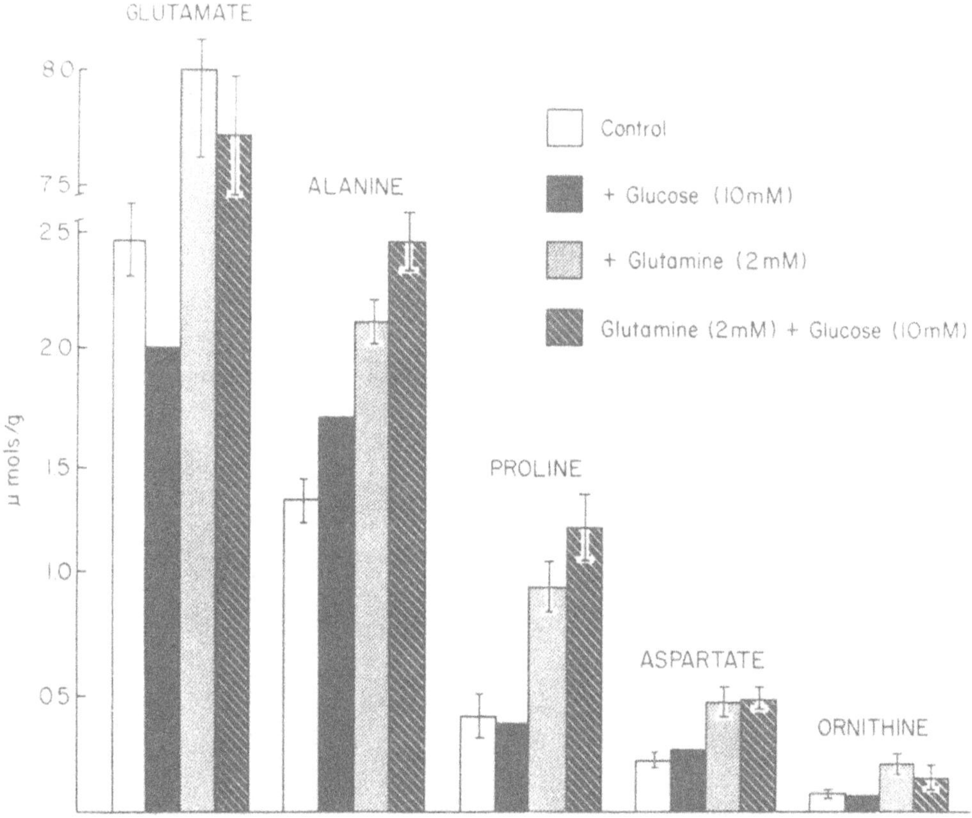

Figure 3. The formation of free amino acids in calvaria when incubated in 2 ml of BSS at 37°, pH 7.4, with the addition of glucose (5 mM) and/or glutamine (2 mM).

In separate studies not detailed here, the addition of glucose (5 mM) to the medium resulted in a 2 to 3 fold increase in lactic acid formation. The activated glycolytic process was associated with both an activated (20%) or deactivated (50%) rate of ammonia production in different experiments *in vitro*. Although glutamine itself did not give rise to lactic acid, increased (30%) or decreased (20%) lactate production from glucose was observed on the addition of glutamine (0.5 - 5 mM) to the medium. The data suggest that glycolysis, long regarded as the predominant metabolic process in bone may be influenced by glutamine metabolism.

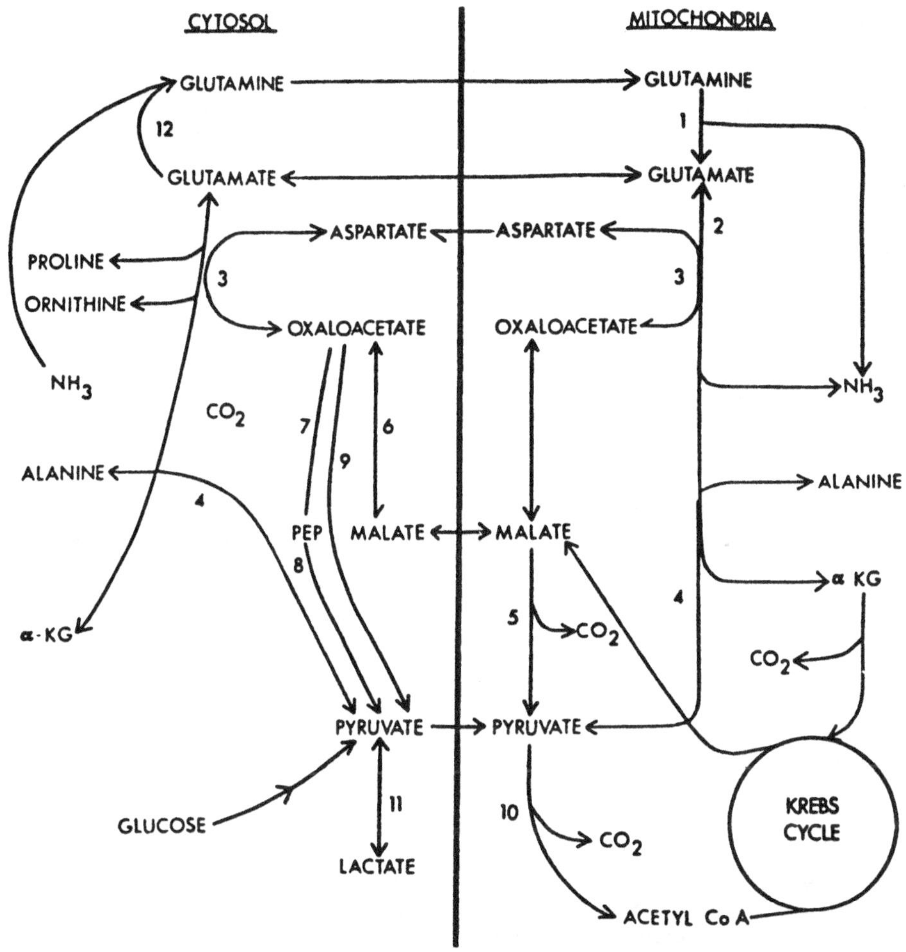

Figure 4. The metabolic fate of glutamine and its relation to glucose metabolism. Enzyme-catalyzed reactions are denoted by (1) phosphate-dependent glutaminase; (2) glutamate dehydrogenase; (3) aspartate aminotransferase; (4) alanine aminotransferase; (5) malic enzyme; (6) malate dehydrogenase; (7) phosphoenolpyruvate carboxykinase; (8) pyruvate kinase; (9) oxaloacetate decarboxylase; (10) pyruvate dehydrogenase; (11) lactic dehydrogenase and (12) glutamine synthetase. Available data indicates that enzymes 1,2, 3,4,6,10, and 11 are present in bone whereas enzyme 12 was not detected.

Amino Acid Formed From Glutamine In Vitro

When calvaria from newborn rats are incubated *in vitro*, glutamine gives rise to glutamate which may, in turn, be utilized for synthesis of other amino acids and proteins. Alanine and aspartate, for example, could be formed in the subsequent metabolism of glutamate via transamination with pyruvate and oxaloacetate (Figure 3). Glutamine may also give rise to ornithine and proline by known metabolic pathways, some of which have been demonstrated in cartilage.[4] Significant increases in alanine, aspartate, ornithine and prline in calvaria incubated with glutamine were noted (Figure 4).

DISCUSSION

Glutamine is transported into bone cells and degraded to ammonia and glutamate by a partcle-bound phosphate-dependent glutaminase (known to be a mitochondrial enzyme in other tissues). Glutamate (formed from glutamine) may subsequently be utilized for the biosynthesis of other amino acids and protein or for the synthesis of tricarboxylic acid cycle intermediates and as a fuel for respiration. The metabolic fate of ammonia, formed in bone from the hydrolysis of glutamine, is more conjectural. It may be rapidly released to the blood. Changing ammonia concentrations within the mitochondria (the site of enzyme-catalyzed deamidation of glutamine and glutamate dehydrogenase) may influence ionic movements within these organelles. Consequently, ammonia production from glutamine in conjunction with the regulatory mechanisms could contribute significantly to the maintenance of a pH gradient, calcium mobilization and other specialized functions of the tissue.

REFERENCES

1. Biltz, R.M., Letteri, J.M., Pellegrino, E.D., Palekar, A., and Pinkus, L.M. Mineral and Electrolyte Metabolism (in press).
2. Kilberg, M.S., Handlogten, M.E., and Christensen, H.N., Characteristics of an amino acid transport system in rat liver for glutamine, asparagine, histidine and closely related analogs, J. Biol. Chem., 255:4011 (1980).
3. Bergmeyer, H.U., in "Methods of Enzymatic Analysis," Acad. Press, New York (1965).
4. Smith, R.J., Reddi, A.H., and Phang, J.M., Changes in proline synthetic and degradative enzymes during matrix-induced cartilage and bone formation, Calcif. Tiss. Intl. 27:275, (1979).

EVOLUTION OF RENAL OSTEODYSTROPHY IN PATIENTS TREATED BY CONTINUOUS AMBULATORY PERITONEAL DIALYSIS

Y. El Shahat, C. Jacobs, B. Issad, J. Rottembourg and M. Legrain
Groupe Hospitalier Pitié-Salpétrière
83, Boulevard de l'Hôpital
75013 - PARIS (France)

INTRODUCTION

To remove the excess of phosphate and correct the deficit of calcium represent the most important goals to be achieved in uremic patients treated by maintenance dialysis methods in order to prevent the multiple complications related to hypersecretion of parathyroid hormone whose stimulation is enhanced by hypocalcemia and hyperphosphatemia (1,2). Despite a general agreement on this statement and ongoing progress in hemodialysis techniques and strategies, this aim remains by far not successfully reached in all patients treated by chronic hemodialysis, whose long survival is all too often complicated by severely disabling bone disease (3). The very principle on which the technique of Continuous Ambulatory Peritoneal Dialysis (CAPD) is based seemed likely to provide a more satisfying solution than hemodialysis for coping with the problem (4,5). A slow but continuous removal of phosphate (Pi) together with a simultaneous supply of calcium (Ca) through the peritoneal route, as well as the "steady" metabolic state resembling the one of a normal subject could prove as more efficient for maintaining a satisfactory calcium-phosphate balance than the "permanently unstable" situation which is the one of the patients treated with maintenance hemodialysis. This assumption depends however on the performances of the peritoneal membrane as regards to its transfer capacities of Ca and Pi. The efficacy of CAPD for the control of serum levels of Ca and Pi and the effect of the method on radiological and histological signs of renal osteodystrophy have been reported thus far only in limited series of patients treated for short periods of time. In the following study we report the clinical, radiological and biological results observed in a series of 40 patients who underwent CAPD as initial mode of treatment of their terminal renal failure over periods ranging between at least 7,5 months up to two years with a cumulative duration of treatment of 48,4 years.

PATIENTS AND METHODS

The study was conducted in 40 patients who commenced CAPD as first mode of therapy of end stage renal disease (ESRD) between August 1978 and December 1980 and who were maintained on that treatment for at least 6 months. There were 21 males and 19 females whose mean age was 64,0 ± 13,6 years (range 28-83 years). Their mean residual creatinine clearance at start of treatment was 4,9 ± 2,5 ml/mn (mean ± SD, range 2.2-7.4 ml/mn). Cause of renal failure was chronic glomerulonephritis in fourteen, chronic interstitial nephritis in twelve, diabetic nephropathy in nine, nephroangiosclerosis in four and remained undetermined in one. The cumulative duration of CAPD treatment was 580 patient-months with an average of 14,5 months per patient (range 7.5-33 months).

Peritoneal Dialysis Technique

CAPD was performed through an indwelling double-cuffed Tenckhoff catheter. The patients performed 4 exchanges per day (7 days a week) of two liters of dialysis fluid contained in plastic bags (Pharmacie Centrale des Hôpitaux, Paris). Composition of dialysis fluid was as follows (mMl/l) : Sodium 133 - Potassium 1 - Calcium 1,75 - Acetate 35 - Glucose 83 (15g/l) or 250 mMl (45g/l). Magnesium concentrations was 0,75 mMl/l between August 1978 and December 1980 and was brought down to 0,5 mMl/l thereafter. Patients exchanged routinely 3 bags of dialysate with the lower glucose concentration and one bag with the higher glucose content, per day.

The dietary prescriptions comprised a daily intake of 1-1,20 g/Kg Body Weight of protein. Quantities of fluid, sodium and potassium were advised according to hydration status, residual renal function and the volume of ultra-filtration that could be achieved. Food intake of calcium and phosphate was not strictly specified, but dietary histories taken from the patients at regular intervals were consistent with an average daily intake of at least 600 mg of calcium and about 800 mg of phosphate. At start of treatment 62 % of the patients were supplemented in aluminium gels (about 1000 mg of Al per day), 65 % in oral calcium (average dose 500 mg per day) and 72,5 % were given 50 µg/day of $25(OH)D_3$.

Biochemical Studies

Concentrations of electrolytes, urea, creatinine, protein, albumin, alkaline phosphatase, total Ca and Pi were determined by auto-analyzer (S.M.A.C. Technicon). Concentrations of magnesium (Mg) in serum and dialysate and of serum aluminium were measured by atomic absorption spectrophotometry. Serum Ca levels were corrected for protein concentration using the modified formula of Parfitt (6) where adjusted serum calcium (mMl/1) =

$$\frac{\text{Measured Serum Calcium (mMl/1)}}{0{,}6 + \dfrac{\text{Total Protein (g/1)}}{19{,}4}}$$

Peritoneal clearances were calculated according to the formula : $C(ml/m) = \frac{D}{P} \times \frac{VD}{t}$ where VD is the total peritoneal drainage volume in 24 hours (ml), and t = 1440 minutes, D and P the concentrations of solutes in the dialysate and serum. The blood sample was drawn usually about two hours after instillation of the first daily bag. The concentrations of solutes in the dialysate were measured in pooled samples of the four dialysate bags used on the day of investigation. Statistical evaluation of the data recorded over time was made using the paired-t-test, with a significance level at $p=0.05$.

Peritoneal mass-transfers of calcium, phosphate and magnesium were carried out in 8 patients (5 males, 3 females) whose age ranged between 44 and 79 years and whose time on CAPD ranged between 5 and 22 months. CAPD technique, dietary prescriptions and determination of serum and dialysate chemistries were made according to the methods described above. The pooled calcium, phosphate and magnesium contents of the four daily bags were measured in order to calculate an overall 24 hours peritoneal balance of these solutes. The PH of the dialysate effluent was brought down to 4,5 through addition of acetic-acid prior to determination of Ca concentration in order to avoid precipitation of calcium phosphate.

Mass-transfers of calcium, phosphate and magnesium were calculated according to the following formula :

$$\text{M.T.} = \left(\begin{matrix}\text{Solute Concentr.}\\ \text{in}\\ \text{Dialysate}\end{matrix} \times \begin{matrix}\text{Volume}\\ \text{Instilled}\\ \text{/24 h}\end{matrix}\right) - \left(\begin{matrix}\text{Solute Concentr.}\\ \text{in peritoneal}\\ \text{effluent}\end{matrix} \times \begin{matrix}\text{Volume}\\ \text{drained}\\ \text{/24 h}\end{matrix}\right)$$

Radiological Studies

Radiological signs of osteomalacia and hyperparathyroid bone disease were assessed in 20 patients for whom comparable skeletal X-Ray films were available at start of CAPD and twelve months thereafter. Bone films were scored by three of us and close attention was paid for detection of unquestionable signs of renal osteodystrophy, such as erosions of the middle phalanx of the second digit of the right hand, Looser zones in pubic rami, occurence or progression of calcifications of digital or pelvic arteries and evidence of asymptomatic rib fractures (7).

RESULTS

Clinical and radiological data

The actuarial survival rate in these 40 patients maintained for at least 6 months on CAPD was 92.2 % at 12 months, 67,4 % at 18 months and 60,8 % at two years. 10 patients died. Causes of death were septicemia in 2, cerebro-vascular accident in 3, cachexia in 1, myocardial infarction in 2, abandonment of treatment in 2. Seven patients had to be transferred to hemodialysis because of recurrent peritonitis in 2, malnutrition in 3, unsatisfactory peritoneal performances in 2.

No spontaneous or traumatic fracture was recorded clinically or on bone X-Ray films over the whole observation period. Bone-pain was claimed at start of treatment by 3 patients but was not mentioned anymore after 6 months of treatment. Backache was reported by 5% of patients at six months and 6% at one year after start of CAPD. Pruritus was claimed by only 5 % of patients at start of treatment, but by 17,5 % at 6 months and 23,5 % of those treated for one year. Frequency of pruritus decreased thereafter being reported by 10 % of patients who were alive on CAPD for 18 months.

Overt radiographic signs of osteomalacia (Looser zones) were present at start of CAPD treatment in 2 patients out of 20 for whom serial X-Ray surveys were analyzed. The radiographic aspect was found unchanged in these two patients 12 months after commencement of treatment. By that time, marked augmentation of pelvic bone radiolucency indicative of evolutive osteomalacia was noticed in one additional patient.

Signs of hyperparathyroid bone disease (as defined above) were evidenced at start of treatment in 7 patients : one year afterwards, radiographic alterations were quoted as stable in 5 patients, improved in 1, deteriorated in 1. Subperiostal erosions in the middle phalanges which were not visible on the initial bone films became apparent in 3 more patients. Some extension of digital vascular calcifications were visible in 3 patients.

Biological Results

No significant modification of the residual clearance of creatinine was recorded in the 34 patients who were followed-up for one year (Table 1). Whereas the peritoneal clearance of creatinine did not vary either during this period of time, peritoneal clearance of phosphate was found higher after 6 months of CAPD than at start of treatment and remained at a stable level thereafter. Whereas no correlation was found at start of CAPD between the peritoneal clearances of creatinine and phosphate, an increasingly positive relationship between these two parameters became apparent over the first 12

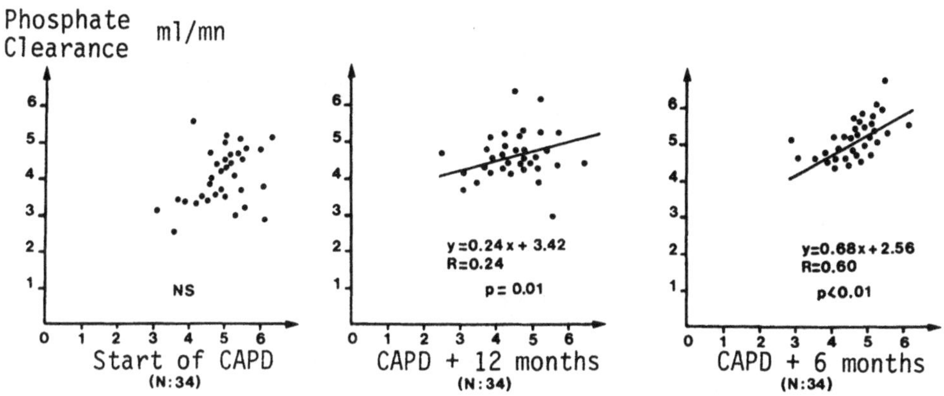

Fig. 1. Correlation between peritoneal clearances of phosphate and creatinine during the course of treatment in 34 patients treated by CAPD.

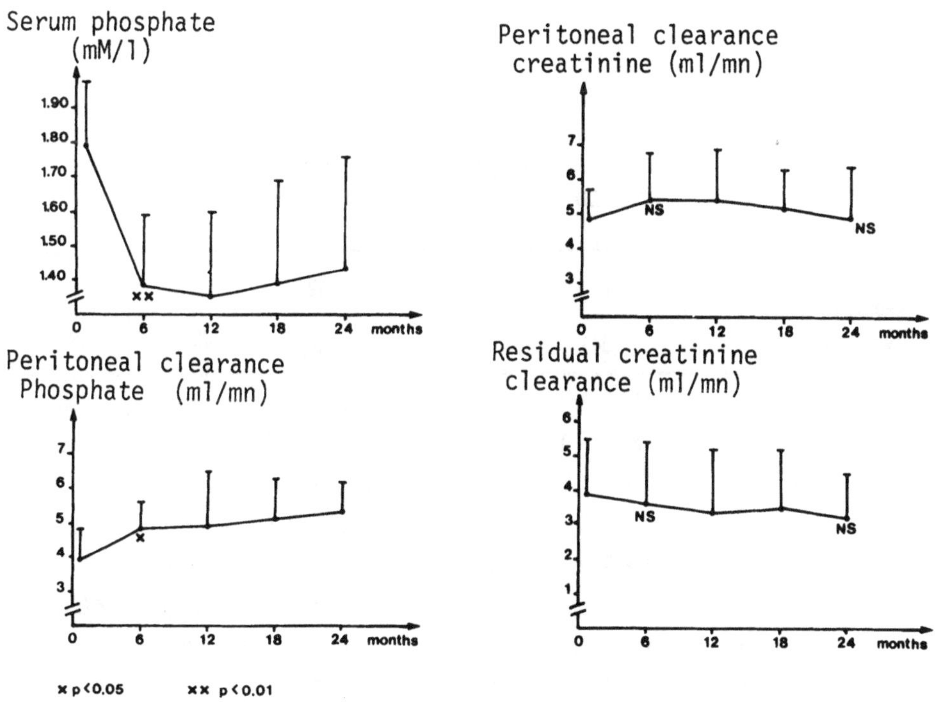

Fig. 2 . Serum phosphate level, peritoneal clearances of phosphate and creatinine and residual creatinine clearance in 8 patients treated for 24 months by CAPD.

RESIDUAL CREATINE CLEARANCE
PERITONEAL CLEARANCES OF CREATININE AND PHOSPHATE
IN 34 PATIENTS TREATED FOR ONE YEAR BY CAPD

TIME ON TREATMENT (Months)	0	6	12
PATIENTS (N)	(34)	(34)	(34)
Residual Creatinine Clearance (ml/mn)	4,6 ± 2,6*	3,7 ± 2,3 (NS)	3,1 ± 2,2 (NS)
Peritoneal Clearances (ml/mn)			
- Creatinine	5,2 ± 1,1	5,01 ± 0,8 (NS)	5,3 ± 1,2 (NS)
- Phosphate	3,9 ± 1,2	4,9 ± 1,6**	4,8 ± 1,7**

* Mean ± SD ** $p < 0.05$ NS : Not Significant

SERUM CHEMISTRIES IN 34 PATIENTS
TREATED FOR ONE YEAR BY CAPD

TIME ON TREATMENT (Months)	0	6	12	P*** 6 Months VS To	P*** 12 Months VS To
PATIENTS (N)	(34)	(34)	(34)		
- Creatinine (mM/l)	812 ± 167*	730 ± 182	758 ± 196	0,05	NS
- Urea (mM/l)	30 ± 5,1	24,2 ± 5,8	23,9 ± 7,5	< 0,001	0,001
- HCO_3^- (mM/l)	20,9 ± 2,3	24,1 ± 2,8	24,6 ± 2,7	< 0,001	< 0,001
- Ca^{++} (mM/l)**	2,4 ± 0,4	2,5 ± 0,3	2,5 ± 0,3	NS	NS
- Pi (mM/l)	1,9 ± 0,7	1,4 ± 0,3	1,3 ± 0,3	0,005	< 0,001
- Mg^{++} (mM/l)	1,1 ± 0,2	1,2 ± 0,2	1,2 ± 0,2	< 0,05	< 0,05
- Alk.Phosphatase (UI/l)	101 ± 55	97 ± 44	89 ± 39	NS	NS
- Total Protein (g/l)	67 ± 7	60 ± 6	60 ± 6	< 0,001	< 0,001
- Albumin (g/l)	35 ± 6	31 ± 4	32 ± 5	< 0,01	0,01

* Mean ± SD ** Corrected for plasma Protein *** paired-t-test

months of treatment (Figure 1). Serum concentrations of creatinine, urea, bicarbonate, total Ca (corrected for protein concentration as mentioned above) Pi, magnesium, alkaline phosphatase, total protein and albumin measured at start of treatment, 6 and 12 months thereafter are presented in Table 2. Serum total Ca and alkaline phosphatase levels did not change significantly over time, the latter remaining slightly above the upper normal range. Mean serum levels of Pi decreased to normal ranges. Serum Mg concentrations were higher at six and 12 months than at start of treatment. This finding entailed subsequently the reduction of Mg concentration in the dialysate from 0,75 to 0,50 mM/liter. In the 21 patients still on CAPD at 18 months after start of treatment, serum Mg concentrations had dropped to 1,01 mM/1 ± 0,2, a value close to the upper normal range (0,98 mM/1). Data recorded in the 8 patients who have been followed-up for 24 months are shown in Figure 2. It is noteworthy that the residual renal function did not decrease significantly over this prolonged period of time. Peritoneal clearances of creatinine and phosphate remained also unchanged at 12 and 24 months as compared to values recorded at 6 months after start of treatment. Mean serum phosphate level was found within the normal range over the whole period.

Determination of the daily cumulative peritoneal mass transfers yielded an average positive balance for calcium (+ 1,5 mM/day ± 1,1 S.D). Wide variations existed among the 8 patients investigated, with values ranging between -0,07 to + 3,3 mM/day. The average negative balance of Pi was 12 mM per day ± 2.7 (range -7,9 to -15,3 mM). With a dialysate magnesium concentration of 0,50 mM/1 the average balance of magnesium was -0,99 ± 0,87 mM/day.

Supplementation of 25(OH)D_3 (average daily dose 50 µg) was maintained in the long run for more than 50 % of the patients. Ca oral supplements and aluminium containing phosphate binders were progressively withdrawn in most of them. Such medications were taken by no more than 4 patients among the 21 who were still treated by CAPD at 18 months. Serum aluminium concentrations decreased from 1,23 µM/1 at start of treatment to 0,72 µM/1 ± 0,31 at six months (p : 0,01) and 0,84 µM/1 ± 0,43 at twelve months.

COMMENTS

Assessment of the efficacy of CAPD for prevention or reversal of clinical and/or radiological manifestations of renal osteodystrophy is still hazardous, since the vast majority of patients submitted to this mode of therapy have thus far been treated for periods shorter than one year (3,8). The data recorded in these series of 40 patients are in accordance with those already reported in the limited literature available to date on the subject. Improvement of clinical and radiological symptoms of osteomalacia have been mentioned with disappearance of bone pain and healing of traumatic or pathologic fractures (9,10). Backache can be related in CAPD patients to the increased lordotic position adopted while carrying the intra-abdominal dialysis fluid and thus demands to be differenciated from osteodystrophic bone pain (11). Improvement of radiological signs of osteitis fibrosa occurs more rarely : amelioration was observed in only one of the seven patients in these series in whom subperiostal erosions of the phalanges were present at start of treatment. Moreover, overt signs of osteitis fibrosa became apparent in 3 out of 20 patients within a one year period of follow-up. Extension of subperiostal bone resorption was also observed in 28 % of the patients reported by Calderaro et al (9). In a series of patients who underwent serial bone biopsies, Gokal et al reported that aggravation of osteitis fibrosa occurs mainly in patients who had been treated previously by maintenance hemodialysis, whereas significant improvement can be achieved in patients in whom CAPD was the initial mode of treatment (12). Persistance or aggravation of hyperparathyroid bone disease is also documented in several series of patients by sustained elevation of serum parathyroid hormone and alkaline phosphatase levels (9,10, 13).

Serum level of total Ca is often found in the high-normal range. However, determination of ionized Ca serum levels have yielded values distributed in the rather lower limit of the normal range (14). Elevation of the serum concentration of Ca can result from a positive peritoneal calcium balance, eventually associated with an improved absorption by the gut, but can also be the result of persistent bone resorption. The hypercalcemic state reported in some CAPD patients (15,16) requires therefore careful analysis since it should lead either to withdrawal of calcium and/or vit.D supplements or to parathyroidectomy in case of uncontrolled hyperparathyroidism. Calderaro et al obtained a negative peritoneal calcium balance in using a dialysate containing 1,5 mM/l of Ca (9), whereas positive balances are achieved when the Ca concentration of the dialysate is raised to 1,75 mM/l (17). Transfer of Ca from the body into the peritoneal effluent however occurs if large quantities of fluid have to be removed from the patients by intensive ultrafiltration (17). Loss of 25(OH)D_3 into the peritoneal effluent and decrease of serum levels down to subnormal values have been documented by several investigators (18,19) justifying therefore a sustained supplementation of vit.D derivatives.

Adequate control of serum phosphate level is obtained in most patients treated by CAPD (14,15,19,20). Several factors contribute to this result. A moderate phosphate intake certainly plays an important role : the data collected in our patients are in agreement with the results reported by Gahl et al who have shown that the average daily protein intake in patients who perform CAPD in their home is actually less than 1 g/Kg body weight instead of the 1,2 to 1,5/Kg body weight that are usually recommended (21). After a slight increase recorded in the first months, peritoneal clearance of phosphate in our patients did not show significant variation over time for periods up to two years. An increasingly positive correlation between the peritoneal clearances of phosphate and creatinine was evidenced over a one year period. The peritoneal membrane seems therefore to behave differently from hemodialysis systems as regards their respective capacities for removal of phosphate and creatinine. Only few data relevant to the clearance of phosphate by hemodialysers are reported in the literature. According to Kerr et al , the phosphate clearance of hemodialysis is roughly predictable from the clearances of urea and creatinine (22). Evaluation of phosphate clearance performed by Gorgels and Tan (23) and also in our Unit for several types of hemodialysers of less than 1.30 sqm surface area have yielded values 20 to 30 % lower than creatinine clearance, ranging between 85 and 110 ml/minute. A 10 to 20 % decrease of both clearances of phosphate and creatinine is moreover recorded between the first and the fourth hour of hemodialysis sessions (unpublished data).

The average weekly peritoneal clearance of phosphate in our CAPD patients would amount to about 50 liters per week, which is less than the circa 70 liters per week than can be provided by 15 hours of hemodialysis. As shown in our peritoneal balance studies, the negative daily peritoneal phosphate balance is only about 12 mM. The contribution of residual renal function appears therefore of critical importance in order to achieve an adequate control of phosphate balance. As reported previously by several authors (24, 25), the peritoneal clearance of creatinine recorded in our patients did not show significant variation over time. Bearing in mind that in advanced renal failure the percentage of filtered phosphate excreted in the urine is around 65 % (26) a residual glomerular filtration of about 3 ml/mn entails an additional renal clearance of phosphate of about 20 liters per week. The total weekly clearance of phosphate reaches thereby a value comparable to the one provided by a conventional hemodialysis strategy.

According to the nomogram presented by Grodstein et al (27), 115 g of glucose are absorbed each day via the peritoneal route by patients undergoing the CAPD regimen employed in this study. This steady supply of glucose enhances the entrance of phosphate into the intra-cellular compartment and contributes therefore to the lowering of serum phosphate concentration.

The reduction of serum phosphate levels to close to normal values insures a permanently low CaxP product thereby preventing the occurence of soft tissue, ocular and vascular calcifications. Withdrawal of aluminium containing phosphate binders could be achieved in more than 80 % of our patients treated by CAPD, an experience also shared by other authors (19,20,28). Six months and one year after start of CAPD mean serum levels of aluminium in our patients dropped down to values observed in non dialysed uremic subjects not submitted to aluminium containing drugs (29). Elevated serum levels of aluminium have however been encountered in a series of patients reported by Gokal et al who have shown that currently available peritoneal dialysis fluid solutions contain about 0,67 mM per liter of aluminium and thus advocate the use of aluminium-free solutions (28).

Much wider experience remains to be gained before a more substantiated response can be given as to the efficacy of CAPD to prevent of improve manifestations of renal osteodystrophy. From the presently available data it may be inferred that acheiving optimal results is highly dependent on commencing CAPD at a sufficient early stage, since the method does not seem likely to be able to reverse or preclude the progression of established severe hyperparathyroid bone disease. A positive peritoneal calcium balance can be achieved in supplying about 14 mM per day of calcium via the dialysis fluid and keeping the ultrafiltration volume moderate. Supplementation of vit.D derivatives remains necessary. Preservation of residual renal function appears of major importance to obtain a satisfactory phosphate balance, considering the high dietary protein requirements that are needed in patients treated by CAPD and the limited amount of phosphate which can be removed through the peritoneal route.

ACKNOWLEDGEMENTS The authors express their thanks to Mrs. F. Aimé, P. Degoulet and C. Devries for their helpful contribution to this study and to Miss E. Goupy for skillful secretarial assistance.

REFERENCES

1. W.J. Johnson, R.S. Goldsmith, J.W. Beabout, J. Jowsey, P.J. Kelly C.D. Arnaud, Prevention and reversal of progressive secundary hyperparathyroidism in patients maintained by hemodialysis, Am.J.Med. 56:827 (1974).
2. E. Slatopolsky, Recommendations for treatment of renal osteodystrophy in dialysis patients, Kidney Int. 7, Supplt.2:253 (1975).
3. C. Jacobs, M. Broyer, F.P. Brunner, M. Brynger, R.A. Donckerwolcke, P. Kramer, N.H. Selwood and A.J. Wing, Combined report on regular dialysis and transplantation in Europe XI. in: Proceed. Europ.Dial.Transpl.Ass. Vol.18, B.H.B. Robinson, ed. Pitman Med. Tunbridge Wells (1981) in Press.
4. R.P. Popovich, J.W. Moncrief, K.D. Nolph, A. Ghods, Z.T. Twardowski and W.K. Pyle, Continuous ambulatory peritoneal dialysis, Ann.Int.Med. 88:449 (1978).
5. D.H. Randerson and P.C. Farrel, Mass transfer properties of the human peritoneum, A.S.A.I.O. Journal, 3:140 (1980).

6. H. Husdan, A. Rapoport and S. Locke, Influence of posture on the calcium serum concentration, Metabolism, 22:787 (1973).
7. A.M. Parfitt, Clinical and radiographic manifestations of renal osteodystrophy, in: Calcium metabolism in renal failure and nephrolithiasis, D.S. David, ed, John Wiley, New York (1977) pp. 145-195.
8. J.W. Moncrief and R.P. Popovich, Continuous ambulatory peritoneal dialysis : worldwide experience, in: Peritoneal dialysis, K.D. Nolph ed. Martinus Nijhoff, The Hague (1981) pp. 178-212.
9. V. Calderaro, D.G. Oreopoulos, H.E. Meema, R. Ogilvie, H. Husdan, R. Khanna, C. Quinton, T. Murray and D. Carmichael, The evolution of renal osteodystrophy in patients undergoing continuous ambulatory peritoneal dialysis, in: Proceed. Europ. Dial.Transpl.Ass. Vol.17, B.H.B. Robinson ed, Pitman Med. Tunbridge-Wells (1980) pp. 533-541.
10. CH. Tielemans, C. Aubry and M. Dratwa, The effects of continuous ambulatory peritoneal dialysis on renal osteodystrophy, in: Proceed.Second Int.Symposium on Peritoneal dialysis, Excerpta Medica, Amsterdam (1981) in Press.
11. D.G. Oreopoulos and R. Khanna, Complications of peritoneal dialysis other than peritonitis, in: Peritoneal Dialysis, K.D. Nolph ed, Martinus Nijhoff, The Hague (1981) pp. 309-343.
12. R. Gokal, H.A. Ellis, J.M. Ramos, J. Dewar, V. Sweeting, M.K. Ward and D.N.S. Kerr, Improvement in secundary hyperparathyroidism in patients on continuous ambulatory peritoneal dialysis, in: Proceed. Second Int. Symposium on peritoneal dialysis, Excerpta Medica, Amsterdam (1981) in Press.
13. R. Khanna, N. Dombros, P. Williams, R.D.G. Blair, S. Vas, H.E. Meema and D.G. Oreopoulous, Three years experience with continuous ambulatory peritoneal dialysis, in: Proceed.Second Int. Symposium on peritoneal dialysis, Excerpta Medica, Amsterdam, (1981) in Press.
14. R. Gokal, R. Fryer, M. MacHugh, M.K.Ward and D.N.S. Kerr, Calcium and phosphate control in patients on continuous ambulatory peritoneal dialysis, in: Continuous ambulatory peritoneal dialysis, M. Legrain, ed. Excerpta Medica, Amsterdam (1980) pp. 283-291.
15. K.D. Nolph, M. Sorkin, J. Rubin, D. Arfania, B. Prowant, L. Fruto and D. Kennedy, Continuous ambulatory peritoneal dialysis : three years experience at one Center, Ann.Int.Med.92:609 (1980).
16. S.B. Kurtz, J.T. MacCarthy and R. Kumar, Hypercalcemia in continuous ambulatory peritoneal dialysis patients, in: Proceed.Second Int. Symposium on peritoneal dialysis, Excerpta Medica, Amsterdam (1981) in Press.
17. A. Parker and K.D. Nolph, Magnesium and calcium mass transfer during continuous ambulatory peritoneal dialysis, Trans.Am.Soc. Art.Int.Org. XXVI :194 (1980).
18. M. Guillot, C. Lavocat, A. Bourdeau, M. Garabedian, C. Sachs, S. Balsan, M.F. Gagnadoux and M. Broyer, Evaluation of 25(OH)D loss in dialysate of children on continuous ambulatory peritoneal dialysis, in: Proceed.Europ.Dial.Transpl.Ass. Vol. 18,

B.H.B. Robinson Ed. Pitman Med. Tunbridge Wells (1981) in Press
19. J.F. De Fremont, P. Fievet, P. Kaczmareck, J.D. Gheerbrandt and A. Fournier, Metabolic tolerance of CAPD, in: Proceed.Second Int. Symposium on peritoneal dialysis, Excerpta Medica, Amsterdam (1981) in Press.
20. D.H. Randerson and P.C. Farrel, Clinical assessment of CAPD, Dial. and Transpl. 10:389 (1981).
21. G.M. Gahl, H.V. Baeyer, R. Averdun, H. Riedinger, B. Borowsak, R. Schurig, H. Becker and M. Kessel, Outpatient evaluation of dietary intake and nitrogen removal in continuous ambulatory peritoneal dialysis, Ann.Int.Med.91:643 (1981).
22. D.N.S. Kerr, N.A. Hoenich, T.H. Frost, C.B. Clayton and D. Jolly, Which dialyser ? Nephron, 12:368 (1974).
23. J. Gorgels and B.H. Tan, An evaluation of the performance of current dialysers in routine use and in vitro, Dial. and Transpl. 5: 68 (1976).
24. P.C. Farrel and D.H. Randerson, Membrane permeability changes in long term CAPD, Trans.Am.Soc.Art.Int.Org. 26:197 (1980).
25. J. Rubin, K. Nolph, D. Arfania, P. Brown and B. Prowant, Follow-up of peritoneal clearances in patients undergoing continuous ambulatory peritoneal dialysis, Kidney Int. 16:619 (1979).
26. S.G. Massry, J.W. Coburn, D.B.N. Lee, J. Jowsey and C.R. Kleeman, Skeletal resistance to parathyroid hormone in renal failure, Ann.Int.Med.78:357 (1973).
27. G.P. Grodstein, M.J. Blumenkrantz, J.D. Kopple, J.K. Moran and J.W. Coburn, Glucose absorption during continuous ambulatory peritoneal dialysis, Kidney Int. 19:564 (1981).
28. R. Gokal, I.S. Parkinson, J.M. Ramos, M.K. Ward and D.N.S. Kerr, Elevated serum aluminium levels in patients on continuous ambulatory peritoneal dialysis, in: Proceed. Second Int. Symposium on peritoneal dialysis, Excerpta Medica, Amsterdam (1981) in Press.
29. M. Boukari , J. Rottembourg, M.C. Jaudon, J.P. Clavel, M. Legrain and A. Galli, Influence de la prise prolongée de gels d'alumine sur les taux sériques d'aluminium chez les patients atteints d'insuffisance rénale chronique, Nouv.Presse Med. 7:85 (1978).

CALCIUM METABOLISM

MEASUREMENTS OF INTRACELLULAR FREE CA^{++}

Antonio Scarpa and George Dubyak

Department of Biochemistry and Biophysics
University of Pennsylvania School of Medicine
Philadelphia, PA

This manuscript reviews the work of this laboratory over the last six years in measuring, non-destructively and kinetically, ionized Ca^{++} in the cytosol of single resting cells and the changes in Ca^{++} following metabolic, electrical, and contractile events. The strategy of this study is to use Ca^{++} indicators with suitable selectivity and sensitivity, to inject them into the cytosol of large cells, and to measure with sensitive microspectrophotometry the absorbance of these indicators in situ as a function of Ca^{++} concentration. This approach, which essentially uses a large cell as a biological cuvet, has been successful both in large neurons and single large muscle cells. We will briefly review five areas: the characteristics of Ca^{++} metallochromic indicators; the experimental set-up to measure free cytosolic Ca^{++} in single cells; the measurement of free Ca^{++} in a resting cell; the kinetics of mitochondrial Ca^{++} uptake and release in single cells in situ; and the intracellular free Ca^{++} transients during contractile events in a single muscle cell.

CA^{++} METALLOCHROMIC INDICATORS

Ca^{++} metallochromic indicators are chemical substances that undergo significant color changes when the concentration of free Ca^{++} in the solution changes. The color difference between the indicator free and the indicator-Ca^{++} complex is often very large and can be used for quantitative determination of the concentration of free Ca^{++} in the solution.

An example of such light absorbance changes of two indicators, arsenazo III[1] and antipyrylazo III[2], in a buffered solution is shown in Figures 1 and 2. Fig. 1 shows the differential spectrum of arsenazo III vs. arsenazo III in the presence of various Ca^{++} concentrations. The presence of Ca^{++} induces a large Ca^{++}-dependent absorbance increase in the spectral area between 570 and 700 nm, and a decrease in absorbance between 450 and 570 nm. By the use of dual wavelength spectrophotometry it is possible to alternatively illuminate at high frequency the cuvet at 685 nm and at 675 nm and to record continuously the differential absorbance. This is shown in the right part of Fig. 1, where the differential absorbance of arsenazo III in the buffered solution is displayed vs. the time. Small additions of Ca^{++} (and not Mg^{++}) produce differential absorbance changes.

Fig. 2 shows the differential spectrum of another Ca^{++} indicator, antipyrylazo III (left side), and the differential absorbance of antipyrylazo III when large concentrations of Mg^{++} and lower concentrations of Ca^{++} are added to the cuvet (right side).

The characteristics of these indicators, together with those of murexide, a less sensitive Ca^{++} indicator which has been used for over twenty years[3], have been published elsewhere in great detail[2, 4-8], and are summarized in Table I. Briefly, both arsenazo III and antipyrylazo III are water soluble Ca^{++} indicators which do not bind to cell structures, nor do they have side effects on cell functions; they respond very rapidly (μsec to a few msec) to changes in ionized Ca^{++}; they have a high Δ_ε, which translates into large differential absorbance changes in the presence of Ca^{++}; they are, under appropriate conditions, Ca^{++}-selective and have Ca^{++}-dependent absorbance spectra in the red area of the spectrum (600-800 nm), where usually aspecific absorbance changes can be minimized. The major difference in these three indicators is their affinity towards Ca^{++}, which should dictate the use of different indicators, depending on the concentration of Ca^{++} free to be measured. In most cases it is preferable that the equilibrium indicator vs. calcium-indicator is toward the indicator in the free form. This translates into linearity between Δ_A and free Ca^{++} concentration and lack of major buffering by the indicator of Ca^{++} in solution or within the cell. The many advantages and the few disadvantages of these indicators, with respect to other ways of measuring ionized Ca^{++}, such as the

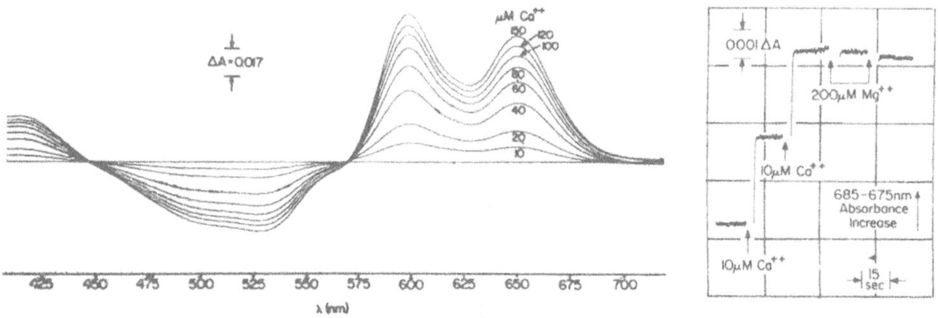

Fig. 1. The differential spectra of arsenazo III vs. arsenazo III plus Ca^{++}. The differential spectra was obtained by adding to the measuring cuvet the concentrations of Ca^{++} indicated in the figure. The reaction mixture contained 0.5 M KCl, 5 mM imidazole buffer, pH 6.8, and 100 μM arsenazo III. The right part of the figure shows an experiment in which the absorbance changes of arsenazo III were measured as a function of the time at 675-685 nm with a dual-wavelength spectrophotometer. Temp. was 22°.

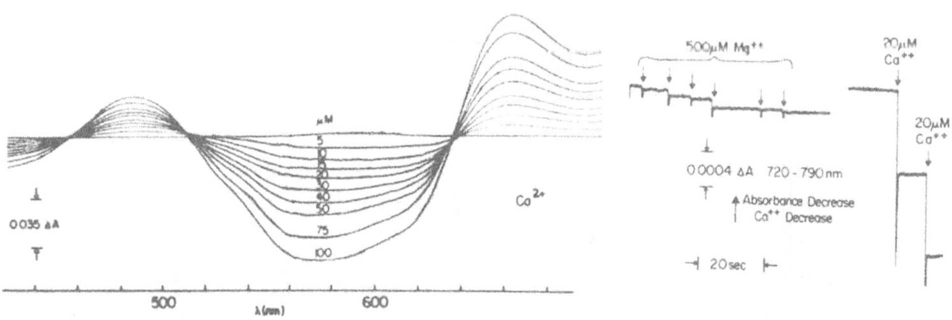

Fig. 2. The differential absorbance spectra of antipyrylazo III in the presence of Ca^{++} (left) and dual-wavelength readout of the differential absorbance of antipyrylazo III following additions of Mg^{++} and Ca^{++}. Experimental conditions identical to those in Fig. 1 were employed, except that 50 μM antipyrylazo III, instead of arsenazo III, was present.

TABLE 1
THE PROPERTIES OF MUREXIDE, ARSENAZO III, AND ANTIPYRYLAZO III

	Murexide	Arsenazo III	Antipyrylazo III
	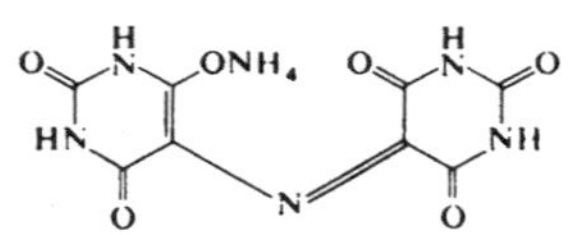	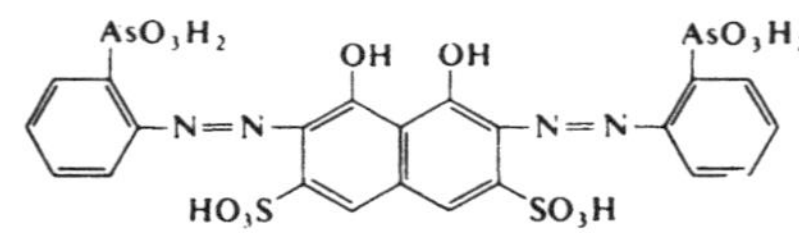	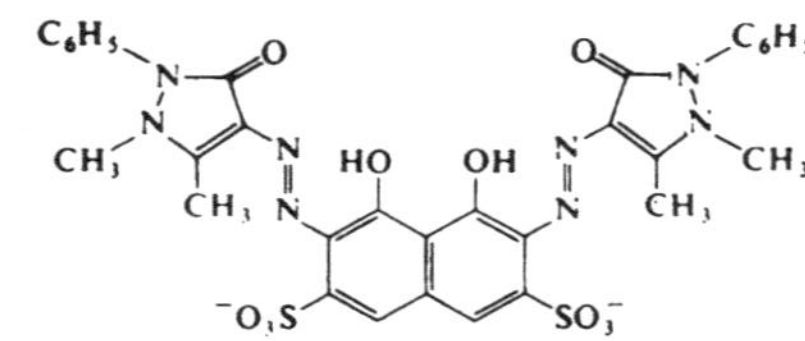
	Ammonium purpurate	*O*-(1,8-Dihydroxy-3,6-disulfonaphthalene-2,7 bisazo)-bisbenzenearsonic acid	bis (4-antipyrylazo)-4,'5-dihydroxy-2,7-naphthalene disulfonic acid
Molecular wt.	284	776	746
Water solubility	>20 mM	>50 mM	>20 mM
Binding to cells and cell fractions	—	—	
Side effects on cell structure and function	—	—	
Indicator-Ca^{2+} complex:			
K_D (at 50 mM and 0.5 M KCl)	1–3 mM	15–60 μM	60–400 μM
$\Delta\epsilon$ ($mM^{-1} \cdot cm^{-1}$)	~6	~25	~7
Relaxation time (τ)	<2 μsec	>2.8 msec	180 μsec
Suitable differential 1 (nm)	540–507	675–685; 650–685	670–690; 720–790

luminescence of the jellyfish protein aequorin[8], or the newly developed Ca^{++} electrodes[9], have been reviewed in great detail[7].

MEASUREMENTS OF CA^{++} INDICATOR ABSORBANCE IN A SINGLE CELL

The above-mentioned Ca^{++} indicators, arsenazo III and antipyrylazo III, can be microinjected into single cells and their differential absorbance can be monitored as a function of the free Ca^{++} concentration. This approach of using cells as "biological cuvets" can be better applied by using giant cells from marine animals.

The single cells used for these measurements were the squid giant axon (400-800 µm in diameter, several cm in length), dissected by established methods from living specimens of Loligo pealei or the large muscle fibers from the Balanus aquila barnacle, and positioned in a chamber containing circulating seawater, as described by Brinley and Mullins[9]. A Ca^{++} metallochromic indicator was microinjected into the axon and it was allowed to distribute uniformly within the axoplasm or sarcoplasm (10-20 min) to reach a concentration ranging from 100 to 1,000 µM. The minute changes in the absorbance of the indicator, which under certain conditions are a linear-function of the ionized Ca^{++}, were measured kinetically in situ with the apparatus schematically illustrated in Fig. 3 and built at the Johnson Research Foundation, University of Pennsylvania[10-11]. The major features of the apparatus consist of a) a light source; b) a rotating wheel containing several interference filters (50% T, 1-5 nm half-band width), driven at variable speeds up to 500 Hz by compressed air directed on the vanes; c) a collimating lens which focuses the light of the lamp after the passage through each filter onto a bundle of minute optical fibers which diverge on a horizontal row at the level of the cell immersed in sea water; d) similar fiber arrangement after the cell connected to the photomultiplier; e) electronic circuitry to generate gates for each filter, individual channel amplifiers and equilization gates, etc. With this instrument it is possible to maintain continuous readout of the indicator absorbance a) at the isosbestic points of the indicator vs. indicator plus Ca; b) at several wavelength pair differentials where the increase or decrease in free Ca^{++} produces changes in the indicator differential absorbance.

For calibration purposes it is possible to impale the giant cell axially with a dialysis capillary permeable to Ca^{++}, EGTA, and other small molecules, so that the cytosolic content of Ca^{++} can be changed at will. The technique of internal dialysis of these cells has been described in detail previously[9, 11].

FREE CA^{++} CONCENTRATION IN THE CYTOSOL OF SQUID AXON AT REST

The measurements of ionized Ca^{++} in the axoplasm of resting axons using arsenazo III depends on the differential absorbance change produced when virtually all the ionized Ca^{++} present in the axoplasm is chelated by the presence in the cytosol of an excess of EGTA. In order to validate this technique, it is necessary to demonstrate that 1) the differential absorbance changes of arsenazo III are linear with ionized Ca^{++} in the range of interest, and 2) chelation of Ca^{++} by EGTA is complete under the experimental conditions selected.

This is shown in Fig. 4. Instead of a squid axon a glass capillary with a lumen comparable to the usual diameter of a squid axon (500 μm) was positioned in the chamber described in Fig. 3 across the optical fibers and a dialysis capillary permeable to Ca^{++} and EGTA was inserted axially. The glass capillary was then flushed with a medium containing artifical axoplasm, a known concentration of arsenazo III, and 2 mM EGTA. The differential absorbance observed with this solution as a function of the time serves as a reference for the 0 Ca^{++} baseline. The capillary was then flushed with solutions containing the indicated ratios of CaEGTA and EGTA to establish a linear relationship between ionized Ca^{++} and differential absorbance. By measuring the ionized Ca^{++} activity with a Ca^{++} electrode under identical conditions, it was found that the values of 2 mM EGTA, 1 mM CaEGTA-2 mM EGTA, and 2 mM CaEGTA-2 mM EGTA indicated in the figure corresponds to 0, 75 nM, and 150 nM, respectively. The vertical arrow in the figure indicates the onset of internal dialysis with an isoosmotic solution of EGTA. When the EGTA diffuses through the porous capillary into the lumen of the glass tube, the residual ionized Ca^{++} is chelated and the differential absorbance returns to the baseline level corresponding to 0 Ca^{++}.

Fig. 5 shows the result of internal EGTA dialysis in four axons. The vertical arrows indicate the points at which the EGTA solution was flashed through the capillary. In the two experiments shown at the top of Fig. 5 dialysis was not continuous, but repetitive short pulses of EGTA were pushed through the capillary. In these experiments a subsequent addition of EGTA confirms that complete chelation of the ionized Ca^{++} by EGTA in the axoplasm did occur.

The collected data from nine axons, based on calibrations similar to that shown in Fig. 4, indicates that the average value of ionized Ca^{++} in resting and metabolically active exons is between 40 and 60 nM[1].

KINETICS OF MITOCHONDRIAL CA^{++} UPTAKE IN SITU

Microspectrophotometric measurements of Ca^{++} indicators *in situ* can be successfully used not only to determine the resting concentrations of ionized Ca^{++} in squid axons, but also the kine-

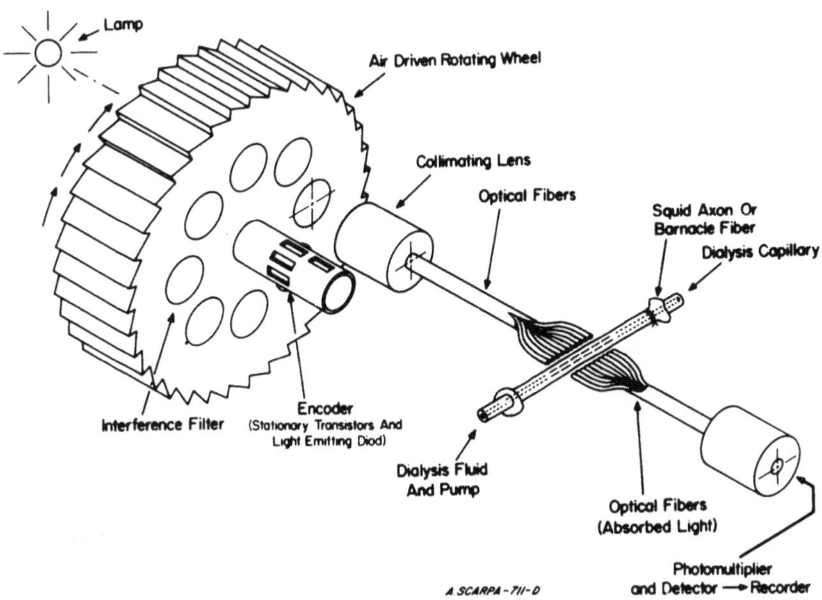

Fig. 3. Schematic representation (not in scale) of the time-sharing multiple wavelength microspectrophotometer for single cells. More details in text.

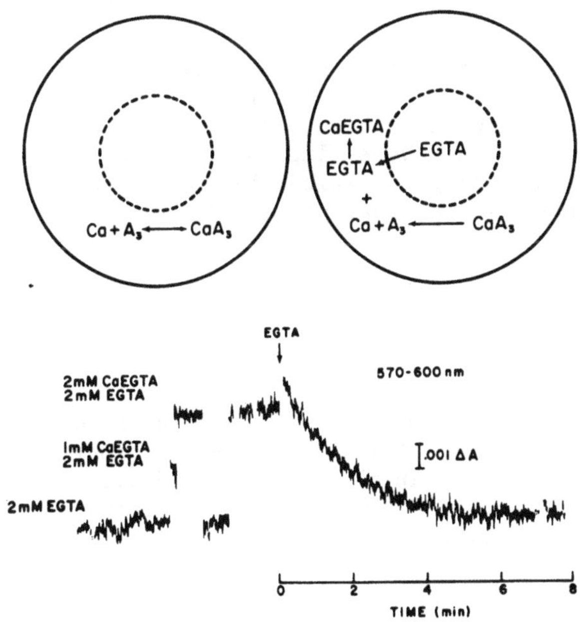

Fig. 4. <u>In vitro</u> calibration of arsenazo III and <u>in vitro</u> dialysis. More details in Ref. 1.

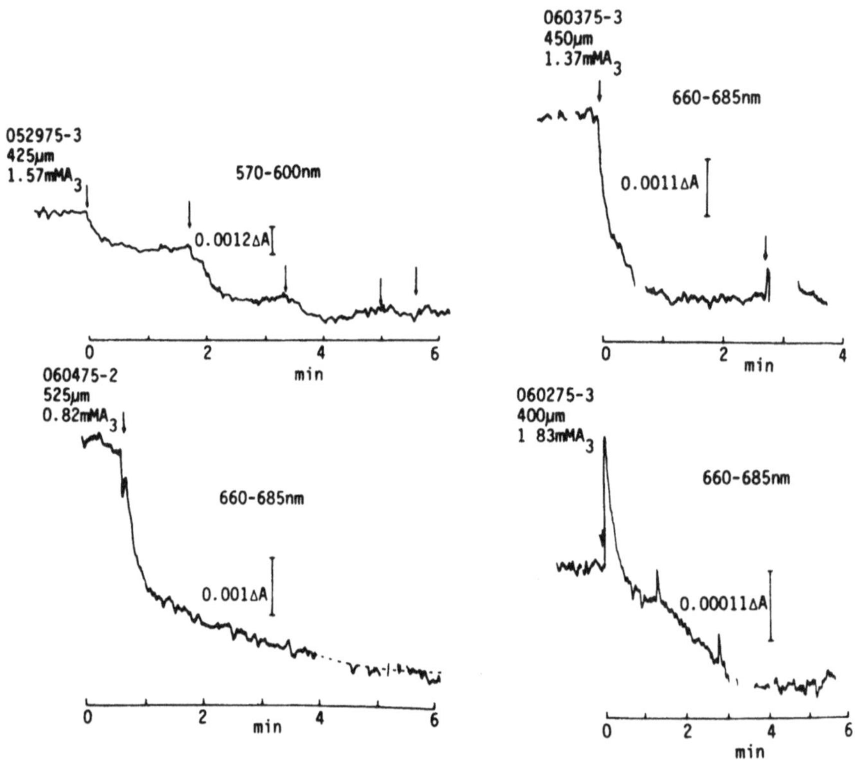

Fig. 5. Determination of cytosolic free Ca^{++} in four different squid axons. Vertical arrows indicate where the axons containing the concentrations of arsenazo III indicated in the figure were flushed with EGTA through the dialysis capillary. Vertical bars indicate the Δabsorbance changes at the dual wavelength indicated. More details in Ref. 1.

tic changes of axoplasmic ionized Ca^{++} in response to metabolic or electrical events. For this series of experiments the axon was dissected, positioned in the chamber, and microinjected with arsenazo III as described previously. Insertion of the dialysis capillary was omitted.

Since the work of Hodkin and Keynes[12], who have shown that excitation of squid axons is accompanied by a net inward calcium flux, it is possible to load the axon with Ca^{++} in a predictable and quantitative fashion by stimulating the axons in the presence of Ca^{++} in the sea water. We have recently shown with both radiochemical and atomic absorbance techniques that the total calcium content of an axon increases linearly upon electical stimulation for over 90 minutes, and that maximal calcium loading can be induced by electrically stimulating the axon 100 times/sec in sea water whose Ca^{++} has been increased to 112 mM. Under these conditions a linear calcium influx corresponding to 14 pmol/cm^2/sec for 500 mμ axons was measured[13].

Under Ca^{++}-loading conditions it is possible to measure changes in ionized free Ca^{++} in the axoplasm by dual wavelength microspectrophotometry. The Ca^{++} buffering capacity of the axon as a function of the time and metabolic conditions can be calculated as the difference between the total Ca^{++} increase in the axon and the value of ionized Ca^{++} measured from the Δ_A of the indicator in situ. Thus, through the use of specific inhibitors it is possible to study kinetically the contribution of intracellular organelles or soluble proteins in buffering cytosolic Ca^{++}. The following three figures show some examples of the application of this technique to the study of the rate and the affinity of the mitochondrial Ca^{++} transport in a single cell in situ.

Fig. 6 shows the time-dependent increase in ionized Ca^{++} in two different axons comparable in size and microinjected with the same concentration of indicator following continuous electrical stimulation (100/sec) in 112 mM Ca^{++} sea water. Following electrical stimulation, ionized Ca^{++} rapidly increased from the resting state, corresponding to 50 nM, to about 3 μM, where it remained relatively constant for over 30 minutes in spite of the continuous Ca^{++} entering the axon during electrical stimulation in high extracellular Ca^{++}. At the end of the experiment the uncoupler FCCP produced a dramatic increase in axoplasmic ionized Ca^{++}. This Ca^{++} increase was due to Ca^{++} release in the cytosol from axoplasmic stores, since the extracellular bathing fluid was shifted from one containing 112 mM Ca^{++} to one containing no Ca^{++} several minutes before FCCP addition. Fig. 6B shows that in a similar axon the addition of FCCP before stimulation produces a minimal increase in ionized Ca^{++}. In the presence of FCCP, however, the axoplasmic Ca^{++} increases almost linearly during electrical stimulation. These results, and several others obtained with various mitochondrial inhibitors, suggest that the cytosolic buffer sensitive to FCCP is identifiable with the mitochondria in the axons, which occupies 1-2% of the axoplasmic volume. The results then indicate that the mitochondria of squid axons are a

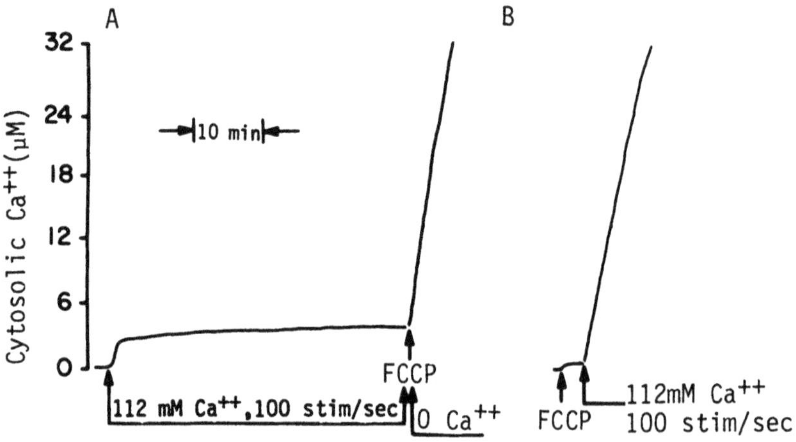

Fig. 6. Time course of the increase of free Ca^{++} in the cytosol of a squid axon electrically stimulated in the presence of high concentrations of Ca^{++}. The axons' sizes were 535 and 520 μm in diameter in A and B, respectively, and both axons were injected with arsenazo III so that their cytosolic concentrations, after diffusional equilibration, were 320 μM. Where indicated, FCCP (carbonyl cyanide p-trifluoromethoxyphenylhydrazone) was superfused. ΔA was continuously monitored at 675-685 nm, as described previously.

powerful Ca^{++} buffering system, but only when the concentration of Ca^{++} in the axoplasm is greater than the resting values.

Fig. 7 shows the results of an experiment in which axons were transiently loaded with smaller amounts of Ca^{++}. This was done through electrical stimulation for shorter periods of time in 3 or 10 mM calcium sea water. After Ca^{++} loading was imposed, the axon was bathed in Ca^{++}-free choline chloride solution to prevent either gain of Ca^{++} by leak across the axolemma or loss of calcium from the axon by the sodium-calcium exchange mechanism[14]. Since the total calcium content remains constant during the recovery period, any decrease in ionized Ca^{++} must reflect uptake by an internal sink. It is evident from the figure that axoplasmic Ca^{++} can be increased from the resting level to approximately 700 nM without any time dependent accumulation by internal buffers. By raising Ca^{++} to higher values (1 and 1.3 μM) the disappearance of Ca^{++} from the axoplasm after Ca^{++} loading became apparent. The conclusion from this and other similar experiments is that mitochondria are not active in sequestering Ca when Ca^{++} concentrations in the axoplasm range from the resting level to 500-700 nM, but that they become active in transporting Ca^{++} when cytosolic Ca^{++} concentrations are higher.

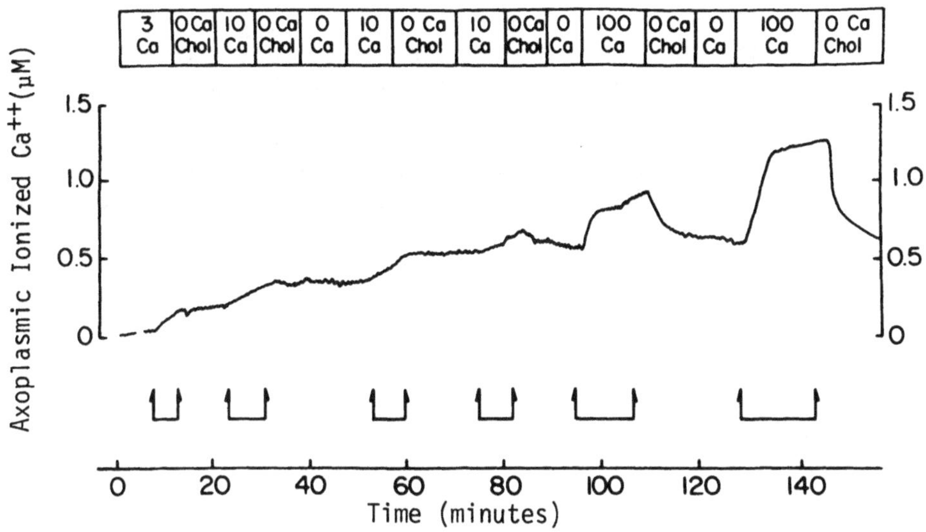

Fig. 7. Continuous recording of the ionized Ca^{++} in squid axons during Ca^{++} loading. The experimental conditions were similar to those of Fig. 6, except that the ΔA was amplified, the electric stimulation was intermittent, and the bathing sea water composition was varied at times. The times between arrows indicate the stimulation intervals (100/sec). The bathing medium at each time is indicated in boxes at the top of the trace. The numbers 0, 3, 10, and 100 indicate the concentration of Ca^{++} (mM) in the artificial seawater. "Chol" indicates that in the bathing medium the Na^{+} of artificial sea water was replaced by choline.

The kinetics of mitochondrial Ca^{++} transport in situ were measured by recording the rate of mitochondrial Ca^{++} uptake after Ca^{++} concentrations in the axoplasm were raised at different levels. Increments of Ca^{++} concentrations in the axoplasm were obtained by loading the axons with Ca^{++} either in the absence or in the presence of a reversible inhibitor (e.g., CN^- in the presence of apyrase). The experimental approach for these experiments and some of the results obtained have been described previously[15], and some of the data are plotted in Fig. 8. As it is technically impossible to impose too many successive cycles of Ca^{++} loading on the same axon, Fig. 8 shows the results of Ca^{++} uptake by mitochondria in situ in two axons, one in which the axoplasmic Ca^{++} concentrations before Ca^{++} uptake were 12-22 and 49 μM (right). The data show that virtually no Ca^{++} uptake occurs in mitochondria within the squid axon until the Ca^{++} concentration in the axoplasm is one order of magnitude greater than the resting value. At higher concentrations the rate increases sigmoidally to reach 180 nmoles/mg/min at 49 μM Ca^{++}. The experiments at higher Ca^{++} concentrations are technically difficult, so that V_{max} for Ca^{++} transport in situ could not be obtained. From these and an extensive number of similar experiments[15], the following considerations can be drawn: a) in spite of the approximation and possible error

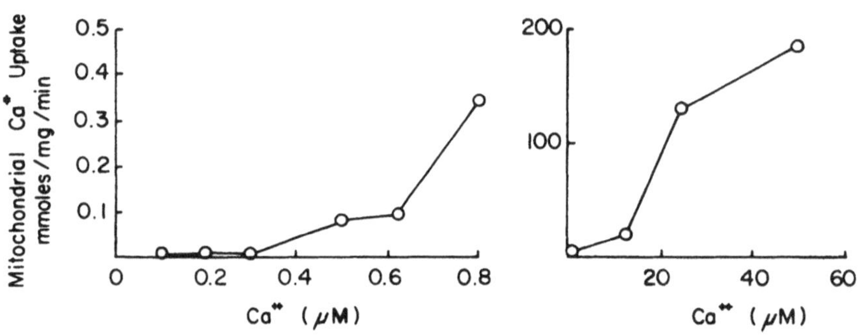

Fig. 8. Plot of the rates of Ca^{++} uptake by mitochondria in squid axons in situ converted to nmol/mg protein as a function of ionized axoplasmic free Ca^{++}. The Ca^{++} concentrations in the axoplasm were low in the experiments on the left, and therefore arsenazo III was used as a Ca^{++} indicator. In the experiments on the right Ca^{++} concentrations in the axoplasm were much greater, and antipyrylazo III was used as indicated. More details may be found in Ref. 15.

intrinsic to this technique, there was good correlation and fitting with points obtained at low and high Ca^{++} concentrations, with different indicators, and with different Ca^{++} loading techniques and/or mitochondrial activation; b) when corrected for mitochondrial content and temperature, these rates are similar (just slightly higher) to those obtained in vitro with isolated mitochondria from various mammalian species[16].

In conclusion, these experiments indicate that in squid giant axons Ca transport by mitochondria in situ occurs only when the concentration of Ca^{++} in the axoplasm is far above physiological resting values. At physiological Ca^{++} concentrations the membrane Ca^{++} pump may be more effective than mitochondria as a Ca^{++} sequestering mechanism, since this process has been shown to be sensitive to Ca^{++} concentrations as low as 10 nM[17]. Furthermore, the remarkable similarity of these rates and amounts of Ca^{++} transport by mitochondria obtained in vitro in squid axons to those obtained with mitochondria isolated from mammalian tissue may extend the significance of these data and conclusions on cytosolic Ca^{++} buffering to mammalian tissues.

MEASUREMENT OF SARCOPLASMIC CA^{++} TRANSIENTS IN SINGLE MUSCLE FIBERS

The use of metallochromic indicators as probes of cellular Ca^{++} homeostasis has recently been applied to investigations of the relationship between sarcoplasmic Ca^{++} concentration and tension development in single barnacle muscle fibers[18]. These single fibers reach 1-1.5 mm in diameter and several cm in length, and are thus readily suitable for the cannulation, micro-injection, and spectrophotometric techniques employed in the squid axon studies. However, the measurement of specific Ca^{++}-induced changes in dye absorbance in muscle fibers is complicated by the large light-scattering changes which accompany even weak isometric contractions. Thus, care must be taken to establish conditions wherein these signals accompanying tension development are predominated by changes in absorbance due to specific Ca^{++}-dye interaction. After extensive studies of spectral characteristics of the indicator in situ, fiber geometry, etc., these problems have been largely overcome.

Fig. 9 illustrates the differential absorbance changes monitored during isometric contractions of a single barnacle muscle fiber before (A) and after (B) injection of 300 µM arsenazo III. In the non-injected fiber no changes in ΔA (665-703 nm) or ΔA (740-780 nm) are observed, regardless of the strength of the isometric contraction. Conversely, after introduction of the indicator, large, graded increases in ΔA (665-703 nm), but not ΔA (740-780 nm) accompany tension development. The changes in differential absorbance at the former, but not the latter, wavelength pair are compatible with the observed effects of Ca^{++} on the arsenazo III absorbance spectrum in vitro (Fig. 1). Such results demonstrate that optical transients predominantly determined by specific changes in metallochromic indicator absorbance can be routinely and reproducibly monitored during isometric contraction-relaxation cycles.

This experimental system can be used to quantitate the tran-

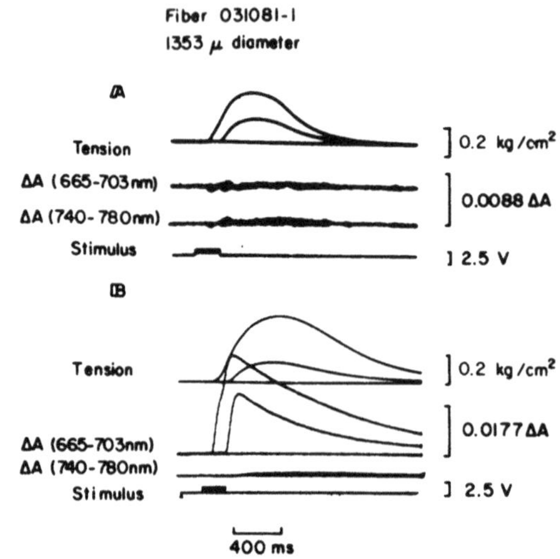

Fig. 9. Differential absorbance changes measured simultaneously with isometric tension in a single barnacle muscle fiber before and after injection of arsenazo III. The fiber was cannulated and mounted in the chamber shown in Fig. 3. A 100 μ platinum wire was advanced down the fiber center to allow passage of uniform depolarizing current pulses. The upper figures illustrate the isometric tension and ΔA transients before injection with dye. The electrode was then withdrawn and the fiber was injected with 280 μM arsenazo III. After the dye had uniformly distributed, the electrode was re-inserted; the lower figures show the changes in ΔA (665-713) and ΔA (740-780 nm) which accompany isometric tension transients in the dye-injected fiber.

sient variations in sarcoplasmic free Ca^{++} that regulate tension development. Since barnacle muscle fibers are characterized by a passive membrane response to depolarizing current pulses[19], the intensity of contraction can be graded by simply varying the amplitude or duration of the current passed through an intracellular electrode running the length of the fiber. Fig. 10 illustrates such graded isometric contractions and the corresponding changes in ΔA (673-713 nm) and ΔA (673-630 nm). In vitro studies using arsenazo III dissolved in a solution approximating the composition of barnacle sarcoplasm (i.e., pH = 7.3; $[Mg^{++}]$ = 6 mM) indicate that 630 nm and 713 nm constitute approximate isosbestic points in the Ca-arsenazo III differential absorbance spectrum. The nearly identical in situ ΔA signals obtained with both wavelength pairs is a further demonsration that their optical transients are not elicited by movement-induced variations in the op-

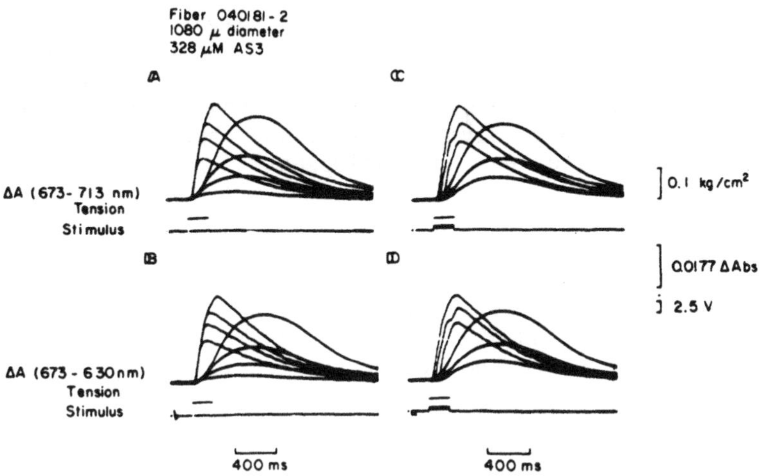

Fig. 10. Differential absorbance and tension transients of an arsenazo III-injected muscle fiber in response to depolarizing current pulses of graded intensity and duration. ΔA (673-713 nm) (Figs. A, C), or ΔA (673-630 nm) (Figs. B, D) was monitored during isometric tension transients resulting from graded depolarizing current pulses of varying intensity (Fig. C, D) or duration (Fig. A, B). In Figs. A and B the stimuli were 25, 50, 100, and 200 ms in duration and 3.0 V in intensity; in Figs. C and D the duration was 200 ms and the intensity ties were 0.5, 1.5, and 3.0 V.

tical path traversing the dye-injected region of the fiber. Under all conditions supra-threshold current pulses elicited abrupt increases in both ΔA (673-713 nm) and ΔA (673-630 nm). Increasing the stimulus intensity (C, D) of constant duration (200 ms) pulses had two effects: 1) the lag times between initiation of current injection and the onset of the optical transient were decreased, and 2) the maximum values of the ΔA signals were increased by similar magnitudes. Increasing the duration of constant amplitude current pulses (A, B) increased both durations and peak magnitudes of rising phases of the optical signals. Regardless of the monitoring wavelength pair or the intensity/duration of the electrical stimuli, the peak ΔA signals preceded the development of maximal tension by 300-400 ms. Using calibration techniques similar to those employed in the squid giant axon studies (Fig. 4), the sarcoplasmic free Ca^{++} levels corresponding to the observed ΔA signals can be calculated. These calibrations indicate that the free Ca^{++} can transiently increase to ∿2.0 μM before the onset of significant tension development. A further 3-fold increase in free $[Ca^{++}]$ is accompanied by a 15-fold increase in contractile intensity. This in situ tension-pCa relationship is quite similar to that obtained with skinned myofibrillar bundles isolated from barnacle fiber[20]. These results unequivocally demonstrate that metallochromic indicators can be used kinetically and quantitatively to resolve the transient changes in sarcoplasmic Ca^{++} that regulate tension development.

ACKNOWLEDGMENTS

The financial support for the experiments shown was provided from grants HL-15835 and HL-18708 from the National Institutes of Health. Many thanks are due to Dan Brannen for the preparation of the manuscript.

REFERENCES

1. R. DiPolo, J. Requena, L.J. Mullins, F.J. Brinley, A. Scarpa, and T. Tiffert, Ionized calcium concentrations in squid axons, J. Gen. Physiol. 67:433 (1976).
2. A. Scarpa, F.J. Brinely, and G. Dubyak, Antipyrylazo III, a 'middle-range' Ca^{++} metallochromic indicator, Biochemistry 17:1378 (1978).
3. A. Scarpa, Spectrophotometric measurement of calcium by murexide, Methods in Enzymology 24:343 (1972).
4. A. Scarpa, F.J. Brinely, T. Tiffer, and G. Dubyak, Metallochromic indicators of ionized Ca^{++}, Ann. N.Y. Acad. Sci. 307:86 (1978).
5. A. Scarpa, Measurement of cation transport with metallochromic indicators, Methods in Enzymology 56:301 (1979).
6. A. Scarpa, Measurements of calcium ion concentrations with metallochromic indicators, in: "Detection and Measurement of Free Calcium Ions in Cells," C. Ashley and F. Campbell, eds., Elsevier/North-Holland, Amsterdam (1979).
7. A. Scarpa, Cell ion measurements with metallochromic indicators, in: "Techniques in Cellular Physiology, P. Baker, ed., Elsevier/North-Holland, Amsterdam, in press.
8. J.R. Blinks, R.G. Prendergast, and D.G. Allen, Photoproteins as biological calcium indicators, Pharmacol. Rev. 28:1 (1976).
9. F.J. Brinley and L.J. Mullins, Sodium extrusion by internally dialyzed squid axons, J. Gen. Physiol. 50:2303 (1967).
10. B. Chance, Principle of differential spectrophotometry with special reference to the dual wavelength method, Methods in Enzymology 24:322 (1972).
11. F.J. Brinley, T. Tiffert, and A. Scarpa, The concentration of ionized Mg^{++} in barnacle muscle fibers, J. Physiol. 266:545 (1977).

12. A.L. Hodgkin and R.D. Keynes, Measurements of labeled calcium in squid giant axons, J. Physiol. (Lond.) 138:253 (1957).
13. F.J. Brinley, T. Tiffert, A. Scarpa, and L.J. Mullins, Intracellular calcium buffering capacity in isolated squid axons, J. Gen. Physiol. 70:355 (1977).
14. M.P. Blaustein and A.L. Hodgkin, The effect of cyanide on the efflux of calcium from squid axons, J. Physiol. (Lond.) 200: 497 (1969).
15. F.J. Brinley, T. Tiffert, and A. Scarpa, Mitochondria and other calcium buffers of squid axons studied in situ, J. Gen. Physiol. 72:101 (1978).
16. A. Scarpa and P. Graziotti, Mechanisms for intracellular calcium regulation in heart. I. Stopped-flow measurements of Ca^{++} uptake by cardiac mitochondria, J. Gen. Physiol. 62: 756 (1973).
17. R. DiPolo, Calcium efflux from internally dialyzed squid giant axons, J. Gen. Physiol. 62:575 (1973).
18. G.R. Dubyak and A. Scarpa, Sarcoplasmic Ca^{++} transients during the contractile cycle of single barnacle muscle fibers: Measurements with arsenazo III-injected fibers, J. Musc. Res. Cell Motil., submitted.
19. C. Edwards, S. Chicibu, and S. Hagiwara, Relation between membrane potential changes and tension in barnacle muscle fibers, J. Gen. Physiol. 48:225-234.
20. C.C. Ashley and D.G. Moisescu, Effect of changing the composition of the bathing solutions upon the isometric tension-pCa relationship in bundles of crustacean myofibrils, J. Physiol. 270:627 (1977).

THE REGULATION OF INTRACELLUALR CALCIUM

Ernesto Carafoli

Laboratory of Biochemistry
Swiss Federal Institute of Technology (ETH)
8092 Zürich Switzerland

INTRODUCTION

The regulation of Ca^{2+} in cells is a complex process, based on the concerted operation of several transport systems located in the plasma membrane and in the intracellular organelles, and on the reversible complexation of Ca^{2+} by soluble cytosolic ligands. The plasma membrane contains a channel for the downhill penetration of Ca^{2+} into the cell from the environment. In excitable cells, the channel is controlled by electrical currents. It also contains 2 systems which are responsible for the pumping of Ca^{2+} out of the cell, a specific ATPase, and a Na^{+}/Ca^{2+} exchanger. Inside cells, Ca^{2+} is transported reversibly by mitochondria and sarco(endo)plasmic reticulum. The former organelle accumulates Ca^{2+} electrophoretically, and releases it through a separate pathway. The latter accumulates Ca^{2+} through a specific ATPase, and releases it through a route which has not yet been identified. The reversible complexation of Ca^{2+} in the cytosol involves the participation of low M_r ligands (e.g., phosphate, adenine nucleotides) and of proteins. Many Ca^{2+}-binding proteins have been described in different cells, e.g., troponin-C, parvalbumin. One which has attracted considerable attention in recent times is calmodulin, a small M_r protein which mediates the interaction of Ca^{2+} with several of its soluble and membrane-bound target enzymatic activities. The schema of Figure 1 summarizes the general concepts of intracellular Ca^{2+} regulation presented in this Introduction. In this paper, however, the discussion will be focused essentially on the pumping systems of the plasma membrane, a field where considerable advances have recently been made. The transport of Ca^{2+} by the intracellular organelles has been extensively reviewed in recent publications (Bygrave,

1978; Carafoli and Crompton, 1978) to which the interested reader is referred.

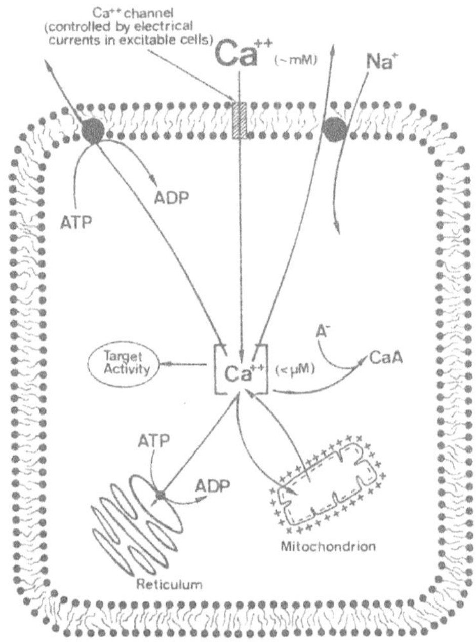

Fig. 1. A scheme of the calcium transporting systems in cells.

THE Ca^{2+}-PUMPING ATPase OF THE PLASMA MEMBRANE

Discovered by Schatzmann and Vincenzi in 1969, this enzyme has recently been purified to homogeneity in a functionally active state from the membrane of erythrocytes (Niggli et al., 1979). The breakthrough which lead to the isolation of the pure enzyme was the discovery that calmodulin activated the pumping of Ca^{2+} into inverted erythrocyte ghosts (Gopinath and Vincenzi, 1977; Jarrett and Penniston, 1977), due to the direct interaction of calmodulin with the Ca^{2+} pumping ATPase. The conclusion was based on the finding (Niggli et al., 1979) that calmodulin was still active on a crude preparation of the Ca^{2+} ATPase solubilized from the membrane by detergents. A calmodulin-affinity chromatography column was thus used as a method of isolation: after extensive washing of the column with excess Ca^{2+}, chelation of Ca^{2+} in the column with EDTA (EGTA) removed a minor protein component enriched in Ca^{2+}-ATPase at least 350 fold with respect to the original ghost material, (Niggli et al, 1979). SDS polyacrylamide gel electrophoresis of the EDTA-eluted peak showed a major monomer of M_r 138,000 and variable propertions of a component having M_r in excess of 200,000

Both components formed acid-labile phosphorylated intermediates upon incubation with ATP, a finding suggesting the existence of mono and dimeric forms of the ATPase.

Some of the most important properties of the purified ATPase are collected in Table 1 (Niggli et al., 1981, a,b; Graf et al., submitted).

Table 1. Properties of the Ca^{2+} pumping ATPase of plasma membranes.

M_r	138,000
Ca^{2+}/ATP stoichiometry	1
K_m	0.4μM
V_{max}	21μMoles ATP per mg of protein per min
Activated by	calmodulin, acidic phospholipids, fatty acids, limited proteolysis
Inhibited by	vanadate
Charge balance	Electroneutral

The high affinity of the ATPase for Ca^{2+} is only seen in the presence of calmodulin: in its absence, the enzyme shifts to a low affinity form (K_m 10μM). Surprisingly, however, the transition from the low to the high affinity form can be induced in the absence of calmodulin by presenting to the purified enzyme an environment of acidic phospholipids or polyunsaturated fatty acids (Niggli et al., 1981 b). Activation of the purified enzyme (i.e., transition to the high affinity form) in the absence of calmodulin can be induced also by a limited proteolytic treatment (Niggli et al., 1981 b) which results in the removal from the enzyme of a polypeptide having M_r of 30-50,000 (Sarkady et al., 1980; Graf et al., submitted).

The purified enzyme can be reconstituted into liposomes. Depending on whether the liposomes do or do not contain acidic phospholipids the reconstituted enzyme exhibits high or low affinity for Ca^{2+} in the absence of calmodulin. The reconstituted enzyme pumps Ca^{2+} with a 1 to 1 stoichiometry to the ATP hydrolyzed: this can be contrasted with the case of the Ca^{2+}-pumping ATPase of sarcoplasmic reticulum, which has a Ca/ATP stoichiometry of 2.

A Ca^{2+}-pumping ATPase has recently been identified in heart sarcolemma (Caroni and Carafoli, 1980). The finding is of interest since it was generally accepted that excitable cells eject Ca^{2+}

through the Na^+/Ca^{2+} exchange, and not (also) through a Ca^{2+}-pumping ATPase. The heart sarcolemma ATPase pumps Ca^{2+} with high affinity (K_m 0.4μM) but at a relatively slow rate (15nmol Ca^{2+} per mg of protein per min). The enzyme is calmodulin-sensitive, and has now been purified on a calmodulin affinity chromatography column (Caroni and Carafoli 1981 a). It is very similar, in its essential properties, to the analogous erythrocyte enzyme. Interestingly, it is regulated also by a phosphorylation-dephosphorylation process which involves c-AMP (Caroni and Carafoli, 1981 b).

ATP-dependent Ca^{2+} pumping systems have recently been described also in other cells: nerve (Di Polo, 1978; Di Polo and Beaugé 1979) corpus luteum (Verma and Penniston 1981) macrophages (Lew and Stossel 1980), adipocytes (Pershadsingh and McDonald, 1980) synaptosomes (Itano and Penniston, personal communication). When measured, the affinity of the enzyme for Ca^{2+} has been found to be high (K_m,< 1μM), and in adipocytes, macrophages and synaptosomes, calmodulin has been found to stimulate. The adipocyte ATPase has been shown to be inhibited by physiological concentrations of insulin (Pershandingh and McDonald, 1979), suggesting that the action of insulin may by related to the regulation of the cellular Ca^{2+} homeostasis.

THE Na^+/Ca^{2+} EXCHANGER OF PLASMA MEMBRANES

The Na^+/Ca^{2+} exchanger has long been known as a system for Ca^{2+} extrusion in excitable tissues (Reuter and Seitz, 1968; Baker et al., 1969; Blaustein and Hodgkin, 1969), and can now be studied on isolated vesicles of heart sarcolemma (Reeves and Sutko, 1978). This simplified system has produced important information on the properties of the exchanger. It has now been established (Pitts, 1979; Caroni et al., 1980; Reeves and Sutko, 1980) that the carrier operates electrogenically with a probable stoichiometry of 3 Na^+ per 1 Ca^{2+}. Charge compensation *in vivo* probably occurs by movements of Cl^- together with Na^+, and/or by movements of K^+ in the same direction as Ca^{2+}.

The exchanger operates with a lower affinity for Ca^{2+} than the Ca^{2+}-pumping ATPase (K_m 1.5μM, Caroni et al., 1980), but its maximal pumping velocity is much higher (up to 20 nmoles per mg of protein per sec). This suggests that the system could become active whenever massive amounts of Ca^{2+} must be transported rapidly out of the cell. ATP has been found to stimulate the exchange of Na^+ for Ca^{2+} in axonal membranes (Baker and Glitsch, 1973; Baker and McNaughton, 1976), and, recently in heart sarcolemmal vesicles (Reinlib et al. 1981). The Na^+/Ca^{2+} exchanger appears to be calmodulin insensitive (Caroni et al, 1980), and is not inhibited by vanadate at concentrations which abolish the Ca^{2+}-ATPase completely (Caroni et al., 1980). Whether the Na^+/Ca^{2+} exchanger exists also in the plasma membrane of non-excitable cells is an open problem. Recent work (Famulski and Carafoli, 1982) indicates that the exchanger may exist in liver plasma membranes.

THE TRANSPORT OF Ca^{2+} IN THE INTRACELLULAR ORGANELLES: A SYNTHETIC SURVEY

Mitochondria

The 2 organelles which handle Ca^{2+} within cells are mitochondria and endoplasmic reticulum (sarcoplasmic reticulum in muscle cells). The properties of the mitochondrial Ca^{2+} uptake system have been established in a long series of studies carried out in a number of Laboratories since the early sixties (for a recent review, see Carafoli, 1982) and are summarized in Table 2. Of particular interest is the affinity of mitochondria for Ca^{2+}, which is now accepted to be expressed by a K_m of between about 2 and about 13μM, depending on the tissue.Mitochondria thus appear capable of buffering Ca^{2+} in a concentration range that lies at the upper border of that presumably existing in most cells. Recent studies of Lehninger (1982) and Nicholls (1981) have shown that the "set-point" at which well coupled mitochondria can maintain extermal (cytosolic) Ca^{2+} is 0.5μM.

Table II The electrophoretic Ca^{2+} uptake by mitochondria

Energy requirements	Respiration or ATP
Inhibitors	Ruthenium red, lanthanides (max. Tm^{3+})
V_{max} (25°)	up to 10nmoles per mg prot. per sec.
Rate at 1μM Ca^{2+}, and 1mM external Mg^{2+} (25°)	0.06nmoles per mg prot. per sec.
K_m (Ca^{2+})	2 - 13μM in different tissues
Tissue specificity	Practically all tissues (exceptions: blowfly flight muscle, yeast)
Mechanism	Electrophoretic, charge uncompensated

A development which has recently generated considerable interest is the finding that mitochondria possess separate routes for Ca^{2+} influx and efflux (Carafoli and Crompton, 1976). Ca^{2+} is thus maintained in mitochondria in a dynamic steady state and is continuously "cycled" across the inner membrane (Carafoli, 1979). The existence of separate uptake and release routes is clearly advantageous from the standpoint of the regulation of extramitochondrial Ca^{2+}, and offers additional possibilities for the control of the transport process. Several mechanisms for the release of the accumulated Ca^{2+} have been described, but only one, a specific Na^+ Ca^{2+} exchange, has been characterized in sufficient detail (Carafoli et al., 1974; Crompton et al., 1976). It appears clear from recent research that mitochondria can be divided in 2 categories, those which release Ca^{2+} in response to Na^+ and those which do not.

The most important properties of the Na^+ induced Ca^{2+} release process are summarized in Table 3.

Table III The Na^+ induced release of mitochondria $Ca2+$

Energy requirements	Faster in energized mitochondria
Inhibitors	Lanthanides (max.La^{3+})
V_{max} (25°)	up to 0.25nmoles per mg prot.per sec
Rate at 1µM Ca^{2+}, and 1mM external Mg^{2+} (25°)	up to 0.25nmoles per mg prot.per sec
K_m (Ca^{2+}- Ca^{2+} exchange)	13µM
K_m (Na^+)	6mM
Tissue specificity	Highest in heart, brain, adrenal cortex, negligible in liver, kidney, lung
Mechanism	Electroneutral

Of interest is the fact that the release is activated half-maximally by about 6mM external Na^+, a value very close to the concentration of ionized Na^+ present in the cytoplasm (Lee and Fozzard, 1975) and the fact that the velocity of Ca^{2+} release is linked to the concentration of external Na^+ by a pronounced sigmoidal releationship. These findings suggest that the process may play an important role in the regulation of the Ca^{2+} balance between mitochondria and the cytosol: indeed, even minor variations of the Na^+ concentration in the ambient surrounding mitochondria could induce a considerable release of Ca^{2+} from the very large reservoir present in the organelles.

As mentioned, some mitochondria are insensitive to Na^+, or only marginally sensitive to it. For them, the activation of the Ca^{2+} releasing process has been suggested to involve alternative mechanisms. Among them, the transition of the redox state of mitochondrial pyridine nucleotides towards increased oxidation, the addition of inorganic phosphate, the addition (or endogenous production) of long chain polyunsaturated fatty acids (see Carafoli, 1982 for a recent review of the problem). At the moment, it is not clear whether any of these Ca^{2+} releasing mechanisms is physiologically significant.

Sarcoplasmic and endoplasmic reticulum

Sarcoplasmic reticulum accumulates Ca^{2+} by way of a specific ATPase, which operates with a very high affinity for Ca^{2+} (K_m, $< 1 \mu M$). During the transport of Ca^{2+}, an acid labile phosphorylated intermediate of the ATPase is formed. Rapid kinetic techniques have permitted to detect many intermediary steps of the transport cycle. The reaction sequence presently favored by most investigators consits of seven steps, during which the enzyme undergoes a conformational change which is supposed to be responsible for the translocation of the Ca^{2+} binding sites to a space no longer accessible to the outer medium. Ca^{2+} is then discharged to the intravesicular space, the overall stoichiometry between ATP hydrolyzed and Ca^{2+} translocated being 0.5.

The ATPase molecule has a M_r of about 105,000, and has been purified and reconstituted in several Laboratories (see De Meis and Inesi, 1982, for a comprehensive review). A recent development of considerable interest is the discovery that the Ca^{2+} ATPase (and the associated Ca^{2+} pumping) are stimulated in heart sarcoplasmic reticulum (Katz and Remtulla, 1978; Le Peuch et al., 1979) by calmodulin. The work by Le Peuch et al., (1979) has shown that the stimulation is not due to the direct interaction of calmodulin with the ATPase, but to a kinase-mediated phosphorylation of a hydrophobic protein of the sarcoplasmic reticulum membrane, phospholamban (Tada et al., 1975). Phospholamban, then, activates the pumping ATPase. Le Peuch et al. (1979) have found that phospholamban is also phosphorylated by a c-AMP-dependent kinase; the two systems, that controlled by calmodulin, and that controlled by c-AMP, apparently operate in parallel. Recent work by Chiesi and Carafoli (1982) has shown that calmodulin is present also in skeletal muscle sarcoplasmic reticulum. Here, however, it may have a different mechanism of action.

One aspect of the transport of Ca^{2+} by sarcoplasmic reticulum that is still obscure is the mechanism by which Ca^{2+} is released. There is no doubt that Ca^{2+} must be released from the vesicels of sarcoplasmic reticulum upon muscle excitation to activate the contraction of the myofibrils. Much research has been devoted to this aspect of the problem, but at the present moment no physiologically plausible mechanism is known.

That endoplasimc reticulum can actively transport Ca^{2+} is now well documented (for a review see Carafoli and Crompton, 1978). The uptake process is probalby similar, in mechanism and regulation, to that of sarcoplasmic reticulum. The total Ca^{2+} loading capacity of endoplasmic reticulum is probably low, but its affinity for Ca^{2+} is high. The studies of Lehninger (1982) and of Nicholls (1981) mentioned in the chapter on mitochondria have shown that endoplasmic reticulum can maintain cytosolic Ca^{2+} at a "set-point" of 0.2μM (as compared to 0.5μM for the case of mitochondria).

CONCLUDING COMMENTS

It has emerged from the preceeding sections that the regulation of intracellular Ca^{2+} is a complex process, which requires the cooperation of various membrane transport systems. One aspect of the problem of intracellular Ca^{2+} homeostasis which was mentioned only in passing in the Introduction of the paper is the role of soluble Ca^{2+} ligands. Of them, calmodulin is undoubtedly the most interesting, not only because of its possible function as a cytosolic Ca^{2+} reservoir, but especially because it activates the pumping of Ca^{2+} by systems located in the plasma membrane, in endoplasmic reticulum, in sarcoplasmic reticulum. It is an easy prediction that the role of calmodulin as a central regulator of the homeostasis of Ca^{2+} in cells will receive increasing attention in the near future.

Whether the contribution of the various membrane transport systems described to the regulation of cellular Ca^{2+} is the same in all cell types is an open problem. Several lines of evidence seem to indicate that this is not the case: the Ca^{2+} transporting ability of sarcoplasmic reticulum in fast muscles is higher than in slow muscles and heart, the Na^{+}-promoted Ca^{2+} releasing route is <u>not</u> active in liver and kidney mitochondria, the permeability of the plasma membrane for Ca^{2+} is certainly lower in erythrocytes than in muscle.

Another important problem is that of the hormonal regulation of the movements of Ca^{2+} across the plasma membrane and in the different cell compartments. The c-AMP-protein kinase system influences (see above) the transporting systems in the plasma membrane and in endo- and sarcoplasmic reticulum. The mitochondrial transporting system has also been indicated as a possible target of hormones like glucagon (Hughes and Barritt, 1977) and insulin (Dorman et al., 1975). Thr problem of whether mitochondrial Ca^{2+} responds to α-adrenergic stimulation is still open (Chen et al., 1978; Blackmore et al., 1978; Blackmore et al., 1979; Althaus-Salzmann et al., 1980).

Table 4. An integrated view of the transport of Ca^{2+} in heart cells.

Membrane system	Ca^{2+} transporting area of heart cells		Ca^{2+} uptake					
			at 10µM Ca^{2+}			at 1µM Ca^{2+} + 1-3mM Mg^{2+}		
	m^2/gm	% of total area (a)	rate (b) (nmol/mg prot./sec)	"total "uptake(a x b)	%of total uptake	rate (b) (nmol/mg prot./sec)	"total" uptake (a x b)	% of total uptake
Sarcolemma	0.10	0.8						
Ca^{2+} ATPase			1.5	1.2	0.4	1.5	1.2	0.7
Na^+/Ca^{2+} exchange			20	16	3.1	10	8	4.9
Sarcoplasmic reticulum	1.5	12.1	20	242	46.5	12	145	88
Mitochondria	10.6	87	3	261	50	0.12	10.4	6.3

The data on the relative distribution of the Ca^{2+}-transporting membrane area are taken from Carafoli and Crompton (1978). For mitochondria, only the inner membrane has been considered. Uptakes are given at 38°. In the case of mitochondria, the rates given by Carafoli and Crompton (1978) have been doubled, on the assumption that the inner membrane represents 50 % of the total protein of heart mitochondrial preparations. For sarcoplasmic reticulum, the rates have been calculated from the data given by Will et al.(1976). The following additional assumption have been made: a) that the degree of contamination of all preparations with extraneous organelles is the same; b) that the protein content for unit of membranes areas is the same in all organelles (from Carafoli et al., 1982).

An integrated picture of the quantitative contribution of the various membrane transporting systems to the overall process of intracellular Ca^{2+} control requires that the kinetic parameters of the transporting systems located in the various membranes be known. It also requires knowledge of the percentage of the total Ca^{2+} transporting area of the cell present in the various membranes. At the moment, this information is only available for the case of heart, and has indeed been used to construct a comprehnsive picture of the process of heart Ca^{2+} homeostasis (Carafoli et al., 1982). The essence of it is that the bulk of intracellular Ca^{2+}, particularly at the low sarcoplasmic levels prevailing under "physiological" conditions, is handled by sarcoplasmic reticulum. Mitochondria play a supporting role, which becomes increasingly important under conditions in which the level of sarcoplasmic Ca^{2+} increases significantly. The plasma membrane, on the other hand, transports only a minor proportion of the total Ca^{2+} handled by heart cells ("trigger" Ca^{2+}).

ACKNOWLEDGEMENTS

The work has been made possible by the financial contribution of the Swiss Nationalfonds (Grant no. 3.634-0.80).

REFERENCES

Althaus-Salzmann, M., Carafoli, E., and Jakob, A.1980 Eur.J.Biochem. 106, 241 - 248.

Baker, P.F., Blaustein, M.P. Hodgkin, A.C. and Steinkardt, R.A. 1969, J.Physiol. (London) 200, 431 - 458.

Baker, P.F., and Glitsch, H.G. 1973 J.Physiol.(London) 233, 43P - 44P.

Baker, P.F., and McNaughton, P.A. 1976 J.Physiol.(London) 259, 103 - 144.

Blackmore, P.F., Dehaye, J.P., and Exton,J.H. 1979 J.Biol.Chem. 253, 4851 - 4858.

Blaustein, M.P., and Hodgkin, A.C. 1969 J.Physiol.(London) 200, 497 - 527.

Bygrave, F.L. 1977 Current Topics in Bioenerg.

Carafoli, E., and Crompton, M. 1978 Current Topics in Membr. and Transport 10, 151 - 216.

Carafoli, E. 1982 in "Membrane Transport of Calcium" E. Carafoli, ed.Acad.Press, New York, in press.

Carafoli, E., and Crompton, M. 1976 Symp.Soc.Exptl.Biol. 30, 89 - 115
Carafoli, E. 1979 FEBS Letters 104, 1 - 5
Carafoli, E., Tiozzo, R., Luger, G., Crovetti, F., and Kratzing, C. 1974 J.Molec.Cell.Cardiol. 6, 361 - 371.
Carafoli, E., Caroni, P., Chiesi, M, and Famulski, R. 1982 in "Metabolic Compartmentation" H. Sies, ed. Acad.Press, New York in press.
Caroni, P., and Carafoli, E. 1980 Nature 283, 765 - 767.
Caroni, P., Reinlib, L., and Carafoli, E. 1980 Proc.Natl.Acad.Sci., USA 77, 6354 - 6358.
Chen, J.L.J., Babcock, D.F., and Lardy, H.A. 1978 Proc.Natl.Acad. Sci, USA 75, 2234 - 2238.
Chiesi, M., and Carafoli, E. 1982 J.Biol.Chem. in press.
Crompton, M., Capano, M., and Carafoli, E. 1976 Eur.J.Biochem. 69, 453,- 462.
DeMeis, L., and Inesi, G. 1982 in "Membrane Transport of Calcium" E.Carafoli, ed., Acad.Press, New York, in press.
DiPolo, R. 1978 Nature 274, 390 - 392.
DiPolo, R., and Beauge, L. 1979 Nature 278, 271 - 273.
Dorman, D.M., Barritt, G.J., and Beaugé , F.L. 1975 Biochem.J. 50, 389 - 395.
Famulski, K., and Carafoli, E., submitted.
Gopinath, R.M., and Vincenzi, F.F. 1977 Biochem.Biophys.Res.Commun. 77, 1203 - 1209.
Graf, E., Verma, A.K., Gorski, J., Lopaschuk, G., Niggli, V., Zurini, M., Carafoli, E., and Penniston, J.T. submitted.
Hughes, B.P., and Barritt, G.J., 1977 Proc.Austr.Biochem.Soc. 10, 36 - 45.
Jarrett, H.W., and Penniston, J.T. 1977 Biochem.Biophys.Res.Commun. 77, 1210 - 1216.
Katz, S., and Remtulla, M.A. 1978 Biochem.Biophys.Res.Commun. 83, 1373 - 1379.
Lee, C.O., and Fozzard, H.G. 1975 J.Gen.Physiol. 65, 695 - 708.
Lehninger, A.L. 1982 in "Calcium and Phosphate Transport Across Membranes" F.Bronner and M. Peterlik, eds.Acad.Press, New York, in press.
Le Peuch, C.J., Haiech, J., and Demaille, S.G. 1979 Biochemistry 18, 5150 - 5157.
Lew, P.D., and Stossel, T.P. 1980 J.Biol.Chem. 255, 5841 - 5846.
Nicholls, D.G. 1982 in "Calcium and Phosphate Transport Across Membranes" F. Bronner and M.Peterlik, eds.Acad.Press, New York in press.
Niggli, V., Penniston, J.T., and Carafoli, E. 1979 J.Biol.Chem. 254, 9955 - 9958.
Niggli, V., Ronner, P., Carafoli, E., and Penniston, J.T. 1979 Arch.Biochem.Biophys. 198, 124 - 130.
Niggli, V., Adunyah, E.S., Penniston, J.T., and Carafoli, E. 1981a J.Biol.Chem. 256, 395 - 401.

Niggli, V., Adunyah, E.S., and Carafoli, E. 1981b J.Biol.Chem. 256, 8588 - 8592.
Pershadsingh, H.A., and McDonald, J.M. 1980 J.Biol.Chem. 255, 4087 - 4093.
Pershadsingh, H.A., and McDonald, J.M. 1979 Nature, 281, 495 - 497.
Pitts, B.J.R. 1979 J.Biol.Chem. 254, 6232 - 6235.
Reeves, J.P., and Sutko, J.L. 1979 Proc.Natl.Acad.Sci, U.S.A. 590 - 594.
Reinlib, L., Caroni, P., and Carafoli, E. 1981 FEBS Letters 126, 74 - 76.
Reuter, H., and Seitz, N. 1968 J.Physiol.(London) 195, 451 - 470.
Sarkady, B., Enyedi, A., and Gardos, G. 1980 Cell Calcium 1, 287 - 297.
Schatzmann, H.J., and Vincenzi, F.F. 1969 J.Physiol(London) 201, 369 - 335.
Tada, M., Kirchberger, M.A., Repke, D.I., and Katz, A.M. 1974 J.Biol.Chem. 249, 6174 - 6180.
Verma, A.K., and Penniston, J.T. 1981 J.Biol.Chem. 256, 1269 - 1275.
Will, H., Blanck, J., Smettan, G., and Wollenberger, A., 1976 Biochim.Biophys.Acta 449, 295 - 303.

CALCIUM AS INTRACELLULAR MESSENGER IN HORMONE ACTION

Howard Rasmussen

Yale University School of Medicine
333 Cedar Street
New Haven, Ct. 06510

Over the past 15 years, our knowledge has grown in two related fields: cellular calcium metabolism and calcium as intracellular messengers (1,2). This knowledge presents us with an apparent paradox. On the one hand is the evidence that the cell has developed an elaborate set of mechanisms for keeping intracellular calcium constant, and on the other that the cell employs changes in cytosolic calcium ion concentration to convey information from its surface to its interior. The paradox is how it can accomplish the latter in the face of the former.

In attempting to answer this question, I shall begin by reviewing briefly the salient facts about cellular calcium metabolism. Then, with these as background, I will consider how Ca^{2+} functions as an intracellular messenger. What I hope to convince you of is that Ca^{2+} is a nearly universal messenger in coupling stimulus to response, that severe constraints are placed on the manner in which it serves this function without causing cell dysfunction, and, that as usual nature has solved this apparent paradox simply and elegantly. Finally, I shall briefly discuss the relationship of the messenger function of Ca^{2+} with that of cAMP. My purpose will be to present the thesis that calcium and cAMP nearly always functions as dual or synarchic messengers in regulating cell function.

CELLULAR CALCIUM METABOLISM

The facts about calcium and cells are dramatic, but not widely appreciated (1). The place to start our consideration of

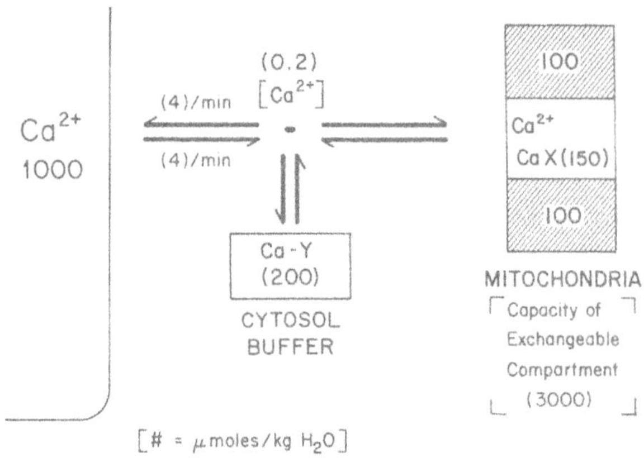

Figure 1.

these facts is with the calcium ion concentration in the cell cytosol (Fig. 1). This is normally in the range of 0.2 μM (2×10^{-7} M). In contrast, the calcium ion concentration in the extracellular fluids surrounding the cell is 1.0 mM (1×10^{-3} M). Thus, there is a 5000-fold concentration gradient of calcium ion across the plasma membrane of the typical mammalian cell (Fig. 1). This is truly a dramatic difference (1). Compare this with the case of Na^+, 15 mM inside, 150 mM outside, or a 10-fold difference in concentration. Two questions are immediately obvious, how and why.

The how is fairly clear. It depends upon three processes in the plasma membrane (1). First, the membrane is not very permeable to Ca^{2+} so that the rate Ca^{2+} enters the cell is normally quite slow, 4 μmoles/kg cell H_2O/minute. However, it is appreciable when one considers the cytosolic calcium ion pool is probably about 0.2 μmole/kg cell H_2O. Hence, the size of this pool would increase dramatically if there were not efficient mechanism for pumping calcium back out of the cell. Two such mechanisms are known. First, Na^+-Ca^+ exchange in which extracellular Na^+ exchanges for intracellular Ca^{2+} (1). This is a process of so-called secondary active transport in which the energy of the Na^+ gradient is used to drive the active transport of Ca^{2+}. Second, a specific Ca^{2+}-dependent-ATPase or pump in which ATP hydrolysis is employed to drive Ca^{2+} out of the cell against its electrochemical gradient.

These two active transport processes are highly efficient, have a considerably greater capacity than 4 µmoles/kg cell H_2O/min, and are, therefore of key importance in maintaining $[Ca^{2+}]_c$ constant. However, there are two other processes which also serve this function. The first is a poorly defined cytosolic buffer system (1). Even though $[Ca^{2+}]_c$ is 0.2 µM, the total calcium content of the cytosol is 50-150 µM (Figure 1). This means over 99 percent of the cytosolic calcium exists in some non-ionic but exchangeable form, and serves a very direct buffering function. The second is an efficient active calcium pump in the inner mitochondrial membrane (Fig. 1). This has an enormous capacity to pump calcium out of the cytosol, and its activity increases as a direct function of $[Ca^{2+}]_c$ so that the slightest rise in $[Ca^{2+}]_c$ leads to a significant increase in mitochondrial calcium uptake. Thus, we can recognize both passive (cytosolic) and an active (mitochondrial) intracellular buffer systems which function to keep $[Ca^{2+}]_c$ constant in the face of sudden alterations in net calcium flux across the plasma membrane.

The why of this elaborate arrangement also appears clear. It was an evolutionary necessity for cells whose energy metabolism is based on a phosphate bond economy. The historical evidence suggests that when the phosphate bond economy developed in the primordial sea, the $[Ca^{2+}]$ was low, but over eons the $[Ca^{2+}]$ of the sea rose to a point where many cellular phosphate esters would precipitate. Hence, it became necessary to exclude calcium from the intracellular soup. In developing an efficient mechanism for accomplishing this task, the cell also exploited the ultimate consequence, the calcium gradient across its membrane, as a means of transferring information from the cell surface to cell interior (2,9). Nonetheless, in doing so, it was necessary to avoid the accumulation of excessive calcium because we now know that excess intracellular calcium is toxic to the cell (10,11). Any process which increases the calcium permeability of the plasma membrane of the cell has a potentially lethal consequence to that cell. In spite of the obvious importance of this aspect of cell calcium, there is only scant information as to the capacity of the cell to handle a calcium load. Based on the available information, it appears, as might be expected, that the mitochondria serve as the main repository of excess Ca^{2+} and that they can continue to function when the exchangeable pool of calcium (largely as a phosphate salt) in the mitochondria increases from 150 to 6000 µmoles/kg H_2O (11,12). This is a 40-fold increase in calcium content, a sizeable safety factor. Nonetheless, as shown by Fleckenstein (11) normal cardiac cells can develop calcium intoxication and die if treated with massive doses of the catecholamine, isoproterenol, for several hours.

The remarkable feature of cellular calcium metabolism in relationship to the intracellular messenger function of calcium is that this ion is employed as an intracellular messenger in the action of many hormones and neurotransmitters without inducing obvious dysfunction of the target cell (2,9). How this is accomplished is the next part of our story.

CALCIUM AS MESSENGER

A useful framework within which to consider the messenger function of Ca^{2+} is that of hormone action as a process of information transfer (2). In this process, one can recognize at least seven sequential steps: 1) recognition of the extracellular messenger by a specific receptor on the cell surface; 2) transduction of this message within the plasma membrane into an intracellular message; 3) transmission of this second message to the cell interior; 4) reception of the intracellular messenger by a specific receptor protein; 5) modulation of the function of response elements by the messenger-receptor complex; 6) response of these elements, and 7) termination of the message.

Dissection of cellular response in terms of these seven steps is applicable to either the Ca^{2+} or cAMP messenger system (6). The basis of each of these steps in each of these systems has been discussed in detail elsewhere (6). The key focus of the present discussion is upon the steps of reception, modulation and response in the Ca^{2+} messenger system.

There are several calcium receptor proteins all of which have an homologous structure (2). The most universal and widely studied is calmodulin (2). Its role in reception, modulation and response will be considered as representative of this class of proteins.

In currently accepted models of cell activation, a rise in the cytosolic concentration of free Ca^{2+} is thought to initiate response by binding to calmodulin. In this view, it is assumed that in the resting cell the $[Ca^{2+}]_c$ is below the level of detectability of calmodulin, and that in the activated cell the $[Ca^{2+}]_c$ rise sufficiently to saturate some or all of the calcium binding sites on calmodulin thereby inducing a conformational change which allows calmodulin to bind to response elements and initiate a response.

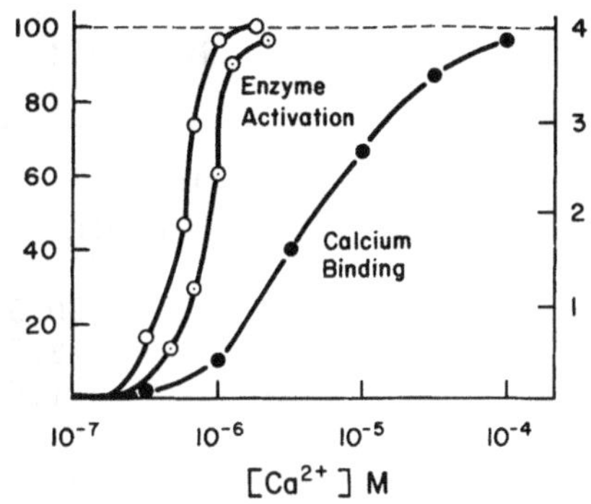

Fig. 2. A plot of binding of calcium to free calmodulin as a function of calcium ion concentration (o——o) (13), and a plot of the calcium-dependent activation of two calmodulin regulated enzymes, the calcium pump in the plasma membrane (●——●) (22), and phosphodiesterase (o——o) (15). These data show that in the presence of a response element (either phosphodiesterase or the calcium pump) the affinity of calcium for calmodulin is markedly enhanced, and highly cooperative.

A plot of calcium binding to calmodulin as a function of the [Ca^{2+}] is shown in Figure 2. These data indicate that free calmodulin binds little calcium when the [Ca^{2+}]is below 5 µM (5x 10^{-6} M)and is fully saturated (4 calciums/mole) when the [Ca^{2+}] is above 100 µM (13). Based on the above model these data would predict that in the resting cell the $[Ca^{2+}]_c$ would be 5 µM and that it would rise to 20-50 µM in the activated state. However, this would present an enormous problem to the cell in terms of the mitochondrial uptake of Ca^{2+} and the load of Ca^{2+} required to maintain the activated state (Table 1).

Table 1 Estimated Cellular Calcium Fluxes at Different Fixed Concentrations of Cytosolic Calcium

$[Ca^{2+}]_c$	(R) 0.2 μM	10 μM	1.0 μM	0.4 μM	(A) 0.3 μM
CELL			FLUX RATE μmoles/kg cell H_2O/min		
Influx	4	100	30	20.5	20.5
Efflux	4	40	24	18.5	18.2
Net	0	60	6.0	1.5	1.8
MITOCHONDRIA					
Influx	0.5	40.5	5.5	1.8	2.0
Efflux	0.5	0.5	0.5	0.5	0.5
Net	0	40.0	5.0	1.3	1.5
CELL DEATH (hrs)	-	1.5	20	75	55

R - Values measured in resting cell; A - Value in activated cell

Fortunately, the system does not operate over this intracellular calcium concentration range. As shown in Figure 2, if the activity of two different calcium-calmodulin modulated enzymes, phosphodiesterase (14-17) and the calcium pump in the plasma membrane (18-20) is plotted as function of $[Ca^{2+}]$, the enzymes are essentially inactive at 0.2 μM Ca^{2+} and fully active at 1.0 μM Ca^{2+}. These are values closer to what is thought to exist within the cell.

MOLECULAR ASPECTS OF MODULATION IN THE Ca^{2+} SYSTEM

There are several possible explanations for the marked difference between the calcium binding curve of calmodulin and the calcium activation curve of phosphodiesterase, a calmodulin activated enzyme, shown in Figure 2. First, it is possible that calmodulin exerts its effect when only 1 or 2 rather than all four calcium binding sites are occupied; second, it is possible that a large excess of calmodulin is present; and third, it is possible that the binding of calcium to calmodulin is influenced in a positively cooperative manner when calmodulin interacts with a response element.

There is no evidence to support the first. On the contrary all present evidence suggests that $Ca_4 \cdot CM$ (calmodulin with all four Ca^{2+} binding sites occupied) is the only form of calmodulin capable of activating capable of activating phosphodiesterase and other response elements (14,15,21).

Both in the _in vitro_ experiments shown in Figure 2, and _in situ_ the concentration of calmodulin greatly exceeds the concentration of response elements. There is approximately 5-10 μM calmodulin, and 0.06 μM phosphodiesterase in a typical cell (22). Hence, one way of enhancing the sensitivity of calcium-calmodulin control is by providing a large molar excess of calmodulin. However, this is not the only way. Equally or of even greater importance, is the evidence that the binding of calcium to calmodulin, and of calmodulin to response elements is an ordered and highly cooperative sequence (14,15,17,21).

From the available data (14-22) it is possible to construct a three step model for the activation of a calmodulin modulated enzyme by Ca^{2+}. Step 1 is the sequential and cooperative binding of two calciums to calmodulin (CM).

Step 1

$$Ca^{2} + CM \rightleftarrows Ca \cdot CM$$

$$Ca^{2+} + CaCM \rightleftarrows Ca_2 \cdot CM$$

The second step is the binding of a response element (RE) to $Ca_2 \cdot$ CM,

Step 2

$$Re + Ca_2 \cdot CM \rightleftarrows Ca_2 \cdot CM \cdot RE$$

and the final step is the binding of the last two calciums leading to the activation of the response element,

Step 3

$$Ca^{2+} + Ca_2 \cdot CM \cdot RE \rightleftarrows Ca_3 \cdot CM \cdot RE$$

$$Ca^{2+} + Ca_3 \cdot CM, RE \rightleftarrows Ca_4 \cdot CM, \cdot RE^*$$

The key features of this arrangement are that the sequence of reactions is ordered, and each ligand binding step enhances the affinity of the next ligand for calmodulin; the first calcium enhances the binding of the second, the binding of the first two calciums greatly enchances the binding of RE to $Ca_2 \cdot CM$, and the binding of RE to $Ca_2 \cdot CM$ enhances the binding of the last two calciums to calmodulin.

There is an extremely important consequence of this arrangement. It is that once the system is activated by a bolus of Ca^{2+}, it will remain activated even though the $[Ca^{2+}]$ falls back toward its basal value. Thus, a transient rise in the $[Ca^{2+}]$ to 1.0 μM will saturate the system, and it will then remain saturated when the $[Ca^{2+}]$ falls back to 0.3-0.4 μM.

AMPLITUDE MODULATION IN THE Ca^{2+} MESSENGER SYSTEM

If we now consider the process of amplitude modulation as it occurs in an idealized cell in response to a hormone, we find that in the resting cell, the $[Ca^{2+}]_c$ is about 0.2 μM, that it rises transiently to 1.0 μM following activation of the cell by the hormone, and then falls back to a value of 0.3-0.4 μM even though the cell remains activated (8,23). Hence, the system behaves in the cell as it does in the test tube.

One important prediction from this behavior is the $[Ca^{2+}]_c$ must fall below its basal or resting values in order for the response to be terminated. From this prediction, it is easy to understand why calmodulin modulates the calcium pump in the plasma membrane (18-20). As long as $Ca_4 \cdot CM \cdot RE^*$ remains high, $Ca_4 \cdot CM \cdot Ca$-ATPase remains high. This arrangement insures that the system can relax back to its resting state rapidly after the activating hormone is removed. However, it puts certain constraints on the cell exhibiting sustained activation. It requires a sustained increase in rate of Ca^{2+} influx into the cell to balance the high rate of efflux. Such a high rate of calcium influx is found in hormonally activated cells exhibiting a sustained response (1-9). In fact, there is net influx under these conditions so there is a net gain of calcium by the cell (9). Most of this extra calcium enters the mitochondria. The fact that the calcium-calmodulin response element complex exhibits ordered, cooperative binding becomes extremely important in determining the magnitude of the net gain in cellular calcium. Based on the known calcium accumulating properties of mitochondria, (1,24,25) it is possible to contrast two situations (Table 1). The the first, a sustained shift in the $(Ca^{2+})_c$ from 0.2 to 1.0 μM would be required to activate the cell and keep it activated over a long period of time. Under this circumstance, there would be a net accumulation of Ca^{2+} into the cell at a rate of 6 μmoles/kg cell H_2O min. This rate would be sufficient to saturate the capacity of the mitochondria to sequester calcium, and thereby lead to cell death within 20 hrs or less. In the second, after an initial rise of $[Ca^{2+}]_c$ to 1.0 μM, the $[Ca^{2+}]_c$ would fall to 0.4 μM and remain at this value during the period of sustained cellular activation. Under this circumstance, the net rate of cellular calcium accumulation would be 1.5 μmoles/kg cell H_2O min, and of mitochondrial calcium accumulation 1.3 μmoles/kg cell H_2O/min. The capacity of the mitochondria to accumulate calcium would not be exceeded for at least 75 hours. It is the latter of the two circumstances which seems to prevail in the Ca^{2+}-activated cell. In other words, the ordered cooperative sequence by which calcium activates calmodulin-regulated enzymes allows the cell to switch from a resting to an activated state by employing a bolus of Ca^{2+} to shift the calmodulin-response element complexes to a state in which they bind Ca^{2+} with a higher affinity. This allows the cell to remain activated when the $[Ca^{2+}]_c$ falls back close to its basal value. This is achieved by having an active mitochondrial calcium pump, and of having the calcium pump in the plasma membrane as a calmodulin response element. This arrangement insures the termination of the response, but requires that during a sustained cellular response the rate of calcium influx remains high. The danger of Ca^{2+} intoxication, posed by this latter property is minimized both by the high rate of calcium efflux and by the fact that the $[Ca^{2+}]_c$ during sustained response is only slightly greater than that found in the resting cell. Viewed in this light, the sustained high rates of calcium cycling across the plasma membrane of the activated cell rather than representing a futile metabolic cycle, are integral aspects of the total process of a calcium-mediated cell activation.

PLASTICITY OF CELLULAR RESPONSE

One additional property of this elegant cellular control device is worthy of comment. Simply by having response elements with differing affinities for $Ca_2 \cdot CM$ (Step 2 in the reaction sequence), one can convert an apparently sterotyped system into a highly plastic one. Under this condition, a small rise in $[Ca^{2+}]_c$ would lead to an activation of only one of several calmodulin-modulated response elements, and a large rise to an activation of all of these response elements. Thus, variable changes in the strength of the extracellular messenger could lead to qualitatively as well as quantitatively different cellular responses depending on the mix of calmodulin response elements activated.

Given this potential for plasticity of response, one might imagine that amplitude modulation is sufficient to meet the operational needs of cellular control devices. However, it appears not to be so. Another form of modulation, <u>sensitivity modulation</u>, can be recognized (1,6). It is of considerable importance in the Ca^{2+} messenger system, and is of particular interest because of the widespread role cAMP playsin this form of modulation in this system (6).

SENSITIVITY MODULATION IN THE CALCIUM MESSENGER SYSTEM

By definition sensitivity modulation is a change in concentration of $Ca_4 \cdot CM \cdot RE^*$ without a change in the $[Ca^{2+}]_c$. The key feature that distinguishes this type of modulation from amplitude modulation is that it is the sensitivity of the response element to the prevailing Ca^{2+} concentration that is altered and not the $[Ca]_c$. Consideration of the reaction sequence involving calcium, calmodulin and their response elements (see above) leads to the conclusion that this could occur either by an increase in calmodulin concentration, an increase in the affinity of calmodulin for the first two calciums, or an increase in the affinity of response element(s) for the complex $Ca_2 \cdot CM$. The last of these appears to be the most important.

If we consider the mechanism of sensitivity modulation in terms of this type of affinity change, we find that a 10-fold increase in the affinity of one response element for $Ca_2 \cdot CM$ would lead to a final $Ca_4 \cdot CM \cdot RE^*$ of 0.025 μM or approximately a 40 percent activation of that particular response element. This would occur without a change in either the calmodulin or calcium concentrations. Nevertheless, calcium is as a necessary reactant in this type of modulation as it is in amplitude modulation.

There are now several well studied examples of this type of modulation in the calcium messenger system. They are all cases in which a rise in [cAMP] leads to the phosphorylation of a component of a calcium-calmodulin modulated response element. In these examples neither the [CM] nor the affinity of CM for the first two calciums are changed. The affinity of $Ca_2 \cdot CM$ for a particular response element is increased, i.e., a covalent modification of the response element alters the apparent affinity of $Ca_2 \cdot CM$ for a response element leading to an increase or decrease in $[Ca \cdot CM \cdot RE^*]$ for that particular response element.

The first specific example of sensitivity modulation is seen in the control of glycogenolysis in skeletal muscle(26,27). The key enzyme in this system is phosphorylase b kinase (Figure 3). This is a multimeric enzyme consisting of four subunits, α, β, γ, δ, of which one, δ , is calmodulin. The γ subunit is the catalytic subunit. Phosphorylation b kinase is a calcium-calmodulin <u>modulated</u> protein kinase. It can be regulated by <u>amplitude modulation</u> when, for example, the calcium ion concentration rises in response to neural stimulation of the muscle. The K_m of activation of the enzyme under these circumstances is 3 μM. It can also be regulated by sensitivity modulation when, for example, the cAMP concentration rises in response to epinephrine. This rise in cAMP activates the cAMP-dependent protein kinase which catalyzes the phosphorylation of the α and β subunits of phosphorylase b kinase. Phosphorylation of these subunits causes a change in its sensitivity to activation by Ca^{2+} from a K_m of 3.0 to one of 0.5 μM (Fig. 3). Such a situation can be characterized as positive sensitivity modulation.

A second example is seen in the contraction of smooth muscle. In the regulation of its contraction and relaxation, the intracellular messengers Ca^{2+} and cAMP act as antagonistic messengers. Contraction is mediated by a rise in $[Ca^{2+}]_c$. This induces an increase in $Ca_2 \cdot CM$ which interacts with the specific response element myosin light chain kinase (MLCK) (28). Phosphorylation of myosin light chain by this calcium-dependent protein kinase initiates the actin-myosin interaction, i.e., contraction. Just as in the phosphorylase system, in this system the calcium-dependent protein kinase (in this case myosin light chain kinase) is a substrate for the cAMP-dependent protein kinase (29-31). However, in contrast to the phosphorylation system, when MLCK becomes phosphorylated by the action of cAMP-dependent protein kinase, its sensitivity to activation by Ca^{2+} decreases (Figure 3). The K_m of Ca^{2+} activation is 0.8 μM for the non-phosphorylation of a protein other than calmodulin alters the interaction of calcium-calmodulin with a response element. However, in this case phosphorylation leads to a decrease in the affinity of calcium for calmodulin, an example of negative sensitivity modulation.

IMPLICATIONS FOR CELLULAR CONTROL

If one considers the examples of phosphorylase b kinase and myosin light chain kinase, the range of $[Ca^{2+}]_c$ necessary to activate calmodulin-sensitive response elements within the cell is from 0.08 to 10 μM (Fig. 3). The implications of these observations go well beyond that of simply underlining the fact that the sensitivity of various response elements to activation by calcium is quite variable. It underscores the previously discussed concept that a given change in the amplitude of a message such as calcium ion will activate different response elements to different extents. Thus, it is possible to envision a graded cellular response. At low external hormone concentrations, the rise in intracellular calcium concentration will activate only a few of several response elements, whereas at high hormone concentrations the greater rise in intracellular calcium concentration will activate many response elements. Furthermore, because the sensitivity of any one response element to activation by calcium-calmodulin can be changed by the action of other hormones, drugs, etc., qualitatively different responses of a particular cell to a particular hormone will occur depending on the history of that particular cell.

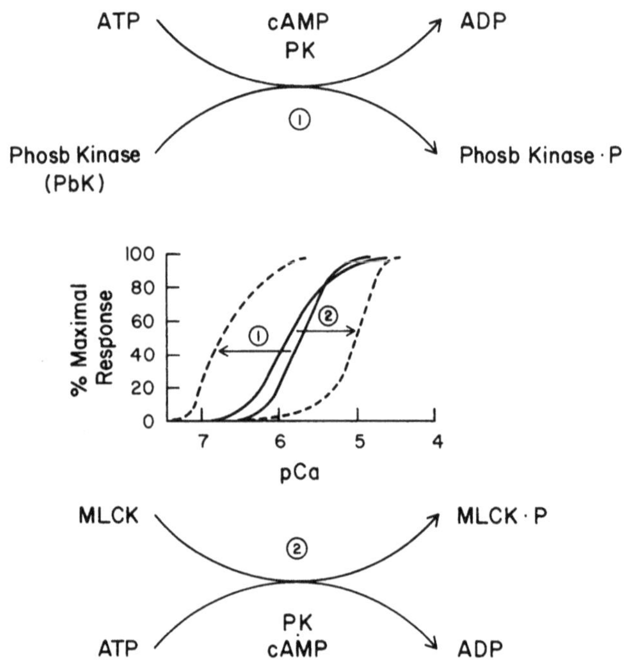

Figure 3. A schematic representation of sensitivity modualtion of the activities of calcium-dependent protein kinases by the cAMP-dependent phosphorylation of these enzymes. The solid lines in the center (above and below the graph) represent the activation of myosin light chain kinase (below), and the activation of phosphorylase b kinase (above). The graph in the center shows that the cAMP-dependent phosphorylation of PbK (1) leads to an increase in sensitivity of PbK to activation by Ca^{2+} (dashed line on left), i.e., an example of positive sensitivity modulation. The cAMP-dependent phosphorylation of myosin light chain kinase (2) leads to a decrease in sensitivity of MLCK to activation by Ca^{2+} (dashed line on right), i.e., an example of negative sensitivity modulation.

AMPLITUDE MODULATION IN THE cAMP MESSENGER SYSTEM

Many of the general features of messenger function in the cAMP messenger system are similar to those in the Ca^{2+} messenger system. One of the most characteristic patterns of change in cAMP concentration is a very rapid but transient rise in [cAMP] to values 3-5 fold above the basal or resting value followed by a fall in [cAMP] during sustained hormonal activation to values only 1.5 fold the basal values seen in the unstimulated cell. (32). Recently it has been shown that during the activation of protein kinase by cAMP the reaction is,

$$4cAMP + R_2C \rightleftarrows 2cAMP_2R + RC$$

$$C + RE \rightleftarrows C{\cdot}RE$$

and that the binding of cAMP to R is a cooperative phenomenon (33). It would thus appear that amplitude modulation in the cAMP messenger system is operationally similar to that in the calcium system, once the system has been shifted from an inactive to an active state, it remains in that state even though the messenger concentration during sustained activation is only slightly above the basal value.

Another similarity between the Ca^{2+} and cAMP messenger system is that cAMP enhances its own termination (hydrolysis) by influencing in a positively cooperative manner the activation of phosphodiesterase (16,17). Also, during sustained hormonal activation when the [cAMP] is back to nearly a basal value, the rate of both cAMP synthesis and hydrolysis are several fold greater than in the unstimulated cell. This increased cycling of messenger is a characteristic of the activated cell whether the messenger is calcium or cAMP.

SYNARCHIC REGULATION

The calcium and cAMP intracellular messenger systems are generally considered as separate or alternative pathways of cell activation by extracellular messengers. This concept persists in spite of detailed and extensive evidence showing that in nearly all animal cells calcium and cAMP act together to regulate cellular response (6). To characterize this nearly universal duality, the term synarchic regulation has been introduced to emphasize their interrelatedness and as a means of focusing attention on the fact that regulation of cell function by dual rather than a single messenger system is the rule rather than the exception (5,6).

The most persuasive evidence in support of the concept of synarchic regulation is that demonstrating interactions between the two systems. These interactions occur at several levels. In many cells, cAMP is involved in either the generation and/or termination of the calcium message. In equally as many, calcium is involved in either the generation and/or termination of the cAMP message. In many circumstances, a cAMP-dependent and a Ca^{2+}-dependent protein kinase catalyze the phosphorylation of the same response element. Most germane to the present discussion is the evidence (discussed above) of their interactions at the step of modulation of cell function. These interactions provide the most elegant molecular evidence in support of the concept of synarchic regulation.

From a consideration of this wealth of evidence, a more adequate model of the actions of either neurotransmitter or

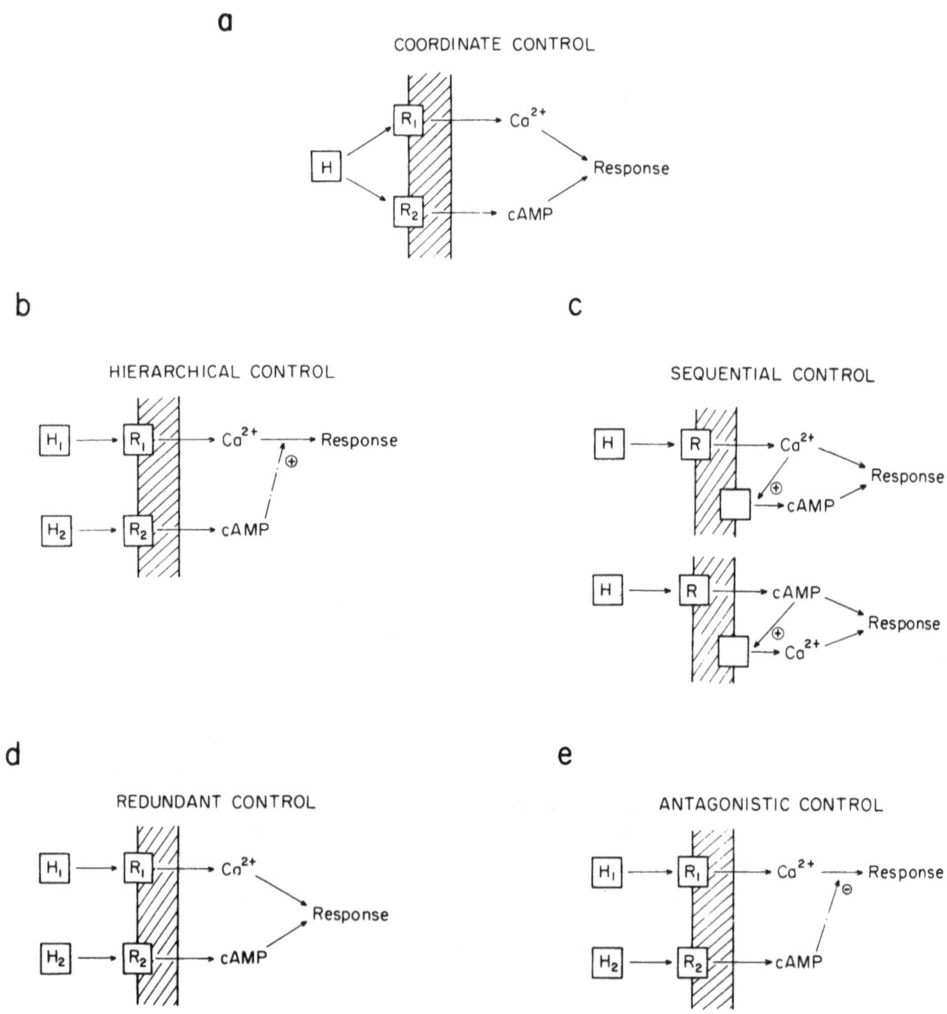

Fig. 4. Patterns of synarchic regulation of cell function in a dual messenger system employing Ca^{2+} and cAMP; a) coordinate, b) hierarchical, c) sequential, d) redundant, and 3) antagonistic control of cell function.

peptide hormone is one in which Ca^{2+} and cAMP function as interrelated messengers in nearly all cells. However, in fulfilling this function the nature of their interaction varies from one cell type to another. It is possible to identify at least five variations on this universal theme: coordinate, hierarchical, redundant, antagonsitic, and sequential (Figure 4).

To coordinate control, the two intracellular messengers are generated simultanteously, and each regulates a critical component of the cellular response. An example is the action of serotonin on fluid and electrolyte secretion in the fly salivary gland.

In hierarchical control, different extracellular messengers or different concentrations of the same messenger, induce the production of the two intracellular messengers, Ca^{2+} and cAMP, and these act in a hierarchical sense. An example in the control of insulin secretion from the beta cell of the Islets of Langerhans. Glucose regulates basal insulin secretion by regulating the calcium messenger system, and glucagon enhances glucose-modulated insulin secretion by enhancing the effect of a given calcium message. It mediates this effect via the generation of intracellular cAMP.

In redundant control, separate extracellular messengers regulate the same cellular process via the separate cAMP and calcium messenger systems. An example is the hormonal control of hepatic gluconeogenesis. Glucagon stimulates this process via the cAMP messenger system; phenylephrine via the Ca^{2+} system.

In antagonistic control, one extracellular messenger acting via the Ca^{2+} system enhances cell response, and another acting via the cAMP system inhibits the calcium mediated response. An example is the contraction of smooth muscle. Acetylcholine induces contraction via the Ca^{2+} messenger system, and epinephrine causes relaxation via the cAMP system.

In sequential control, a single extracellular messenger gives rise to one of the two intracellular messengers, and this intracellular messenger induces a rise in the concentration of the other. An example is the regulation of adrenal medullary secretion by acetylcholine. The interaction of acetylcholine with its receptor initiates the secretory response by increasing the calcium ion concentration in the cell cytosol $[Ca^{2+}]_c$. This increase in $[Ca^{2+}]_c$ produces an activation of adenylate cyclase, and, thereby, an increase in $[cAMP]_c$. This rise in $[cAMP]_c$ is transient because the calcium message also activates phosphodiesterase, the enzyme that catalyzes the hydrolysis of cAMP. Nonetheless, this transient spike of cAMP plays a critically important role in the trophic effects of acetylcholine in this tissue.

CONCLUSION

Major advances in our understanding of cellular calcium metabolism and of the messenger functions of calcium and cAMP in cell activation have led to an appreciation that these two messengers usually function together to regulate cell function. To emphasize this duality of messenger function in the term synarchic regulation has been chosen.

A consideration of messenger function within the synarchic system has led to the distinction between two mechanisms by which these messengers binding to their respective specific intracellular receptor proteins modulate the behavior of specific response elements within the cell. These two mechanisms are that of increasing the amplitude of a particular messenger, or of increasing the sensitivity of activation of a particular response element by a fixed concentration of messenger.

The present discussion of the physiological role of modulation as a critical step in intracellular information transfer leads to the conclusion that there are a large number of discrete cellular processes whose activities are all controlled by the same intracellular messenger via the same intracellular receptor protein each with its distinctive and variable sensitivity to activation by that intracellular messenger. This means that cellular responses, even those that are highly specialized, are not stereotyped but plastic in character, and that this plasticith underlies the organizational elegance of intracellular control.

The characteristics and molecular basis of modulation of cell function by intracellular messengers have been considered. The key molecular feature which underlies modulation is that the messenger receptor proteins possesses two types of ligand binding sites; one for the particular intracellular messenger, and one for a variety of other protein response elements. Binding of ligand to the messenger-binding sites alters protein conformation and, thereby, ligand binding at the other type of site. Likewise, binding of a response element (protein) at the second type of site alters the conformation of the receptor protein and, thereby, the characteristics of the binding interactions between messenger and receptor protein at the first type of site.

Finally, the operation of the calcium messenger in the context of the known properties of cellular calcium metabolism has been discussed. The feature of greatest interest is the very precise coupling of cytosolic events with those occuring at the plasma membrane, and the fashion in which the calcium messenger system functions so as to minimize the danger of excessive cellular calcium accumulation. A particular feature of the calcium messenger system in relationship to cellular calcium metabolism is the apparent paradox arising from two considerations: on the one hand, the cell has developed an extremely elaborate set of mechanisms for maintaining cellular calcium homeostatsis and for keeping the $[Ca^{2+}]_c$ constant; and on the other, it employs changes in the $[Ca^{2+}]_c$ as a major means of communicating information from cell surface to cell interior. The paradox is how it achieves the latter in the face of the former. The present discussion provides a resolution of this paradox and emphasizes that for precise control of cellular response by changes in $[Ca^{2+}]_c$, it is absolutely essential that very elaborate mechanisms exist for regulating the $[Ca^{2+}]_c$ because very small changes in $[Ca^{2+}]_c$ have such profound effects upon cellular behavior. Without these precise controls Ca^{2+} could not serve its messenger function.

REFERENCES

1. Borle, A. (1981) Control, modulation and regulation of cell calcium. Rev. Physiol. Biochem. Pharmacol. 90: 14-152.
2. Rasmussen, H. and Waisman, D.M. (1981) The messenger function of calcium in endocrine systems. Bioch. Actions of Hormones VIII: 1-115.
3. Katz, B. Nerve, Muscle and Synapse. (1966) McGraw-Hill, New York.
4. Douglas, W.W. and Rubin, R.P. (1961) The role of calcium in the secondary response of the adrenal medulla to acetylcholine J. Physiol. London 159: 40-57.
5. Rasmussen, H. (1980) Calcium and cAMP in stimulus-response coupling. Ann. N.Y. Acad. Sci. 356: 346-353.
6. Rasmussen, H. Calcium and cAMP as Synarchic Messengers. John Wiley and Sons, New York (1981).
7. Berridge, M.J. (1975) The interaction of cyclic nucleotides and calcium in the control of cellular activity. Adv. Cyclic Nuc. Res. 6: 1-98.
8. O'Doherty, J., Youmans, S.J., Armstrong, W.McD and Stark, R.J. (1980) Calcium regulation during stimulus-secretion coupling: continuous measurement of intracellular calcium activities. Science 209: 510-513.
9. Borle, A. and Uchikawa, T. (1978) Effects of parathyroid hormone on the distribution and transport of calcium in cultural kidney cells. Endocrinology 102: 1725-1732.
10. Schanne, F.A.X., Kane, A.B., Young, E.E. and Farber, J.L. (1979) Calcium dependence of toxic cell death: A final common pathway. Science 206: 206-208.
11. Fleckenstein, A. (1974) Drug-induced changes in cardiac energy Adv. Cardiol. 12: 183-197.
12. Wrogemann, K. and Pena. S.D.J. (1976) Mitochondrial calcium overload: a general mechanism for cell necrosis in muslce disease. Lancet I: 672:673.

13. Crouch, T.H. and Klee, C.B. (1980) Positive cooperative binding of calcium to bovine brain calmodulin. Biochemistry 19: 3692-3698.
14. Wang, J.H., Sharma, R.K., Huang,C.Y. and Chau, V. and Chock, P.B. (1980) On the mechanism of activation of cyclic nucleotide phosphodiesterase by calmodulin. Ann. N.Y. Acad. Sci. U.S.A. 356: 190-204.
15. Huang, C.Y., Chau, V., Chock, P.B., Wang, J.H. and Sharma, R. K. (1981) Mechanism of activation of cyclic nucleotide phosphodiesterase: requirement of the bindingof four Ca^{2+} to calmodulin for activation. Proc. Natl. Acad. Sci. USA 18: 871-874.
16. Wang, J.H.,Teo, T.S. Ho, H.C. and Stevens, F.C. (1975) Bovine heart protein activator ofcyclic nucleotide phosphodiesterase. Adv. Cyclic Nucl. Res. 5: 179-194.
17. Cheung, W.Y., Lynch. T.J., Wallace, R.W. and Tallant, E.C. (1981) cAMP renders Ca^{2+}-dependent phosphodiesterase refractory to inhibition by a calmodulin-binding protein (calcineuria). J. Biol. Chem. 256: 4439-4443.
18. Penniston, J.T., Graf, E. and Itano, T. (1980) Calmodulin regulation of the Ca^{2+} pump of erythrocyte membranes. Ann. N.Y. Acad. Sci. 356: 245-257.
19. Vincenzi, F.F., Hinds, T.R. and Raess, B.V. (1980) Calmodulin and the plasma membrane calcium pump. Ann. N.Y. Acad. Sci. 256: 233-244.
20. Waisman, D.M., Gimble, J., Goodman, D.B.P. and Rasmussen, H. (1981) Studies of the Ca^{2+} transport mechanism of human inside-out plasma membrane vesicles. 1. Regulation of the Ca^{2+} pump by calmodulin. J. Biol. Chem. 256: 409-414.
21. Blumenthal, D.K. and Stuff, J.T. (1980) Activation of skeletal muscle myosin light kinase by calcium and calmodulin Biochemistry 19: 5608-5614.
22. Scharff, P. (1981) Calmodulin and its role in cellular activation. Cell Calcium 21: 1-28.
23. Berridge, M.J. and Lipke,H. (1979) Changes in calcium transport across Calliphora salivary glands induced by 5-hydroxytryptamine and cyclic nucleotides. J. Exp. Bio. 78: 137-158.
24. Nicholls, D.G. (1978) The regulation of extramitochondrial free calcium ion concentration by rat liver mitochondria. Biochem. J. 1979: 511-522.
25. Murphy, E. Catt, K. Rich, T.L. and Williamson, J.R. (1980). Hormonal effects on calcium homeostasis in isolated hepatocytes. J. Bio. Chem. 255: 6600-6608.
26. Bronstrom, C.O. and Hunkeler, R.L. and Krebs, E.G. (1971). The regulation of skeletal muscle phosphorylase kinase by Ca^{2+}. J. Biol. Chem. 246: 1961-1967.
27. Shenolikar, S., Cohen, P.T.W., Cohen, P. Nairn, A.C. and Perry, S.V. (1979) The role of calmodulin in the structure and regulation of phosphorylase kinase from rabbit skeletal muscle. Eur. J. Biochem. 100: 327-329.

28. Hartshorne,D.J. and Persechini, A.J. (1980) Phosphorylation of myosin as a regulatory component in smooth muscle. Ann. N.Y. Acad. Sci. 356: 130-141.
29. Adelstein, R.S., Conti, M.A. and Pato, M.D., (1980) Regulation of myosin light chain kinase by reversible phosphorylation and calcium-calmodulin. Ann. N.Y. Acad. Sci 356: 142-150.
30. Kerrick, W.G.L., Hoar, P.E. and Cassidy, P.S. (1980) Calcium-activated tension: the role of myosin light chain phosphorylation. Fed. Proc. 39: 1558-1563.
31. Silver, P.J., Holroyde, M.J., Solaro, J. and Disalvo, J. (1981) Ca^{2+}, calmodulin and cyclic AMP-dependent modulation of actin-myosin interactions in aorta. Biochim. Biophys. Acta 674: 65-70.
32. Rasmussen, H. (1970) Cell communication, calcium ion and cyclic adenosine monophosphate. Science 170: 404-412.
33. Smith, S.B., White,H.D., Siegel,J.B. and Krebs, E.G. (1981) Cyclic AMP-dependent protein kinase I: cyclic nucleotide binding, structural changes, and release of catalytic subunits. Proc.Natl. Acad. Sci. USA 78: 1591-1595.

EFFECTS OF DIURETICS ON CALCIUM METABOLISM

Wadi N. Suki

Baylor College of Medicine and The Methodist Hospital
Houston, Texas

INTRODUCTION

In addition to their known effects on sodium metabolism diuretic agents also exert profound effects on calcium metabolism. A substantial body of data bearing on this subject, some of which conflicting, has now accumulated in the literature. The purpose of this review is to discuss the results of studies on the effects of low-ceiling and high-ceiling diuretics on serum calcium, urinary calcium, bone calcium and the transport of calcium in the gut. The review will include studies in normal humans and experimental animals, and during various pathological states.

Changes in the Serum Calcium

Within 2 h after the intravenous administration of chlorothiazide to normal subjects the total and ionized serum calcium concentrations rise only to return to control values 2 h later (1). This effect is not observed in hypoparathyroid patients, but in hyperparathyroid patients the elevation of serum calcium is sustained, and in hypoparathyroid patients the response is restored by the infusion of PTH. These observations suggest that the acute effect of chlorothiazide is dependent upon the presence of PTH and that the elevation in ionized calcium concentration shuts off PTH secretion in normal persons and thereby limits the duration of this phenomenon. The mechanism of this effect is not clear, but it could not have been mediated by changes in urinary calcium since calcium excretion actually rose following chlorothiazide (1), and the effect occurred too soon for it to have been due to changes in intestinal absorption of calcium. More likely it is a PTH-dependent action on bone.

When hydrochlorothiazide is given daily for 25 days to normal subjects both the total and ionized serum calcium concentrations rise and remain elevated (2). The rise in ionized calcium excludes the possibility that the concomitant increase in total serum protein concentration alone is responsible for the rise in total calcium concentration in the serum. Furthermore, PTH concentration in the serum correlated negatively with the ionized calcium concentration, an observation that excludes a role for stimulation of parathyroid hormone in bringing about the rise in calcium. The exact mechanism of this effect on ionized serum calcium is obscure.

A number of observations on the effects of various thiazide diuretics on the serum calcium in pathological states have been reported. It appears that significant elevations of the serum calcium follow the administration of these agents to patients undergoing chronic hemodialysis (3), patients with osteoporosis (4) or hypoparathyroidism receiving vitamin D (5-7), or to patients with hyperparathyroidism (4,7-10). The fact that serum calcium would rise in patients without significant residual renal function, such as in those undergoing hemodialysis (3), or without significant changes in the urine calcium, such as in hypoparathyroid patients (5-7), has led to the suggestion that thiazides exert a PTH or vitamin D-dependent effect on bone. This presumed effect formed the basis for the proposal that thiazides may serve as a provocative test for occult hyperparathyroidism (10). In most of these studies, however, the ultrafilterable or ionized calcium concentrations were not measured and therefore it is difficult to draw absolute conclusions from these observations. When ultrafilterable and ionized calcium concentrations were actually measured in normocalcemic renal stone formers and in hyperparathyroid patients (11) no significant changes were observed although the total calcium did rise. Similar observations of increased total and protein-bound calcium have also been made in hypertensive patients, without evidence of any disturbance in calcium metabolism, who became hypercalcemic while receiving thiazide diuretics (12,13). These observations shed considerable doubt on the usefulness of thiazides as a provocative test for the diagnosis of occult hyperparathyroidism. The prevalence of hypercalcemia among patients treated with thiazides, however, is threefold than in the general population (14) and the majority of those who develop hypercalcemia will be found to have adenomas of the parathyroid glands (14,15). This may be because hyperparathyroidism is often manifested as hypertention or renal stones, two conditions which are frequently treated with thiazides.

Because of the observations that thiazides will raise the serum calcium, we have administered chlorthalidone to hypoparathyroid patients not receiving vitamin D and found that this long-acting thiazide-type diuretic will raise the total and ionized serum calcium into the normal range and sustain this elevation for many months supplemented only with oral calcium preparations (16). Elevations of the serum calcium by thiazides in hypoparathyroid patients has also been observed by other workers (5-7). Whether this effect is brought about by increased intestinal absorption of calcium or by bone resorption has not been established at this time.

The effects of the more potent diuretics, such as ethacrynic acid and furosemide, on the serum calcium are simpler than those of the thiazides. In normal subjects these agents cause only modest reductions or no change in the total or ionized serum calcium (7,17). Apparently, the serum calcium is maintained normal, despite the increased urinary calcium, by the stimulation of parathyroid hormone secretion (17). In the absence of parathyroid hormone, therefore, it may be anticipated that the serum calcium would fall. The development of hypocalcemia in hypoparathyroid patients given furosemide indeed has been reported (18). In hypercalcemic patients, the administration of furosemide intravenously in large doses results in significant and beneficial reductions in the serum calcium (19). This has become now an established method for treating acute symptomatic hypercalcemia.

Changes in Urinary Calcium

The administration acutely of thiazide diuretics to man (1,20) and animals (21,22) results in very small elevations in the urine calcium despite the marked natriuresis that ensues. This is thought to be due to the fact that thiazides inhibit sodium transport in the distal tubule where the absorption of sodium and calcium is dissociated (23). In other studies, however, thiazide diuretics administered acutely resulted in a fall in the urine calcium excretion (24,25). This has been attributed to direct tubular enhancement of calcium absorption (25) and recent studies utilizing free-flow micropuncture and in situ microperfusion clearly show enhanced calcium absorption in the distal convoluted tubule (26). This effect may be explained by increased sodium entry and calcium exit, by a sodium-calcium antiport in the basolateral cell membrane, caused by inhibition with chlorothiazide of sodium absorption in the distal convoluted tubule cells and lowering of intracellular sodium concentration (26). However, other cellular effects of the thiazide diuretics such as stimulation of calcium uptake by renal cortical microsomes may also play a role (27).

The more chronic administration of these drugs significantly reduces the excretion of calcium (28-30), an effect that has been effectively utilized in treating hypercalciuric stone formers (31-33). This effect was proposed by us to be due to the extracellular volume depletion which ensues and which enhances fluid, sodium and calcium absorption in the nephron (34). Other workers, however, have suggested that parathyroid hormone was required for this action of thiazides since it could not be reproduced in hypoparathyroid patients (6,7). However, hypoparathyroid rats do respond to thiazides with a reduction of their urinary calcium excretion (34-36). In phosphate-depleted dogs thiazides also reduced calcium excretion inspite of hypercalcemia and presumed suppression of PTH (37). Furthermore in acute clearance and micropuncture studies PTH was not necessary for the effect of thizaides to dissociate sodium and calcium excretion (38,39). Finally, we have clearly shown that when vitamin D is withdrawn and dietary salt is restricted, urinary calcium excretion in hypoparathyroid patients will be considerably reduced (16). In fact, this treatment is now utilized in our hypoparathyroid patients to reduce the potential for hypercalciuria, nephrolithiasis and nephrocalcinosis. When all the evidence is weighed, it would appear that the effect of salt depletion coupled with a direct tubular effect explains the hypocalciuric action of prolonged thiazide administration. Whether the direct tubular effect of thiazide on calcium transport in man requires the presence of parathyroid hormone is not, as yet, settled.

Acutely, the potent diuretics ethacrynic acid and furosemide produce major calciuresis parallel in its magnitude to the increase in sodium excretion (20,22). It is this property of these agents that has led to their use in the treatment of hypercalcemic emergencies (19). This effect is thought to be due to the fact that these agents inhibit chloride transport in the thick ascending limb of Henle's loop (40) where both active and passive calcium transport has been demonstrated (41-43). Furosemide inhibits the potential-driven calcium transport in the medullary and cortical segments of the thick ascending limb (42,43).

Chronic administration of furosemide produces sustained hypercalciuria (44, 45) and secondary hyperparathyroidism (17). This observation has not been uniform however (46).

Effects on Bone

It has been suggested that thiazides increase the serum calcium by a PTH-dependent action on bone. One possible mechanism that might account for this action is inhibition by thiazides of cyclic AMP phosphodiesterase as has been shown for preparations of this enzyme made from beef heart (47). However, neither basal nor post-PTH levels of cAMP in rat calvaria were increased after thiazide addition in vitro, and bone cAMP after systemic administration of PTH was actually depressed by thiazides (48). These observations argue against a PTH-dependent effect on bone mediated via inhibition of phosphodiesterase. Furthermore, in the latter studies, the concentration of chlorothiazide necessary for half-maximal inhibition of the enzyme was much higher (3×10^{-3} M) than is likely to be achieved with ordinary diuretic doses.

Indirect studies of bone turnover gleaned from urinary hydroxyproline excretion and from studies with radioisotopic calcium show a decrease of hydroxyproline excretion in man and in the rat, and an increase in ^{45}Ca entry into bone in the rat (49,50). However, in the thyroparathyroidectomized dog hydroxyproline excretion was increased by hydrochlorothiazide, and histomorphometric studies showed a 21% increase in the number of osteocytes, both changes suggesting enhanced osteocytic osteolysis (51). The reasons for the discrepancy between these and previous observations are obscure.

There are no studies on the acute or chronic effects of the high-ceiling diuretics on bone.

Changes in Intestinal Calcium Absorption

Studies of intestinal absorption of calcium, utilizing a variety of methodologies done in man and in experimental animals, show a decrease (36,52,53), an increase (32,54), or no change (53). These variations may be explained on the basis of the differences in methodology, underlying clinical or experimental disorder, and the duration of therapy with thiazides. It remains to be established, therefore, whether low-ceiling or high-ceiling diuretics exert any direct effect on intestinal calcium transport whether acutely or chronically.

References

1. Popovtzer, M.M.; Subryan, V.L.; Alfrey, A.C.; Reeve, E.B., and Schrier, R.W.: The acute effect of chlorothizaide on serum-ionized calcium. Evidence for a parathyroid hormone-dependent nechanism. J. Clin. Invest. 55:1295-1302 (1975).
2. Stote, R.M.; Smith, L.H.; Wilson, D.M.; Dube, W.J.; Goldsmith, R.S., and Arnaud, C.D.: Hydrochlorothiazide effects on serum calcium and immunoreactive parathyroid hormone concentrations. Studies in normal subjects. Ann. Intern. Med. 77:587-591 (1972).
3. Koppel, M.H.; Massry, S.G.; Shinaberger, J.H.; Hartenbower, D.L., and Coburn, J.W.: Thiazide-induced rise in serum calcium and magnesium in patients on maintenance hemodialysis. Ann. Intern. Med. 72:895-901 (1970).
4. Parfitt, A.M.: Chlorothiazide-induced hypercalcemia in juvenile osteoporosis and hyperparathyroidism. New Engl. J. Med. 281:55-59 (1969).
5. Parfitt, A.M.: Thiazide-induced hypercalcemia in vitamin D-treated hypoparathyroidism. Ann. Intern. Med. 77:557-563 (1972).
6. Parfitt, A.M.: The interactions of thiazide diuretics with parathyroid hormone and vitamin D. Studies in patients with hypoparathyroidism. J. Clin. Invest. 51:1879-1888 (1972).
7. Brickman, A.S.; Massry, S.G., and Coburn, J.W.: Changes in serum and urinary calcium during treatment with hydrochlorothiazide. Studies on mechanisms. J. Clin. Invest. 51:945-954 (1972).
8. Torsti, P. and Lamberg, B.A.: Effect of two-day treatment with chlorothiazide on urinary excretion of calcium, phosphate and sodium in hyper- and hypocalcemia. Acta Med. Scand. 175:suppl. 412, p. 181-191 (1964).
9. Paloyan, E.; Forland, M., and Picklman, J.R.: Hyperparathyroidism coexisting with hypertension and prolonged thiazide administration. J. Am. Med. Ass. 210: 1243-1245 (1969).
10. Adams, P.; Chalmers, T.M.; Hill, L.F., and Truscott, B. Mc N.: Idiopathic hypercalciuria and hyperparathyroidism. Br. Med. J. IV:582-585 (1970).

11. Jørgensen, F.S.; Transbøl, I., and Binder, C.: The effect of bendroflumethizaide on total, ultrafilterable and ionized calcium in serum in normocalcaemic renal stone formers and in hypoparathyroidism. Acta Med. Scand. 194:323-326 (1973).
12. Duarte, C.G.; Winnacker, J.L; Becker, K.L., and Pace, A.: Thiazide-induced hypercalcemia. New Engl. J. Med. 284:828-830 (1971).
13. Mohamadi, M.; Bivins, L., and Becker, K.L.: Effect of thiazide on serum calcium. Clin. Pharmacol. Therap. 26:390-394 (1979).
14. Christensson, T.; Hellstrom, K., and Wengle, B.: Hypercalcemia and primary hyperparathyroidism. Prevalence in patients receiving thiazides as detected in a health screen. Archs Intern. Med. 137:1138-1142 (1977).
15. Yendt, E.R.; Guay, G.F., and Garcia, D.A.: The use of thiazides in the prevention of renal calculi. Can. Med. Ass. J. 102:614-620 (1970).
16. Porter, R.H.; Cox, B.G.; Heaney, D.; Hostetter, T.H.; Stinebaugh, B.J., and Suki, W.N.: Treatment of hypoparathyroid patients with chlorthalidone. New Engl. J. Med. 298:577-581 (1978).
17. Coe, F.L.; Canterbury, J.M.; Firpo, J.J., and Reiss, E.: Evidence for secondary hyperparathyroidism in idiopathic hypercalciuria. J. Clin. Invest. 52:134-142 (1973).
18. Gabow, P.A.; Hanson, T.J.; Popovtzer, M.M., and Schrier, R.W.: Furosemide-induced reduction in ionized calcium in hypoparathyroid patients. Ann. Intern. Med. 86:579-581 (1977).
19. Suki, W.N.; Yium, J.J.; Minden, M. von; Saller-Hebert, C.; Eknoyan, G., and Martinez-Maldonado, M.: Acute treatment of hypercalcemia with furosemide. New Engl. J. Med. 283:836-840 (1970).
20. Demartini, F.E.; Briscoe, A.M., and Ragan, C.: Effect of ethacrynic acid on calcium and magnesium excretion. Proc. Soc. Exp. Biol. Med. 124:320-324 (1967).
21. Duarte, C.G.: Effects of chlorothiazide and amipramizide (MK 870) on the renal excretion of calcium, phosphate and magnesium. Metabolism 17:420-429 (1968).
22. Eknoyan, G.; Suki, W.N., and Martinez-Maldonado, M.: Effects of diuretics on urinary excretion of phosphate, calcium and magnesium in thyroparathyroidectomized dogs. J. Lab. Clin. Med. 76:257-266 (1970).
23. Edwards, B.R.; Baer, P.G.; Sutton, R.A.L., and Dirks, J.H.: Micropuncture study of diuretic effects on sodium and calcium reabsorption in the dog nephron. J. Clin. Invest. 52:2418-2427 (1973).
24. Duarte, C.G. and Bland, J.H.: Calcium, phosphorus and uric acid clearances after intravenous administration of chlorothiazide. Metabolism 14:211-219 (1965).
25. Costanzo, L.S. and Weiner, I.M.: On the hypocalciuric action of chlorothiazide. J. Clin. Invest. 54:628-637 (1974).
26. Costanzo, L.S. and Windhager, E.E.: Calcium and sodium transport by the distal convoluted tubule of the rat. Am. J. Physiol. 235:F492-F506 (1978).
27. Dan, T. and Gemba, M.: Effects of diuretics on calcium uptake and

release in renal microsomes. Biochem. Pharmacol. 29:2339-2343 (1980).
28. Lamberg, B.A. and Kuhlbäck, B.: Effect of chlorothiazide on the excretion of calcium in urine. Scand. J. Clin. Invest. 11:351-357 (1959).
29. Lichtwitz, A.; Parker, R.; DeSeze, S.; Hioco, D., and Miravet, L.: L'effect hypocalciurique des sulfamides diuretiques. Sem. Hôp. Paris 37:2350-2361 (1961).
30. Higgins, B.A.; Nassim, J.R.; Collins, J., and Hilb, A: Effect of bendrofluazide on urine calcium excretion. Clin. Sci. 27:457-462 (1964).
31. Nassim, J.R., and Higgins, B.A.: Control of idiopathic hypercalciuria. Br. Med. J. 1:675-681 (1965).
32. Yendt, E.R.; Gagne, R.J.A., and Cohanim, M.: The effects of thiazides in idiopathic hypercalciuria. Am. J. Med. Sci. 251:449-460, 1966.
33. Yendt, E.R.; Guay, G.F., and Garcia, D.A.: The use of thiazides in the prevention of renal calculi. Canad. Med. Assoc. J. 102:614-620 (1970).
34. Suki, W.N.; Eknoyan, G.; Samaan, N.; Dichoso, C.; Johnson, P.C., and Martinez-Maldonado, M.: Idiopathic hypercalciuria. Its diagnosis, pathogenesis and treatment; in Becker, Cornell Seminars in Nephrology (Wiley, New York 1973).
35. Jorgensen, F.S.: The effect of bendroflumethiazide (Centyl) on the renal excretion of calcium and sodium in normal, parathyroidectomized, thyroidectomized and thyroparathyroidectomized rats. Acta Pharmacol. Toxicol. 30:296-307 (1971).
36. Rizzoli, R.; Hugi, K.; Fleisch, H., and Bonjour, J-P.: Effect of hydrochlorothiazide on 1,25-hydroxyvitamin D_3-induced changes in calcium metabolism in experimental hypoparathyroidism in rats. Clin. Sci. 60:101-107 (1981).
37. Meyer-Sabellek, W.; Brautbar, N.; Moser, S.; Montcalm, A., and Massry, S.G.: Effect of thiazides on the hypercalciuria of phosphate depletion. J. Lab. Clin. Med. 96:830-837 (1980).
38. Costanzo, L.S.; Moses, A.M.; Rao, K.J., and Weiner, I.M.: Dissociation of calcium and sodium clearances in patients with hypoparathyroidism by infusion of chlorothiazide. Metabolism 24:1367-1373 (1975).
39. Quamme, G.A.; Wong, N.L.M.; Sutton, R.A.L., and Dirks, J.W.: Interrelationship of chlorothiazide and parathyroid hormone: a micropuncture study. Am. J. Physiol 229:200-205 (1975).
40. Burg, M.B.; Stoner, L.; Cardinal, J., and Green, N.: Furosemide effect on isolated perfused tubules. Am. J. Physiol. 225:119-124 (1973).
41. Rocha, A.S.; Magaldi, J.B., and Kokko, J.P.: Calcium and phosphate transport in isolated segments of rabbit Henle's loop. J. Clin. Invest. 59:975-983 (1977).
42. Suki, W.N.; Rouse, D.; Ng, R.C.K., and Kokko, J.P.: Calcium transport in the thick ascending limb of Henle. Heterogeneity of

transport in the medullary and cortical segments. J. Clin. Invest. 66:1004-1009 (1980).
43. Bourdeau, J.E., and Burg, M.B.: Voltage dependence of calcium transport in the thick ascending limb of Henle's loop. Am. J. Physiol. 236:F357-F364 (1979).
44. Pecchini, F.; Andreucci, V.E., and Savi, M.: Effetto del furosemide sulla calciuria. G. Clin. Med. 48:191-200 (1967).
45. Warshaw, B.L.; Anand, S.K.; Kerian, A., and Lieberman, E.: The effect of chronic furosemide administration on urinary calcium excretion and calcium balance in growing rats. Pediatr. Res. 14:1118-1121 (1980).
46. Toft, H., and Roin, J.: Effect of frusemide administration on calcium excretion. Br. Med. J. 1:437-438 (1971).
47. Moore, P.F.: The effects of diazoxide and benzothiadiazide diuretics upon phosphodiesterase. Ann. N.Y. Acad. Sci. 150:256 (1968).
48. Marcus, R.; Orner, F.; Arvesen, G., and Lundquist, C.: Thiazide diuretics do not potentiate cAMP response to parathyroid hormone. Metabolism 27:701-710 (1978).
49. Middler, S.; Pak, C.Y.C.; Murad, F., and Bartter, F.C.: Thiazide diuretics and calcium metabolism. Metabolism 22:139-146 (1973).
50. Jørgensen, F.S., and Neilsen, S.P.: Effects of long-term administration of bendroflumethiazide on bone metabolism in the rat. Acta Pharmacol. Toxicol. 31:521-528 (1972).
51. Malluche, H.H.; Meyer-Sabellek, W.; Singer, F.R., and Massry, S.G.: Evidence for a direct effect of thiazides on bone. Min. Elec. Metab. 4:89-96 (1980).
52. Yendt, E.R., and Couhanim, M.: Prevention of calcium stones with thiazides. Kidney Intl. 13:397-409 (1978).
53. Ehrig, U.; Harrison, J.E., and Wilson, D.R.: Effect of long-term thiazide therapy on intestinal calcium absorption in patients with recurrent renal calculi. Metabolism 23:139-145 (1974).
54. Jørgensen, F.S., and Transbøl, I.: The effect of bendroflumethiazide on the intestinal absorption of calcium in normocalcaemic renal stone formers and in hyperparathyroidism. Acta Med. Scand. 195:33-36 (1974).

EFFECTS OF CHLOROTHIAZIDE ADMINISTRATION AND DIETARY CALCIUM RESTRICTION ON PARATHYROID FUNCTION, VITAMIN D METABOLISM AND INTESTINAL CALCIUM ABSORPTION IN THE RAT

Murray J. Favus, Fredric L. Coe, Satish C. Kathpalia, Asher Porat, Prabir K. Sen and Louis M. Sherwood

Department of Medicine, Michael Reese Hospital and Medical Center
Chicago, Illinois 60616 U.S.A.

Thiazide diuretic agents reduce urine calcium excretion by stimulating distal nephron calcium reabsorption and by reducing extracellular fluid volume (1-3). In patients with idiopathic hypercalciuria, thiazide administration lowers urinary calcium excretion. In addition, circulating $1,25(OH)_2D_3$ and intestinal calcium absorption rates can also be reduced to normal in those patients with hypercalciuria arising from defective tubular calcium reabsorption (4,5). Its effects upon serum $1,25(OH)_2D_3$ and intestinal calcium absorption could be due to the reversal of secondary hyperparathyroidism (6). The physiological adaptation to dietary calcium restriction involves an increase in $1,25(OH)_2D_3$ synthesis which, in turn, enhances the intestinal calcium active transport process (7-9). Since this sequence of events is thought to be initiated by an increase in parathyroid hormone (PTH) secretion, we investigated whether thiazide can prevent the intestinal adaptive response to low calcium diet (LCD).

MATERIALS AND METHODS

Male Sherman rats weighing 150 g were housed in metabolic cages and fed either normal chow (1.2% calcium, .9% phosphorus, .24% magnesium and 2.5 IU D_3 per g) or a low calcium diet (LCD, .02% calcium, .34% phosphorus, .24% magnesium and 2.5 IU D_3 per g) for 21 days. Chlorothiazide (CTZ) was added to the diet in half of the rats receiving chow and half of those fed LCD. The animals ingested 20 g of food per day which delivered 25 mg of CTZ per kg body weight.

Rates of calcium uptake were measured in vitro by the everted gut sac technique using segments prepared from duodenum (proximal 5 cm), jejunum (middle 30 cm), ileum (distal 12 cm) and descending colon (10). The incubation medium was a Krebs-Ringer bicarbonate buffer (pH 7.4) containing 1.25 mM calcium, 11 mM D-glucose and .3 μCi of ^{45}Ca per ml.

The unidirectional transepithelial fluxes of calcium were measured across descending colon segments under conditions of electrochemical neutrality by previously described techniques (10). The exposed tissue area was 0.69 cm^2, and the buffer was the same as that used for the gut sac studies.

$1,25(OH)_2D_3$ was measured on one ml of serum pooled from 2 to 4 rats. Following ether extraction and purification using Sephadex LH-20 and microsilica (HPLC) column chromatography, samples were assayed in triplicate using the chick intestinal cytosol receptor method of Eisman et al (11). Initial specific binding ranged from 30 to 42%, least detectable dose was 2 pg per assay tube. Overall recovery was 55±8%.

The radioimmunoassay for PTH was performed in duplicate on 2.0 ml serum aliquots using the double antibody technique (12). The antiserum recognizes intact 1 to 84 PTH and carboxyl terminal fragments. Serum and urine chemistries were measured by conventional Auto Analyzer and flame photometric methodologies.

RESULTS

Twenty-one days of LCD increased calcium uptake by everted sacs of duodenum, ileum and descending colon as expected (Figure 1). CTZ failed to alter calcium uptake during LCD and did not change uptake rates during normal calcium intake (Figure 1). The increased calcium uptake during LCD was due to a stimulation of calcium active transport, and CTZ did not alter the increase in the absorptive flux (Jms) stimulated by LCD (Figure 2). LCD also increased serum PTH and $1,25(OH)_2D_3$ (Figure 3). CTZ administration prevented the secondary hyperparathyroidism in response to LCD, but serum $1,25(OH)_2D_3$ rose to levels achieved in the absence of the drug (Figure 3). CTZ had no effect on serum PTH or $1,25(OH)_2D_3$ when given with normal chow. Serum PTH and $1,25(OH)_2D_3$ were positively correlated over the range of dietary calcium intake studied (Figure 4). CTZ disrupted this relationship because serum $1,25(OH)_2D_3$ rose during LCD plus CTZ and PTH did not ($r = .381$, NS, Figure 4).

Serum calcium was unchanged by LCD or CTZ (Figure 5). LCD raised serum phosphorus in the absence and presence of CTZ. Serum PTH varied inversely with serum calcium ($r = .231$, $df = 58$, $p<.025$). CTZ treated animals tended to have higher serum calcium levels, suggesting that CTZ prevented secondary hyperparathyroidism during LCD by raising serum calcium.

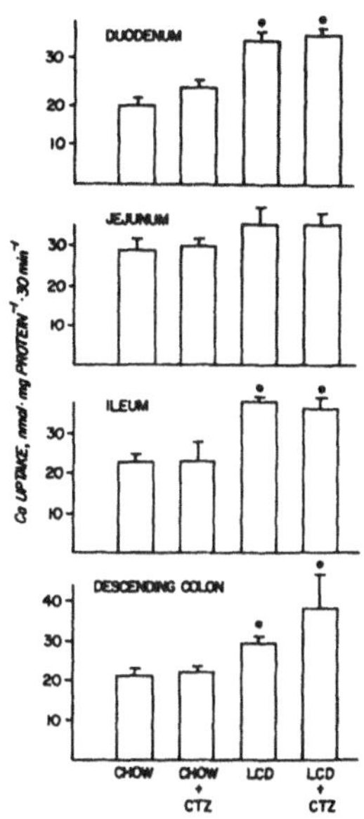

Figure 1. Effect of 21 days of low calcium diet (LCD) and chlorothiazide (CTZ) administration on calcium transport by everted gut sacs of small and large intestine. For each group there were 8 chow, 9 chow = CTZ, 7 LCD and 9 LCD + CTZ rats. Values are mean±SEM. Asterisk indicates values greater than chow with or without CTZ, p<.01.

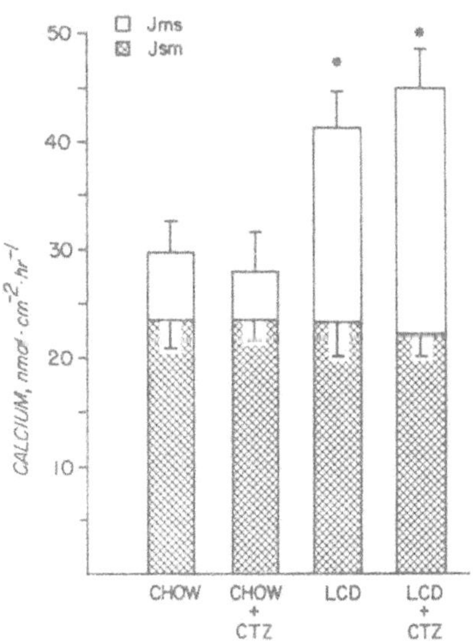

Figure 2. Effects of low calcium diet (LCD) and chlorothiazide (CTZ) on the unidirectional fluxes of calcium across descending colon. Height of each bar is the absorptive flux, Jms. Hatched area of bar is secretory flux, Jsm. Net absorption is Jms-Jsm. Values are mean± SEM for Jms and Jsm. Asterisk indicates significant increase in Jms above chow with or without CTZ.

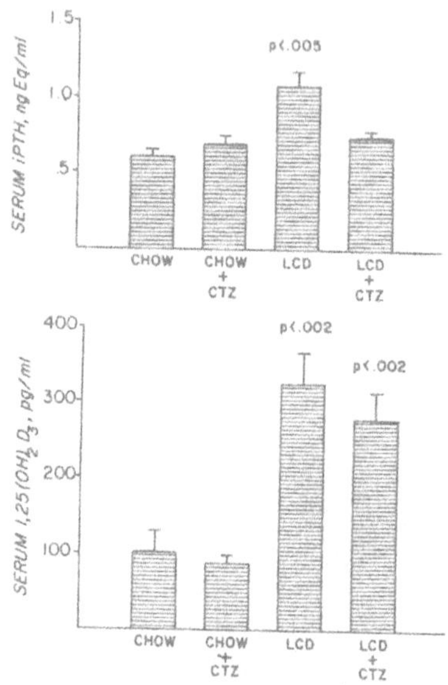

Figure 3. Response of serum immunoreactive parathyroid hormone, iPTH (top panel) and $1,25(OH)_2D_3$ (bottom panel) to low calcium diet (LCD) and chlorothiazide (CTZ for 21 days. Values are mean±SEM. iPTH was measured in 18 sera of all groups but chow (15) and LCD (15). $1,25(OH)_2D_3$ was measured in 7 sera pools from the LCD group and 6 pools for each of the other groups.

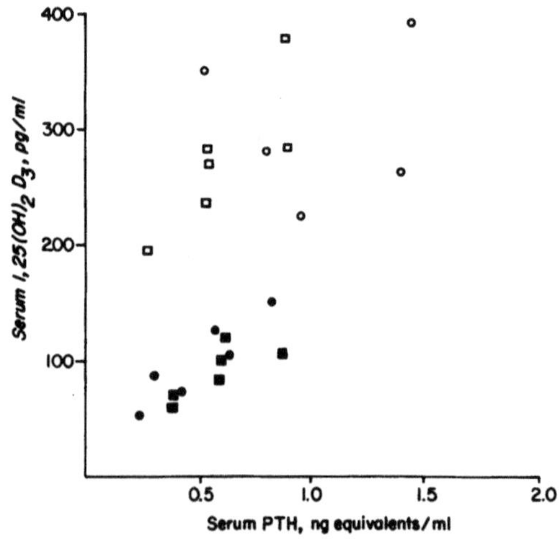

Figure 4. Paired immunoreactive parathyroid hormone (PTH) and $1,25(OH)_2D_3$ levels in serum pooled from 2 to 4 rats fed chow (●), low calcium diet (LCD) (○), chow plus chlorothiazide (CTZ) (■) or LCD plus CTZ (□). For chow and LCD, n = 11, slope = 202±68, p<.016, r = .703. For chow plus CTZ and LCD plus CTZ, n = 12, slope = 196±150, NS, r = .381.

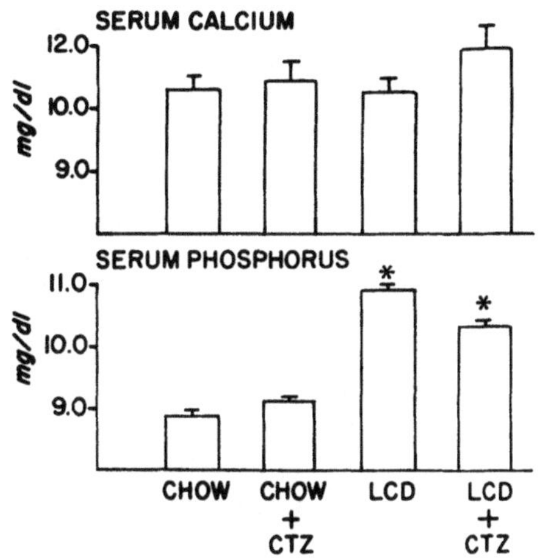

Figure 5. Effects of 21 days of low calcium diet (LCD) and chlorothiazide (CTZ) on serum calcium (top panel) and serum phosphorus (bottom panel). Values are mean±SEM for 18 animals per group. Asterisk indicates significant elevation above chow with or without CTZ, $p<.01$.

DISCUSSION

The increase in the efficiency of intestinal calcium absorption during low calcium intake is mediated by $1,25(OH)_2D_3$. Under these conditions, increased renal 25-OH-1-hydroxylase activity (13) leads to a rise in circulating $1,25(OH)_2D_3$ and accumulation of $1,25(OH)_2D_3$ in intestinal mucosa (8, 14-16). As a result, calcium active transport is enhanced (9,14). The present study shows that the $1,25(OH)_2D_3$ and intestinal response to LCD is not influenced by thiazide.

PTH is thought to be the major stimulus for the rise in circulating $1,25(OH)_2D_3$ during LCD (17). Increased $1,25(OH)_2D_3$ and intestinal calcium transport can increase during LCD in the absence of the parathyroid glands (14-16,18). Presumably hypocalcemia is the stimulator of the 25-OH-1-hydroxylase under these conditions (18). In our study, serum PTH doubled in response to LCD, and thiazide abolished this response. That CTZ permits a normal response of $1,25(OH)_2D_3$ and intestinal calcium absorption yet interferes with a rise in serum PTH supports previous observations that intestinal adaptation can occur without the development of secondary hyperparathyroidism. Hypocalcemia and hypophosphatemia, known stimulators of $1,25(OH)_2D_3$ production, were not present in our study and cannot explain the increase in $1,25(OH)_2D_3$. CTZ alone is unlikely to be the signal for increased $1,25(OH)_2D_3$ production, since the drug had no effect in animals fed normal chow. The signal for vitamin D adaptation to LCD under these conditions is unknown and requires further investigation. Our observations also suggest that different mechanisms may regulate $1,25(OH)_2D_3$ during LCD and in patients with renal idiopathic hypercalciuria.

REFERENCES

1. A.S. Brickman, S.G. Massry and J.W. Coburn, Changes in serum and urinary calcium during treatment with hydrochlorothiazide: Studies on mechanisms, J. Clin. Invest. 51:1879 (1972).

2. L.S. Constanzo and I.M. Weiner, On the hypocalciuric action of chlorothiazide, J. Clin. Invest. 54:628 (1974).

3. N. Breslau, A.M. Moses and I.M. Weiner, The role of volume contraction in the hypocalciuric action of chlorothiazide, Kidney Int. 10:164 (1976).

4. D.E. Barilla, R. Tolentino, R.A. Kaplan and C.Y.C. Pak, Selective effectives of thiazide on intestinal absorption of calcium in absorptive and renal hypercalciurias, Metabolism 27:125 (1978).

5. J.E. Zerwekh and C.Y.C. Pak, Selective effects of thiazide therapy on serum 1α,25-dihydroxyvitamin D in renal and absorptive hypercalciuria, Metabolism 29:13 (1980).

6. F.L. Coe, J.M. Canterbury, J.J. Firpo and E. Reiss, Evidence for secondary hyperparathyroidism in idiopathic hypercalciuria, J. Clin. Invest. 52:134 (1973).

7. R. Nicolaysen, N. Eeg-Larsen and O.J. Malm, Physiology of calcium metabolism, Physiol. Rev. 33:424 (1953).

8. I.T. Boyle, R.W. Gray and H.F. DeLuca, Regulation by calcium of in vivo synthesis of 1,25-dihydroxycholecalciferol and 21,25-dihydroxycholecalciferol, Proc. Nat. Acad. Sci. 68:2131 (1971).

9. M.W. Walling and S.S. Rothman, Apparent increase in carrier affinity for intestinal calcium transport following dietary calcium restriction, J. Biol. Chem. 245:5007 (1970).

10. M.J. Favus, S.C. Kathpalia, F.L. Coe and A.E. Mond, Effects of diet calcium and 1,25-dihydroxyvitamin D on colon calcium active transport, Am. J. Physiol. 238:G75 (1980).

11. J.A. Eisman, A.J. Hamstra, B.E. Kream and H.F. DeLuca, A sensitive, precise and convenient method for determination of 1,25-dihydroxy-vitamin D in human plasma, Arch. Biochem. Biophys. 176:235 (1976).

12. A.B. Schneider, S.A. Wells, J.C. Gunnells, J.B. Leslie and L.M. Sherwood, Regulation of function of transplanted parathyroid glands in man, Am. J. Med. 63:710 (1977).

13. H.L. Henry, R.J. Midgett, and A.W. Norman, Regulation of 25-hydroxy-vitamin D_3-1-hydroxylase in vivo, J. Biol. Chem. 249:7584 (1974).

14. M.J. Favus, M.W. Walling, and D.V. Kimberg, Effects of dietary calcium restriction and chronic thyroparathyroidectomy on the metabolism of (^{3}H)-25-hydroxyvitamin D_3 and active transport of calcium by rat intestine, J. Clin. Invest. 53:1139 (1974).

15. M.R. Hughes, P.F. Brumbaugh, M.R. Haussler, J.E. Wergedal and D.J. Baylink, Regulation of serum 1α,25-dihydroxyvitamin D_3 by calcium and phosphate in the rat, Science 190:578 (1975).

16. J.I. Rader, D.J. Baylink, M.R. Hughes, E.F. Safilian and M.R. Haussler, Calcium and phosphorus deficiency in rats: Effects on PTH and 1,25-dihydroxyvitamin D_3, Am. J. Physiol. 236:E118 (1979).

17. M. Garabedian, M.F. Holick, H.F. DeLuca, and I.T. Boyle, Control of 25-hydroxycholecalciferol metabolism by the parathyroid glands, Proc. Nat. Acad. Sci. 69:1673 (1972).

18. U. Trechsel, J.A. Eisman, J.A. Fischer, J.-P. Bonjour, and H. Fleisch, Calcium-dependent, parathyroid hormone-independent regulation of 1,25-dihydroxyvitamin D, Am. J. Physiol. 239:E119 (1980).

ACKNOWLEDGEMENT

The authors gratefully acknowledge the technical assistance of Vrishali Tembe, Peggy Imanaka and Elin Angeid-Backman and the secretarial efforts of Janice Penson. This work was supported by grant AM 20585 from the NIH.

CALCIUM FLUXES ACROSS MEMBRANES ISOLATED FROM SMALL INTESTINAL EPITHELIUM

Heini Murer and Bruno Hildmann

Institute of Physiology, University of Zurich, Zurich
Switzerland and Max Planck Institut für Biophysik
Frankfurt, Germany

INTRODUCTION

Studies using intact tissue preparations revealed that transepithelial transports of calcium in the small intestine is dependent on the presence of sodium (1-5). These observations suggest that transcellular transport of calcium is coupled to transcellular sodium flux (for review see: 2).

Due to the presence of a high affinity Ca-ATPase in basallateral membranes isolated from small intestinal epithelium (6,7), Ca might also be transported transcellularly in a sodium independent manner.

In view of the intra-/extracellular concentration differences for Ca, transport of Ca from the cytosol into the serosal interstitium represents an energy requiring "uphill" movement, whereas influx into the cell from the lumen is a downhill movement.

In this short review we will briefly summarize experiments performed in different laboratories, in order to characterize in studies with isolated vesicles the cell surface membrane mechanisms involved in small intestinal transcellular transport of calcium. These studies showed that the basic membrane mechanisms found in the small intestinal epithelium are similar to those found in proximal tubular epithelium (2,8-11).

The important interplay between plasma membrane bound mechanisms, mitochondria and binding-protein(s) and other intracellular membranes will not be discussed in this overview (for review see: 2, 12, 13).

TRANSMEMBRANE TRANSPORT OF CALCIUM

In general, plasma membranes of mammalian cells contain two types of Ca-transport mechanisms: 1) Ca/Mg-ATPase with high affinity transport sites for Ca and 2) Na/Ca-exchange systems (14). Studies with intact epithelia as well as biochemical studies have suggested that these two mechanisms are also involved in transepithelial calcium flux in small intestine as briefly mentioned above (2,4,5,6, 7). Furthermore, a basal-lateral localization of these mechanisms is to be expected.

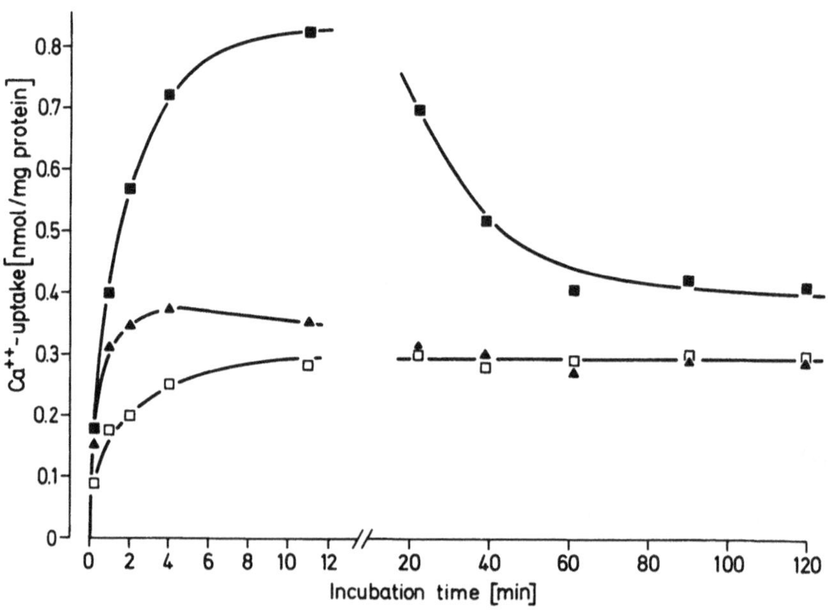

Fig. 1. ATP-driven transport of Ca into rat small intestinal basal-lateral membrane vesicles. The membranes were suspended in 300 mmol/l mannitol, 20 mmol/l HEPES, adjusted to pH 7.4 by Tris, 100 mmol/l KCl, 5 mmol/l Mg Cl_2. The incubation medium contained the same solutes and in addition 1 µg/ml oligomycin, 2 mmol/l ouabain, 0,05 mmol/l Ca Cl_2 and 5 mmol/l Mg-ATP (■,▲) or no ATP (□). In one condition A 23 187 was added to a concentration of 2 µg/ml to the membrane suspension (▲). This figure is taken from reference 8.

Isolated basal-lateral membrane vesicles contain an ATP driven Ca-transport mechanism (2,8,22). The presence of inside out vesicles in a plasma membrane preparation is a prerequisit that ATP can reach its site on the Ca-transport system during incubation with ATP added only to the incubation medium. Uptake in such vesicle fractions will represent an extrusion system in the intact cell. As can be seen from figure 1, the addition of ATP to a membrane fraction isolated by a Percoll-centrifugation method (15) leads to an acceleration of initial Ca-uptake as compared to the situation without ATP and to accumulation of Ca above the equilibrium uptake. As the addition of the ionophore A 23 187 prevents the accumulation of Ca, addition of ATP promotes transmembrane Ca-flux rather than increased Ca-binding. Copurification of the ATP driven Ca-transport mechanism with classical basal-lateral membrane markers could be demonstrated (figure 2). Inhibitors of mitochondrial Ca-transport did not affect ATP driven Ca-transport in isolated basal-lateral membrane preparations (8). Thus, it is reasonable to assume that the ATP driven Ca-uptake associated with the isolated basal-lateral membrane fraction is indeed a property of the basal-lateral membrane. Furthermore, ATP dependent Ca-uptake is stimulated by calmodulin (22).

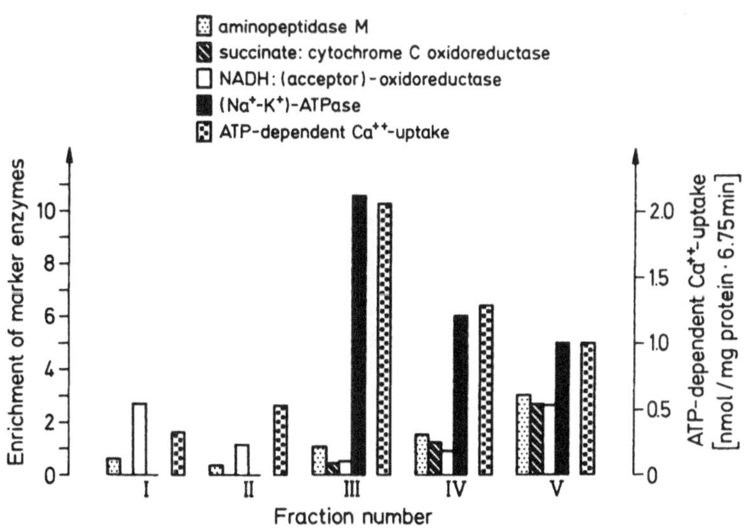

Fig. 2. Distribution of marker enzymes and ATP-dependent Ca-uptake in subfractions of a heavy microsomal fraction separated by a Percoll gradient. A crude plasma membrane fraction was separated in a 35 ml-Percoll gradient (15) and divided (continued)

into five fractions, designated I - V from the top of 7,5 ml /I, II, IV, V) and 5 ml (III).
The marker enzymes of brush-border membranes (aminopeptidase M), mitochondrial inner membrane (succinate: cytochrome C oxidoreductase), endoplasmic reticulum (NADH: acceptor-oxidoreductase in the presence of KCN) and basal-lateral plasma membrane (Na-K-ATPase) as well as ATP dependent Ca-transport were assayed in each fraction. * = no detectable activity in membrane fraction. Incubation media for Ca-uptake containing: 300 mmol/l mannitol, 20 mmol/l HEPES/Tris, 100 mmol/l KCl, 5 mmol/l ATP or ADP, 5 mmol/l Mg Cl_2, 1 µg/ml oligomycin and 50 µmol/l Ca Cl_2. This figure is taken from reference 8.

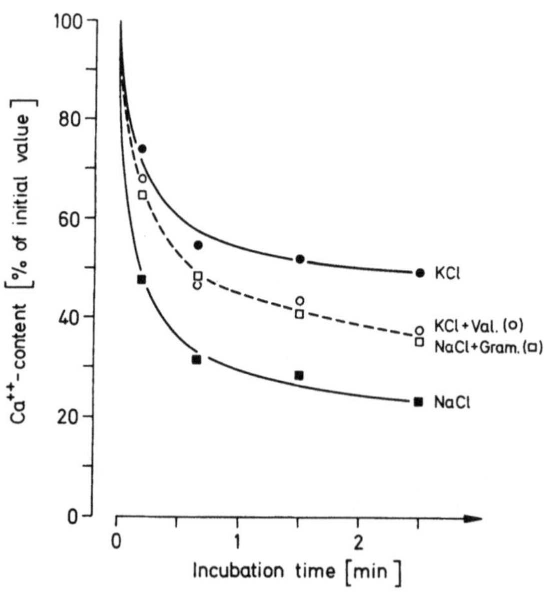

Fig. 3. Efflux of Ca from basal-lateral plasma membrane vesicles of rat small intestine, effect of Na^+. Membranes were preincubated for 1 hour at 25°C with 0,1 mmol/l ^{45}Ca Cl_2 in 300 mmol/l mannitol, 20 mmol/l HEPES/Tris, pH 7.4, 100 mmol/l (continued)

choline chloride, 5 mmol/l Mg Cl_2. Efflux of Ca was initiated by the addition of 10 µl 20 mmol/l EGTA in 300 mmol/l mannitol, 20 mmol/l HEPES/Tris pH 7.4, 5 mmol/l Mg Cl_2 and 1 mol/l NaCl (■,□) or KCl (●,○) to 130 µl of membrane suspension. Valinomycin (○) or gramicidin (□), dissolved in ethanol were added to a concentration of 20 µg/ml to the membrane suspension 5 min before the start of efflux, the respective controls (●,■) received the same amount of ethanol (2%). This figure is taken from reference 8.

Evidence for a Na/Ca-exchange mechanism is also available from studies with basal-lateral membrane vesicles (2,8). ATP driven Ca-uptake was maximal in a KCl medium, i.e. in the complete absence of sodium. Increased sodium concentrations in the medium decreased ATP driven Ca-transport and prevented at high sodium concentrations ATP dependent intravesicular accumulation. This suggests a sodium dependent pathway for Ca in the same vesicular structure that contained the ATP driven Ca-transport mechanism (2,8). Further evidence for a Na/Ca exchange mechanism comes from experiments on the efflux of Ca from preloaded vesicles in the presence of different transmembrane ion gradients (2,8). Efflux of Ca was faster in the presence of an inwardly directed sodium gradient than with a potassium gradient. Increased sodium permeability of the membranes brought about by the addition of ionophores, lead to a decrease of the sodium effect (figure 3). These results can be explained by a Na/Ca exchange mechanism, because increasing sodium influx into the vesicle by pathways different from a Na/Ca-exchanger must lead to a reduction of sodium gradient accelerated efflux. For energetic reasons, an electrogenic nature and a high stoichiometry between Na- and Ca-flux - at least 3 - should be expected. Conclusive experiments on the stoichiometry of the Na/Ca-exchanger have not been carried out with basal-lateral membranes isolated from small intestine.

Results from investigations on Ca-influx across the brush-border membrane into the enterocyte in intact tissue preparations are in agreement with a passive entry mechanism (5,16,17,18). Evidence for mediated Ca-transport across the brush-border membrane was also obtained with membrane vesicles isolated from small intestine (19) and chicken duodenum (20). A clear interpretation of the experiments with rat brush-border membrane vesicles (19) is difficult, due to the high amount of calcium binding to the membrane surface. It seems to be easier to differentiate transport and binding of calcium in chicken intestinal brush-border membrane preparations (20). Similar to the studies with rat membrane vesicles (19), experiments in our laboratory on rabbit duodenal brush-border membrane vesicles revealed that at Ca-concentrations of 0,1-0,5 mmol/l the Ca-equilibrium uptake is 5-20 fold as large as that expected from the intravesicular volume estimated by the D-glucose space (B. Hildmann and H. Murer, unpublished observation). Since binding of Ca to the external vesicle surface can be expected to be minimized by the EGTA-wash-procedure used in these studies, these observations indicate that large amounts of Ca are bound to the vesicle interior.

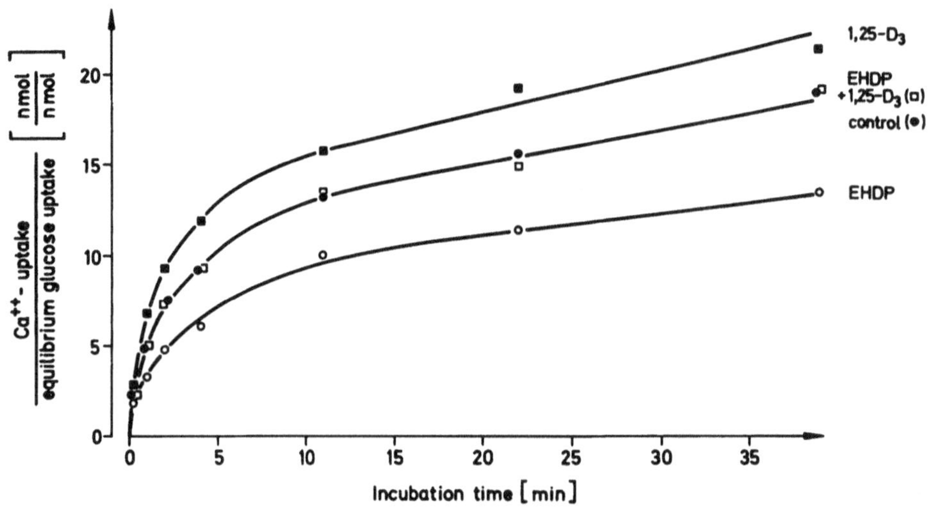

Fig. 4. Ca-uptake by rabbit duodenal brush-border membranes. The rabbits were treated in vivo as described by Danisi et al. (21) and as indicated in the figure. Membrane vesicles were suspended in 300 mmol/l mannitol, 20 mmol/l HEPES/Tris, pH 7.4, 100 mmol/l KCL. 40 µl were added to 200 µl of incubation medium containing the same buffer and in addition 0,5 mmol/l Ca Cl_2 and 0,2 mmol/l ^{3}H-D-glucose. As equilibration of Ca occurs very slowly, Ca-uptake was referred to glucose equilibrium uptake to obtain a Ca-uptake rate. Glucose equilibrium uptake after 20 min of incubation was equal in the four different membrane preparations. This figure is taken from reference 2.

As postulated from results obtained with intact epithelium (16,17, 18), alteration by 1,25 $(OH)_2$ vitamin D_3 treatment of passive Ca-influx into isolated duodenal brush-border membrane vesicles could be observed. In chicken preparations the apparent v_{max} of the saturable Ca-influx was doubled after repletion of vitamin D deficient chicken with a pharmacological dose of 1,25 $(OH)_2$ vitamin D_3 (20). Similar results have been reported for rat small intestinal brush-border vesicles (19). In agreement with the findings on rat (19) and chicken brush-border membranes (20) our experiments with rabbit duodenal brush-border membranes isolated (figure 4) from animals with different 1,25 $(OH)_2$ vitamin D_3 levels revealed a decrease of Ca-uptake in brush-border membranes from 1,25 $(OH)_2$ vitamin D_3 deficient rabbits and a restoration to the control level after administration of 1,25 $(OH)_2$ vitamin D_3 (2). However, due to large binding of calcium in the case of rabbits and rats, it cannot be excluded entirely that accelerated uptake of Ca is due to increased binding of Ca to the inner membrane surface or components near to it. This criticism is not valid for the experiments with chicken brush-border membranes, because apparently only little amounts of Ca are bound in the vesicle interior in the chicken preparation (20). Altogether these findings indicate that 1,25 $(OH)_2$ vitamin D_3 induces events leading to altered cellular uptake of calcium across the brush-border membrane. Presently available evidence suggests an altered lipid composition but not de nuovo protein synthesis as a cellular mechanism involved in this regulation (for review see ref. 2).

CONCLUSIONS

In concordance with studies on intact epithelial preparations, studies with basal-lateral and brush-border membrane vesicles revealed that transcellular calcium fluxes in the small intestine are coupled to transcellular sodium flux, i.e. secondary active via coupling to the primary active sodium flux. There exists also a primary active transport mediated by the Ca-ATPase. The relative transport capacities of the two different transport mechanisms are at the present unknown.

ACKNOWLEGMENTS

The work presented and/or discussed in this review was in part supported by the Swiss National Science Foundation, Grant No. 3.451.079.

REFERENCES

1. A.W. Norman, Calcium and phosphorus absorption, in: "Vitamin D", D.E.M. Lawson, ed., Academic Press, London, New York, San Francisco (1978)
2. H. Murer and B. Hildmann, Transcellular transport of calcium and inorganic phosphate in the small intestinal epithelium, Amer. J. Physiol. 240:G 409-G 416 (1981).
3. H.N. Nellans and D.V. Kimberg, Cellular and paracellular calcium transport in rat ileum. Effects of dietary calcium, Amer. J. Physiol. 235:E 726-737 (1978).

4. H.W. Nellans and D.V. Kimberg, Intestinal calcium transport: Absorption secretion and vitamin D., in: "Int. Rev. Physiol.; Gastro. Physiol." R.K. Crane, ed., 19:227-261 (1979).
5. D.L. Martin and H.F. De Luca, Influence of sodium on calcium transport by the rat small intestine, Amer. J. Physiol. 216: 1351-1359 (1969).
6. W.E.J.M. Ghijsen and C.H. van Os, Ca^{2+} stimulated ATPase in brush-border and basolateral membranes of rat duodenum with high affinity sites for Ca^{2+} ions, Nature, 279:802-803 (1979).
7. W.E.J.M. Ghijsen, M.D. De Jong and C.H. van Os, Dissociation between Ca^{2+} ATPase and alkaline phosphatase activities in plasma membranes of rat duodenum, Biochim. Biophys. Acta, 599:538-551 (1980).
8. B. Hildmann, A. Schmidt and H. Murer, Ca^{++} transport across basal-lateral plasma membranes from rat small intestinal epithelial cells, J. Membrane Biol. in press (1981).
9. K.J. Ullrich, G. Rumrich and S. Klöss, Active Ca^{2+} reabsorption in the proximal tubule of the rat kidney. Dependence on sodium and buffer transport, Pflügers Arch. 365: 223-228 (1976).
10. H. Murer and R. Kinne, The use of isolated membrane vesicles to study epithelial transport processes, J. Membrane Biol. 55:81-95 (1980).
11. P. Gmaj, H. Murer and R. Kinne, Calcium ion transport across plasma membranes from rat kidney cortex, Biochem. J. 172: 57-62 (1978).
12. D.D. Bikle, E.M. Askew, D.T. Zolock, R.L. Morrissey and R.H. Herman, Calcium accumulation by chick intestinal mitochondria. Regulation by vitamin D_3 and 1,25 dihydroxyvitamin D_3, Biochim. Biophys. Acta, 598:561-574 (1980).
13. H. Rasmussen and M.C. Gustin, Some aspects of the hormonal control of cellular calcium metabolism, Annals N.Y. Acad. Sci. 307:391-401 (1978).
14. E. Carafoli and M. Crompton, The regulation of intracellular calcium, in: "Current Topics in Membranes and Transport", F. Bronner and A. Kleinzeller, ed., Academic Press, New York, San Francisco, London, 10: 151-216 (1978).
15. V. Scalera, C. Storelli, C. Storelli-Joss, W. Haase and H. Murer, A simple and fast method for the isolation of lateral basal plasma membranes from rat small intestinal epithelial cells, Biochem. J. 186: 177-181 (1980).
16. H.F. De Luca, H.E. Paaren and H.K. Schnoes, Vitamin D and calcium metabolism, in: "Topics of Current Chemistry", 83: 2-65 (1979).

17. M.J. Fauran-Clavel, J. Oustrin and F. Fauran, Effects of 1,25 dihydroxyvitamin D_3 on calcium uptake, into rat intestine after chronic oral cadmium administration, Experientia, 36: 1147-1149 (1980).
18. J.M. Donnell and M. Smith, Influence of cholecalciferol (vitamin D_3) on the initial kinetics of the uptake of calcium by rat small intestinal mucosa, Biochem. J. 134: 667-669 (1973).
19. A. Miller and F. Bronner, Calcium uptake in isolated brush-border vesicles from rat small intestine, Biochem. J. 196: 391-400 (1981).
20. H. Rasmussen, O. Fontaine, E.E. Max and D.B. P. Goodman, The effect of 1-α hydroxyvitamin D_3 administration on calcium transport in chick intestine brush-border vesicles, J. Biol. Chem. 254: 2993-2999 (1979).
21. G. Danisi, J.Ph. Bonjour and R.W. Straub, Regulation of Na^+-dependent phosphate influx across the mucosal border of duodenum by 1,25 dihydroxy-cholecalciferol, Pflügers Arch. 388: 227-232 (1980).
22. W.E.J.M. Ghijsen, H.R. De Jonge and C.H. van Os, Effects of calmodulin on Ca-ATPase and ATP dependent Ca^{++} uptake in basolateral plasma membranes of rat duodenum. Abstract: European Intestinal Transport Group, Berlin, September (1981).

PARATHYROID HORMONE METABOLISM AND ITS EXTRASKELETAL EFFECTS

THE PARATHYROID HORMONE MOLECULE:

BIOLOGICAL IMPLICATIONS OF STRUCTURE

Michael Rosenblatt

Endocrine Unit
Massachusetts General Hospital
Boston, Mass 02114

Analysis of the relation of structure to hormonal function for parathyroid hormone (PTH) has provided important insights into the physiological roles served by certain regions of the hormone molecule and the initial events and mechanisms by which hormonal messages are translated into physiological actions. Chemical synthesis of multiple segments of the hormone has now been achieved. Thus far approximately 80 analogues or fragments of PTH have been synthesized. Taken together, these synthetic fragments comprise (with considerable overlap) the entire structure of pre-proparathyroid hormone (Pre-ProPTH) and multiple analogues of the active core.

THE PRECURSOR-SPECIFIC REGION OF THE HORMONE

Parathyroid hormone is initially biosynthesized in a precursor form termed Pre-ProPTH, a single-chain protein of 115 amino acids (Figure 1). At the NH_2-terminus of Pre-ProPTH, there is a 25-amino acid region representative of a class of precursor-specific sequences found in secreted proteins, enzymes, and peptide hormones known as leader, or signal, sequences.

These sequences are believed to serve a specialized and essential role in intracellular transport; they are thought to promote binding of nascent peptide—polysome complexes to rough endoplasmic reticulum (RER) and transfer of nascent peptides across the RER membrane.

Blobel and Sabatini[1] and later Milstein et al.[2] suggested that the first step in transmembrane transport of pre-hormones is binding

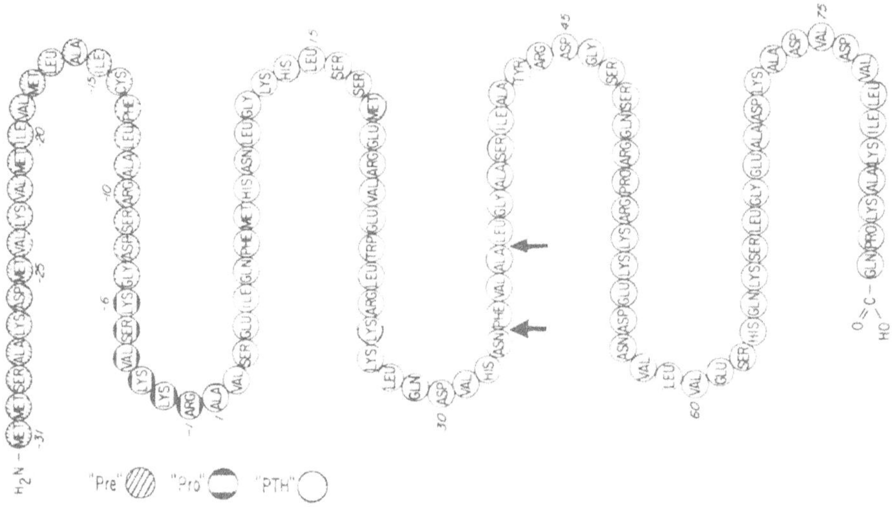

Fig. 1. The complete amino acid sequence of bovine Pre-ProPTH. The cross-hatched residues indicate the leader sequence (positions -31 to -7). The shaded region is the hexapeptide specific to ProPTH (positions -6 through -1). The open residues comprises the native form of the hormone, the sequence 1—84. The region 28—48 is recognized by enzymes(s) that metabolize the hormone *in vivo*; arrows marked the principal sites of hormone cleavage *in vivo*.

of the leader sequence to RER at specific recognition sites. It is this interaction of the leader sequence with a membrane receptor that is thought to determine whether a nascent protein remains intracellular or is secreted. For PTH, the leader sequence is removed concomitantly with translation: when biosynthesis is completed, the prohormone remains sequestered within the RER cisterna.

Using a chemically synthesized peptide representing the precursor-specific region of Pre-ProPTH,[3] we have obtained evidence strongly supporting the presence of a common, perhaps universal, RER apparatus which processes pre-hormones.[4] Processing was defined as (a) conversion of the pre-hormone to authentic hormone or prohormone and (b) translocation of the protein product into the interior of microsomal vesicles. Our studies examined processing of the precursor forms of several hormones of unrelated function from different species and different tissues: prolactin, placental lactogen, growth hormone, and PTH. We demonstrated competitive inhibition of processing of these several pre-hormones by the chemically synthesized precursor-specific region of Pre-ProPTH (Fig. 2). Diminished processing of pre-hormones was specific, dose-related, occurred in

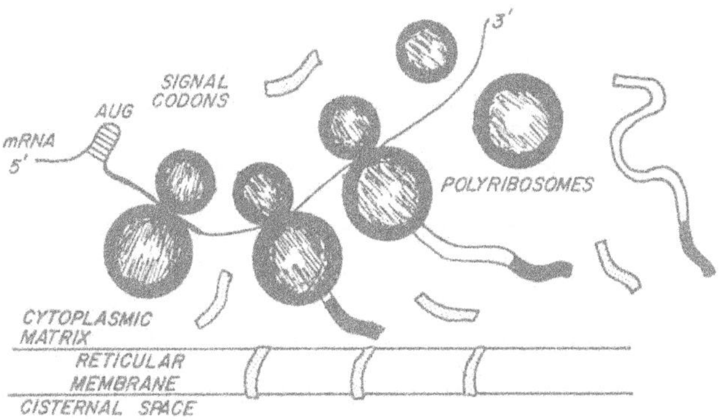

Fig. 2. Schematic representation of the effects of synthetic precursor-specific region of Pre-ProPTH on pre-horhone processing. According to the signal hypothesis,[1,2] an intracellular membrane receptor binds the leader sequence of a pre-hormone, an event which commits the nascent protein to translocation across the membrane, removal of the leader sequence, and ultimately to secretion by the cell. Competing synthetic precursor-specific peptide of Pre-ProPTH inhibits these processing events.[3,4]

the micromolar concentration range of added synthetic peptide, and was accompanied by accumulation of pre-hormone.[4]

The role of the prohormone-specific hexapeptide has not yet been elucidated. The "pro" segment is present at the amino-terminus from the time of removal of the leader sequence (upon entry into the RER cisternal space) until packaging of the mature hormone into secretory granules in the Golgi apparatus (approximately 15 min). It does not appear to have the same functions possessed by other prohormone-specific sequences. It neither appears to promote PTH tertiary conformation after biosynthesis, as the connecting peptide does for insulin; nor does it serve to separate biologically active, but functionally different, hormones linked in the same precursor molecule, as occurs in the pro-ACTH-endorphin molecule. Presumably, the prohormone-specific segment facilitates intracellular transport or packaging of the hormone.

THE SECRETED FORM OF THE HORMONE

The principal secreted form of the hormone contains 84 amino acids. PTH's critical role in the physiology of calcium homeostasis results from its multiple actions on kidney and bone. Expression of hormone action is linked to a number of biochemical events at the surface and within target-tissue cells. PTH interacts with hormone-specific receptors on the plasma membrane of target-tissue cells.

This interaction initiates a cascade of intracellular events: the generation of cAMP, phosphorylation of specific intracellular proteins by PTH-activated kinases, intracellular entry of calcium, and activation of intracellular enzymes which ultimately contribute to or cause directly a full spectrum of ensuing metabolic consequences.

The NH_2-terminal one-third of this molecule (positions 1—34) contains all the structural requirements necessary for full biological activity in multiple assay systems, in terms of calcium and phosphate metabolism. This region has been synthesized and found to be nearly equipotent, on a molar basis, to native PTH in vitro and in vivo.[5,6] Also, binding of bPTH-(1—34) to renal membrane receptors is equal, on a molar basis, to binding of bPTH-(1—84).[7,8]

No physiological function has yet been established for the remaining major (COOH-terminal) portion of the PTH (positions 35—84). Indeed, substantiation that regions other than the NH_2 terminus of the molecule are devoid of PTH-like agonist activity and are unable to bind to PTH receptors has been achieved through synthesis of middle and COOH-terminal segments of the hormone: bPTH-(28—48),[9] hPTH-(44—68),[10] and hPTH-(53—84).[11]

It appears as if the COOH-terminal 2/3 of the molecule merely serves to prolong the half-life of the hormone in circulation. However, the COOH-terminal portion of the molecule actually may contain structural determinants critical to a number of PTH actions outside the arena of calcium metabolism that have only recently begun to be investigated (discussed below).

THE ACTIVE CORE OF THE PTH MOLECULE

Structure/activity studies of the fully active portion of PTH, the sequence 1—34, have determined the minimum structural elements necessary for bioactivity. Tregear et al.[5] synthesized multiple fragments of the active region and evaluated their potency in vitro and in vivo. Stepwise shortening at the COOH-terminus results in a progressive decline in activity in vitro and in vivo until position 27 is deleted, after which point no further activity remains. Since the time of these studies, more-sensitive in vitro techniques employing highly purified canine renal membranes for the in vitro renal adenylate cyclase assay have been developed, and extremely weak agonist activity has been shown for the fragments 1—26 and 1—25. The decline in potency observed with progressive truncation of the COOH-terminus correlates with a reduction in binding affinity.[8] Stepwise deletions at the NH_2 terminus also cause decline in bioactivity, but at much more rapid rate. Tregear et al.[5] showed that the simple deletion of position 1 caused a 90% loss of potency. Removal of two residues, yielding the fragment bPTH-(3—34), caused complete loss of activity in the cyclase assay. The fragment bPTH-(3—34) is either nearly or completely inactive in all _in vitro_ and _in vivo_ systems tested.[5,12,13]

These studies delineate the minimum sequence required for biological activity: the region 2—25. Simultaneous addition of bPTH-(1—12) and bPTH-(13—34) failed to stimulate a PTH-like response, demonstrating that the sequence must be intact and continuous to be active.[13] These studies also reveal the importance of position 1 for bioactivity, and directed further effort toward exploring modifications of position 1.[14]

ANALOGUES OF ENHANCED BIOLOGICAL ACTIVITY

From these studies, several structural modifications that enhance bioactivity have been identified; all of them are confined to either the NH_2 or COOH terminus. Substitution of a D-alanine at position 1 yielded an analogue 300% as active _in vivo_ as bPTH-(1—34).[13] _In vitro_, the analogue was only 55% as active as bPTH-(1—34),[13] suggesting that resistance to degradation _in vivo_ might be responsible for enhanced activity and not increased receptor affinity. Simple conversion of the COOH terminus to a carboxyamide increases activity to 250% that of PTH both _in vitro_ and _in vivo_.[13] Substitution of tyrosine for phenylalanine at position 34 increased activity to 140% that bPTH-(1—34).[15] Combination of both modifications in the same analogue produced a compound, [Tyr-34]bPTH-(1—34)-amide, 300% as active as bPTH-(1—34) _in vitro_.[16] Most recently, we[17] have shown that the analogue [Nle-8,Nle-18,D-Tyr-34]bPTH-(1—34)amide is more than four times as active as bPTH-(1—34) _in vitro_, and is therefore the most potent PTH analogue yet synthesized.

A recently synthesized photolabile PTH analogue may provide additional guidance for design of analogues of enhanced bioactivity.[18] Addition of aromatic nitro azides to lysine side-chains causes a 2- to 3-fold increase in bioactivity.

INHIBITORS OF PTH

For PTH, "binding" and "activation" regions of the molecule appear largely separable. The amino acids at positions 1 and 2 are critical for stimulation of adenylate cyclase, whereas the minimum structural determinants required for receptor binding reside within the region 3—34 (Fig. 3). Following this rationale, activity-enhancing modifications were imposed on the region 3—34 in an attempt to increase affinity for receptors without restoring agonist properties.

We synthesized an analogue of the region 3—34, [Nle-8,Nle-18,-Tyr-34]bPTH-(3—34)amide, that lacks agonist activity and is a potent

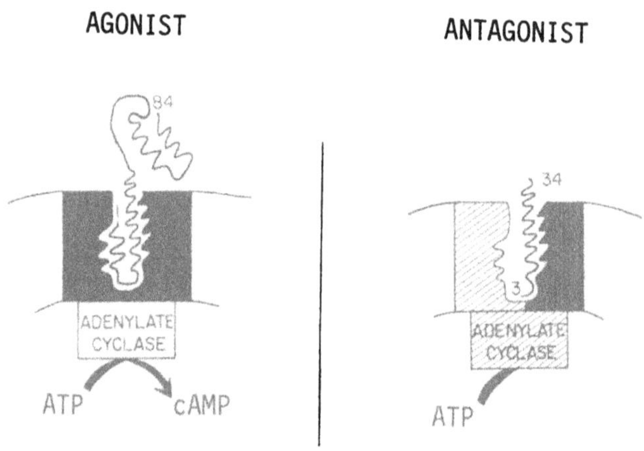

Fig. 3. Schematic representation of interactions with the PTH receptor. For agonist forms of the hormone, such as native PTH-(1—84), the 1—34 region alone is sufficient to fully activate adenylate cyclase. Inhibitory analogues containing the 3—34 sequence can occupy the receptor without activating adenylate cyclase.

inhibitor of PTH-stimulated adenylate cyclase activity in vitro: using canine renal cortical plasma membranes, the analogue caused approximately 50% inhibition of PTH action when present at concentrations equimolar to PTH.[19] The analogue could inhibit completely PTH action. The inhibitory constant (K_i=1.24 x 10^{-8}M) was derived by Eadie-Hofstee plots, and the analogue demonstrated kinetics characteristic of a pure competitive inhibitor. Similar studies were undertaken in bone, and comparable data were obtained.[20]

Although these in vitro studies provide direction for the eventual design of in vivo inhibitors of PTH, the importance of assessing inhibitory potency in multiple biological systems cannot be overemphasized. Preliminary evaluation of [Nle-8,Nle-18,Tyr-34]bPTH-(3—34)amide in the chick and rat has failed to confirm either inhibitory or agonist properties for this analogue.[21] Studies in the dog reveal possible inhibitory effects, but also definite weak partial agonist properties.[22] The analogue possessed agonist-like effects on serum calcium and on urinary phosphate and cyclic AMP excretion. The potency of the compound was estimated to be less than 1% that of bPTH-(1—84). These agonist properties precluded potential use of the analogue as an inhibitor in vivo. The reasons for the discrepancy between agonist and antagonist responses in vitro and in vivo remain to be elucidated. Possible explanations for the discrepant observations include alteration in (damage to) receptor properties during preparation of membranes for in vitro studies (which impairs their capacity to respond to weak agonists), or accelerated clearance or metabolism of analogues *in vivo*. In addition, it must be considered that all mineral-ion transport responses to PTH may not be coupled to the receptor-linked adenylate cyclase that is studied *in vitro*. Along these lines Herrmann-Erlee and co-workers (personal communication) have demonstrated for the first time inhibition of a PTH-mediated metabolic response other than cyclic AMP generation: at a ratio of antagonist to agonist of 10:1, the analogue completely inhibited PTH-stimulated calcium release from embryonic bone *in vitro*.

Although the ideal inhibitory analogue of PTH has not yet been prepared, this early line of investigation appears promising. Further refinements in structure and more extensive *in vivo* evaluation using multiple assay systems will be required to produce inhibitors of clinical utility.

THE BINDING CORE OF THE PTH MOLECULE

Fragments of the inhibitory analogue [Nle-8,Nle-18,Tyr-34]-bPTH-(3—34)amide have been used in delineating the principal binding domain of the PTH molecule. The fragments 5—34, 7—34, 10—34, 15—34, 20—34, and 25—34 displayed progressive decline in binding affinity for the renal receptor with increasing NH_2-terminal deletions.[23] A smaller fragment, 28—34, did not compete for renal binding sites.

Deletion of the COOH-terminal region 28—34 causes a large decline in binding affinity: binding of bPTH-(1—27)amide was reduced by a factor of 50,000--100,000 compared with [Nle-18,Nle-18, Tyr-34]bPTH-(1—34)amide.[24] Increasing NH_2-terminal deletions of bPTH-(1—27)amide caused progressive declines in binding affinity, until position 15 is reached: bPTH-(15—27)amide cannot bind to renal receptors.

These studies identified at least two binding domains within the molecule which are relatively small (10 amino acids or smaller) when compared with the entire 84-amino acid sequence. The region 25—34 is the sequence containing the principal structural determinants for receptor interaction (Fig. 4).

ANALOGUES THAT ARE SELECTIVE IN THEIR SPECTRUM OF BIOLOGICAL ACTIONS

Another area of analogue design is directed at synthesizing compounds whose spectrum of biological activity is narrowed or altered. For instance, an analogue whose sole biological activity is to promote phosphaturia without causing hypercalcemia might be of great value in the treatment of chronic renal failure. Preliminary evidence suggests such possibilities.

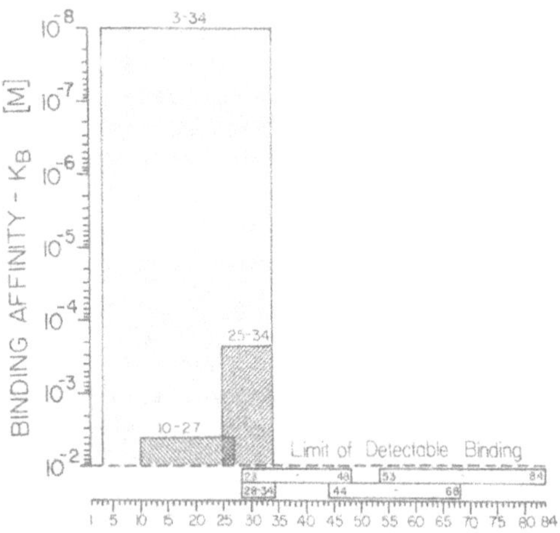

Fig. 4. Delineation and relative importance of binding domains of PTH. On the horizontal axis is plotted position number of amino acids in the sequence of the native hormone, PTH-(1—84). Binding affinity (K_B) to renal receptors is plotted on the vertical axis. The contribution to binding of the fully active 1—34 sequence (stippled) by the mid-region, 10—27, and COOH-terminal region, 25—34 (cross-hatched), is shown. Despite its shorter sequence, the contribution of the 25—34 domain to binding is 20-fold greater than the 1—27 region, and hence appears to be the principal binding domain. Because there is no increase in binding affinity attributable to residues COOH-terminal to position 34, the binding of PTH-(1—84) is not shown. Similarly, PTH-(3—34) (vertical line) has a binding affinity equal to PTH-(1—34); hence, deletion of the NH_2-terminal two residues does not decrease affinity for the renal receptor. Previously evaluated peptides representing regions of PTH 28—34, 28—48, 44—68, and 53—84 all have no demonstrable binding. These peptides are depicted as open boxes below the limit of detectable binding and overlying their sequence.[24]

The analogue [desamino Ala-1]bPTH-(1—34) is identical with bPTH-(1—34), except that it lacks the NH_2-terminal NH_2 group. Parsons et al.,[13] using an in vivo rat assay, found that the effects of I.V. administration of the desamino analogue were markedly different from those of bPTH-(1—34). Whereas bPTH-(1—34) raises plasma phosphate, presumably reflecting mobilization of phosphate from bone, the desamino analogue causes a fall in plasma phosphate and is considerably more phosphaturic than bPTH-(1—34). These experiments provide the first evidence that it may be possible to direct structure in order to selectively obtain only one or a limited number of hormonal effects of PTH. Successful design of such analogues depends ultimately on the nature of the PTH receptor in each target tissue. If PTH receptors in kidney and bone are identical, it seems unlikely that simple structural modification of PTH will produce analogues whose actions on these organs diverge. Currently, indirect comparison of receptors has yielded somewhat contradictory information. Whereas bPTH-(1—84) and bPTH-(1—34) are both active in renal systems, some investigators have found bPTH(1—84) to be nearly inactive and bPTH-(1--34) to be markedly active in a bone system.[25] Others have found that bPTH-(1—84) is somewhat active in bone,[26] or that the characteristics of the presumed receptors in bone and kidney are nearly identical.[20]

CLEAVAGE OF THE PTH MOLECULE IN VIVO

PTH is cleaved in vivo. Detailed analysis of metabolism of the hormone and the implications for clinical application of PTH radioimmunoassays have been discussed previously.[27] The important issue in this field is centered on the physiologic significance of metabolism. Cleavage may generate biologically active fragments of PTH and thus represent an activation process for expression of PTH action on certain target organs such as bone.[25] If such cleavage occurs before hormone interaction with target tissue, the hormone fragments produced could constitute the predominant, if not the sole, mediator of all or of certain PTH actions. Alternatively, cleavage of PTH may be principally a catabolic step, the first step in a pathway leading to removal of hormone from blood and tissue fluids. Even if the principal role of cleavage is hormone degradation as opposed to potentiation, cleavage may represent an important control point in regulating levels of active hormone in vivo.

Preliminary evidence suggests that a region of the PTH molecule encompassing the cleavage site may contain all the structural determinants necessary for recognition by the enzymes that mediate cleavage (Fig. 1). The liver appears to mediate the predominant cleavage of PTH in vivo, although the kidney also metabolizes the hormone. D'Amour et al.[28] found that the region PTH-(28—48) contains a critical recognition sequence for PTH hormone uptake and metabolism by the liver.

PTH ACTIONS UNRELATED TO CALCIUM AND PHOSPHATE METABOLISM

The clustering of structures critical to PTH effects on calcium and phosphate metabolism at the NH_2 terminus raises important teleological issues concerning the function of the remaining COOH portion of the hormone, and may indicate physiological roles as yet undetermined for PTH. A number of biological actions of the hormone on tissues not conventionally regarded as PTH target tissues have been described.

High circulating levels of PTH have been implicated as contributing to the genesis of anemia in uremia. Surgical correction of primary or secondary hyperparathyroidism is often accompanied by restoration of a normal hematocrit. Preliminary in vitro studies[29] show that PTH-(1—34) and PTH-(1—84) increase osmotic fragility and hemolysis of erythocytes. In addition, PTH appears to be a potential bone-marrow toxin, causing inhibition of erythropoiesis.[30] Intact PTH-(1--84) (in concentrations comparable to that found in uremic sera) inhibits human peripheral blood erythroid-colony formation (BFU-E) in vitro; neither PTH-(1—34) nor PTH-(53—84) possesses this property. Hence, either the complete sequence or the large COOH-terminal fragments that accumulate in uremia are needed for this effect. The mechanism for inhibition of erythropoiesis has not yet been determined. There is evidence that response to erythropoietin is impaired,[31] and that large amounts of calcium entering bone-marrow cells may suppress proliferation of erythroid colonies.[32] In addition, changes in the bone marrow microenvironment resulting from exposure to PTH may inhibit erythropoiesis.

In further exploring possible PTH-mediated effects in uremia, Bogin et al.[33] examined the interaction of PTH with heart tissue. Rat heart cells grown in culture increased their rate of beating and died prematurely. This effect was observed for both PTH-(1—84) and PTH-(1—34), but not for PTH-(53—84), and appears related to calcium entry into cells.

Liver, too, may be a target tissue for PTH action and not merely the site of hormone degradation. Hruska et al.[34] have shown that PTH-(1—84) stimulated hepatic release of glucose and gluconeogenesis in vivo when used in concentrations comparable to those attained in uremia. These data correlate with in vitro data demonstrating PTH-stimulated increases in cAMP in rat liver cells and homogenates.[35,36] Again, the entire hormone sequence was required; PTH-(1—34) was devoid of this activity.

Along similar lines, Arber et al.[37] have employed a highly sensitive cytochemical assay based on renal distal convoluted-tubule cells to study the biological effects of PTH and its fragments. PTH-(1—84) causes a peak in glucose-6-phosphate dehydrogenase (G6PD) activity at 8 minutes, and a second comparable peak at 14 minutes. PTH-(1—34) causes a G6PD at only 8 minutes. PTH-(53—84) also stimulates G6PD activity, but only at the later time. The physiological significance of this finding for a COOH-terminal PTH fragment and the relation of PTH action to G6PD have not yet been clarified.

SUMMARY AND FUTURE DIRECTIONS

Peptide synthesis and the application of a wide range of biological assays have permitted intensive and detailed study of structure/activity relations for PTH. Several discrete regions of the molecule have been identified that are responsible for independent physiological functions. It was determined that these separate functions are displayed in an almost linear fashion along the primary sequence of the hormone — a conceptual framework that has greatly facilitated the synthesis of PTH analogues. The NH_2-terminal region of Pre-ProPTH contains a leader sequence. Despite differences between the PTH leader sequence and other precursor-specific sequences, this region of the molecule possesses biological properties related to intracellular transport and metabolism which appear to be universal for precursor forms of many, if not all, peptide hormones and secreted proteins. In contrast, the NH_2-terminal portion of the native molecule, the region 1—34, has an amino acid sequence which is homologous to that of several peptide hormones, including ACTH, α-MSH, β-MSH, and β-lipotropin, yet the biological "message" conveyed by this peptide sequence appears unique to PTH. This message can be further subdivided into distinct domains: two domains responsible for receptor binding and one critical to activation of adenylate cyclase have been identified.

Directions have now been established for the design of hormone inhibitors, for analogues of enhanced bioactivity, and perhaps for analogues possessing an altered spectrum of biological properties. Although the use of PTH analogues has thus far concentrated on studies of the mode of hormone action, metabolism, and mineral-ion transport, the mode and regulation of hormone biosynthesis, post-translation modification, and secretion are areas of investigation just beginning to be examined. The rapid advances that are occurring in techniques for peptide synthesis, purification, and analysis; in the variety, sensitivity, and specificity of the increasing number of bioassays; and in the elucidation of peptide and protein conformation may provide important new directions for analogue design. Extension of these investigations of structure and function over the next several years should yield a more sophisticated understanding of the mode of hormone action. In such studies lies the promise of generating highly refined and perhaps clinically useful analogues of PTH.

ACKNOWLEDGEMENTS

Many of the studies described in this review were performed collaboratively with investigators and supporting staff of the Endocrine Unit, Massachusetts General Hospital. Their efforts are gratefully acknowledged, as is partial support from Grant No. AM11794 from the N.I.A.M.D.D.K.D.

REFERENCES

1. G. Blobel and D.D. Sabatini, Ribosome-membrane interaction in eukaryotic cells, Biomembranes. 2:193 (1971).
2. C. Milstein, G.G. Brownlee, T.M. Harrison and M.B. Mathews, A possible precursor of immunoglobulin light chains, Nature New Biol. 239:117 (1972).
3. M. Rosenblatt, J.F. Habener, G.A. Tyler, G.L. Shepard, and J.T. Potts, Jr., Chemical synthesis of the precursor-specific region of pre-proparathyroid hormone, J. Biol. Chem. 254:1414 (1979).
4. J.A. Majzoub, M. Rosenblatt, B. Fennick, R. Maunus, H.M. Kronenberg, J.T. Potts, Jr. and J.F. Habener, Synthetic pre-proparathyroid hormone leader sequence inhibits cell-free processing of placental, parathyroid, and pituitary pre-hormones, J. Biol. Chem. 255:11478 (1980).
5. G.W. Tregear, J. van Rietschoten, E. Greene, H.T. Keutmann, H.D. Niall, B. Reit, J.A. Parsons and J.T. Potts, Jr., Bovine parathyroid hormone: minimum chain length of synthetic peptide required for biological activity, Endocrinology 93:1349 (1973).
6. M. Rosenblatt, Parathyroid hormone: chemistry and structure—activity relations, Pathobiol. Annu. (in press).
7. R.A. Nissenson and C.D. Arnaud, Properties of the parathyroid hormone receptor-adenylate cyclase system in chicken renal plasma membranes, J. Biol. Chem. 254:1469 (1979).
8. G.V. Segre, M. Rosenblatt, B.L. Reiner, J.E. Mahaffey and J.T. Potts, Jr., Characterization of parathyroid hormone receptors in canine renal cortical plasma membranes using a radio-iodinated sulfur-free hormone analogue: correlation of binding with adenylate cyclase activity, J. Biol. Chem. 254:6980 (1979).
9. M. Rosenblatt, G.V. Segre and J.T. Potts, Jr., Synthesis of a fragment of parathyroid hormone, bPTH-(28—48): an inhibitor of hormone cleavage in vivo, Biochemistry 16:2811 (1977).
10. M. Rosenblatt, H.T. Keutmann, G.W. Tregear and J.T. Potts, Jr., Synthesis of a fragment of human parathyroid hormone, bPTH-(44—68), J. Med. Chem. 20:1452 (1977).
11. M. Rosenblatt, G.V. Segre, G.W. Tregear, G.L. Shepard, G.A. Tyler and J.T. Potts, Jr., Human parathyroid hormone: synthesis, chemical, biological, and immunological evaluation of the carboxyl-terminal region, Endocrinology 103:978 (1978).
12. M.P.M. Herrmann-Erlee, J.N.M. Heersche, J.W. Hekkelman, P.J. Gaillard, G.W. Tregear, J.A. Parsons and J.T. Potts, Jr., Effects on bone in vitro of bovine parathyroid hormone and synthetic fragments representing residues 1—34, 2—34, and 3—34, Endocrine Res. Commun. 3:21 (1976).

13. J.A. Parsons, B. Rafferty, D. Gray, B. Reit, J.M. Zanelli, H.T. Keutmann, G.W. Tregear, E.N. Callahan and J.T. Potts, Jr., Pharmacology of parathyroid hormone and some of its fragments and analogues, in: "Calcium-Regulating Hormones: Proceedings of the Fifth Parathyroid Conference," R.V. Talmage, M. Owen and J.A. Parsons, eds., Excerpta Medica, Amsterdam (1975).
14. G.W. Tregear and J.T. Potts, Jr., Synthetic analogues of residues 1—34 of human parathyroid hormone: influence of residue number 1 on biological potency in vitro, Endocrine Res. Commun. 2:561 (1975).
15. M. Rosenblatt, D. Goltzman, H.T. Keutmann, G.W. Tregear and J.T. Potts, Jr., Chemical and biological properties of synthetic sulfur-free analogues of parathyroid hormone, J. Biol. Chem. 251:159 (1976).
16. M. Rosenblatt and J.T. Potts, Jr., Design and synthesis of parathyroid hormone analogues of enhanced biological activity, Endocrine Res. Commun. 4:115 (1977).
17. M. Rosenblatt, M.D. Coltrera, G.L. Shepard, D.A. Gray, J.A. Parsons and J.T. Potts, Jr., Sulfur-free parathyroid hormone analogues containing D-amino acids: biological properties in vitro and in vivo, Biochemistry (in press).
18. M.D. Coltrera, J.T. Potts, Jr. and M. Rosenblatt, Identification of a renal receptor for parathyroid hormone by photoaffinity radiolabeling using a synthetic analogue, J. Biol. Chem. (in press).
19. M. Rosenblatt, E.N. Callahan, J.E. Mahaffey, A. Pont and J.T. Potts, Jr, Parathyroid hormone inhibitors: design, synthesis, and biologic evaluation of hormone analogues, J. Biol. Chem. 252:5847 (1977).
20. S.R. Goldring, J.E. Mahaffey, M. Rosenblatt, J.-M. Dayer, J.T. Potts, Jr. and S.M Krane, Parathyroid hormone inhibitors: comparison of biological activity in bone- and skin-derived tissue, J. Clin. Endocrinol. Metab. 48:655 (1979).
21. D.A. Gray, J.A. Parsons, J.T. Potts, Jr., M. Rosenblatt and R.W. Stevenson, In vivo testing of a parathyroid hormone antagonist, [Nle-8,Nle-18,Tyr-34]bPTH-(3—34)amide, Br. J. Pharmacol. (submitted).
22. G.V. Segre, G. Tully, M. Rosenblatt, J. Laugharn, B. Reit and J.T. Potts, Jr., Evaluation of an in vitro parathyroid hormone (bPTH) antagonist in intact dogs, Calcif. Tissue Int. 28:171 (1979) (Abstr).
23. M. Rosenblatt, G.V. Segre, G.A. Tyler, G.L. Shepard, S.R. Nussbaum and J.T. Potts, Jr., Identification of a receptor-binding region in parathyroid hormone, Endocrinology, 106:545 (1980).
24. S.R. Nussbaum, M. Rosenblatt and J.T. Potts, Jr., Parathyroid hormone-renal receptor interactions: demonstration of two receptor-binding domains, J. Biol. Chem. 255:10183 (1980).

25. K.J. Martin, J.J. Freitag, M.B. Conrades, K.A Hruska, S. Klahr and E. Slatopolsky, Selective uptake of the synthetic amino terminal fragment of bovine parathyroid hormone by isolated perfused bone, J. Clin. Invest. 62:256 (1978).
26. D. Goltzman, Examination of the requirement for metabolism of parathyroid hormone in skeletal tissue before biological action, Endocrinology 102:1555 (1978).
27. G.V. Segre, H.D. Niall, J.F. Habener and J.T. Potts, Jr., Metabolism of parathyroid hormone: physiologic and clinical significance, Am. J. Med. 56:774 (1974).
28. P. D'Amour, P.M. Huet, G.V. Segre, and M. Rosenblatt, Charactersitics of bovine parathyroid hormone extraction by the dog liver in vivo, Am.J. Physiol. (in press).
29. S.G. Massry, E. Bogin, D. Meytes, G. Bristol, J. Smith and P.P. Dukes, Effect of parathyroid hormone (PTH) on red blood cells (RBC) and on erythropoiesis, Clin. Res. 28:535A (1980). 30.
30. D. Meytes, E. Bogin, A. Ma, P.P. Dukes and S.G. Massry, Effect of parathyroid hormone on erythropoiesis, J. Clin. Invest. 67:1263 (1981).
31. A.J. Erslev, T. Connelly and J. Caro, The role of parathyroid hormones in erythropoiesis, in: "Proceedings of The Conference on Aplastic Anemia: A Stem Cell Disease," A.S. Levine, ed., U.S. Dept. of Health and Human Services, National Institutes of Health, N.I.H. Publication No. 81-1008 (1981).
32. J. Misiti and J.L. Spivak, Erythropoiesis in vitro, J. Clin. Invest. 64:1573 (1979).
33. E. Bogin, S.G. Massry and I. Harary, Effect of parathyroid hormone on rat heart cells, J. Clin. Invest. 67:1215 (1981).
34. K.A. Hruska, J. Blondin, R. Bass, J. Santiago, L. Thomas, P. Altsheler, K. Martin and S. Klahr, Effect of intact parathyroid hormone on hepatic glucose release in the dog. J. Clin. Invest. 64:1016 (1979).
35. J.M. Canterbury, G. Levy, E. Ruiz and E. Reiss, Parathyroid hormone activation of adenylate cyclase in liver, Proc. Soc. Exp. Biol. Med. 147:366 (1974).
36. M.A. Moxley, N.H. Bell, S.R. Wagle, D.O. Allen and J. Ashmore, Parathyroid hormone stimulation of glucose and urea production in isolated liver cells, Am. J. Physiol. 227:1058 (1974).
37. C.E. Arber, J.M. Zanelli, J.A. Parsons, L. Bitensky and J. Chayen, Comparison of the bioactivity of highly purified human parathyroid hormone and of synthetic amino- and carboxyl-region fragments, J. Endocrinol. 85:55P (1980).

FUNCTIONAL PROPERTIES OF PARATHYROID HORMONE RECEPTORS IN KIDNEY AND BONE

A.P. Teitelbaum, N.B. Pliam, C. Silve, S.R. Abbott, R.A. Nissenson, and C.D. Arnaud

Medical Service, Veterans Administration Medical Center, San Francisco, CA 94121; and the Department of Medicine, University of California, San Francisco CA 94143

INTRODUCTION

It is well established that the renal and skeletal actions of parathyroid hormone (PTH) contribute to the maintenance of calcium and phosphate homeostasis. Considerable evidence exists for the involvement of cAMP in mediating some of the effects of PTH in the kidney: 1) *in vivo* administration of the hormone rapidly increases urinary cAMP and subsequently induces phosphaturia[1]; 2) cAMP mimics this response[1,2]; and 3) renal plasma membranes contain PTH-responsive adenylate cyclase activity[3]. The role of cAMP in PTH regulation of bone metabolism is less clear. Although it has been shown that PTH stimulates production of cAMP in whole bone[4] and in cultured bone cells[5], evidence exists both for and against the involvement of cAMP in PTH-induced bone resorption, osteocytic osteolysis, inhibition of bone formation, and skeletal lactate production[6].

The initial biochemical event leading to the actions of PTH is presumably the interaction of the hormone with its receptor. Specific, high affinity PTH binding sites, which appear to be coupled to adenylate cyclase activity, have been identified in chicken[7], canine[8,9], and human[9] renal plasma membranes. However, to our knowledge, skeletal PTH receptors have not previously been demonstrated. In the present studies, we used [^{125}I]-labeled bovine PTH(1-34) to study PTH binding in bone cells isolated from fetal chicken calvaria. The characteristics of these skeletal PTH receptors are virtually identical with respect to specificity of binding and stimulation of cAMP production to those we have found for renal PTH receptors.

Guanyl nucleotides markedly potentiate the renal adenylate cyclase response to PTH[10-13]. This action may be mediated via a nucleotide-dependent regulatory protein, shown in other systems to interact with and modulate the function of both receptors and adenylate cyclase[14,15]. As part of an investigation to determine the mechanism of the enhancement of PTH action by guanyl nucleotides, we studied their effect on the PTH-receptor interaction in plasma membranes from canine kidney.

METHODS

The synthetic amino-terminal bovine and human sequences of PTH, bPTH(1-34) and hPTH(1-34) [Brewer et al.[16]] were donated by Beckman Bioproducts. Synthetic hPTH(1-34) [Niall et al.[17]] was donated by Peninsula Labs. Bovine PTH(1-34) was the gift of Dr. J. Zanelli. [^{8}Nle,^{18}Nle,^{34}Tyr]-substituted bPTH(1-34)amide and bPTH(3-34)amide were generously supplied by Drs. M. Rosenblatt and J.T. Potts, Jr. Glucagon and arginine vasopressin (AVP) were purchased from Sigma Co.; insulin from Eli Lilly Corp.; the amino-terminal 24 amino acid sequence of adrenocorticotrophic hormone [ACTH(1-24)] from Biochem Inc.; calcitonin was the gift of Armour Pharmaceutical Co.

Renal Plasma Membrane Preparation

Plasma membrane fractions were isolated from the kidney cortex of adult mongrel dogs or from the whole kidneys of 8-10 week old female chickens by the method of Fitzpatrick et al.[18] as modified by DiBella[19]. Canine kidney tissue was disrupted by three 5 sec. low speed bursts of a Polytron homogenizer prior to processing. Membrane fractions were enriched 6-10 fold (relative to homogenate) in Na^{+}-K^{+} ATPase activity. Plasma membrane fractions were stored in aliquots at -80°C; PTH binding and adenylate cyclase activities were stable for at least 6 months.

Chicken Bone Cell Isolation

Bone cells were isolated from the calvaria of 18 day chicken embryos by the method of Peck et al.[6] as modified by Nijweide et al.[20]. Briefly, calvaria were incubated twice with collagenase (2 mg/ml) (Millipore Corp., Worthington Division) for 1 hr at 37°C in Hank's balanced buffered salt solution, and centrifuged at 200 x g for 5 min. The supernates from the two incubations were pooled and resultant cells formed monolayers in culture dishes. Medium 199 containing 10% chicken serum was used as the growth medium.

Radioiodination of bPTH(1-34)

An electrolytic procedure[21] was used to prepare [^{125}I]-bPTH-(1-34). The preparation was purified by receptor adsorption[7] prior to use in binding assays. Specific activity varied between 80 and 120 μc/μg.

PTH Binding Assays

Renal plasma membranes. Incubations contained 25 mM Tris HCl (pH 7.5), 2 mM $MgCl_2$, [^{125}I]-bPTH(1-34)(100,000 cpm/ml), 0.1% bovine serum albumin (BSA), unlabeled hormone or diluent (10 mM acetic acid, 0.1% BSA) and 25-50 μg membrane protein. Reactions were carried out at 30°C. Bound and free hormone were separated on 0.2 μm cellulose acetate filters[7].

Bone cells. Confluent cells were incubated at room temperature with serum-free Medium 199 containing 20,000 cpm/ml [^{125}I]-bPTH-(1-34) unlabeled hormone or diluent and 0.1% BSA. The reaction was terminated by aspirating the medium. Cells were washed 4 times with ice-cold Hank's salt solution and scraped off the dishes for determination of bound radioactivity. Scatchard analysis[22] was performed on equilibrium binding data to yield affinity and concentration of receptors.

Adenylate Cyclase Activity

Assays contained 25 mM Tris HCl, 2 mM $MgCl_2$, 0.1 mM [α-^{32}P]-ATP, 1 mM 1-methyl, 3-isobutylxamthine (IBMX), 0.3 mg/ml creatine phosphokinase, and 10 mM creatine phosphate. [^{32}P]-cAMP was isolated by the double column procedure of Salomon et al.[23].

cAMP Assay

Confluent cells were incubated for 5 min. at room temperature with Medium 199, 1 mM IBMX, hormone or diluent and 0.1% BSA. Cell cAMP was extracted with 4 washes of absolute ethanol. Samples were evaporated on a Brinkmann sample concentrator, resuspended in 50 mM sodium acetate (pH 4.0), and cAMP measured using the competitive protein binding assay of Gilman[24].

Autoradiographs

[^{125}I]-bPTH(1-34), approximately 200 fmole, was incubated with one half calvarium (with or without excess unlabeled bPTH(1-34) (243 nM) for 60 min., washed and processed by the method of Hradek et al.[25]. The grains so obtained were quantitated by the method of Goldfine et al.[26].

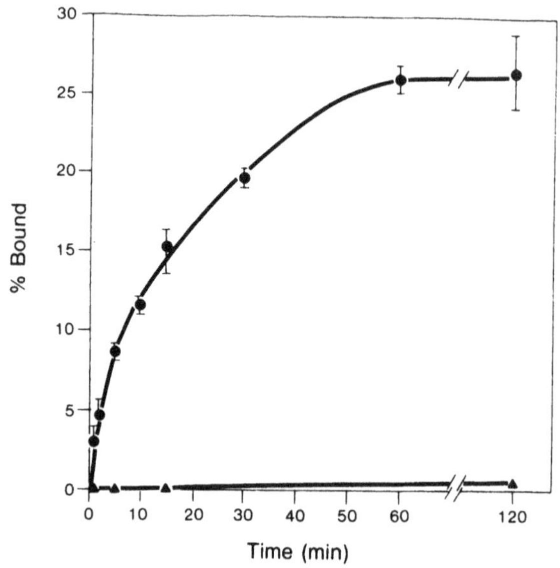

Figure 1. Time course for [^{125}I]-bPTH(1-34) binding to renal plasma membranes. Binding was measured after addition of 0.5 mg/ml membrane protein in the absence (●) or presence (▲) of 0.75 μM unlabeled bPTH(1-34). Each point is the mean ± S.E. of triplicate determinations.

RESULTS

Specific binding of [^{125}I]-bPTH(1-34) to canine renal plasma membranes reached apparent steady-state after 60 min. (Fig. 1). Total binding was 25% of the radioactivity added; non-specific binding was < 1%. The forward rate constant, calculated by the method of Rodbard[27] was 0.04 nM-min. When 100 μM Gpp(NH)p was present, apparent steady-state was reached after 30 min. (not shown) and the forward rate constant was 0.005 nM-min.

Unlabeled bPTH(1-34), bPTH(1-84), [^{8}Nle,^{18}Nle,^{34}Tyr]bPTH(1-34)-amide and hPTH(1-34) (Niall sequence)[17] were equipotent competitors for PTH receptors (Fig. 2A). The concentration of these peptides required to displace 50% of [^{125}I]-bPTH(1-34) from receptors was 2 nM, compared with 80 nM for hPTH(1-34) synthesized according to the amino acid sequence determined by Brewer[16]. The order of potency of these peptides was the same for stimulation of adenylate cyclase (Fig. 2B) and for PTH binding. The binding affinity of [^{8}Nle,^{18}Nle,^{34}Tyr]bPTH(3-34)amide, a competitive antagonist of PTH, was approximately 20 nM. This peptide did not stimulate adenylate cyclase when added alone to renal plasma membranes and was a potent inhibitor of bPTH(1-34) activation of the enzyme. The potency of peroxide-treated bPTH(1-34) was only 1% of that of the untreated peptide (not shown). This residual activity might have been due to incomplete oxidation of the peptide.

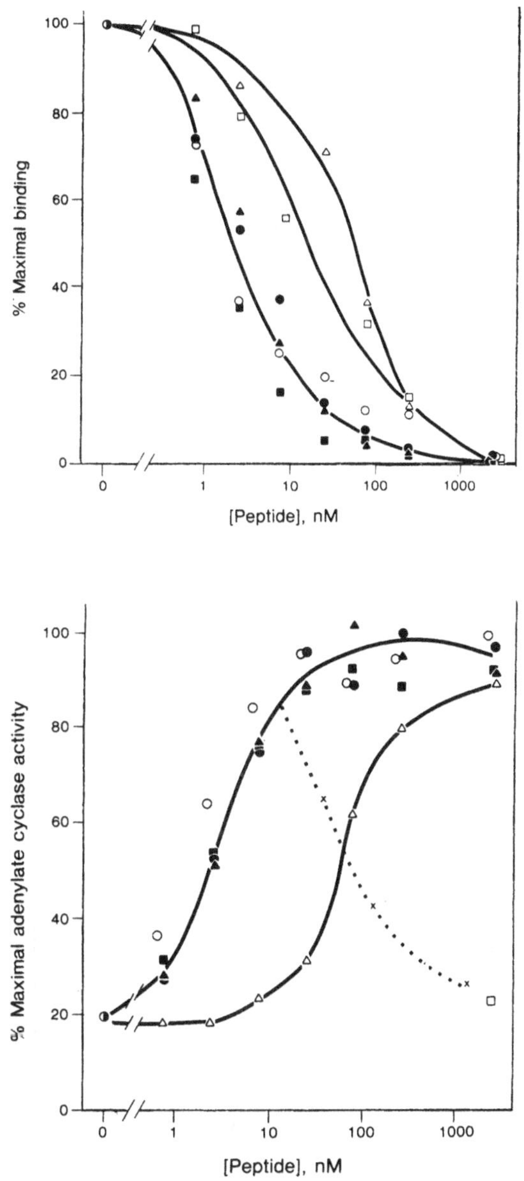

A

B

Figure 2. Effect of various PTH peptides on [^{125}I]-bPTH(1-34) binding and adenylate cyclase in renal plasma membranes. A: competitive displacement of [^{125}I]-bPTH(1-34) by bPTH(1-34) (●); bPTH(1-84) (o); hPTH(1-34), Brewer sequence (Δ), hPTH(1-34), Niall sequence (▲); bPTH(1-34)A and bPTH(3-34)A (□). B: stimulation of adenylate cyclase by the same PTH peptides as in A. (x---x) bPTH(1-34) (12.5 nM) was incubated with several concentrations of bPTH(3-34)A. Each data point represents the mean of at least 3 measurements.

Several peptide hormones, structurally unrelated to PTH (glucagon, calcitonin, AVP and insulin) when tested up to 10 μg/ml, did not compete with [^{125}I]-bPTH(1-34) for receptors (not shown). A higher concentration (17 μM) of ACTH(1-24) which shares a sequence homology with the binding region of PTH, inhibited labeled hormone binding 50% and decreased by 18% the stimulation of adenylate cyclase by PTH (10 nM). Of the non-PTH peptides tested, only glucagon significantly stimulated adenylate cyclase activity (1.6-fold relative to basal activity), but to a much lesser extent than bPTH(1-34).

Gpp(NH)p, a stable analog of GTP, enhances both basal and PTH-stimulated adenylate cyclase activity[10-13]. In canine renal cortical plasma membranes, 10^{-4} M Gpp(NH)p increases the sensitivity of the PTH response 100-fold (not shown). The effect of 100 μM Gpp(NH)p on PTH binding is shown in Figure 3. Specific binding of PTH was decreased by the nucleotide. In both cases (±Gpp(NH)p), a single class of PTH binding sites was obtained (inset). Gpp(NH)p reduced the affinity of canine renal PTH receptors 3-4 fold, but the number of receptors was not decreased. This concentration of

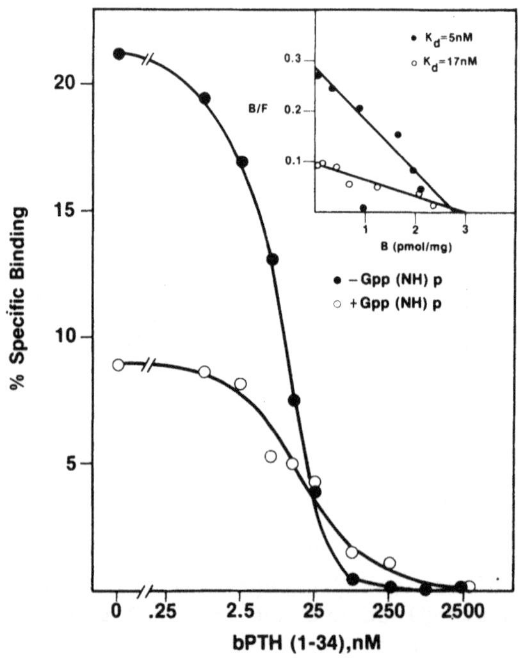

Figure 3. Effect of Gpp(NH)p on PTH receptor affinity. [^{125}I]-bPTH-(1-34) was incubated with canine renal plasma membranes in the absence and presence of 100 μM Gpp(NH)p for 60 min. Determination of Kd was by Scatchard analysis (inset). The data shown are from a representative experiment; each data point represents the mean of duplicate determinations.

Gpp(NH)p had a dramatic effect on the slow dissociation rate ($t\frac{1}{2} \simeq$ 200 min.) of [^{125}I]-bPTH(1-34) (not shown); the reverse rate constant for PTH binding was increased more than 200-fold by the nucleotide.

The potentiation by guanyl nucleotides of the PTH effect on chicken renal adenylate cyclase activity is obscured at high nucleotide concentrations (10^{-4}M) because of the large increment in basal activity. Therefore, we tested the effect of 10^{-6} Gpp(NH)p on PTH binding in these membranes. No change in dissociation rate ($t\frac{1}{2} \simeq$ 4 min.) or binding affinity was seen in the presence of the nucleotide (not shown). Figure 4 shows that Gpp(NH)p alters the linear relationship between the fraction of occupied PTH receptors and adenylate cyclase activity. These data indicate that Gpp(NH)p enhances the coupling of occupied receptors to the enzyme by increasing the fractional response to the hormone at any given level of receptor occupancy.

The time course for binding of [^{125}I]-bPTH(1-34) to primary cultures of chicken bone cells is shown in Figure 5. Apparent steady-state was reached after 60 min. and remained constant until 90 min. Specific binding ranged from 5 to 10% of the radioactivity added. Cellular binding of labeled PTH was only partially reversible (not shown); 90 min. after addition of a 1000-fold molar excess of unlabeled bPTH(1-34) to cells preincubated (for 1 hr.) with [^{125}I]-bPTH(1-34), only 60% of the radioactivity was released from receptors.

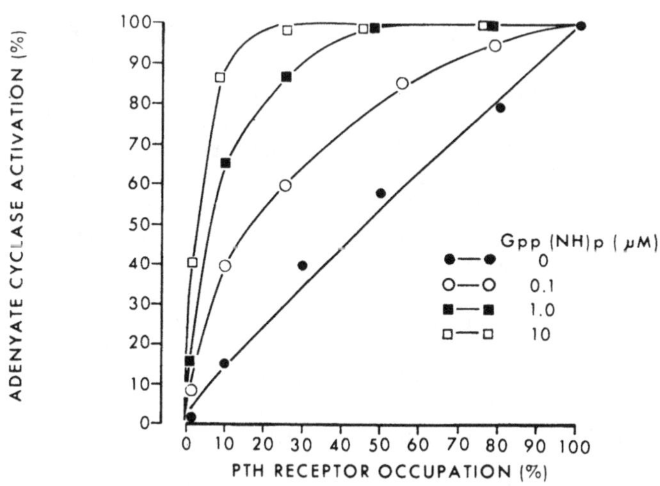

Figure 4. Effect of Gpp(NH)p on the relationship between PTH receptor occupancy and PTH-stimulation of adenylate cyclase in chicken renal plasma membranes. PTH binding and adenylate cyclase were measured under identical experimental conditions. 100% PTH receptor occupancy was determined from Scatchard analysis of competitive displacement data.

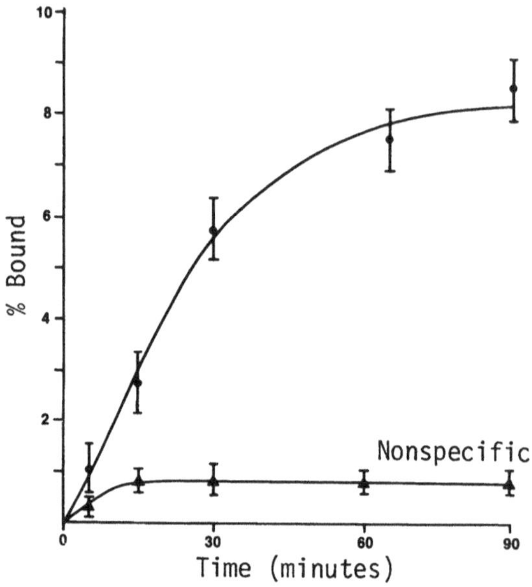

Figure 5. Time course for [^{125}I]-bPTH(1-34) binding to cultured bone cells from embryonic chick calvaria. Binding was measured in the absence (●) or presence (▲) of excess unlabeled bPTH(1-34) (0.25 μM). Culture dishes contained 0.8-1.0 mg cell protein. Each point is the mean ± S.E. (n = 3).

Figure 6A shows that the affinity of bPTH(1-34) for binding sites in bone cells was approximately 1 nM. Scatchard analysis revealed a single class of PTH receptors. Assuming equal distribution of binding sites among the cell populations, we calculated that there are approximately 10,000 receptors per cell. Bovine PTH(1-84) was as effective as bPTH(1-34) in displacing labeled PTH from receptors, whereas hPTH(1-34) (Brewer sequence) was 30-fold less potent (not shown). Glucagon, calcitonin, and insulin did not compete for PTH receptors when tested at 1 μg/ml (not shown).

The PTH peptides tested stimulated cAMP accumulation with the same order of potency with which they competed for PTH receptors. The concentration of peptide which half-maximally increased cellular cAMP levels was 3 nM for bPTH(1-34) (Figure 6B) and bPTH(1-84), and 90 nM for hPTH(1-34) (Brewer sequence) (not shown).

Autoradiographs of intact fetal chick calvariae incubated with [^{125}I]-bPTH(1-34) for 60 min. in the absence or presence of excess unlabeled bPTH(1-34) showed specific binding of the hormone to the plasma membranes of osteoblasts (not shown). However, a quantitative analysis of the grain distribution in the cells demonstrated that a fraction of PTH was significantly internalized, as was suggested by the presence of grains associated with coated

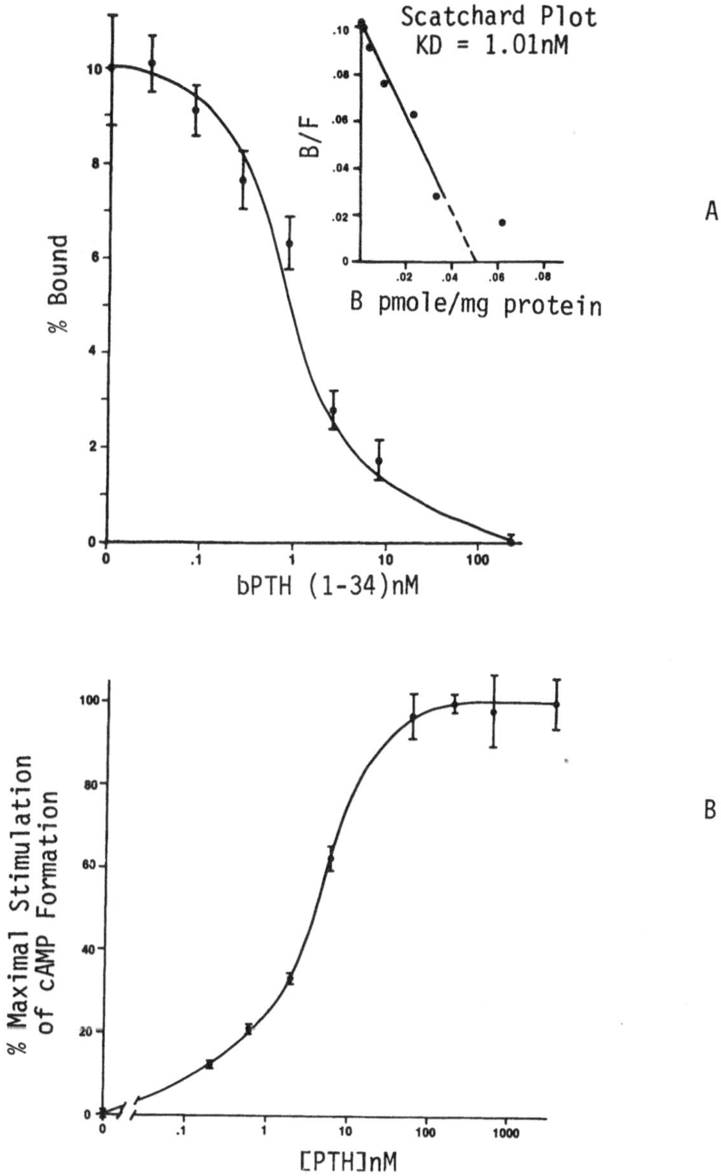

Figure 6. A: Specific [^{125}I]-bPTH(1-34) binding to bone cells from embryonic chick calvaria in the presence of varying concentrations of unlabeled bPTH(1-34). Incubations were for 60 min. at room temperature. B: Bovine PTH(1-34) stimulation of cyclic AMP accumulation in cultured bone cells from embryonic chick calvaria after 5 min. of incubation. Half maximal cyclic AMP accumulation was obtained in the presence of 3 nM bPTH(1-34). Each point is the mean ± S.E. (n = 3).

pits and coated vesicles. Electron micrographs of the bone cells isolated from these calvaria reveal that the majority of these cells are osteoblast-like, containing single nuclei and well-developed rough endoplasmic reticulum.

Table 1 compares PTH receptor binding and adenylate cyclase activation in renal plasma membranes from several species with PTH receptors and cAMP production in cultured chicken bone cells. The K_d and K_m values measured in all four systems are similar. The lower receptor number calculated for bone cells reflects normalization to whole cell protein rather than plasma membrane protein.

Table 1. Comparison of PTH receptor-adenylate cyclase systems in chicken, canine, and human renal plasma membranes and in chicken bone cell cultures.

Renal Plasma Membranes	Adenylate Cyclase	PTH Receptors	
	Km, nM	Kd, nM	Bmax^Δ
Chicken	5 - 12	7 - 10	4 - 6
Canine	3 - 9	3 - 8	2 - 3
Human	5 - 12	6 - 7	2 - 3
	cAMP Production		
Chicken Bone Cells	3*	0.6 - 1	0.05

*Concentration of bPTH(1-34) required to stimulate cAMP production half maximally, nM.

ΔNumber of PTH binding sites, pmole/mg protein.

DISCUSSION

The amino-terminal 34 amino acid sequence of PTH contains the structural requirements necessary for all of known renal and skeletal biological actions of the hormone[28]. Therefore, [^{125}I)-labeled synthetic bPTH (1-34) is a valid tracer for the study of PTH receptors in target tissues. In these studies, we have shown that the binding sites for PTH in mammalian and avian kidney and in avian bone cells have similar biochemical characteristics with respect to affinity and specificity for the hormone. These receptors appear to be functionally coupled to adenylate cyclase and may thus be involved in those PTH actions which are mediated by cAMP.

We found that bPTH(1-34) and bPTH(1-84) were equipotent in binding to PTH receptors. Furthermore, these peptides stimulated cAMP production in bone cells to a similar degree, over the same concentration range, after only 5 min. of incubation. Thus, it is unlikely that the intact hormone, bPTH(1-84), has a different time course of activation of avian skeletal adenylate cyclase than the amino-terminal fragment. Martin et al.[29] have shown that bPTH(1-34) is extracted by isolated, perfused canine tibiae and stimulates production of cAMP, but that bPTH(1-84) is neither taken up nor increases cAMP levels. The data obtained in the perfused bone system are consistent with the notion that production of an active PTH fragment is required for skeletal adenylate cyclase activation. This hypothesis is supported by data obtained in vivo which indicate that PTH is cleaved in the liver and kidney between amino acids 34 and 39, conceivably producing a biologically active fragment[30]. However, PTH metabolism was shown not to be required for its action in both kidney[31,32] and bone[33], but rather that cleavage of the hormone inactivates it. Our data in bone cells are also inconsistent with the idea that the intact molecule must be metabolized to a smaller fragment prior to activation of skeletal adenylate cyclase.

In several hormone-receptor systems, the enchanced coupling of occupied receptor to adenylate cyclase, promoted by guanyl nucleotides, is accompanied by decreased hormone binding[33]. However, in a few systems in which guanyl nucleotides potentiate hormone action, no effects of these agents on hormone binding were observed[13,34]. We found that although Gpp(NH)p enhances PTH responsiveness in both canine and chicken renal plasma membranes, membrane binding of PTH was affected only in the canine system. The reasons for this difference are unclear and may be explained by a species variation in the coupling mechanism. We have previously postulated a post-receptor locus of action of guanyl nucleotides on coupling in chicken renal membranes[13]. Alternatively, this difference might be explained on the basis of the GTP levels in the two systems. Several lines of evidence are consistent with the notion that endogenous guanyl nucleotide levels are higher in chicken than canine renal membranes: 1) basal adenylate cyclase activity in chicken renal membranes is 6 times greater than in the canine system, 2) the dissociation rate of [^{125}I]-bPTH(1-34) is 50 times greater in chicken than in canine renal membranes, and 3) guanyl nucleotides have no effect on this rate in chicken, but enhance 200-fold the dissociation rate in the canine system.

Investigation of the mechanisms involved in transmission of the hormonal signal to activation of adenylate cyclase will increase our understanding of diseases in which responsiveness to PTH is reduced, e.g., pseudohypoparathyroidism. It is of interest that recent studies in vitro have shown that PTH-responsive adenylate cyclase activity was impaired in renal plasma membranes isolated from a patient with this disease, and that this activity was restored by exogenous GTP.[36]

Furthermore, a reduced level of nucleotide dependent regulatory protein was found in the platelets of such patients[37]. Whether a defect in the coupling of PTH receptors to adenylate cyclase also exists in the bone cells of pseudohypoparathyroid patients remains to be determined. The ability to study PTH receptors in bone and kidney will permit a more complete assessment of the biochemical lesions contributing to the reduced PTH response in these patients.

ACKNOWLEDGEMENTS

This work was supported in part by the Veterans Administration and by Grant AM 21614 from the National Institutes of Health.

REFERENCES

1. L.R. Chase and G.D. Aurbach, Parathyroid function and the renal excretion of 3'5'-adenylic acid, Proc Natl Acad Sci USA 58:525 (1967).
2. N.I. Kaminsky, A.E. Broadus, J.G. Hardman, D.J. Jones, Jr., J.H. Ball, E.W. Sutherland and G.W. Liddle, Effects of parathyroid hormone on plasma and urinary adenosine 3'5'-monophosphate in man, J Clin Invest 49:2387 (1970).
3. L. Chase and G. Aurbach, Renal adenyl cyclase: anatomically separate sites for PTH and vasopressin, Science 159:545 (1968).
4. L.R. Chase, S.A. Fedak and G.D. Aurbach, Activation of skeletal adenyl cyclase by parathyroid hormone in vitro, Endocrinology 84:761 (1969).
5. W.A. Peck, Cyclic AMP as a second messenger in the skeletal actions of parathyroid hormone: A decade-old hypothesis, Calcif Tiss Int 29:1 (1979).
6. W.A. Peck and S. Klahr, Cyclic Nucleotides in bone and mineral metabolism, Adv Cyclic Nucleotide Res 11:89 (1979).
7. R.A. Nissenson and C.D. Arnaud, Properties of the parathyroid hormone receptor-adenylate cyclase system in chicken renal plasma membranes, J Biol Chem 254:1469 (1978).
8. G.V. Segre, M. Rosenblatt, B.L. Reiner, J.E. Mahaffey and J.T. Potts, Jr., Characterization of parathyroid hormone receptors in canine renal cortical plasma membranes using a radioiodinated sulfur-free hormone analogue, J Biol Chem 254:6980 (1979).
9. R.A. Nissenson, A.P. Teitelbaum, S.R. Abbott, N. Pliam, C. Silve, L. Zitzner, K. Nyiredy and C.D. Arnaud, Parathyroid hormone receptors in kidney and bone: Relation to adenylate

cyclase activation, in: "Hormonal Control of Calcium Metabolism," D.V. Cohn, R.V. Talmage, J.L. Matthews, Eds., Excerpta Medica, Amsterdam, pp.44-54 (1981).

10. N.H. Hunt, T.J. Martin, V.P. Michelangi and J.A. Eisman, Effect of guanyl nucleotides on parathyroid hormone-responsive adenylate cyclase in chick kidney, J Endocrinol 69:401 (1976).
11. V.P. Michelangeli, N.H. Hunt and T.J. Martin, States of activation of chick kidney adenylate cyclase induced by parathyroid hormone and guanyl nucleotides, J Endocrinol 72:69 (1977).
12. D. Goltzman, E.N. Callahan, G.W. Tregear and J.T. Potts, Jr., Influence of guanyl nucleotides on parathyroid hormone stimulated adenylyl cyclase activity in renal cortical membranes, Endocrinology 103:1352 (1978).
13. R.A. Nissenson, K.O. Nyiredy and C.D. Arnaud, Guanyl nucleotide potentiation of parathyroid hormone-stimulated adenylate cyclase in chicken renal plasma membranes: A receptor-independent effect, Endocrinology 108:1949 (1981).
14. T. Pfeuffer, GTP-binding proteins in membranes and the control of adenylate cyclase activity, J Biol Chem252:7224 (1977).
15. E.M. Ross, A.C. Howlett, K.M. Ferguson and A.G. Gilman, Reconstitution of hormone-sensitive adenylate cyclase activity with resolved components of the enzyme, J Biol Chem 253:6401 (1978).
16. H.B. Brewer, Jr., T. Fairwell, R. Ronan, G.W. Sizemore and C.D. Arnaud, Human PTH: amino acid sequence of the amino-terminal residues 1-34, Proc Natl Acad Sci USA 69:3585 (1972).
17. H.D. Niall, R.T. Sauer, J.W. Jacobs, H.T. Keutmann, G.V. Segre, J.L.H. O'Riordan, G.D. Aurbach, and J.T. Potts, Jr., The amino-acid sequence of the amino-terminal 1-37 residues of human PTH, Proc Natl Acad Sci USA 71:384 (1974).
18. D.F. Fitzpatrick, G.R. Davenport, L. Forte, E.J. Landon, Characterization of plasma membrane proteins in mammalian kidney, J Biol Chem 244:3561 (1969).
19. F.P. DiBella, T.P. Dousa, S.S. Miller, C.D. Arnaud, Parathyroid receptors of renal cortex: Specific binding of biologically active, ^{125}I-labeled hormone and relationship to adenyl cyclase activation, Proc Natl Acad Sci 71:723 (1974).
20. P.J. Nijweide, A. Van Der Plas and J.P. Scherft, Calcif Tiss Int (in press).
21. P.J. Sammon, J.S. Brand, W.F. Neuman and L.G. Raisz, Metabolism of labeled parathyroid hormone, Endocrinology 92:1596 (1973).
22. G. Scatchard, The attraction of proteins for small molecules and ions, Ann NY Acad Sci 51:660 (1949).
23. Y. Salomon, C. Landos and M. Rodbell, A highly sensitive adenylate cyclase assay, Analytical Biochem 58:541 (1974).
24. A.G. Gilman, A protein binding assay for adenosine 3'-5'-cyclic monophosphate, Proc Natl Acad Sci USA 67:305 (1970).
25. R.H. Renston, D.G. Maloney, A.L. Jones, G.T. Hradek, K.Y. Wong, I.D. Goldfine, Bile secretory apparatus: Evidence for a vesicular transport mechanism for proteins in the rat, using

horseradish peroxidase and ^{125}I insulin, Gastroenterology 78: 1373 (1980).
26. I.D. Goldfine, A.L. Jones, G.T. Hradek, K.Y. Wong and J.S. Mooney, Entry of insulin into human cultured lymphocytes: Electron microscope autoradiographic analysis, Science 202: 760 (1978).
27. D. Rodbard, Mathematics of hormone-receptor interaction, in: "Advances in Experimental Medicine and Biology" 36:289, Plenum Press (1973).
28. J.T. Potts, T.M. Murray, M. Peacock, H.D. Niall, G.W. Tregear, H.T. Keutmann, D. Powell and L.J. Deftos, Parathyroid hormone: sequence, synthesis, immunoassay studies, Am J Med 50:639 (1971).
29. K.J. Martin, J.J. Freitag, M.B. Conrades, K.A. Hruska, S. Klahr and F. Slatopolsky, Selective uptake of the synthetic amino-terminal fragment of bovine parathyroid hormone by isolated perfused bone, J Clin Invest 62:256 (1978).
30. G.V. Segre, P.D'Amour, J.T. Potts, Jr., Metabolism of radio-iodinated bovine PTH in the rat, Endocrinology 99:1645 (1976).
31. D. Goltzman, A. Peytremann, E.N. Callahan, G.V. Segre and J.T. Potts, Jr., Metabolism and biological activity of parathyroid hormone in renal cortical membranes, J Clin Invest 57:8 (1976).
32. A.P. Teitelbaum, N. Schneider and W.F. Neuman, On the relation between peripheral cleavage of parathyroid hormone and its biological activity in kidney, Metab Bone Dis Rel Res 2:25 (1979).
33. D. Goltzman, Examination of the requirement for metabolism of parathyroid hormone in skeletal tissue before biological action. Endocrinology 102:155 (1978).
34. E.M. Ross and A.G. Gilman, Biochemical properties of hormone-sensitive adenylate cyclase, Ann Rev Biochem 49:533 (1980).
35. A.R. LaBarbera, N.D. Richert and R.J. Ryan, Nucleotides do not modulate rat luteocyte human chorionic gonadotropin responsiveness by inhibiting human chorionic gonadotropin binding, Arch Biochem Biophys 200:177 (1980).
36. M.K. Drezner and W.M. Burch, Jr., Altered activity of the nucleotide regulatory site in the parathyroid hormone-sensitive adenylate cyclase from the renal cortex of a patient with pseudohypoparathyroidism, J Clin Invest 62:1222 (1978).
37. Z. Farfel and H.R. Bourne, Deficient activity of receptor-cyclase coupling protein in platelets of patients with pseudo-hypoparathyroidism, J Clin Endocrinol Metab 51:1202 (1980).

ASSESSMENT OF BIOLOGICALLY ACTIVE PARATHYROID HORMONE IN HYPERPARATHYROID MAN

R.A. Nissenson, S.R. Abbott, K. Pua, L. Zitzner,
A.P. Teitelbaum, and O.H. Clark

Medical and Surgical Services, Veterans Administration Medical Center, San Francisco, CA 94121; and the Departments of Medicine and Surgery, University of California, San Francisco, CA 94143

INTRODUCTION

The ability to measure peptide hormone levels in serum by radioimmunoassay (RIA) has revolutionized clinical endocrinology. It has become evident, however, that many peptide hormones circulate in multiple forms[1], and that region-specific RIAs may fail to recognize one or more of these hormonal species. Furthermore, inasmuch as antigenic determinants bear no necessary relationship to regions of the hormone molecule required for biologic action, RIA measurements do not always reflect levels of biologically active hormone.

Nowhere are these problems more evident than in the case of parathyroid hormone (PTH). It is well established that circulating PTH is immunochemically heterogeneous[2,3] due to renal and hepatic cleavage of intact PTH(1-84)[4], as well as to secretion of PTH fragments by the parathyroid gland[5]. The predominant circulating form of PTH, at least in patients with hyperparathyroidism, is a fragment(s) recognized by antisera directed against either the carboxyl-terminal or middle region of PTH[6]. This fragment(s) appears to lack antigenic determinants of the amino-terminal region of PTH, and thus is biologically inactive.

To evaluate the quantity and molecular forms of endogenous, biologically active human PTH, we have developed a highly sensitive biologic assay for PTH based on the activation of canine renal cortical adenylate cyclase in the presence of the potentiating guanosine triphosphate analog, 5'-guanylimidodiphosphate [Gpp(NH)p][7]. In the present report, we describe the properties of this assay, and its use to evaluate secreted and circulating, biologically active PTH in hyperparathyroid man.

METHODS

Adenylate cyclase activity was measured by the conversion of [α-^{32}P]ATP to [^{32}P]cAMP. Standard incubations were carried out in a final volume of 0.1 ml containing 25 mM Tris-HCl (pH 7.5), 2.0 mM $MgCl_2$, 0.1% BSA, 0.1 mM [α-^{32}P]ATP (100-300 cmp/pmol), an ATP-regenerating system consisting of 30 μg creatine phosphokinase and 10 mM creatine phosphate, and 1.0 mM 1-methyl, 3-isobutylxanthine, a potent inhibitor of cyclic nucleotide phosphodiesterase. The hydrolysis-resistant GTP analog, Gpp(NH)p (100 μM), was also added. This nucleotide was found to markedly augment the sensitivity of adenylate cyclase to PTH. For measurement of biologically active PTH in serum, we added either PTH standards [purified hPTH(1-84)] in 10 μl normal human serum containing no detectable PTH bioactivity, or 10 μl test serum.

Immunochemical measurements of PTH were carried out in a nonequilibrium RIA system[8] using three different PTH antisera. Antiserum GP-FM was raised in guinea pigs immunized with the supernatant of a trichloracetic acid extract of adenomatous and hyperplastic human parathyroid glands[9]. This supernatant contains predominantly carboxyl-region (C-region) PTH fragments. GP-FM has high affinity for PTH(1-84) as well as PTH(53-84), but does not bind PTH(1-34). Antiserum GP-1M was raised in guinea pigs immunized with crude porcine PTH and has high affinity for PTH(1-84) and PTH(44-68), but low affinity for PTH(1-34)[10]. In addition to these C-region RIAs, we used antiserum CH-12 which was raised in a chicken immunized with crude bPTH. CH-12 has high affinity for PTH(1-84), at least 30-fold lower affinity for PTH(1-34), and no affinity for C-region PTH fragments[10].

Abnormal parathyroid glands were identified at surgical operations to correct primary or secondary hyperparathyroidism. A blood sample (2-4 ml) was obtained from a vein draining the abnormal parathyroid gland or glands using a 5 ml syringe with a 25-gauge needle. At the same time, a peripheral venous sample of blood was obtained. Both samples were placed in glass tubes on ice. Within 1 h, serum was separated by centrifugation and was subsequently stored at -20°C. Parathyroid venous effluent sera were fractionated by gel filtration chromatography on columns of Bio-Gel P-150, as described by Flueck et al.[5]. Column effluent fractions were lyophilized and resuspended in 10 mM acetic acid for bioassay.

RESULTS

Development of the PTH Bioassay

Over the past few years, it has become apparent that hormonal activation of adenylate cyclase requires the presence of a membrane component in addition to hormone receptor and catalytic adenylate cyclase. This additional component is a guanyl nucleotide-dependent protein (termed N protein) which serves to couple receptor occupancy to enzyme activation[11]. Figure 1 demonstrates the influence of the hydrolysis-resistant GTP analog 5'-guanylimidodiphosphate [Gpp(NH)p] on PTH-stimulated canine renal cortical adenylate cyclase activity. The concentration of bPTH(1-34) required to stimulate adenylate cyclase half-maximally was reduced from 80 to 10 ng/ml by 1.0 μM Gpp(NH)p, and was decreased further to 0.7 ng/ml (or 110-fold) in the presence of a maximally effective concentration of Gpp(NH)p (100 μM). At this higher nucleotide concentration, as little as 30 pg/ml bPTH(1-34) produced significant enzyme stimulation. The nucleotide produced shifts in the dose-response curves for bPTH(1-84) and hPTH(1-84) stimulation of adenylate cyclase that were equivalent to that for the synthetic bovine 1-34 peptide (not shown). The molar potency of bPTH(1-34) was identical to those of bPTH(1-84) and hPTH(1-84), in both the presence and absence of Gpp(NH)p.

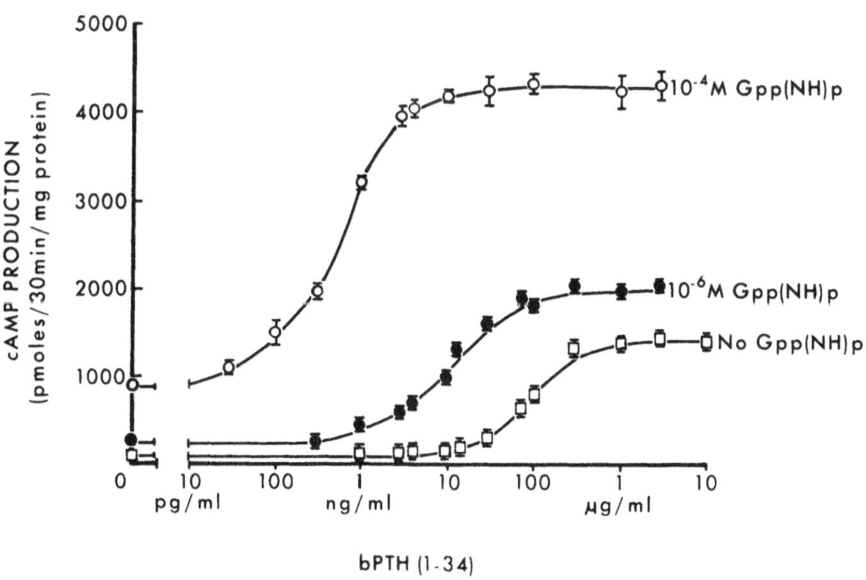

Figure 1. Potentiation of bPTH(1-34) stimulation of adenylate cyclase in renal cortical plasma membrane by Gpp(NH)p. Each point is the mean ± SE of three determinations.[7]

The marked augmentation of PTH sensitivity elicited by Gpp(NH)p suggested to us that guanyl nucleotide-amplified renal adenylate cyclase might provide the basis for a biological assay for PTH in human serum. This possibility was reinforced by the relative PTH specificity of the biological response (Table 1). In the experiment shown, a near-maximal concentration of bPTH(1-34) (3.0 ng/ml) produced 3-fold stimulation of adenylate cyclase; 2-fold stimulation was elicited by 0.3 ng/ml bPTH(1-34). In contrast, epinephrine, glucagon, PGE_1, and human calcitonin failed to activate adenylate cyclase at concentrations as high as 0.1 μg/ml. At higher concentrations (10 μg/ml), epinephrine, PGE_1, and glucagon produced 42%, 35%, and 14% stimulation of adenylate cyclase, respectively. ACTH and arginine vasopressin were inactive at concentrations up to 100 μg/ml.

Table 1. Effect of various agents on canine renal cortical adenylate cyclase in the presence of 100 μM Gpp(NH)p.[7]

Agent	Conc. (ng/ml)	Adenylate cyclase activity (pmol cAMP/mg protein . 30 min)[a]
None		590
bPTH(1-34)	0.3	1070
	1.0	1500
	3.0	1800
	100	1850
Epinephrine	100	622
	1,000	790
	10,000	838
PGE_1	100	659
	1,000	740
	10,000	795
Glucagon	100	541
	1,000	583
	10,000	673
Human calcitonin	100	521
	1,000	552
	10,000	602

[a] Mean of duplicate determinations which agreed within 5%.

Measurement of Biologically Active PTH in Peripheral Serum

We utilized this guanyl nucleotide-amplified renal adenylate cyclase assay to measure biologically active PTH in peripheral serum of 8 patients with chronic renal failure and markedly elevated C-region immunoreactive PTH (Table 2). For patient 1, the bioassay value obtained was validated by the loss of measurable PTH bioactivity in the presence of the PTH antagonist, [^{8}Nle,^{18}Nle,-^{34}Try]bPTH(3-34)amide (6 μg/ml) and after parathyroidectomy (not shown). Of the eight sera examined, five contained biologically active PTH at concentrations ranging from 0.3-4.8 ng-eq hPTH(1-84) /ml. Biologically active PTH was undetectable in the three other sera. When measured against the same hPTH(1-84) standard, C-region immunoreactive PTH (antiserum GP-FM) was consistently found to be present at a much higher concentration (10- to 100-fold, in most cases) than biologically active PTH in the same serum sample. In contrast, values obtained with the intact PTH RIA agreed more closely with bioassay values determined with the same serum sample, although in each case, the RIA value was somewhat greater.

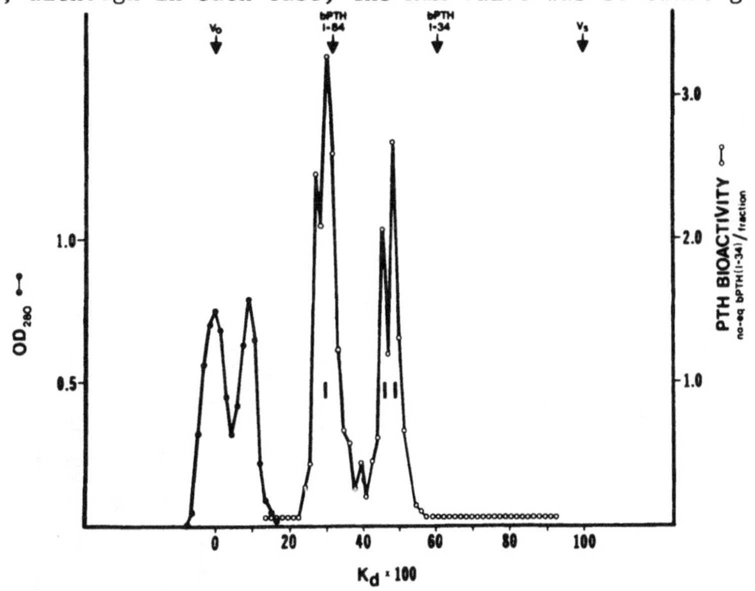

Figure 2. Parathyroid venous effluent serum (1.0 ml) from a patient with primary hyperparathyroidism was fractionated on a Bio-Gel P-150 gel filtration column. Effluent fractions (each 5.6 ml) were concentrated by lyophilization, and PTH bioactivity determined with the guanyl nucleotide-amplified renal adenylate cyclase assay. The major peaks of biologic activity are designated I and II. Kd (distribution coefficient) was calculated as (elution volume of substance - Vo)/(Vs-Vo).

Table 2. Serum concentrations of biologically active and immunoreactive PTH in eight patients with chronic renal failure[7].

Patient No.	Serum PTH [ng-eq hPTH(1-84)/ml]			Serum PTH (µl-eq/ml)
	Bioassay	Intact RIA (CH-12)[a]	C-Region RIA (GP-FM)[b]	by C-Region RIA (GP-1M)[c]
1	4.8	5.3 (1.1)[d]	12 (2.5)[e]	3,400
2	0.8	2.3 (2.9)	56 (70)	12,000
3	0.8	1.0 (1.3)	26 (33)	3,100
4	0.7	0.80 (1.1)	8.0 (11)	5,600
5	0.3	0.80 (2.7)	48 (160)	7,300
6	<0.3	0.81 (>2.7)	26 (>87)	1,400
7	<0.3	0.55 (>1.8)	11 (>37)	1,700
8	<0.3	1.3 (>4.3)	78 (>260)	8,400

[a] Normal value, <0.15 ng-eq hPTH(1-84)/ml

[b] Normal value, <0.4 ng-eq hPTH(1-84)/ml

[c] Normal value <40 µl-eq ml

[d] The ratio of intact RIA (CH-12) to bioassay results is in parentheses.

[e] The ratio of C-region RIA (GP-FM) to bioassay results is in parentheses.

Biologically Active PTH in Parathyroid Venous Effluent Serum

We used the guanyl nucleotide amplified renal adenylate cyclase assay to determine whether hyperfunctioning human parathyroid glands secrete multiple forms of biologically active PTH. Parathyroid venous effluent sera, obtained at the time of parathyroidectomy, were fractionated on Bio-Gel P-150 gel filtration columns, and effluent fractions were assessed for PTH bioactivity. Figure 2 illustrates the results of one such experiment. Two major peaks of biologically active PTH were found. One of these (peak I) eluted in the position expected for intact PTH(1-84), while the other (peak II) eluted in a position intermediate between PTH(1-84) and PTH(1-34). Two lines of evidence indicate that the activities in peaks I and II were due specifically to species of PTH. First, serial dilutions of both peaks produced adenylate cyclase activation curves which were parallel to those produced by authentic PTH. Secondly, the PTH antagonist, [^{8}Nle,^{18}Nle,^{34}Tyr]bPTH(3-34)amide abolished the biologic activity due to both both peaks. Gel filtration of purified human PTH(1-84) resulted in a single peak of bioactivity which coeluted with peak I.

Table 3 summarizes gel filtration data obtained on 5 patients to date. In each case, 2 peaks of PTH bioactivity were observed corresponding in elution position to peaks I and II in Figure 2. The relative proportion of peaks I and II, which varied considerably from sample to sample, did not relate in any obvious way to the preoperative indices of hyperparathyroidism (serum calcium or immunoreactive PTH). The data indicate that hyperfunctioning human parathyroid glands may secrete a biologically active PTH fragment in addition to PTH(1-84).

DISCUSSION

The guanyl nucleotide-amplified canine renal cortical adenylate cyclase assay described here has several advantages over earlier PTH bioassay methods. The absolute detection limit of this assay (3 pg hPTH(1-84)/0.1 ml incubation volume) is at least 2-3 orders of magnitude lower than that afforded by previous adenylate cyclase assays. In addition, the assay shows a high degree of specificity for PTH. When several non-PTH agents were tested, ACTH(1-24) and human calcitonin were shown to be totally inactive. Epinephrine, glucagon, and PGE_1 were inactive at concentrations less than 100 ng/ml and produced only slight stimulation of adenylate cyclase at higher doses. Even at these higher concentrations, adenylate cyclase activation was only a fraction (< 20%) of that produced by a near-maximal concentration of bPTH(1-34) (3 ng/ml). Inasmuch as the normal serum concentrations of glucagon[12], epinephrine[13], and PGE_1[14] are reported to be between

Table 3. Summary of Data on 5 Patients to Date.

			Pre-Operative		Gel Filtration of Parathyroid Venous Serum		
Patient	Diagnosis	Parathyroid Pathology	Serum Calcium (mg/dl)	Serum iPTH[a] (μl-eq/ml)	Peak I (Kd[b])	Peak II (Kd)	%Total PTH bioactivity in Peak II
1	1°HPT	adenoma	11.5	520	0.30	0.48	41
2	"	"	10.9	48	0.29	0.48	98
3	"	"	10.4	170	0.28	0.46	64
4	"	"	11.2	-	0.29	0.47	17
5	2°HPT (CRF[c])	hyperplasia	8.4	2500	0.31	0.49	41

[a] measured with a C-region antiserum GP-1M; normal < 40 μl-eq/ml

[b] Kd = gel filtration distribution coefficient

[c] chronic renal failure

0.01-0.20 ng/ml, it is unlikely that these agents could have interfered with our measurements of biologically active PTH in serum. This conclusion is strongly supported by the elimination of bioactivity in peripheral chronic renal failure serum produced by the competitive PTH antagonist, [^{8}Nle,^{18}Nle,^{34}Tyr]bPTH(3-34)-amide and by the total loss of PTH bioactivity in peripheral serum after parathyroidectomy. Another significant advantage offered by this bioassay is its relative convenience; daily assay of 10-20 test samples at multiple dilutions may be carried out and the final results obtained within 1-2 days.

The present study demonstrates that biologically active PTH circulates in concentrations in excess of 300 pg-eq hPTH(1-84)/ml in some patients with severe hyperparathyroidism. This finding is consistent with recent data obtained using the cytochemical PTH bioassay, demonstrating that 4 of 13 patients with hyperparathyroidism had peripheral biologially active PTH concentrations in excess of 300 pg/ml (range, 34-11,000 pg/ml; normal range, 2.9-29 pg/ml)[15]. A comparison of biologically active and C-region immunoreactive PTH levels in the peripheral serum of 8 patients with hyperparathyroidism secondary to chronic renal failure revealed that, in 7 cases, at least 90% of the circulating immunoreactive PTH was biologically inert. In contrast, values for biologically active PTH and intact immunoreactive PTH agreed reasonably well. These findings are consonant with previous observations which demonstrate the predominance of C-region immunoreactive PTH fragments (presumed to be biologically inactive) relative to intact PTH in chronic renal failure serum[16]. They further suggest that whereas measurement of circulating C-region immunoreactive PTH may be a valid index of chronic PTH hypersecretion (i.e., degree of parathyroid hyperplasia) in patients with chronic renal failure, intact PTH RIAs may be more useful in assessing levels of circulating biologically active hormone.

We have also obtained evidence that hyperfunctioning human parathyroid glands secrete a biologically active PTH fragment in addition to the intact hormone. Thus, parathyroid venous effluent serum from all patients studied (4 with primary hyperparathyroidism and 1 with chronic renal failure and secondary hyperparathyroidism) contained 2 peaks of activity in the adenylate cyclase assay. That these 2 peaks activated adenylate cyclase through the PTH receptor was demonstrated by the complete inhibition of their activity produced by the competitive PTH antagonist, [^{8}Nle,^{18}Nle,-^{34}Tyr]bPTH(3-34)amide. One of these peaks (peak I) was presumably intact PTH(1-84), whereas the other (peak II) behaved upon gel filtration as a smaller peptide. Murray et al.[17] reported that bovine parathyroid glands contained a biologically active PTH fragment which they identified as PTH(1-65). In preliminary experiments, we have found that bovine parathyroid gland extracts contain a biologically active PTH fragment which elutes from Bio-Gel P-150 columns beyond the position of peak II. This suggests that peak II may represent PTH from which < 20 carboxyl-terminal residues have been cleaved.

We cannot rule out the possibility that some cleavage of intact PTH may have occurred post-secretion (e.g., during sample handling and storage). However, the results of the control experiment with exogenous human PTH(1-84) make it extremely unlikely that this could account for all of the activity in peak II. Further studies will be required to determine whether this PTH fragment can be identified in human parathyroid gland extracts, and whether significant quantities circulate in patients with hyperparathyroidism.

ACKNOWLEDGEMENTS

The authors gratefully acknowledge the expert secretarial assistance of Ms. Susan Festa. This work was supported by N.I.H. grant AM 27755 (to R.A. Nissenson) and by a grant from the University of California Academic Senate Committee on Research (to R.A. Nissenson).

REFERENCES

1. D. Rabinowitz and J. Roth, Eds., "Heterogeneity of Polypeptide Hormones," Academic Press, Inc., New York (1974).
2. S.A. Berson and R.S. Yalow, Immunochemical heterogeneity of parathyroid hormone in plasma, J Clin Endocrinol Metab 28:1037 (1968).
3. C.D. Arnaud, G.W. Sizemore, S.B. Oldham, J.A. Fischer, H.S. Tsao and E.T. Littledike, Human parathyroid hormone: glandular and secreted molecular species, Am J Med 50:630 (1971).
4. K.J. Martin, K.A. Hruska, J.J. Freitag, S. Klahr and E. Slatopolsky, The peripheral metabolism of parathyroid hormone, N Engl J Med 30: 1092 (1979).
5. J.A. Flueck, F.P. DiBella, A.J Edis, J.M. Kehrwald and C.D. Arnaud, Immunoheterogeneity of parathyroid hormone in venous effluent serum from hyperfunctioning parathyroid glands, J Clin Invest 60: 1367 (1977).
6. C.D. Arnaud, R.S. Goldsmith, P.J. Bordier and G.W. Sizemore, Influence of immunoheterogeneity of circulating parathyroid hormone on results of radioimmunoassays of serum in man, Am J Med 56:785 (1974).
7. R.A. Nissenson, S.R. Abbott, A.P. Teitelbaum, O.H. Clark and C.D. Arnaud, Endogenous biologically active human parathyroid hormone: measurement by a guanyl nucleotide-amplified renal adenylate cyclase assay, J Clin Endocrinol Metab 52:840 (1981).

8. C.D. Arnaud, H.S. Tsao and T. Littledike, Radioimmunoassay of human parathyroid hormone in serum, J Clin Invest 50:21 (1971).
9. F.P. DiBella, J.B. Gilkinson, J. Flueck and C.D. Arnaud, Carboxyl-terminal fragments of human parathyroid hormone in parathyroid tumors: unique new source of immunogens for the production of antisera potentially useful in the radioimmunoassay of parathyroid hormone in human serum, J Clin Endocrinol Metab 46:604 (1978).
10. J.C. Gallagher, B.L. Riggs, C.M. Jerpbak and C.D. Arnaud, The effect of age on serum immunoreactive parathyroid hormone in normal and osteoporotic women, J Lab Clin Med 95:373 (1980).
11. E.M. Ross and A.G. Gilman, Biochemical properties of hormone-sensitive adenylate cyclase, Ann Rev Biochem 49:533 (1980).
12. R. Rizza, C. Verdonk, J. Miles, F.J. Service, J. Gerich, Effect of intermittent endogenous hyperglucagonemia on glucose homeostasis in normal and diabetic man, J Clin Invest 63:1119 (1979).
13. E. Endert, Determination of noradrenaline and adrenaline in plasma by a radioenzymatic assay using high pressure liquid chromatography for the separation of the radiochemical products, Clin Chim Acta 96:233 (1979).
14. A.R. Wharton, B.J. Sweetman, J. A. Oates, Application of high performance liquid chromatography and gas chromatography-mass spectrometry to analysis of prostaglandin E_1 in biological media, Anal Biochem 98:455 (1979).
15. D. Goltzman, B. Henderson, N. Loveridge, Cytochemical bioassay of parathyroid hormone, J Clin Invest 65:1309 (1980).
16. R.S. Goldsmith, J. Furszyter, W.J. Johnson, A.E. Fournier, G. W. Sizemore and C.D. Arnaud, Etiology of hyperparathyroidism and bone disease during chronic hemodialysis. III. Evaluation of parathyroid suppressibility, J Clin Invest 52:173 (1973).
17. T.M. Murray, S.A. Muzzafar, J.A. Parsons and H.T. Keutmann, A biologically active hormonal fragment isolated from bovine parathyroid glands (BPTH 1-65), Biochemistry 14:2705 (1975).

EFFECT OF PARATHYROID HORMONE ON PHOSPHOLIPID METABOLISM

Saulo Klahr, Jeremiah Morrissey, and Keith Hruska

Renal Division, Department of Medicine
Washington University School of Medicine
and Jewish Hospital
St. Louis, Missouri

INTRODUCTION

Until recently it has been generally assumed that the major, if not the only, role of lipids in biological membranes is to provide a semipermeable barrier between intracellular and extracellular environments. Within the concept of membrane models, such as the "fluid-mosaic" model (1), active and facilitated transport and other events vital to cell or organelle function are mediated by proteins extending into or through the lipid bilayer with the possibility that lipids surrounding these proteins play some ill-defined regulatory role. However, it now appears that the view of lipids as inert building blocks of biomembranes is incomplete, and that lipids may participate directly in many functional processes. Recent years have seen a dramatic increase in knowledge about the physicochemistry of membrane lipids mainly due to the development of sensitive calorimetric, X-ray and neutron diffraction and a variety of spectroscopic methods. A number of reviews have appeared recently (2-6).

Most, although not all, membrane lipids are based on the glycerol molecule, a simple three carbon structure with a hydroxyl (OH) group attached to each of the carbons. Membrane lipids usually have two long chain fatty acids replacing two hydroxyl groups of the glycerol molecule, the third position being occupied by a polar group (Fig. 1). Often this is a group that carries or can accept an electric charge and is, therefore, soluble in water. Since the two fatty acid chains are insoluble in water, they are thought to project from the glycerol chain in a direction opposite to that taken by the polar group (Fig. 1).

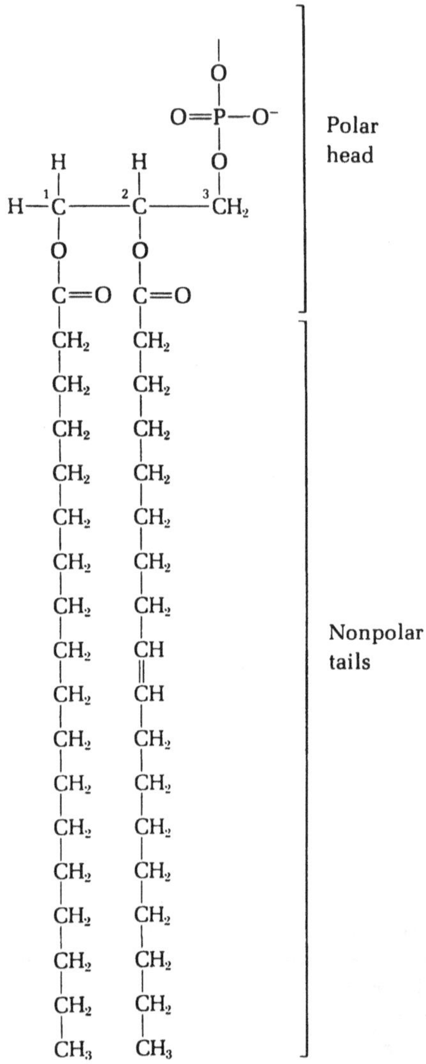

Fig. 1. General structure of phospholipids. The phosphate group attached to the third carbon represents the polar head. The two fatty acids attached to carbons 1 and 2 represent the non-polar portion of the molecule. The fatty acid in the 2 position is usually unsaturated.

Membrane lipids differ among themselves in the identity of the fatty acids or of the polar group, or both (7). Thus, in the phosphoglycerides or phospholipids, the most numerous class, the molecule may contain any two of more than half a dozen fatty acids. Usually a phospholipid from a biologic membrane contains a saturated and an unsaturated fatty acid, the latter generally lies in the middle position on the glycerol chain between the saturated acid at one end and the polar group at the other. As yet, no good explanation has been provided for this particular arrangement, or indeed why the two fatty acids should almost always be of different types. The polar groups of the phospho-

Phosphoglyceride	*Alcohol component*
Phosphatidyl ethanolamine	$HO\,CH_2CH_2NH_2$
Phosphatidyl choline	$HO\,CH_2CH_2\overset{+}{N}(CH_3)_3$
Phosphatidyl serine	$HOCH_2CHNH_2COOH$
Phosphatidyl inositol	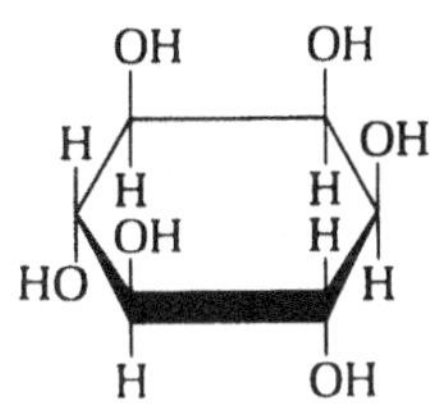
Phosphatidyl glycerol	$HO\,CH_2CHOHCH_2OH$

Fig. 2. Alcohols contributing the polar groups of the major phospholipids. These alcohols are attached to the phosphoric acid in the polar head of the phospholipid (see Figure 1).

lipids are no less diverse than are the fatty acids. All of them, as the name implies contain a phosphate group, but additional groups are also present and these can often be fairly complicated. All phosphoglycerides possess a polar head and two nonpolar hydrocarbon tails. For this reason, they are called amphipathic or polar lipids. The name of the common phosphoglycerides and the structure of the polar head groups are shown in Figure 2.

The most abundant phospholipids in higher plants and animals are phosphatidylethanolamine and phosphatidylcholine which contain, respectively, the amino alcohols ethanolamine and choline esterified to the phosphoric acid to form a phosphodiester. In phosphatidylserine, the hydroxyl group of serine is esterified to the phosphoric acid. In phosphatidylinositol, the six carbon sugar alcohol inositol is attached. In phosphatidylglycerol, a molecule of glycerol is esterified to the phosphoric acid.

Phosphoglycerides are the most polar of the lipids. All of them have a negative charge at the phosphate group at pH 7. The pK' of this group is in the range of 1-2. The polar groups of phosphatidylinositol, phosphatidylglycerol, and the phosphatidyl sugars have no electrical charge but are highly polar. The polar groups of phosphatidylethanolamine and phosphatidylcholine have a positive charge at pH 7 since their amino groups have pK' values of about 10 and 13 respectively. These two phosphoglycerides are, therefore, dipolar zwitterions at pH 7 and have no net electric charge. The polar group of phosphatidylserine contains an alpha amino group, pK' 10, and a carboxyl group, pK' 3. The phosphatidylserine molecule does contain a total of two negative groups and one positive group at pH 7 giving it a net negative charge. These variations in the size, shape, polarity and charge of the polar heads play a very significant role in the structure of micelles, monolayers and bilayers of lipids, as well as in membrane systems. Phosphoglycerides may be hydrolyzed by specific phospholipases which have become important tools in the determination of phosphoglyceride structures (Figure 3). Phospholipases of the class A specifically hydrolyze the fatty acid from the 2 position. The resulting product is called a lysophosphatide. Lysophosphatides are not normally found in cells or tissues in any quantity. They are toxic and injurious to membranes. Phospholipase B is specific for removing the second or both fatty acids. Phosphatidylcholine on treatment with phospholipase B yields glycerol-3-phosphoryl choline. Phospholipase C hydrolyses the bond between phosphoric acid and glycerol while phospholipase D removes the polar group to leave a phosphatidic acid. Phosphoglycerides, as well as other complex lipids, are readily separated and identified by thin layer chromatography or by chromatography on silicic acid columns.

Biosynthesis of phosphoglycerides

Phosphoglycerides or phospholipids are formed by a branching biosynthetic pathway starting from phosphatidic acid (Fig. 4). Phosphatidic acid occurs in only trace amounts in cells but it is an important intermediate common to the biosynthesis of both triacylglycerols and phosphoglycerides. The partition of phosphatidic acid between these two pathways is crucial in the regulation of lipid synthesis. To form the triacylglycerols (trigly-

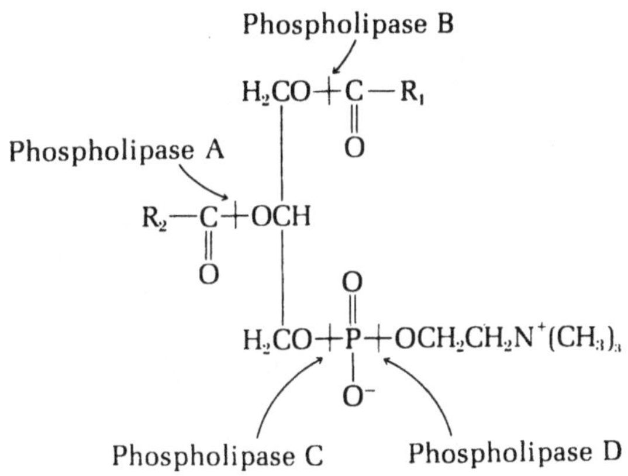

Fig. 3. Sites of action of phospholipases on a phospholipid (phosphatidylcholine) (see text for a complete description).

cerides) phosphatidic acid undergoes hydrolysis by a specific phosphatase to form diacylglycerols. The central importance of phosphatidic acids and of cytidine nucleotides in the biosynthesis of phosphoglycerides was first discovered by Kennedy (8). These reactions take place largely in the endoplasmic reticulum. Phosphatidic acid is first converted by a reversible reaction with CTP into cytidine diphosphate diacylglycerol, which is the common precursor of all phosphoglycerides formed by this pathway (see Fig. 4). In subsequent reactions the cytidine monophosphate moiety is displaced from CDP diacylglycerol by one of the three alcohols, serine, inositol or glycerol phosphate to form phosphatidylserine, phosphatidylinositol, and 3-phosphatidylglycerol-1-phosphate respectively. Enzymatic decarboxylation of the serine residue of phosphatidylserine leads to formation of phosphatidylethanolamine.

Phosphatidylinositol is the precursor of two derivatives, phosphatidylinositol monophosphate and phosphatidylinositol di-

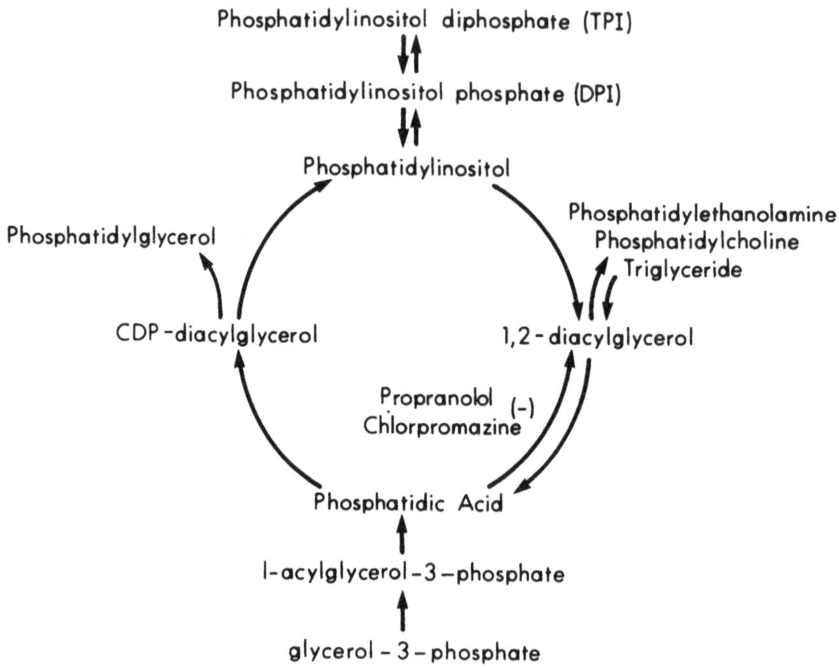

Fig. 4. General scheme of phospholipid synthesis.

phosphate, also called diphosphoinositide (DPI) and triphosphoinositide (TPI), which are formed by successive phosphorylations by ATP of free hydroxyl groups in the inositol residue (9). These phosphorylated forms of phosphatidylinositol are particularly abundant in the mitochondrial membrane and in brain tissue. The rapid metabolic turnover of the phosphate groups in the inositol residue suggests that phosphoinositides may be involved in membrane transport phenomena. Although phosphoinsotides comprise a small fraction of total renal membrane phospholipids, they are highly polar and significant changes in their metabolism may result in dramatic changes in the physicochemical properties of the membranes in which they are located. Phosphoinositol metabolism has been reported to be increased by cholinergic agents, 1-histamine receptor stimulation, vasopressin, serotonin, and alpha-1-agonists in several different tissues (10,11). The stimulatory effect involves an initial hydrolysis of phosphatidylinositol by phospholipase C and subsequent phosphatidylinositol resynthesis through phosphatidic acid. Thus, the turnover of phosphatidylinositol is stimulated. The hormones that stimulate phosphoinositide turnover share a common property of action to increase cytosolic calcium. Several studies have suggested that the mechanism of increasing cytosolic calcium is related to phosphatidylinositol turnover (9,12), and it has been proposed that all hormones which increase cytosolic calcium also increase phosphatidylinositol turnover (9).

EFFECTS OF PTH AND CYCLIC NUCLEOTIDES ON RENAL PHOSPHOLIPIDS

Lo et al (13) first reported that parathyroid hormone increased the incorporation of ^{32}Pi (inorganic phosphorus) into phosphatidic acid and phosphatidylinositol in cat renal cortical slices. Incorporation was not observed into any other phospholipids and the effects were seen as early as 1 minute for phosphatidic acid and 10 minutes for phosphatidylinositol. 8-bromo-adenosine-3',5'-monophosphate did not mimic the effects of PTH. Concentrations of parathyroid hormone (1 x 10^{-8} M to 1 x 10^{-7} M) which increased the incorporation of ^{32}Pi into phosphatidic acid and phosphatidylinositol maximally did not alter tissue cyclic AMP levels. From these observations Lo et al suggested that the incorporation of ^{32}Pi into phospholipids in cat kidney cortical slices was independent of cyclic AMP. This rapid PTH induced increase in the incorporation of ^{32}Pi into phosphatidic acid and phosphatidylinositol could be the result of: 1) a primary increase in phosphatidic acid or 2) more rapid phosphatidylinositol breakdown and resynthesis. Baricos et al (14) reported that dibutyrylcyclic AMP or cyclic AMP decreased the labeling by ^{32}P of DPI but not TPI in rabbit kidney cortical slices. Caffeine, an inhibitor of phosphodiesterase, potentiated the effect of cyclic AMP. Addition of cyclic GMP to the incubation medium decreased the labeling of DPI and, to a lesser extent, of TPI. Parathyroid hormone added alone also decreased the ^{32}Pi labeling of DPI but not TPI. Prelabeling experiments with ^{32}P revealed that kidney slices incubated in medium containing cyclic AMP had decreased labeling of DPI when compared to control renal slices. The authors interpreted these results to suggest an increased rate of DPI breakdown in the presence of elevated concentrations of cyclic AMP. Recently, Farese et al (15) have shown that PTH rapidly increases the concentrations of phosphatidylinositol, diphosphoinositide and triphosphoinositide in rabbit kidney cortex. The levels of diphosphoinositide increased after 15 minutes of PTH exposure by 57% and the levels of triphosphoinositide by 103% (Fig. 5). In addition to increasing DPI and TPI, PTH also increased the levels of phosphatidic acid from 202 $\pm$ 34 to 438 $\pm$ 54 ngms per 100 mg of tissue. These effects of PTH were blocked by cycloheximide which also was shown in vivo to block the phosphaturic effect of PTH (Fig. 6). This increase in renal phosphoinositides after PTH treatment was quite similar to that previously reported by Farese et al after ACTH treatment in the adrenal cortex (16). Both effects occur rapidly, are accompanied by increases in phosphatidic acid and phosphatidylinositol and are

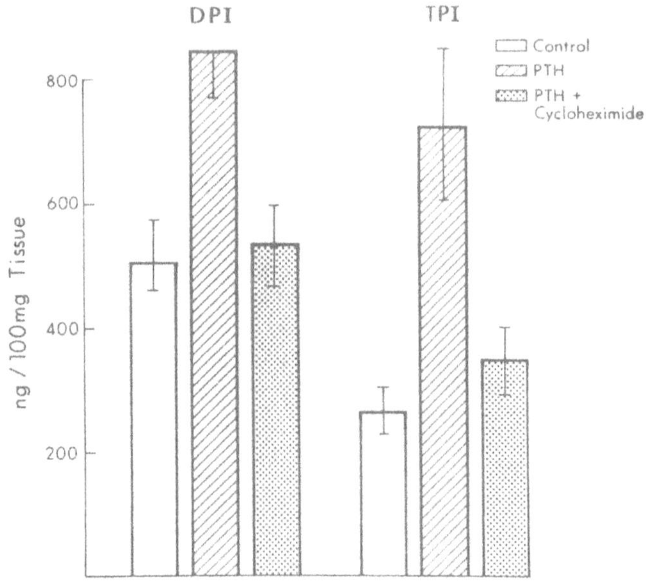

Fig. 5. Effect of cycloheximide on the parathyroid hormone (PTH) induced changes in renal phospholipids. DPI = diphosphoinositide; TPI = triphosphoinositide. Adapted from reference 15.

blocked by cycloheximide. Meltzer et al (17) have confirmed the observations of both Lo and Farese et al. These investigators studied the effect of PTH and 8-bromo cyclic AMP on renal phosphoinositide metabolism using isolated renal cortical tubules from dogs. PTH stimulated the rate of ^{32}Pi incorporation into phosphatidylinositol, phosphatidic acid, diphosphoinositide and triphosphoinositide. PTH also caused an increase of approximately 50% in the tissue levels of diphosphoinositide, phosphatidylinositol and phosphatidic acid by 5 minutes of incubation. By 30 minutes of incubation the levels of ^{32}Pi incorporated were similar in PTH and controls but the actual levels of phosphatidylinositol remained elevated. In addition, they found in tubules preincubated with [2-^{3}H] myo-

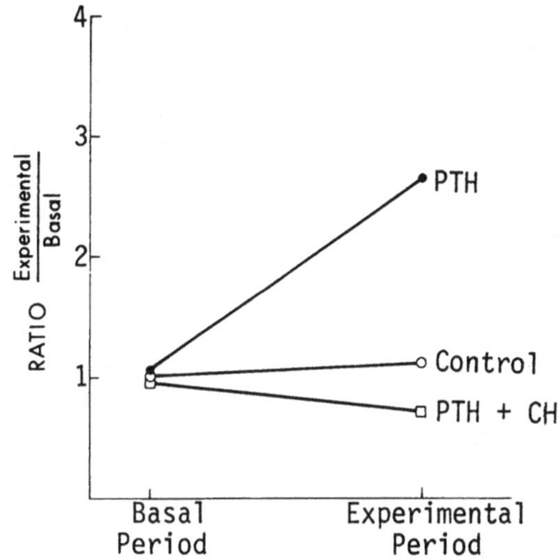

Fig. 6. Effect of cycloheximide administation on the phosphaturia produced by PTH in the rabbit. CH = cycloheximide. Adapted from reference 15.

inositol that PTH stimulated and accelerated initial decrements in ^{3}H labeled phosphatidylinositol. In tubules preincubated with ^{14}C-arachidonic acid PTH decrease the rate of ^{14}C-PGE and ^{14}C-arachidonic acid released into the incubation medium. The hormone did not stimulate an increase in ^{14}C labeling of phosphatidic acid. In contrast to data recently published by Bidot-Lopez et al (18) showing that dibutyryl cyclic AMP had effects on phosphoinositides similar to PTH, Meltzer et al (17) were unable to demonstrate an effect of 8-bromo cyclic AMP, at concentrations of 10^{-6} to 10^{-4} M on phosphoinositide metabolism. The reason for this discrepancy is not immediately apparent. The data of Farese et al would suggest that PTH stimulates phosphoinositide metabolism via cyclic AMP. The data of Meltzer et al suggest that the two effects may occur independently and that the stimulation of phosphoinositide metabolism produced by PTH may not require increases in cyclic AMP. These results would be in agreement to those reported by Lo and his associates. The results of all these studies demonstrate that PTH stimulates the turnover of phosphoinositides. They indicate that the stimulation of turnover occurs through a mechanism that results in a net increase in the content of renal phosphoinositides. The mechanism involved seems to be different from the stimulation of phosphatidylinositol turnover seen in platelets where phospholipase C activation by thrombin results initially in hydrolysis of phosphoinositide (19). The results with PTH also appear to differ from the effects produced by cholinergic stimuli and alpha-adrenergic stimuli in other tissues which are also characterized by an initial stimulation of breakdown and subsequent increase in resynthesis of phosphatidylinositol (Fig. 7).

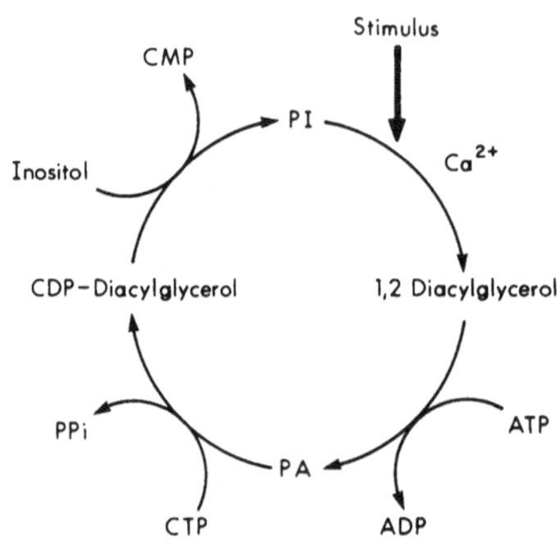

Fig. 7. The cycle of phosphatidylinositol (PI) breakdown and resynthesis. The stimulus is shown to increase the breakdown of PI to 1,2-diacylglycerol which is then converted to phosphatidic acid (PA) which, in turn, is converted to cytidine diphosphate diacylglycerol. In this example the turnover of the cycle is accelerated but the actual levels of PI are not increased.

The increased levels of phosphoinositides and phosphatidic acid produced by PTH may have dramatic effects on the membranes in which these phospholipids are contained. An area in which changes in phosphoinositide metabolism may relate to known effects of PTH is that of cellular metabolism of calcium. PTH is known to increase cytosolic calcium and stimulate calcium transport in renal tubular cells. Recent studies have demonstrated a calcium ionophoric property of phosphatidic acid (20). Mechanisms whereby acidic phospholipids may selectively increase membrane permeability to calcium have also recently been demonstrated (21,22). Finally, the ability of acidic phospholipids to bind calcium has also been demonstrated. Thus, the effect of PTH on phosphoinositide metabolism may be related to the action of the hormone on calcium transport across cell membranes, particularly in the kidney.

EFFECTS OF Ca^{++} ON PARATHYROID GLAND PHOSPHOLIPIDS

Recent studies by Morrissey and Hruska (23) in our laboratory have demonstrated that membrane phospholipids of the parathyroid gland are affected by changes in extracellular calcium. Incubation of bovine parathyroid cells in a medium containing ^{32}Pi resulted in the labelling of several phospholipids. The incorporation of ^{32}Pi into phosphatidylinositol was stimulated by an increase in extracellular calcium from 0.5 to 3.0 mM. On the other hand, the incorporation of ^{32}Pi into phosphatidylcholine was not affected by this change in Ca^{++} concentration in the medium. Densitometric scanning of the autoradiogram revealed that ^{32}Pi incorporation was greater in phosphatidylinositol, phosphatidic acid and phosphatidylethanolamine/phosphatidylglycerol. Studies demonstrated that the increase in the ratios of phosphatidylinositol to phosphatidylcholine observed in the membranes of dispersed parathyroid cells correlated well with the decrease in parathyroid hormone secretion observed as the calcium concentration was increased progressively from 0.5 to 2 mM. The increase in ^{32}Pi incorporated into phosphatidylinositol could be due to stimulation of the "PI cycle" resulting from enhanced phospholipid turnover with no change in or an actual decrease in net phosphatidylinositol levels (15). Alternatively, the greater ^{32}Pi incorporation could be due to increased levels of phosphatidylinositol as a consequence of increased synthesis and/or decreased degradation of the phospholipid (15). Glycerol incorporation, on the other hand, is an index of de novo phospholipid synthesis. Incubation of bovine parathyroid cells with ^{14}C-glycerol resulted in the labelling of phosphatidylinositol, as the major phospholipid species, and neutral lipid. There was no radioactive glycerol incorporated into phosphatidylcholine. When parathyroid cells were incubated in a medium containing 2 mM Ca^{++} there was a mean increase of 50% in ^{14}C-glyerol incorporation into phosphatidylinositol as compared to cells incubated with 0.5

mM Ca^{++} in the medium. These results reveal a profound effect of the calcium ion concentration on the metabolism of phosphatidylinositol in bovine parathyroid cells. The time course of and dose-response curve of phosphatidylinositol metabolism in response to calcium are similar to the effects of calcium on parathyroid hormone secretion. The increased glycerol incorporation into cellular phosphatidylinositol seen with an increase in the calcium ion concentration of the medium suggest that the formation of the phospholipid is increased in the parathyroid cell. Whether this is due to an increase in the synthetic rate, decreased degradation, or both, is not known at present.

The factors by which changes in phosphatidylinositol metabolism may influence parathyroid hormone secretion are many and include the following: Phosphatidylinositol is located in cell membranes along the entire protein secretory route for parathyroid hormone, i.e. endoplasmic reticulum, Golgi apparatus, secretory granuli and plasma membrane (9). An increase in phosphatidylinositol synthesis may reduce the level of fusogenic lipids such as 1,2-diacylglycerol for secretory-granule plasma-membrane merger (24). The increase in phospholipid may participate in formation of lipofuscin bodies for degradation of hormone (25). The phosphatidylinositol content of the plasma membranes may control the calcium flux of the cell and hence influence the cytosolic levels of calcium (9) which in turn control hormone secretion. Phosphotidylinositol metabolism also entails changes in arachidonic acid metabolism. Bovine parathyroid cells have recently been found to produce cyclooxygenase products in a calcium-dependent manner (26). Whether cyclooxygenase or lipooxygenase metabolites of arachidonic acid control hormone secretion requires further study. Lastly, lipid sensitive protein kinase activities may modulate protein secretion (27).

POTENTIAL MECHANISMS BY WHICH CHANGES IN PHOSPHOLIPID METABOLISM MAY AFFECT CALCIUM TRANSPORT OR HORMONAL SECRETION

Recent observations indicate that all biological membranes appear to contain lipids which adopt non-bilayer phases, particularly the hexagonal phase, in isolation. It has been shown that phosphoethanolamine isolated from human erythrocytes, endoplasmic reticulum, sarcoplasmic reticulum and rat liver mitochondria all exhibit hexagonal phases at 37° in the presence of excess of aqueous buffer (22). These observations suggest that this major lipid component commonly constituting 30-40 moles percent of the lipid phospholipids does not contribute to the integrity or stability of the membrane bilayer. The ability of lipids to adopt non-bilayer structures may be of importance to three types of membrane transport. These include facilitated transbilayer transport of polar molecules, transport involving membrane fusion phenomena such as exo- and endocytosis, as well as transport processes arising from the different membrane morphology allowed by non-bilayer lipid interaction. Changes in lipid composition of membranes may regulate the activity of proteins and enzymes present in such membranes (6).

Takai et al (27,28) have described a new species of cyclic nucleotide-independent, multifunctional protein kinase which is selectively activated by the simultaneous presence of calcium and phospholipids. Subsequent studies revealed that in addition to phospholipid, a small quantity of diacylglycerol, particularly which contains an unsaturated fatty acid, greatly enhances the reaction velocity with a concomitant decrease in the calcium concentration giving rise to maximum enzyme activation. Since the first product of phosphatidylinositol breakdown is expected to be a diacylglycerol with an unsaturated fatty acid such as arachidonic or oleic acid, it is conceivable that the activation of this newly found protein kinase may be directly related to phosphatidylinositol turnover. This protein kinase has been referred to as protein kinase C. Hokin and Hokin (29) presented the first evidence that phospholipid, particularly phosphatidylinositol, turns over very rapidly in response to various extracellular messengers. Subsequent studies have shown that this phospholipid turnover can be stimulated in virtually any type of tissue stimulated by a variety of extracellular messengers including alpha-adrenergic and muscarinic cholinergic stimulators. It is well known that phosphatidylinositol in mammalian tissues is composed of mainly unsaturated fatty acids such as arachidonic and oleic acids particularly in the position 2. Hence, external messengers which increase the degradation of phosphatidylinositol to diacylglycerol may activate protein kinase C and may serve as substrates to produce unsaturated fatty acids which are in turn converted to prostaglandins. Unsaturated fatty acids, as well as prostaglandins, have been shown to stimulate guanylate cyclase activity and the increased phosphatidylinositol turnover appears to occur in parallel with a rise in cyclic GMP in many tissues. It should be emphasized that the mechanisms reported by Takai et al for protein kinase C activation may occur without a net increase in the intracellular calcium concentration since the small quantity of diacylglycerol which results from phosphatidylinositol hydrolysis would sharply increase affinity of the newly found protein kinase system for this divalent cation.

ACKNOWLEDGMENTS

Work from our laboratory reported in this paper was supported by USPHS NIAMDD Grant AM-09976. Dr. Hruska is an Established Investigator of the American Heart Association. We would like to thank Ms. Pat Verplancke for her secretarial assistance.

REFERENCES

1. S.J. Singer and G.L. Nicolson, The fluid mosaic of the structure of cell membranes, Science 175:720 (1972).
2. S.J. Singer, The molecular organization of membranes, Annual Rev. Biochem. 43:805 (1974).
3. Melchior and J.M. Stein, Thermotropic transitions in membranes, Annual Rev. Biophys. Bioenergetics 5:205 (1976).
4. J.I. Korenbrot, Ion transport in membrane incorporation of biological ion-translocating proteins in model membrane systems, Ann. Rev. Physiol. 39:19 (1977).
5. C. Tanford and J.A. Reynolds, Characterization of membrane protein in detergent solutions, Biochim. Biophys. Acta 457:133 (1977).
6. H. Sandermann, Jr., Regulation of membrane enzymes by lipids, Biochim. Biophys. Acta 515:207 (1978).
7. A.L. Lehninger, "Biochemistry", Worth Publishers, Inc., New York, (1970), pp. 194-198.
8. E.P. Kennedy, The metabolism and function of complex lipids, Harvey Lectures 57:143 (1962).
9. R.H. Michell, Inositol phospholipids and cell surface receptor function, Biochim. Biophys. Acta 415:81 (1975).
10. M.E.M. Tolbert, A.C. White, K. Aspry, J. Cutts, and J.N. Fain, Stimulation of vasopressin and -catecholamines of phosphatidylinositol formation in isolated rat liver parenchymal cells, J. Biol. Chem. 255:1938 (1980).
11. J.N. Fain and J.A. Garcia-Sainz, Role of phosphatidylinositol turnover in $alpha_1$ and of adenylate cyclase inhibition in $alpha_2$ effects of catecholamines, Life Sciences 26:1183 (1980).
12. M.J. Berridge and J.N. Fain, Inhibition of phosphatidylinositol synthesis and the inactivation of calcium entry after prolonged exposure of the Blowfly salivary to 5-hydroxytryptamine, Biochem. J. 178:59 (1979).
13. H. Lo, D.C. Lehotay, D. Katz, and G.S. Levey, Parathyroid hormone-mediated incorporation of ^{32}P-orthophosphate into phosphatidic acid and phosphatidylinositol in renal cortical slices, Endocr. Res. Comm. 3:377 (1976).
14. W.H. Baricos, M.W. Hurst, and C.G. Huggins, Effects of cyclic nucleotides and related agents on renal polyphosphoinositide metabolism, in: "Cyclitols and Phosphoinositides", W.W. Wells and F. Eisenberg, Jr., eds., Academic Press, New York, p. 223 (1978).
15. R.V. Farese, P. Bidot-Lopez, A. Sabir, J.S. Smith, B. Schinbeckler, and R. Larson, Parathyroid hormone acutely increases polyphosphoinositides of the rabbit kidney cortex by a cycloheximide-sensitive process, J. Clin. Invest. 65:1523 (1980).

16. R.V. Farese, A.M. Sabir, and S.L. Vandor, Adrenocorticotropin acutely increases adrenal polyphosphoinositides, J. Biol. Chem. 254:6842 (1979).
17. V. Meltzer, S. Weinreb, E. Bellorin-Font and K.A. Hruska, Characterization of the effect of parathyroid hormone on renal phosphoinositide metabolism, Biochim. Biophys. Acta, In press.
18. P. Bidot-Lopez, R.V. Farese, and M.A. Sabir, Parathyroid hor mone and adenosine-3',5'-monophosphate acutely increase phospholipids of the phosphatidate-polyphosphoinositide pathway in rabbit kidney cortex tubules in vitro by a cycloheximide-sensitive process, Endocrinology 108:2078 (1981).
19. S. Rittenhouse-Simmons and D. Deykin, The mobilization of arachidonic acid in platelets exposed to thrombin or ionophore A23187, J. Clin. Invest. 60:495 (1977).
20. J.W. Putney, Jr., S.J. Weiss, C.M. Van De Walle, and R.A. Haddas, Is phosphatidic acid a calcium ionophore under neurohumoral control?, Nature 284:345 (1980).
21. D.E. Green, M. Fry, and G.A. Blondin, Phospholipids as the molecular instruments of ion and solute transport in biological membranes, Proc. Natl. Acad. Sci. USA 77:257 (1980).
22. P.R. Cullis, B de Kruijff, M.J. Hope, R. Nayar, and S.L. Schmid, Phospholipids and membrane transport, Can. J. Biochem. 58:1091, (1980).
23. J. Morrissey, and K. Hruska, Effect of cations on parathyroid secretion and phospholipid metabolism, Abstract, The Endocrine Society, 63rd Annual Meeting, 579 (1981).
24. D. Allan and R.H. Michell, The possible role of lipids in control of membrane fusion during secretion, Symp. of the Soc. for Exptl. Biol. 33:323 (1980).
25. H. Rohr, and B. Krassig, Elektronenmikroskopische untersuchungen ube den sekretionsmedus des parathormones, Zeitschrift fur Zellforschung 85:271 (1968).
26. E.M. Brown, and S.L. Swartz, Production of prostaglandins by bovine parathyroid tissue in vitro, Prog. Abst. Am. Soc. Bone and Min. Res. 33A (1981).
27. Y. Takai, A. Kishimoto, Y. Iwasa, Y. Kawahara, T. Mori, and Y. Nishizuka, Calcium-dependent activation of a multifunctional protein kinase by membrane phospholipids, J. Biol. Chem. 254:3692 (1979).
28. A. Kishimoto, Y. Takai, T. Mori, U. Kikkaw, and Y. Nishizuka, Activation of calcium and phospholipid-dependent protein kinase by diacylglycerol, its possible relation to phosphatidylinositol turnover, J. Biol. Chem. 255:2273 (1980).
29. L.E. Hokin and M.R. Hokin, Effects of acetylcholine on the turnover of phosphoryl units in individual phospholipids of pancreas slices and brain cortex slices, Biochim. Biophys. Acta 18:102 (1955).

EFFECTS OF PARATHYROID HORMONE ON GLOMERULAR ULTRAFILTRATION IN THE RAT

I. Ichikawa, N. Schor and B.M. Brenner

Laboratory of Kidney and Electrolyte Physiology
Brigham and Women's Hospital, Children's Hospital Medical Center and Harvard Medical School, Boston, MA

INTRODUCTION

Parathyroid hormone, which influences a spectrum of renal tubule transport processes, is thought to exert its actions via the intermediacy of cyclic AMP. Of interest to those concerned with glomerular function, several groups of workers (1-4) have found in rats and rabbits that glomeruli also possess an adenylate cyclase enzyme system which is sensitive to parathyroid hormone.

Using radiolabelled PTH, Sraer et al. (5) demonstrated that activation of the glomerular adenylate cyclase system is a consequence of PTH binding to specific glomerular receptors.

We recently undertook a series of experiments in the Munich-Wistar rat to determine the functional role of PTH in the mammalian glomeruli (6).

RESULTS

In defining the effects of circulating endogenous PTH on the glomerular microcirculation, we compared the results from 14 rats which had undergone acute thyroparathyroidectomy (TPTX) 2 1/2 hours prior to study with 8 other rats which underwent sham neck surgery. In the TPTX group fractional excretion of phosphate averaged 1.4%, a value well below that of non-TPTX controls and was taken as evidence for the effective removal of functioning parathyroid tissue. Before describing our findings on the determinants of glomerular ultrafiltration, some of the key aspects of this ultrafiltration process will be briefly reviewed: The rate of fluid transport across the glomerular capillary wall is governed by the imbalance between transcapillary hydraulic and oncotic pressures. The rate of ultrafiltration for the entire capillary network of a single nephron is therefore given by the equation:

$$\text{SNGFR} = K_f \times \overline{P}_{UF}$$

The mean net driving force in the glomerulus ($\overline{P}_{UF}$) is determined by the glomerular transcapillary hydraulic pressure difference, plasma oncotic pressure and glomerular plasma flow rate. It is important to recognize that in addition to these three determinants, which set the value of $\overline{P}_{UF}$, SNGFR is also a function of the ultrafiltration coefficient (K_f), the fourth and final determinant of GFR.

Using micropuncture techniques, these determinants were directly measured in our experiments and the results are shown in Figure 1. Values in this and subsequent figures denote means plus/minus one standard error. As shown in the upper panel, the mean value for initial glomerular plasma flow rate, Q_A, for TPTX rats was essentially the same as that in the non-TPTX group. As with total kidney GFR,

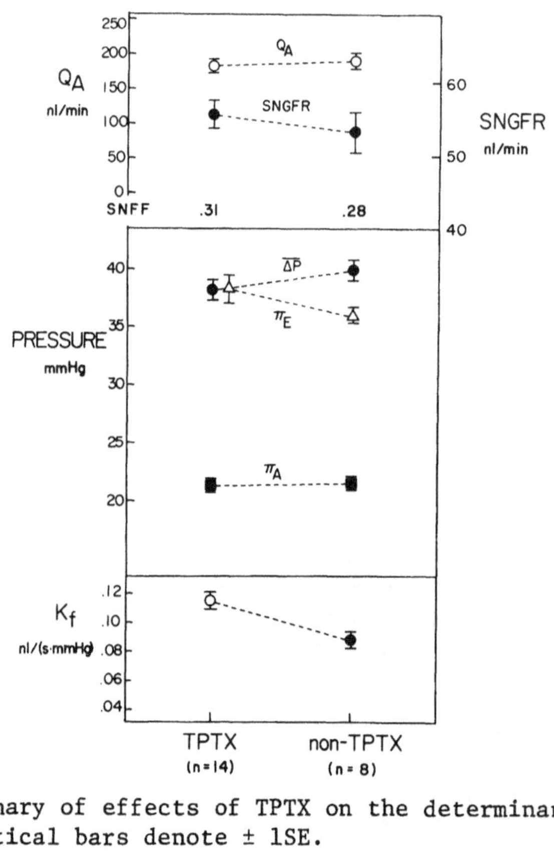

Fig. 1. Summary of effects of TPTX on the determinants of SNGFR. Vertical bars denote ± 1SE.

superficial SNGFR was, on average, slightly but insignificantly higher in the TPTX group, as was single nephron filtration fraction (SNFF). As shown in the middle panel, mean glomerular transcapillary hydraulic pressure difference ($\overline{\Delta P}$) was not significantly different between groups, nor were mean values for systemic (Π_A) and efferent arteriolar oncotic pressures (Π_E). Of note, however, whereas the mean value for Π_E was always less than $\overline{\Delta P}$ in non-TPTX rats, these values were essentially equal in the TPTX group, denoting achievement of filtration pressure equilibrium by the end of the glomerular capillary in TPTX group. As is clear from the bottom panel, this was largely due to significantly higher values of K_f obtained in TPTX rats than those in non-TPTX rats.

To ascertain whether these high K_f values obtained in TPTX rats are a specific consequence of PTH deficiency, we infused 1 U/KgBW/min of synthetic bovine 1-34 fragment PTH into 7 of these same TPTX rats. Although not shown here, 60-100 min infusion of this PTH fragment resulted in a slight but significant reduction in total kidney GFR, on average, from 1.4 to 1.2 ml/min in association with normalization of fractional excretion of phosphate.

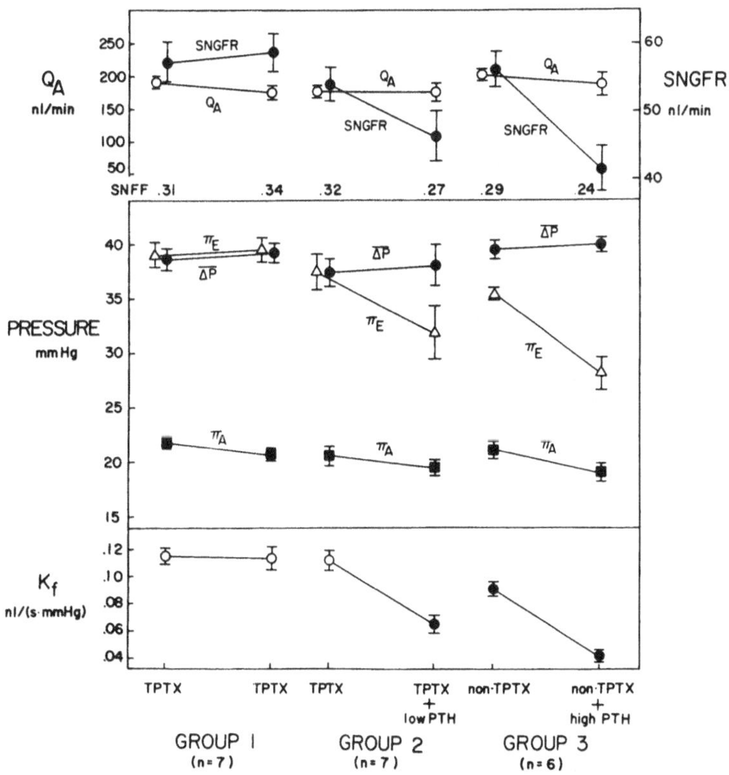

Fig. 2. Summary of changes in single nephron function in TPTX and non-TPTX rats treated with sham solution or low or high dose of PTH. Vertical bars denote ± 1SE.

The effects on glomerular dynamics of PTH infusion are shown in Figure 2. Thus, whereas glomerular plasma flow, Q_A, was essentially unaffected by PTH, SNGFR decreased, and in proportion to the fall in total kidney GFR. Single nephron filtration fraction, SNFF, therefore decreased in each rat, on average from 0.32 to 0.27 following PTH infusion. As shown in the middle panel on the right, we found near constancy of $\overline{\Delta P}$, and systemic oncotic pressure, Π_A, whereas efferent oncotic pressure, Π_E, declined in each rat, on average from 37 to 32 mmHg, indicating achievement of filtration pressure disequilibrium. As shown in the bottom panel, the value for K_f thus calculated was substantially lower in each rat given PTH than the value for the same rats obtained prior to PTH infusion.

In sham-PTH treated TPTX rats, as shown on the left, we failed to detect similar changes in K_f or the other quantities measured. To determine whether these PTH effects on K_f are dose-dependent, we infused a 10-fold higher dose of PTH into 6 non-TPTX rats. As also shown in Figure 2, the quantitative effects on glomerular dynamics in this group given a higher dose of PTH were similar to those obtained with lower dose of PTH, but included more pronounced effects on SNGFR, SNFF, Π_E and K_f. Once again, however, reduction in SNGFR was found to be the consequence primarily of the reduction in K_f. Values for K_f in the present study were relatively high when plasma PTH levels were presumed to be low or absent, and tended to decline with exogenous PTH administration. These observations raise the attractive possibility that the reductions in GFR commonly associated with hyperparathyroid states may be due, at least in part, to PTH excess.

Of interest are the findings from recent studies in rats that several other hormones and vasoactive substances are also capable of reducing K_f. Those include; angiotensin II (7), antidiuretic hormone (8), prostaglandins E_1, E_2 and I_2 (9,10), acetylcholine (9), Bradykinin (9), histamine (11) and dibutyryl cyclic AMP (dBcAMP) (8). Of interest also are the findings that all of these substances but angiotensin II have been shown to activate the adenyalte cyclase system in rat and rabbit glomeruli (1-4,12-14). Given the fact that cyclic AMP has been demonstrated to be a potent stimulus for renal renin release (15-18), it seemed reasonable to speculate that these hormonal substances, including PTH, regulate K_f by virtue of their capacity to enhance intrarenal angiotensin II formation via cyclic AMP production with angiotensin II playing the role of a common mediator for the reduction in K_f. This speculation was indeed supported in a recent study performed by Schor et al. (19).

In this study, initial micropuncture measurements were performed in a group of 7 Munich-Wistar rats during infusion of 5 U/KgBW/min of PTH, and the results were compared with 7 control rats given vehicle alone. As shown in Table 1, glomerular transcapillary hydraulic pressure difference, $\overline{\Delta P}$, rose slightly but

Table 1. Summary of Single Nephron Function in Rats Given PTH Before and During Saralasin Infusion

	$\overline{\Delta P}$ mmHg	SNGFR --nl/min--	Q_A	R_{TA} x10^{10} dyn·s·cm^{-5}	K_f nl/(s·mmHg)
SHAM	37	39.5	119	3.9	0.081
	±1	1.9	6	0.1	0.010
PTH	40*	35.1	100	5.1*	0.047*
	1	1.8	7	0.4	0.004
PTH + Saralasin	39	41.7	115	4.1	0.076*
	1	1.8	6	0.3	0.005

* $P<0.05$ vs. preceding group

significantly. Mild declines in SNGFR and Q_A were also observed, the latter due to an increase in total renal arteriolar resistance (R_{TA}). PTH also led to an impressive lowering of K_f. These observations therefore essentially duplicate our previous observations with exogenous PTH administration (6). After these measurements while PTH infusion was continued, infusion of saralasin, a competitive angiotensin II antagonist was begun in each rat. After a 30 min equilibration period, all measurements and collections were repeated. The results are also shown in Table 1. In the presence of saralasin, the effects of PTH on SNGFR, Q_A, $\overline{\Delta P}$, R_{TA} and K_f were largely reversed.

A similar K_f-reversing effect of saralasin was observed in rats treated with dBcAMP, a nucletide derivative known to mimic the action of cyclic AMP in a variety of tissues. Thus, as shown for a second group of rats we studied (Table 2), dBcAMP administration alone led to a small but significant increase in $\overline{\Delta P}$. SNGFR and Q_A declined by some 25% and 30%, respectively, the latter again due to a marked increase in total renal arteriolar resistance, R_{TA}. These effects are identical to those obtained by us with dBcAMP previously (8) as was the finding also shown in Table 2, that dBcAMP infusion led to a marked decline in K_f. In the presence of saralasin, the effects of dBcAMP on $\overline{\Delta P}$, Q_A, SNGFR, R_{TA} and K_f were completely reversed (Table 2).

These results indicate that the actions of PTH and its intermediate, cyclic AMP, on the glomerular ultrafiltration coefficient, K_f, are channeled through an action of angiotensin II. It has been shown by us recently that the K_f-lowering effects of prostaglandin E_2 and I_2 are also mediated by the intermediate action of angiotensin II (19).

Table 2. Summary of Single Nephron Function in Rats Given dBcAMP before and during Saralasin Infusion

	$\overline{\Delta P}$ mmHg	SNGFR --nl/min--	Q_A	R_{TA} x10^{10} dyn·s·cm^{-5}	K_f nl/(s·mmHg)
SHAM	37	39.5	119	3.9	0.081
	±1	1.9	6	0.1	0.010
dBcAMP	40*	30.2*	84*	5.8*	0.035*
	1	2.5	7	0.5	0.002
dBcAMP + Saralasin	35*	46.5*	142*	3.0*	0.087*
	1	2.7	10	0.2	0.008

* $P<0.05$ vs. preceding group

DISCUSSION

How, then, does angiotensin II cause this reduction in K_f. It is important to recognize that the glomerular ultrafiltration coefficient, K_f, is the product of total glomerular capillary filtering surface area (S) and capillary hydraulic conductivity (k):

$$K_f = S \times k$$

Selective alterations in k are not likely to be revealed in in vivo studies of glomerular function and, to date at least, permselective alterations of the glomerular wall in response to a variety of K_f-lowering agents have not been found.

On the other hand, considerable evidence has been amassed to suggest that the reduction in K_f seen with many agents largely reflects a decrease in S, particularly by virtue of the actions of these agents to promote mesangial cell contractility. It has been shown that glomeruli isolated from rat renal cortex are capable of contracting spontaneously (20) as well as in response to angiotensin II (21). Osborne et al. (22) localized radiolabelled angiotensin II predominantly in mesangial areas of glomeruli by autoradiographic methods. More recently, Ausiello et al. (23) found that rat mesangial cells grown in culture undergo intense contraction in response to angiotensin II and antidiuretic hormone. In addition, Hornych et al. (24) have shown markedly constricted glomerular capillary tufts in rats treated acutely with angiotensin II infusion, and Avasthi et al. (25) demonstrated reduction of total endothelial fenestral area in chronically salt depleted rats. The fall in K_f with ADH and angiotensin II may therefore be a reflection of the tendency of these peptides to promote glomerular mesangial cell contraction, which in turn brings about a reduction in total filtering surface area.

Since a variety of acute and chronic pathophysiological conditions characterized by a low level of GFR are often associated with high local/circulating levels of many of the humoral and vasoactive substances that we have been discussing, including PTH, it is reasonable to speculate that the reduced GFR in these conditions are due to reductions in K_f, in turn mediated by mesangial contraction triggered by angiotensin II.

REFERENCES

1. J. Sraer, R. Ardaillou, N. Loreau and J.D. Sraer, Evidence for parathyroid-hormone sensitive adenylate cyclase in rat glomeruli, Mol. Cell Endocrinol. 1:285 (1974).

2. M. Imbert, D. Chabardes and F. Morel, Hormone sensitive adenylate-cyclase isolated rabbit glomeruli, Mol. Cell Endocrinol. 1:295 (1974).

3. V.E. Torres, R.E. Northrup, R.M. Edwards, S.B. Shah and T.P. Dousa, Modulation of cyclic nucleotides in isolated rat glomeruli, J. Clin. Invest. 62:1334 (1978).

4. D. Schlondorff, P. Yoo and B.E. Alpert, Stimulation of adenylate cyclase in isolated rat glomeruli by prostaglandins, Am. J. Physiol. 235:F458 (1978).

5. J. Sraer, J.D. Sraer, D. Chansel, H. Jueppner, D. Hesch and R. Ardaillou, Evidence for glomerular receptors for parathyroid hormone, Am. J. Physiol. 235:F96 (1978).

6. I. Ichikawa, H.D. Humes, T.P. Dousa and B.M. Brenner, Influence of parathyroid hormone on glomerular ultrafiltration in the rat, Am, J. Physiol. 234:F393 (1978).

7. R.C. Blantz, K.S. Konnen, and B.J. Tucker, Angiotensin II effects upon the glomerular microcirculation and ultrafiltration coefficient of the rat, J. Clin. Invest. 56:419 (1976).

8. I. Ichikawa and B.M. Brenner, Evidence for glomerular actions of ADH and dibutyryl cyclic AMP in the rat, Am. J. Physiol. 233:F102 (1977).

9. C. Baylis, W.M. Deen, B.D. Myers and B.M. Brenner, Effects of some vasodilator drugs on transcapillary fluid exchange in renal cortex, Am. J. Physiol. 230:1148 (1976).

10. N. Schor, I. Ichikawa and B.M. Brenner, Mechanism of intermittent glomerular perfusion in the rat, Clin. Res. 28:56A (1980).

11. I. Ichikawa and B.M. Brenner, Mechanisms of action of histamine and histamine antagonists on the glomerular microcirculation in the rat, Circ. Res. 45:737 (1979).

12. H.E. Abboud, S.V. Shah and T.P. Dousa, Effects of biogenic amines and prostaglandins on cAMP and cGMP in isolated glomeruli, Clin. Res. 27:406A (1979).

13. N. Beck, R.V. Patak, Effects of prostaglandin E_2 (PGE_2) on cyclic AMP (cAMP) generation in isolated dog glomeruli, Clin. Res. 26:540A (1978).

14. R. Patak and N. Beck, Prostagcyclin (PGI_2) and angiotensin II (Ang-II) interaction on cyclic AMP (cAMP) generation in the isolated dog glomerulus (GL), Clin. Res. 27:426A (1979).

15. W.B. Campbell, R.M. Fraham and E.K. Jackson, Role of renal prostaglandins in sympathetically mediated renin release in the rat, J. Clin. Invest. 64:448 (1979).

16. A.M. Michelakis, J. Caudle and G.W. Liddle, In vitro stimulation of renin production by epinepnrine, norepinephrine, and cyclic AMP* (33647), Proc. Soc. Exp. Biol. Med. 130:748 (1969).

17. T. Okahara, Y. Abe and K. Yakamoto, Effects of dibutyrl cyclic AMP and propranolol on renin secretion in dogs, Proc. Soc. Exp. Biol. Med. 156:213 (1977).

18. N. Wimer, D.S. Chokshi and N.G. Walkenhorst, Effects of cyclic AMP, sympathomimetic amines, and adrenergic receptor antagonists on renin secretion, Circ. Res. 29:239 (1971).

19. N. Schor, I. Ichikawa and B.M. Brenner, Mechanisms of activity of various hormones and vasoactive substances on glomerular ultrafiltration in the rat, Kidney Int. 20:442, 1981.

20. M.B. Bernik, Contractile activity of human glomeruli in culture, Nephron 6:1 (1969).

21. J.D. Sraer, J. Sraer, R. Ardaillou and D. Mimoune, Evidence for renal glomerular receptors for angiotensin II, Kidney Int. 6:241 (1974).

22. M.J. Osborne, B. Droz, P. Myer and F. Morel, Angiotensin II: Renal localization in glomerular mesangial cells by autoradiography, Kidney Int. 8:245 (1975).

23. D.A. Ausiello, J.I. Kreisberg, C. Roy and M.J. Karnovsky, Contraction of cultured rat glomerular cells of apparent mesangial origin after stimulation with angiotensin II and arginine vasopressin, J. Clin. Invest. 65:754 (1980).

24. H. Hornych, M. Beaufils and G. Richet, The effects of exogenous angiotensin on superficial and deep glomeruli in the rat kidney, Kidney Int. 2:336 (1972).

REGULATION MECHANISMS OF THE RENAL PHOSPHATE HANDLING IN RENAL FAILURE - WHAT IS THE ROLE OF PTH ?

H. Fleisch, J. Caverzasio, and J.-P. Bonjour

Department of Pathophysiology
University of Berne
Berne, Switzerland

INTRODUCTION

It has been known for a long time, that plasma inorganic phosphate (Pi) increases in renal failure. Since 1954 it has been realized that this increase occurs only at a glomerular filtration rate (GFR) below approximately 25 ml/min (1). Above this value plasma Pi remains constant in spite of a decrease in GFR and with an unchanged urinary Pi. As a consequence, fractional excretion (FE) will have to increase or conversely fractional tubular reabsorption (TRP%) must decrease (1).

MECHANISMS

The mechnisms leading to this altered handling have become subject of intense debates. Several possibilities have been proposed: a) Changes in single nephron GFR (SNGFR), b) secondary hyperparathyroidism, and c) PTH independent mechanisms, such as renal adaptation to Pi needs.

a) Single nephron GFR

SNGFR can increase dramatically in renal failure (2,3) which will lead to an increased filtered load of Pi per nephron. At least in early renal failure, the change in the fractional excretion may be explained by an increase in SNGFR and not by an intrinsic decrease in TmPi per nephron. This is supported by the finding that reabsorption of Pi in the isolated proximal tubule in vitro is not changed after unilateral nephrectomy (4). On the other hand, an acute decrease of GFR has been found not to change the percent TRP in experimental uraemia (5). Thus, the role played by this parameter remains still unclear.

It must be realized that the increase in the maximum tubular Pi reabsorption per unit volume of glomerular filtrate i.e. TmPi/GFR (6) because of the change in SNGFR does not exactly reflect the TmPi per nephron. SNGFR may also affect micropuncture data. On the other hand, the effect on Pi can be dissociated from the effect on Na reabsorption (7,8), speaking for a specific effect on Pi handling.

Whatever the major part of the change in Pi handling is due to, it is likely that there is also an intrinsic decrease in reabsorption of Pi which is not due to an increase load per nephron of the remaining nephrons. If such is the case, two main mechanisms are invoked: secondary hyperparathyroidism and PTH independent mechanisms.

b) Secondary hyperparathyroidism

It has been known for over 40 years that renal failure is accompanied by an enlargement of the parathyroid glands (9,10). Moreover, its was also shown that renal failure in man is accompanied by clinical secondary hyperparathyroidism (11). This has been confirmed later by measurements of circulating plasma PTH (12,13).

The cause of this PTH increase is still subject of dispute. Bricker and Slatopolsky have proposed (13-17) that a retention of Pi in renal failure will lead to a decrease in ionized calcium which in turn will stimulate PTH secretion. The weakness of this theory is that in early renal failure no hyperphosphataemia occurs, to the contrary sometimes a tendency to hypophosphataemia was found (18). The absence of hyperphosphataemia is not surprising, if it realized that in the presence of a constant TmPi a decrease in GFR by 50 % will increase plasma Pi only slightly, and if Pi intake is kept small, then only by a negligible amount (6). Furthermore, the transient hyperphosphataemia, if present, is unlikely to be large enough to decrease ionized calcium sufficiently to influence PTH secretion. Indeed, it can be calculated from the association constants that a change of 1 mg% Pi alters ionized Ca only by about 0.01 mg% (19). On the other hand it is possible, although not proven, that a retention of Pi alters plasma ionized Ca concentration by other mechanisms rather than by calcium binding.

Another possibility may prevail which is based on observations with humans (20) and then strengthened by the experiments of Massry et al. (21-25) and others (26). According to these authors, secondary hyperparathyroidism is due to a decrease of ionized calcium because of a skeletal resistance in renal failure to the bone resorbing effect of PTH. This resistance would lead to a decreased release of calcium from bone thus causing hypocalcaemia which in turn would stimulate PTH secretion. Under certain conditions, this resistance can be corrected partially by $1,25(OH)_2D_3$ (23) and completely by the administration of both $1,25(OH)_2D_3$ and $24,25(OH)_2D_3$ (25). Thus, the resistence may be secondary to a failure of the vitamin D metabolism. However, it is not certain whether in early renal failure $1,25(OH)_2D$ is actually decreased when PTH is already high. Furthermore, in rats with acute renal failure one observes a skeletal resistance even when $1,25(OH)_2D_3$ and $24,25(OH)_2D_3$ in plasma are still normal (27). In this model Pi retention seems to play the important role (28). Thus, the cause of the skeletal resistance is not yet ascertained.

A third possibility may exist namely PTH is increased because of an improper degradation. It is well established that PTH is broken down in the kidney and the liver (29) and that this breakdown is impaired in subjects with renal failure (30).

The increase in PTH and the well known fact that PTH decreases the tubular reabsorption of Pi, made it tempting to relate the decrease in reabsorption of Pi in renal failure to secondary hyperparathyroidism, an old hypothesis (1,11) propagated lately by Bricker and Slatopolski (13-17). This mechanism has been termed the "trade-off hypothesis", whereby the price to pay for maintaining Pi homeostasis, is secondary hyperparathyroidism (15). For this theory speaks the fact that the change in handling of Pi can be normalized if hyperparathyroidism is corrected by parathyroidectomy (5). The handling of Pi can also remain normal if hyperparathryroidism is prevented by lowering Pi intake proportionally to the degree of renal failure (13,31). However, this may not always completely be the case (8), even when PTH is normalized (32).

c) PTH independent mechanisms - renal adaptation to Pi needs

In 1975 it was first shown that in renal failure parathyroidectomized animals too can decrease their tubular reabsorption of Pi, and must thus be able to do this independently of PTH (33). This finding has since been confirmed in the rat and the dog by various investigators (3,8,34,35). Further evidence has been obtained by micropuncture techniques showing that an increase in fractional delivery exists along the late proximal tubule, which is independent of PTH (36). The change in the handling of Pi in renal failure of non-TPTX animals and in man might thus be regulated by yet another mechanism than secondary hyperparathyroidism.

In the last 5 years a new concept has emerged which advanced our understanding on how Pi is handled by the kidney. Thus it has been realized that the kidney is able to adapt independently of PTH its tubular Pi reabsorption according to variations in the dietary Pi intake (37,38). Later on it was shown that this adaptation also occurs when bone mineralization (39) or when growth rate become altered (40). Not only the basic Pi handling but also the phosphaturic response to PTH depends strongly on the state of this adaptation mechanism (39). Thus, the kidney is able to adapt its handling of Pi and its response to PTH to the need of the organism (41).

It was therefore tempting to interpret the change in renal handling of Pi in renal failure to an adaptation phenomenon to a reduced renal mass, a theory proposed by Bonjour et al. (42). This theory would also explain the increased sensitivity of the tubule to PTH in its Pi handling, both in vivo (8) and in vitro (43). It would appear, that this increase in sensitivity is probably not due to a higher production of cAMP but to the response of the uraemic kidney to this nucleotide (8). However, since the sensitivity to PTH is also increased in uraemia if dietary Pi is reduced (26), some other mechanism may still be involved.

Relative importance of PTH and PTH independent mechanisms

Thus, both interpretations are based on facts. On one hand, there is a hyperparathyroidism in renal failure, and PTH decreases tubular reabsorption. On the other hand, a change in Pi handling also occurs in thyroparathyroidectomized animals. The question therefore is not whether one or the other mechanisms can operate, but which of the two is the more important one.

At this stage, a definitive answer to this question is still difficult to give. Indeed, while the regulatory factor of the first hypothesis, namely PTH, can be measured in plasma and can be removed by parathyroidectomy the same does not apply for the adaptation, because the regulatory factor, if any, is still unknown. However, some indication on the relative importance of the two mechanisms is given if the handling of PTH intact and parathyroidectomized animals are compared in normal state and renal failure (Fig. 1) (35). Two elements can be considered:

a) Effect of nephrectomy. If PTH represents the main mechanism, then this intervention should bring about a larger decrease in tubular reabsorption in normals than in TPTX animals. As seen in Fig. 1 this seems not to be the case, to the contrary, the effect of nephrectomy shows a tendency to be even larger in the TPTX animals.

b) Effect of parathyroidectomy. If PTH is important in renal failure, this intervention should produce a larger increase in tubular reabsorption in this condition since in renal failure PTH is higher than in animals with normal kidneys. This again is not the case, rather a tendency prevails that points in the opposite direction.

It should be mentioned here that the argument stating that the change in renal failure is completely due to PTH, because parathyroidectomy brings the decreased tubular reabsorption value back to normal, is misleading. Indeed, parathyroidectomy should not bring back the handling of Pi to normal values, but to values of parathyroidectomized animals or subjects without renal failure. This, however, is not the case, since the handling of Pi only reaches values comparable to levels of parathyroid intact animals. Thus, to the contrary, this result would actually indicate the presence of another mechanism rather than PTH.

Finally, recent results which show that doses of cimetidine which will bring back PTH levels in blood to normal in renal failure if anything lead to a decrease in plasma Pi and a decrease in tubular reabsorption of Pi (44), would also speak against a major role of PTH.

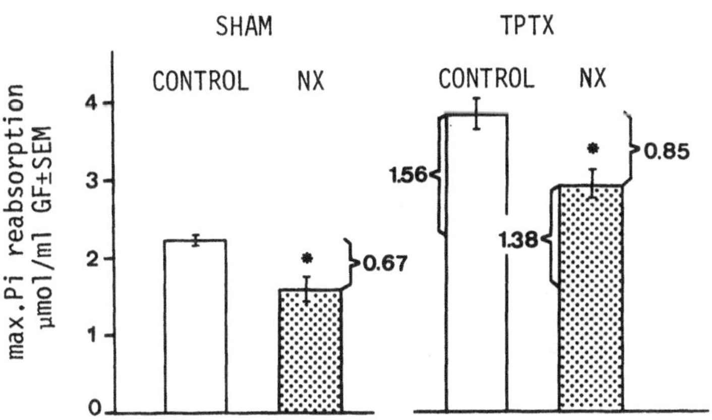

Fig. 1. Effect of renal failure and parathyroidectomy on the renal handling of Pi in the rat (from Ref. 35).

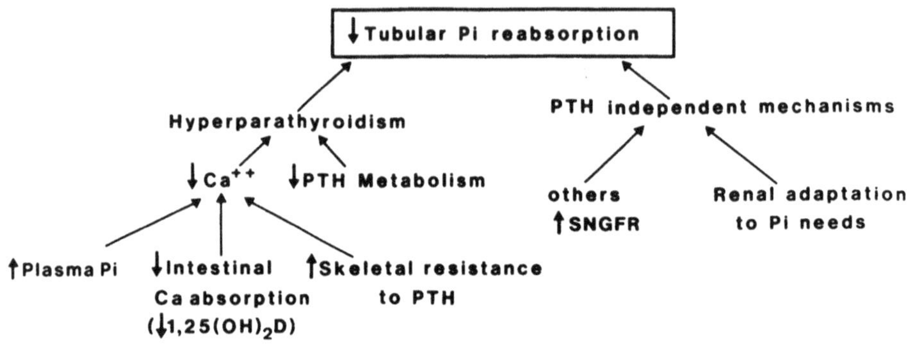

Fig. 2. Possible mechanisms leading to altered renal handling of Pi in renal failure

CONCLUSION

Various mechanisms may be involved in the change in the renal handling of Pi during the course of renal failure (Fig. 2). It would appear that PTH is actually not the main mediator which causes the change in renal Pi handling, but that other mechanisms, possibly renal adaptation to Pi needs, are just as important, if not more so.

ACKNOWLEDGEMENTS

This work has been supported by the Swiss National Science Foundation (grant 3.824.79) and by the Ausbildungs- und Förderungsfonds der Arbeitsgemeinschaft für Osteosynthese (AO), Chur, Switzerland.

REFERENCES

1. R. Goldman, and S. H. Bassett, Phosphorus excretion in renal failure, J. Clin. Invest. 33:1623 (1954).
2. N. Bank, W. S. Su, and H. S. Aynedjian, A Micropuncture study of renal phosphate transport in rats with chronic renal failure and secondary hyperparathyroidism, J. Clin. Invest. 61:884 (1978).
3. S.- F. Wen, and R. W. Stoll, Renal phosphate adaptation in uraemic dogs with a remnant kidney, Clin. Sci. 60:273 (1981).
4. P. C. Brazy, J. W. McKeown, R. H. Harris, and V. W. Dennis, Comparative effects of dietary phosphate, unilateral

nephrectomy, and parathyroid hormone on phosphate transport by the rabbit proximal tubule, Kidney Int. 17:788 (1980).

5. E. Slatopolsky, L. Gradowska, C. Kashemsant, R. Keltner, C. Manley, and N. S. Bricker, The control of phosphate excretion in uremia, J. Clin. Invest. 45:672 (1966).

6. B. Morgan, "Osteomalacia Renal Osteodystrophy and Osteoprosis", C. C. Thomas, Springfield, Illinois (1973).

7. C. H. Espinel, Effect of proportional reduction of sodium intake on the adaptive increase in glomerular filtration rate/nephron and potassium and phosphate excretion in chronic renal failure in the rat, Clin. Sci. and Mol. Med. 49:193 (1975).

8. M. L. Purkerson, D. B. Rolf, J. Yates, E. Slatopolsky, and S. Klahr, Factors that influence urinary phosphate excretion in rats with reduced renal mass. Evidence for increased sensitivity to parathyroid hormone, Min. Electr. Met.4:258 (1980).

9. A. M. Pappenheimer, and S. L. Wilens, Enlargement of the parathyroid glands in renal disease, Am. J. Pathol. 11:73 (1935).

10. A. M. Pappenheimer, The effect of experimental reduction of kidney substance upon the parathyroid glands and skeletal tissue, J. exp. Med. 64:965 (1936).

11. F. Albright, and E. C. Reifenstein, jr., "The Parathyroid Glands and Metabolic Bone Disease", The Williams & Wilkins Company, Baltimore (1948).

12. S. A. Berson, and R. S. Yalow, Parathyroid hormone in plasma in adenomatous hyperparathyroidism, uremia, and bronchogenic carcinoma, Science 154:907 (1966).

13. E. Slatopolsky, S. Caglar, J. P. Pennell, D. D. Taggart, J. M. Canterbury, E. Reiss, and N. S. Bricker, On the pathogenesis of hyperparathyroidism in chronic experimental renal insufficiency in the dog, J. Clin. Invest. 50:492 (1971).

14. E. Slatopolsky, A. M. Robson, I. Elkan, and N. S. Bricker, Control of phosphate in uremic man, J. Clin. Invest. 47:1865 (1968).

15. N. S. Bricker, On the pathogenesis of the uremic state. An Exposition of the "Trade-off Hypothesis", N. Engl. J. Med. 286:1093 (1972).

16. N. S. Bricker, L. G. Fine, M. Kaplan, M. Epstein, J. J. Bourgoignie, and A. Light, "Magnification phenomenon" in chronic renal disease, N. Engl. J. Med. 299:1287 (1978).

17. E. Slatopolsky, W. E. Rutherford, K. Hruska, K. Martin, and S. Klahr, How important is phosphate in the pathogenesis of renal osteodystrophy? Arch. Intern. Med. 138:848 (1978).

18. J. W. Coburn, M. H. Koppel, A. S. Brickman, and S. G. Massry, Study of intestinal absorption of calcium in patients with renal failure, Kindney Int. 3:264 (1973).
19. W. G. Robertson, Personal communication.
20. J. M. Evanson, The response to the infusion of parathyroid extract in hypocalcaemic states, J. Clin. Sci. 31:63 (1966).
21. S. G. Massry, J. W. Coburn, D. B. N. Lee, J. Jowsey, and C. R. Kleeman, Skeletal Resistance to parathyroid hormone in renal failure, Ann. Intern. Med. 78:357
22. S. G. Massry, A. I. Arieff, J. W. Coburn, G. Palmieri, and C. R. Kleeman, Divalent ion metabolism in patients with acute renal failure: Studies on the mechanism of hypocalcemia, Kidney Int. 5:437 (1974).
23. S. G. Massry, R. Stein, J. Garty, A. I. Arieff, J. W. Coburn, A. W. Norman, and R. M. Friedler, Skeletal resistance to the calcemic action of parathyroid hormone in uremia: Role of $1,25(OH)_2D_3$, Kidney Int. 9:467 (1976).
24. S. G. Massry, S. Dua, J. Garty, and R. M. Friedler, Role of uremia in the skeletal resistance to the calcemic action of parathyroid hormone, Min. Electr. Met. 1:172 (1978).
25. S. G. Massry, S. Tuma, S. Dua, and D. A. Goldstein, Reversal of skeletal resistance to parathyroid hormone in uremia by vitamin D metabolites, J. Lab. Clin. Med. 94:152 (1979).
26. M. A. Kaplan, J. M. Canterbury, G. Gavellas, D. Jaffe, J. J. Bourgoignie, E. Reiss, and N. S. Bricker, The calcemic and phosphaturic effects of parathyroid hormone in the normal and uremic dog, Metabolism 27:1785 (1978).
27. P. J. Somerville, and M. Kaye, Resistance to parathyroid hormone in renal failure: Role of vitamin D metabolites, Kidney Int. 14:245 (1978).
28. P. J. Somerville, and M. Kaye, Evidence that resistance to the calcemic action of parathyroid hormone in rats with acute uremia is caused by phosphate retention, Kidney Int. 16:552 (1979).
29. K. J. Martin, K. A. Hruska, J. J. Freitag, S. Klahr, and E. Slatopolsky, The peripheral metabolism of parathyroid hormone, N. Engl. J. Med. 20:1092 (1979).
30. K. A. Hruska, A. Korkor, K. Martin, and E. Slatopolsky, Peripheral metabolism of intact parathyroid hormone, J. Clin. Invest 67:885 (1981).
31. E. Slatopolsky, S. Caglar, L. Gradowska, J. Caterbury, E. Reiss, and N. S. Bricker, On the prevention of secondary hyperparathyroidism in experimental chronic renal disease using "proportional reduction" of dietary phosphorus intake, Kidney Int. 2:147 (1972).

32. M. A. Kaplan, J. M. Canterbury, G. Gavellas, D. Jaffe, J. J. Bourgoignie, E. Reiss, and N. S. Bricker, Interrelations between phosphorus, calcium, parathryoid hormone, and renal phosphate excretion in response to an oral phosphorus load in normal and uremic dogs, Kidney Int. 14:207 (1978).
33. R. S. Swenson, J. R. Weisinger, J. L. Ruggeri, and G. M. Reaven, Evidence that parathyroid hormone is not required for phosphate homeostasis in renal failure, Metabolism 24:199 (1975).
34. J. Caverzasio, H. J. Gloor, H. Fleisch, and J.P. Bonjour, Parathyroid hormone-independent adaptation of tubular phosphate transport to renal mass reduction, Kidney Int. 17:886 (1980).
35. J. Caverzasio, H. J. Gloor, H. Fleisch, and J.-P. Bonjour, Parathyroid hormone-independent adaptation of the renal handling of phosphate in response to renal mass reduction, Kidney Int., in press.
36. N. L. M. Wong, G. A. Quamme, J. H. Dirks, and R. A. L. Sutton, Phosphate handling by the remnant dog kidney in the presence and absence of the contralateral normal kidney, Min. Electr. Metab. 2:280 (1979).
37. U. Troehler, J.-P. Bonjour, and H. Fleisch, Inorganic phosphate homeostasis. Renal adaptation to the dietary intake in intact and thyropharathyroidectomized rats. J. Clin. Invest. 57:264 (1976).
38. T. H. Steele, and H. F. DeLuca, Influence of dietary phosphorus on renal phosphate reabsorption in the parathyroidectomized rat. J. Clin. Invest. 57:867 (1976).
39. J.-P. Bonjour, U. Troehler, C. Preston, and H. Fleisch, Parathyroid hormone and renal handling of Pi: effect of dietary Pi and diphosphonates, Am. J. Physiol. 234:F497 (1978).
40. J. Caverzasio, J.-P. Bonjour, and H. Fleisch, Adaptation of tubular phosphate transport: Relation between phosphate requirement, as influenced by growth, and supply, in: "Phosphate and Minerals in Health and Disease", Proc. 4th Int. Workshop on Phosphate and Other Minerals, Strasbourg 1979, S. G. Massry, E. Ritz, and H. Jahn, eds., Plenum Press, New York and London (1980).
41. J.-P. Bonjour, and H. Fleisch, Tubular adaptation to the supply and requirement of phosphate, in: "Renal Handling of Phosphate", S. G. Massry and H. Fleisch, eds., Plenum Publishing Company, New York (1980).
42. J.-P. Bonjour, J. Caverzasio, H.-J. Gloor, and H. Fleisch, Adaptation of the renal handling of phosphate in chronic renal failure: Evidence for a parathyroid hormone-independent mechanism, in: "Advances in Basic and Clinical

Nephrology", Proc. of the 8th Int. Congress of Nephrology, Athens 1981, W. Zurukzoglu, M. Papadimitriou, M. Pyrpasopoulos, M. Sion, C. Zamboulis, eds., Karger, Basel (1981).

43. N. Yanagawa, B. Houston, and L. G. Fine, Altered parathyroid hormone (PTH) sensitivity of the uremic proximal tubule: Evidence for regulation of hormone-receptor interaction, Kidney Int. 19:118 (1981).

44. A. I. Jacob, J. M. Canterbury, G. Gavellas, P. W. Lambert, and J. J. Bourgoignie, Reversal of secondary hyperparathyroidism by cimetidine in chronically uremic dogs, J. Clin. Invest. 67:1753 (1981).

INTERACTIONS BETWEEN LIVER AND PARATHYROID HORMONE

Kevin Martin, Keith Hruska, and Eduardo Slatopolsky

Renal Division
Department of Medicine
Washington University School of Medicine
St. Louis, Missouri

Heterogeneity of Circulating PTH

In the past decade advances have been made in the understanding of the metabolism of parathyroid hormone and the interpretation of the findings of fragments of parathyroid hormone in peripheral blood. Early studies[1,2] with radioimmunoassay gave different results in patients with primary hyperparathyroidism. It was thought that the radioimmunoassay for parathyroid hormone measured in blood the peptide secreted by the parathyroid glands. However, Berson and Yalow[3] demonstrated that parathyroid hormone in plasma of patients was heterogeneous and differed immunologically from the hormone extracted from parathyroid glands of humans. Using different antisera they clearly demonstrated the presence of fragments of the PTH molecule with various half lives such that some fragments rapidly become undetectable after parathyroidectomy while other fragments had prolonged half lives in circulation. They also demonstrated that the half life of immunoreactive PTH was markedly prolonged in patients with uremia. Subsequently it became apparent that intact PTH and the biologically active amino-terminal fragments have short half lives in the circulation (less than 5 minutes) while carboxy-terminal fragments have much longer half lives (30 to 40 minutes). A major question has been whether these hormonal fragments are secreted by the parathyroid glands or are the results of metabolism of intact PTH by peripheral organs. Several years ago Habener and collaborators[4] suggested that intact PTH was secreted by the parathyroid glands and peripheral metabolism of PTH was critical in the generation of circulating PTH fragments. Later studies in vivo and in vitro by several investigators[5-7] have provided firm evidence for direct glandular secretion of PTH fragments. However, there is also substantial evidence that peripheral metabolism of intact PTH also contributes to the circulating PTH fragments. The appearance of PTH fragments in blood after injection or infusion of purified intact PTH intravenously provides firm evidence that PTH fragments are produced and returned to the circulation by peripheral organs.[8] The major organs involved in the peripheral metabolism of PTH are the liver, kidney and bone.

Degradation of PTH by Liver

Evidence for the importance of the liver in the metabolism of parathyroid hormone was presented by Fang and Tashjian.[9] These investigators demonstrated in rats that partial hepatectomy markedly prolongs the disappearance of iPTH from blood. They also demonstrated that incubation of PTH with the rat liver homogenate led to a rapid loss of the calcium mobilizing, phosphaturic and immunological activities of the hormone. Subsequently, Canterbury and collaborators[10] using an isolated perfused rat liver model, demonstrated cleavage of intact PTH by the liver and production of PTH fragments similar, on gel filtration, to those seen in the peripheral circulation. After 15 minutes of perfusion of the isolated liver they found in addition to the intact PTH, which was added to the perfusate, the presence of two other peaks of i-PTH, one with a molecular weight of approximately 7000 daltons and a second with a molecular weight of approximately 3500 daltons. Chromatographic studies indicate that peak 1 contained intact hormone with both amino terminal and carboxy terminal immunoreactivity and was biologically active. Peak 2 consisted of only carboxy-terminal immunoreactivity and was biologically inactive. And peak 3 contained predominantly amino terminal immunoreactivity and was biologically active. Moreover, they demonstrated that the rate of metabolism of PTH seems to be regulated by the concentration of calcium in the medium. At high concentrations of calcium (greater than 11 mg/100 ml) PTH metabolism was retarded. On the other hand, at low concentrations of calcium (less than 5 mg/100 ml) the rate of metabolism was greatly increased. Thus, the cleavage system of the liver exhibits features that may play important physiological homeostatic roles. Subsequent studies by Newman and collaborators[11] demonstrated that the liver is the principle site of PTH deposition and suggested that nephrectomy had only minor effects on the rate of peripheral degradation of the hormone. Their studies demonstrated that the intact hormone was the principal form found in liver extracts and the uptake of parathyroid hormone was greatly influenced by the biologic activity of the preparation. In other words, when biologically inactive hormone was administered to the animals the uptake of the hormone was markedly reduced. On the other hand, when pure preparation of biologically active PTH was used in the studies, there was a significant degree of degradation. Subsequently, the same investigators demonstrated a significant binding of electrolytically iodinated PTH to membranes obtained from hepatocytes.[12] Studies by d'Amour and collaborators[13] and Segre and collaborators[14] have suggested that the cleavage of intact PTH by the liver is mediated by the Kupffer cells and that the liver appears to be the major source of the carboxy-terminal fragments found in the circulation. These authors[14] studied the proteolysis of intact hormone by isolated rat Kupffer cells and hepatocytes. They demonstrated when intact parathyroid hormone was incubated with Kupffer cells this peptide disappeared with a T½ of 12 ± 4 min, coincident with the appearance of PTH fragments from both the amino- and carboxy-terminal portions of the intact hormone. On the other hand, metabolism of PTH by hepatocytes was minimal. They also suggested that the metabolism of parathyroid hormone by Kupffer cells results in the appearance of fragments in the media that are immunochemically indistinguishable from and chemically identical with those found in plasma when the intact hormone is injected intravenously. Whether the Kupffer cells of the liver are solely responsible for PTH metabolism remains controversial since cellular effects of PTH on liver such as gluconeogenesis, and glycogenolysis are more readily attributable to hepatocytes and it is, therefore, possible that these cells may also contribute to the metabolism of PTH. Martin and collaborators[15] examined the uptake of PTH by the liver in vivo in dogs with indwelling hepatic venous catheters following either single injections or constant infusions of bovine PTH 1-84 and synthetic b-PTH 1-34. After a single injection of b-PTH 1-84 hepatic arteriovenous (AV) differences for i-PTH was 39% at 2 minutes after the injection but decreased to 0% by 25 minutes despite high levels of iPTH in the arterial circulation. Chromatographic studies of arterial and hepatic venous samples obtained when hepatic AV difference for i-PTH were demonstrable (2 minutes) revealed hepatic uptake of intact hormone and addition of a smaller carboxy terminal fragment, eluting just after the intact hormone to the hepatic venous blood (Figure 1). Gel filtration of samples obtained 20-30 minutes after injection of bovine PTH 1-84, when no hepatic AV difference for i-PTH was demonstrable, revealed no detectable intact hormone in the circulation. Levels of carboxy-terminal fragments of the hormone at the time were identical in arterial and hepatic venous samples (Figure 2). In additional experiments no hepatic AV difference was observed after the injection of synthetic bovine PTH 1-34 (Figure 3). As is illustrated in Figure 3, the kidney demonstrated an AV difference after injection of synthetic bPTH 1-34. These studies suggest that the uptake of iPTH by the liver is selective for the intact hormone and indicates that the liver does not remove either amino-terminal or carboxy-terminal fragments from the circulation. On the other hand, this organ is a source of carboxy-terminal iPTH fragments found in the circulation. Recently, Hruska and collaborators[16] further characterized

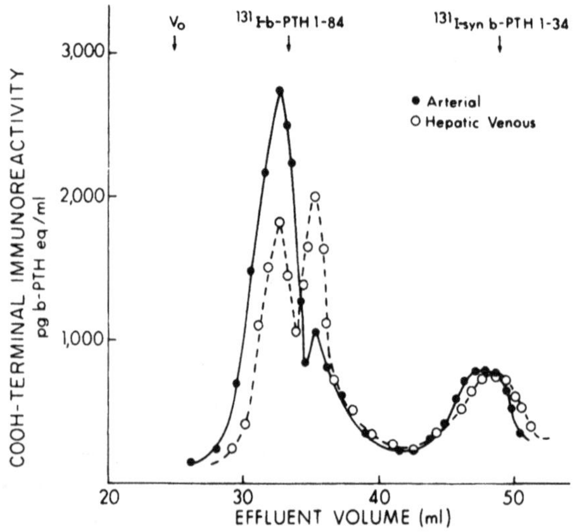

Fig. 1. Elution pattern of COOH-terminal i-PTH in arterial (•) and hepatic venous (o) plasma obtained from a dog 5 min. after injection of b-PTH 1-84. COOH-terminal i-PTH was determined with the CH9 antiserum preincubated with excess syn b-PTH 1-34. Gel filtration was performed on a 1.5 x 50 cm column of Bio-Gel P-10. (From K. Martin et al, J. Clin. Invest. 58: 781, 1976).

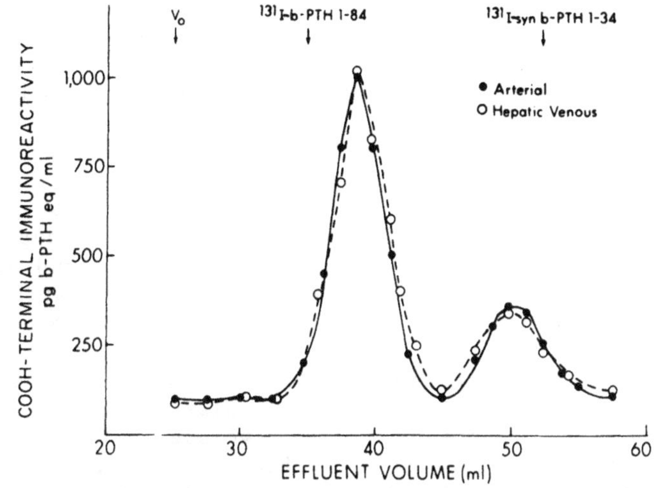

Fig. 2. Elution pattern of COOH-terminal i-PTH in arterial (●) and hepatic venous (o) plasma obtained from a dog 20 min. after injection of b-PTH 1-84. COOH-terminal i-PTH was determined with the CH9 antiserum preincubated with excess syn b-PTH 1-34. Gel filtration was performed on a 1.5 x 50 cm column of Bio-Gel P-10. (From K. Martin et al, J. Clin. Invest. 58: 781, 1976.)

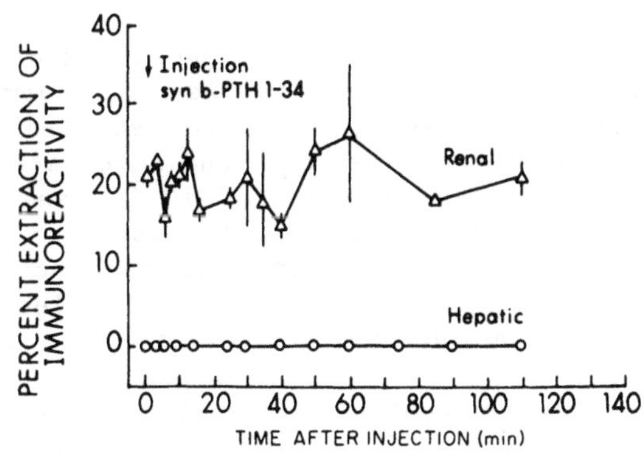

Fig. 3. Hepatic (o) and renal (Δ) extraction of NH_2-terminal i-PTH after a single injection of syn b-PTH 1-34. Each point represents the mean ±SE of the percent extraction seen in five dogs in which simultaneous renal and hepatic venous plasma samples were obtained. (From K. Martin et al, J. Clin. Invest. 58: 781, 1976.)

the contribution of the liver in the metabolism of intact parathyroid hormone. Studies performed in awake dogs demonstrated that the metabolic clearance rate (MCR) of intact PTH was found to be very rapid, 21.6 ± 3.1 ml/kg/min. The liver accounted for the greatest fraction of the MCR of intact PTH, approximately 60%. The renal uptake of intact PTH accounted for approximately 30% of the metabolic clearance rate of intact PTH. The MRC of biologically inactive PTH was markedly decreased to approximately 8.8 ± 1 ml/kg/min. These results suggest that high rates of hepatic PTH uptake are decreased by inactivation of the hormone and are compatible with the hypothesis that part of the demonstrated PTH uptake is due to binding to sites specific for biologically active hormone. This hypothesis was in part confirmed by recent studies of Newman and Schneider[12] which demonstrated binding of biologically active PTH to hepatocyte plasma membranes and a marked activation of the adenylate cyclase (cAMP production increased over 5 fold). Dogs with chronic renal failure have a significant decrease in the MCR of intact PTH from 21.6 ± 3.1 ml/kg/min in normal dogs, to 11.3 ± 1.3 ml/min/kg in the dogs with reduced renal function. Of interest is that the hepatic clearance of parathyroid hormone was also greatly affected in the uremic animals. The hepatic clearance of intact parathyroid hormone decreased by approximately 30% in the animals with chronic renal insufficiency. However, the contribution of the hepatic metabolism of parathyroid hormone to the total metabolic clearance rate greatly increased since there was (as is expected) a remarkable decrease in the renal degradation of intact PTH in the animals with chronic renal insufficiency.

Effects of PTH on Liver Metabolism

Moxley and collaborators[17] studied the effect of parathyroid hormone on activation of adenylate cyclase on plasma membranes from rat liver and on gluconeogenesis in isolated rat hepatocytes. These authors demonstrated that the adenylate cyclase was stimulated by PTH at a concentration of 10^{-9} M and above. The concentrations of cyclic AMP in hepatocytes was increased by 134% by parathyroid hormone. Glucose production was increased by 21% by parathyroid hormone in comparison to 124% by glucagon. Similarly ^{14}C glucose formation from ^{14}C-alanine was increased by 31%. These authors[17] also demonstrated that PTH has a glycogenolytic effect and glycogen content in hepatocytes was reduced by 28% by parathyroid hormone. Urea production also was increased when hepatocytes were incubated with parathyroid hormone in a concentration of 10^{-6} M. The doses of PTH employed to demonstrate the above-mentioned effects were clearly pharmacologic but this was also the case in studies related to the effect of PTH on gluconeogenesis and cyclic AMP production by renal tubules and slices.[18,19] Hruska and collaborators[20] characterized further the effect of parathyroid hormone on hepatic glucose in the dog.

The studies performed in vivo with indwelling catheters in awake dogs demonstrated that bovine PTH 1-84 stimulated glucose release in dogs from basal values of 31 ± 8 to 68 ± 9 mg/min/kg after bolus injection of PTH. The amino terminal PTH fragment synthetic b-PTH 1-34 had no effect. Bovine PTH 1-84 also increased incorporation of ^{14}C from infused ^{14}C-alanine into glucose. The administration of bovine PTH 1-84 stimulated hepatic glucose release in part through increased gluconeogenesis in vivo. Other studies also have shown that PTH inhibits glycogen synthesis in the isolated perfused rat liver.[21] Thus, studies in vitro as well as in vivo suggest that the liver may represent an important target organ of PTH. Additional studies will be needed to clarify the potential role of PTH in carbohydrate intolerance observed in uremic patients. However, recent studies by Bevilacqua and collaborators[22] in awake dogs with indwelling portal, hepatic venous and arterial catheters did not show an increase in glucose production or release after the administration of bovine PTH 1-84. At the present time there is no apparent explanation for the discrepancy in results between the two above-mentioned investigators.

Besides the effect of cyclic AMP, glucose and urea production, other effects of PTH on liver metabolism also have been demonstrated. PTH has been shown to increase the uptake of calcium by liver cells[23] and release inorganic phosphate.[24] PTH also has been shown to increase the uptake of amino acid.[17,19] In addition, parathyroidectomy reduces the initiation of DNA synthesis and mitosis which is normally induced in liver parenchymal cells by partial hepatectomy.[25]

In conclusion, it would seem, therefore, that there is a remarkable relationship between parathyroid hormone and liver. The Kupffer cells have a primary role in the degradation of parathyroid hormone and PTH has a significant biological effect on liver hepatocytes. The relationship between degradation of the hormone and metabolism by the liver requires further clarification.

ACKNOWLEDGMENTS

Work from our laboratory reported in this paper was supported by USPHS NIAMDD Grant AM-09976. Dr. Hruska is an Established Investigator of the American Heart Association.

REFERENCES

1. S.A. Berson, and R.S. Yalow, Parathyroid hormone in plasma in adenomatous hyperparathyroidism, uremia and bronchogenic carcinoma, Science 154:907 (1966).

2. E. Reiss, and J.M. Canterbury, A radioimmunoassay for parathyroid hormone in man, Proc. Soc. Exptl. Biol. 128:501 (1968).
3. S.A. Berson, and R.S. Yalow, Immunochemical heterogeneity of parathyroid hormone in plasma, J. Clin. Endocrinol. Metab. 28:1037 (1968).
4. J.F. Habener, D. Powell, T.M. Murray, G.P. Mayer, and J.T. Potts, Jr., Parathyroid hormone: secretion and metabolism in vivo, Proc. Natl. Acad. Sci. USA 68:2986 (1971).
5. J.C. Flueck, F.P. Di Bella, A.J. Edis, J.M. Kehrwald, and C.D. Arnaud, Immunoheterogeneity of parathyroid hormone in venous effluent serum from hyperfunctioning parathyroid glands, J. Clin. Invest. 60:1367 (1977).
6. G.P. Mayer, J.A. Keaton, J.G. Hurst, and J.F. Habener, Effects of plasma calcium concentration on the relative proportion of hormone and carboxyl fragments in parathyroid venous blood. Endocrinology 104:1778 (1979).
7. D.A. Hanley, K. Takatsuki, J.M. Sultan, A.B. Schneider, and L.M. Sherwood, Direct release of parathyroid hormone fragments from functioning bovine parathyroid glands in vitro, J. Clin. Invest. 62:1247 (1978).
8. J.F. Habener, G.P. Mayer, P.C. Dee, and J.T. Potts, Jr., Metabolism of amino and carboxyl-sequence immunoreactive parathyroid hormone in the bovine: Evidence for peripheral cleavage of hormone, Metabolism 25:385 (1976).
9. V.S. Fang, A.H. Tashjian, Jr., Studies on the role of the liver in the metabolism of parathyroid hormone. I. Effects of partial hepatectomy and incubation of the hormone with tissue homogenates, Endocrinology 90:1177 (1972).
10. J.M. Canterbury, L.A. Bricker, J.S. Levey, P.L. Kozlovskis, E. Ruiz, J.E. Zull and E. Reiss, Metabolism of bovine parathyroid hormone: immunological and biological characteristics of fragments generated by liver perfusion, J. Clin. Invest. 55:1245 (1975).
11. W.F. Neuman, M.W. Neuman, K. Lane, L. Miller, and P.J. Sammon, The metabolism of labeled parathyroid hormone. V. Collected biological studies, Calcif. Tissue Res. 18:271 (1975).
12. W.F. Neuman and N. Schneider, The parathyroid hormone-sensitive adenylate cyclase system in plasma membranes of rat liver, Endocrinology 107:2082 (1980).
13. P. D'Amour, G.V. Segre, S.I. Roth, and J.T. Potts, Jr., Analysis of parathyroid hormone and its fragments in rat tissues: chemical identification and microscopical localization, J. Clin. Invest. 63:89 (1979).
14. G.V. Segre, A.S. Perkins, L.A. Witters, and J.T. Potts, Jr., Metabolism of parathyroid hormone by isolated rat Kupffer cells and hepatocytes,
15. K. Martin, K. Hruska, A. Greenwalt, S. Klahr, and E. Slatopolsky, Selective uptake of intact parathyroid hormone

in the liver: differences between hepatic and renal uptake, J. Clin. Invest. 58:781 (1976).

16. K.A. Hruska, A. Korkor, K. Martin, and E. Slatopolsky, Peripheral metabolism of intact parathyroid hormone: role of liver and kidney and the effect of chronic renal failure. J. Clin. Invest. 67:885 (1981).

17. M.A. Mosely, N.H. Bell, S.R. Wagle, D.O. Allen, J. Ashmore, Parathyroid hormone stimulation of glucose and urea production in isolated liver cells, Am. J. Physiol. 227:1058 (1974).

18. K. Kurokawa, T. Ohno, and H. Rasmussen, Ionic control of renal gluconeogenesis. II. The effect on Ca^{2+} and H^{+} upon the response to parathyroid hormone and cyclic AMP. Biochem. Biophys. Acta 313:32 (1973).

19. W.G. Guder and O.H. Wieland, Metabolism of isolated kidney tubules. Additive effects of parathyroid hormone and free-fatty acids on renal gluconeogenesis, Eur. J. Biochem. 31:69 (1972).

20. K. Hruska, J. Blondin, R. Bass, J. Santiago, L. Thomas, P. Altsheler, K. Martin, and S. Klahr, Effect of intact parathyroid hormone on hepatic glucose release in the dog, J. Clin. Invest. 64:1016 (1979).

21. D.A. Hems, C.S. Harmon, and P.D. Whitton, Inhibition by parathyroid hormone og glycogen synthesis in the perfused liver, Fed. Eur. Biochem. Soc. Lett. 58:167 (1975).

22. S. Bevilacqua, E. Barret, E. Ferrannini, R. Gusberg, A. Stewart, D. Richardson, D. Smith, and R. DeFronzo, Lack of effect of parathyroid hormone on hepatic glucose metabolism in the dog, Metabolism 30:469 (1981).

23. A.B. Chausmer, B.S. Sherman, S. Wallach, The effect of parathyroid hormone on hepatic cell transport of calcium, Endocrinology 90:663 (1972).

24. R.A. Meyer, M.H. Meyer, Soft tissue phosphate loss accompanying the hyperphosphaturic effect of parathyroid hormone in rats, Endocrinology 94:1331 (1974).

25. R.H. Rixon, J.F. Whitfield, Parathyroid hormone: a possible initiator of liver regeneration, Proc Soc Exp Biol Med 141:93 (1972).

PARATHYROID HORMONE AND THE HEART

Shaul G. Massry

Division of Nephrology, Department of Medicine
University of Southern California
2025 Zonal Avenue, Los Angeles, California USA

Evidence is rapidly accumulating supporting the proposal originally made by Massry in 1977 that parathyroid hormone is a major uremic toxin (1). This hypothesis implied that PTH has a multifarious extraskeletal actions affecting the functions of many organs Several observations from our laboratory (1-12) and many of the presentations in this Workshop provide strong support for a wide extraskeletal effect of PTH.

Myocardiopathy is encountered in uremia (13) and certain old experimental data suggested that excess PTH in uremia may be associated with myocardial disease (14,15). Cardiac lesions predictably occurred in rats after bilateral nephrectomy or bilateral ureteral ligation; administration of PTH enhanced the development of these lesions and parathyroidectomy either ameliorated or completely prevented their evolution. To evaluate the role of PTH in the myocardiopathy of uremia, we examined the interaction between the hormone and the heart.

We first examined the effect of PTH on the beating rate of rat heart cells grown in culture utilizing the method of Harary and Farley (16). Both intact PTH (1-84) and its amino-terminal fragment (1-34) produced significant increments in the beating rate within 30 seconds of their addition to the media (Figure 1). Thereafter, the beating rates of the cells in the medium containing PTH was significantly lower than that of the control cells, and the PTH treated cells ceased to beat earlier than the control ones. There was a dose-response relationship between both 1-34 and 1-84 PTH and their effect on beating rate (Figure 2).

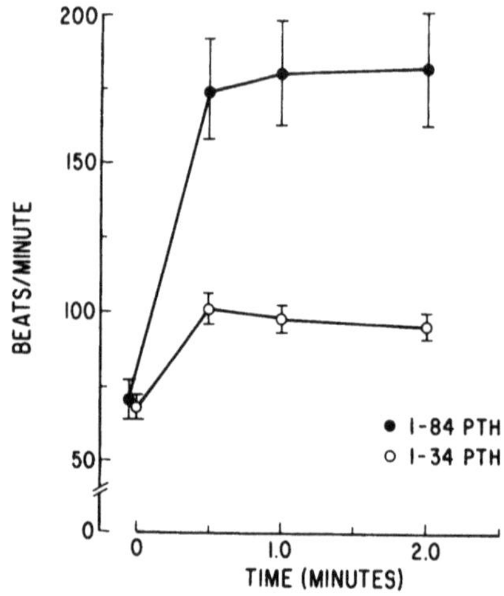

Figure 1. The effect of the intact molecule of PTH (1-84) and its amino-terminal fragment (1-34) on beating rates of heart cells in relation to time, after the addition of the hormone to the medium containing the cells. ●, 1-84 PTH; O, 1-34 PTH. By permission from (8).

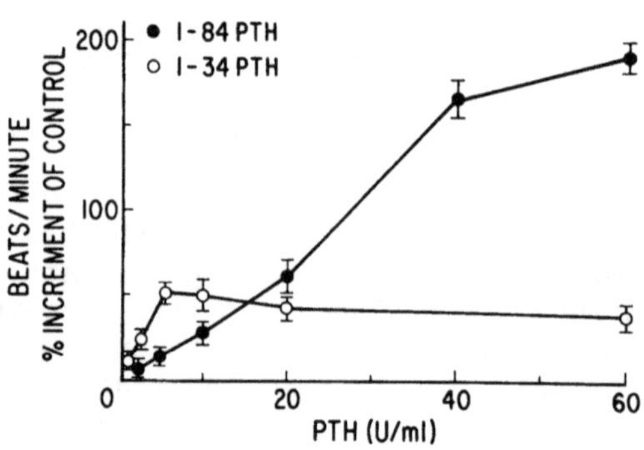

Figure 2. Dose-response curves for the effects of intact molecules of PTH (1-84) and its amino-terminal fragment (1-34) on the beating rates of the heart cells. ●, 1-84 PTH; O, 1-34 PTH. By permission from (8).

It is of interest that the effect of 1-84 PTH was significantly ($p<0.01$) smaller than that of 1-34 PTH at the lower doses and significantly ($p<0.01$) greater at the higher doses. The effect of both moities of PTH on the heart cells was reversible, and the stimulation of beating rate disappeared after removal of PTH from the medium. The carboxy-terminal fragment (53-84) in high concentration did not stimulate the beating of the heart cells, and inactivation of 1-34 or 1-84 PTH abolished their effect.

Figure 3 demonstrates that the addition of 1-34 PTH to medium produced a significant ($p<0.01$) increment in cyclic AMP production by the heart cells within 30 seconds. Thereafter, cyclic AMP production fell but remained significantly ($p<0.01$-0.05) higher than baseline levels for the entire 60 minutes of the study.

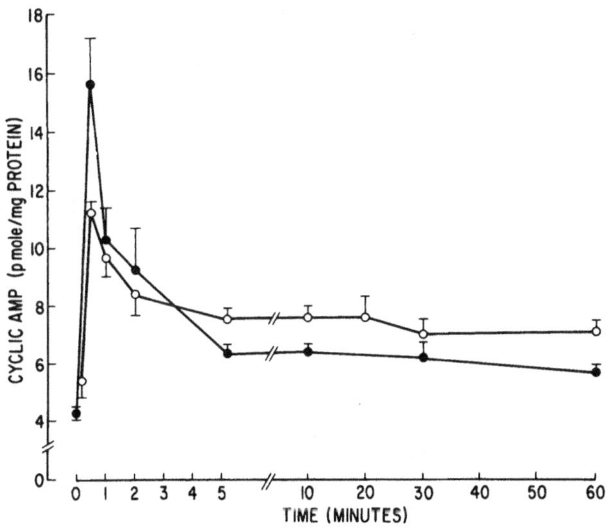

Figure 3. The effect of 1-34 PTH on cyclic AMP production by heart cells. Each line represents one experiment and each point denotes the mean±SE of three studies.

The basal beating rate of the heart cells was calcium dependent. It was lowest (33±7.2 beats/min) at 0.2 mM calcium and increased as the concentration of calcium was raised to 0.4 mM (58±4.2 beats/min) 0.6 mM (73±3.8 beats/min) and 1.3 mM (110±4.1 beats/min). Addition of 1-34 PTH produced significant ($p<0.01$)

increments in beating rate at all concentrations of calcium. The beating rate at a lower calcium concentration in the presence of PTH was not different from that observed with the next higher calcium concentration but without PTH, as if PTH magnified the concentration of calcium.

Both α- and β-adrenergic agonists produced significant ($p<0.01$) stimulation of the beating rate of the heart cells. These effects occurred within 30 seconds and plateaued, thereafter. Addition of 1-84 PTH to those already stimulated cells produced within 30 seconds further significant ($p<0.01$) stimulation of the beating rate (Figure 4). These additive effects were also demonstrable when the sequence of addition of adrenergic agonists and PTH to the media was reversed. Both α and β-adrenergic blockers did not affect the stimulation of the beating rate by 1-84 PTH, whether the blockers were added to the medium before or after the addition of 1-84 PTH (Figure 4).

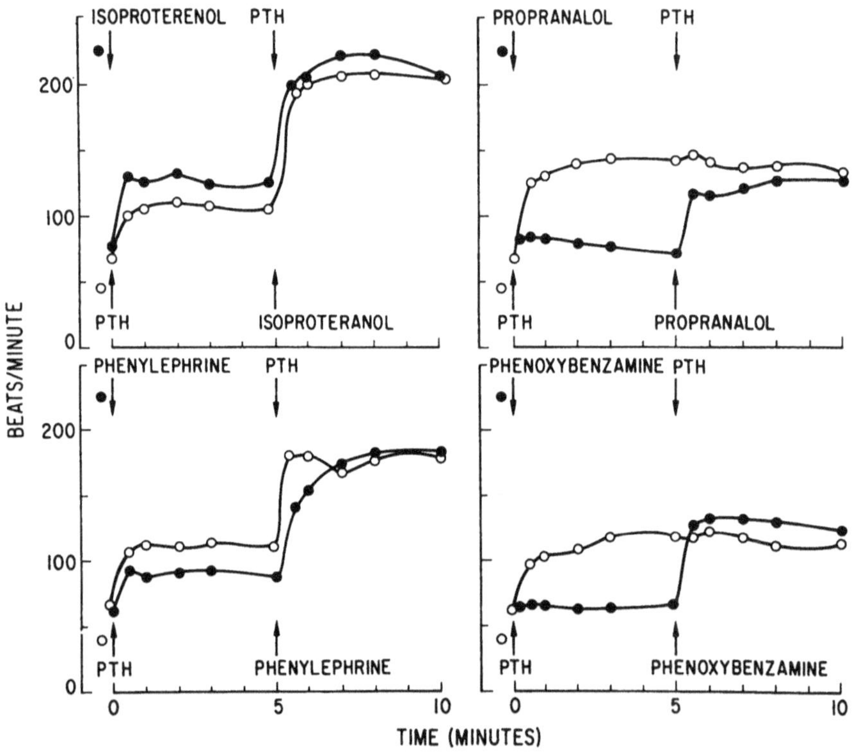

Figure 4. Representative studies depicting the interaction between PTH and α-(phenylphrine) and β-(isoproterenol) adrenergic agents and between PTH and α-(phenoxybenzamine) and β-(propranolol) adrenergic blockers and beating rates of heart cells. By permission from (8).

The simultaneous addition of suboptimal doses of 1-84 PTH and the β-adrenergic agonist isoproterenol produced significantly ($p<0.01$) greater increments in beating rate than the sum of the increments obtained by PTH or isoproterenol alone. In contrast, simultaneous addition of PTH and the α-adrenergic agonist phenylephrine did not produce greater stimulation of the beating rate than the sum of the stimulation produced by PTH and phenylephrine alone. Thus, it appears that the action of PTH is synergistic with that of the β-adrenergic agonists and additive to that of the α-adrenergic agonists.

Calcium ionophore A23187 produced stimulation of the beating rate of the heart cells similar to that observed with 1-84 PTH, and addition of calcium ionophore to cells already stimulated by PTH produced no further stimulation of the beating rate (Figure 5). Furthermore, the stimulation of the beating rate of the heart cells by PTH or calcium ionophore alone or together was not different.

Addition of verapamil to the medium was associated with gradual but significant decline in the beating rates of the heart cells. The subsequent addition of 1-84 PTH to the medium already containing verapamil did not produce stimulation of heart cells. When verapamil was added to PTH-stimulated heart cells the beating rate declined within one minute to the original baseline values and continued to fall gradually during the ensuing five minutes (Figure 5).

Figure 6 depicts the effects of uremic sera with and without PTH on the beating rates of the heart cells. Uremic sera from nephrectomized rats with intact parathyroid glands produced significant ($p<0.05$-0.01) stimulation of the beating rate for 12-20 hours. Thereafter, the beating rate started to decline and was significantly lower than that of control cells. These observations are similar to those seen during the addition of either 1-34 or 1-84 PTH to the medium. In contrast, uremic sera from Nx-parathyroidectomized (PTX) rats did not affect the beating rate of the heart cells; the latter was similar in the presence of both control serum and serum from PTH-uremic rats. Finally, uremic serum obtained from PTX-uremic rats treated with 1-84 PTH produced significant ($p<0.05$-0.01) stimulation of the heart cells for 10-20 hours, followed by slowing of the beating rate. These observations are similar to those noted after the addition of 1-34 or 1-84 PTH or in the presence of serum from uremic rats with intact parathyroid glands.

The observations described above demonstrate that a) the heart is a target organ for PTH and may have receptors for the hormone, b) PTH increases beating of the heart cells (chronotropic effect) and prolonged exposure to the hormone causes early death of the cells, c) this chronotropic effect of PTH appears to be due to calcium entry into heart cells, d) the locus of action through

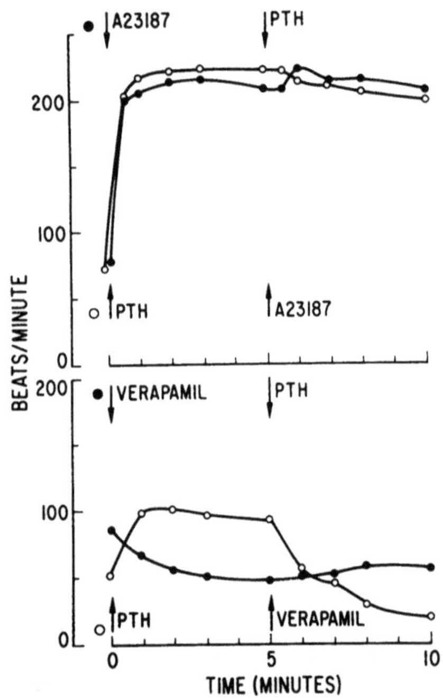

Figure 5. Representative studies on the interaction between PTH and calcium ionophore A23187 (upper panel) and PTH and verapamil (lower panel) on the beating rates of the heart cells. By permission from (8).

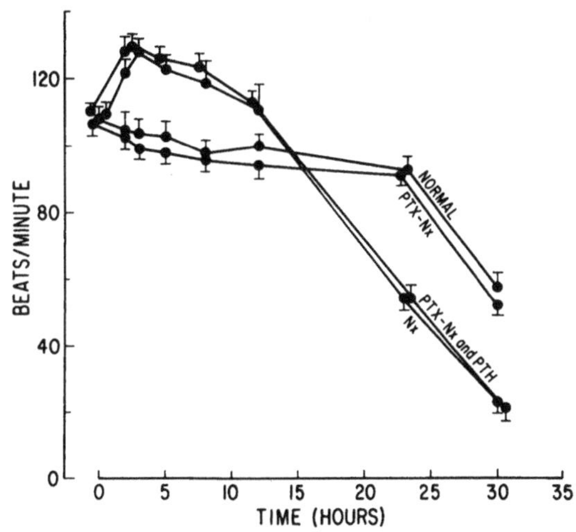

Figure 6. Representative experiment depicting the effect of sera from normal rats, nephrectomized (Nx) rats, parathyroidectomized-nephrectomized rats (PTX-Nx), and PTX-Nx rats treated with PTH (PTX-Nx and PTH). Each point represents the mean±SE of seven studies. By permission from (8).

PTH induces calcium entry is different from that for catecholamines, and e) uremic serum has no effect unless it contains PTH.

In an effort to understand the mechanism of action of PTH on the myocardium, we examined the effect of PTH on the function of isolated heart mitochondria. The hormone inhibited mitochondrial respiration in the presence of malate or β-hydroxybutyrate but not succinate as substrates. It also inhibited phosphorylation and uncoupled oxidative phosphorylation. These effects of PTH were dose dependent (Figure 7) and occurred only in the presence of calcium (Figure 8). A change in calcium concentration from zero to 2 mM did not affect mitochondrial function. PTH also stimulated mitochondrial ATPase. The inhibitory effect of PTH on mitochondrial respiration and on oxidative phosphorylation would result in decreased ATP synthesis and, hence, reduced availability of ATP. Such a sequence of events may provide an explanation for a potential long-term adverse effect of the hormone on the myocardium.

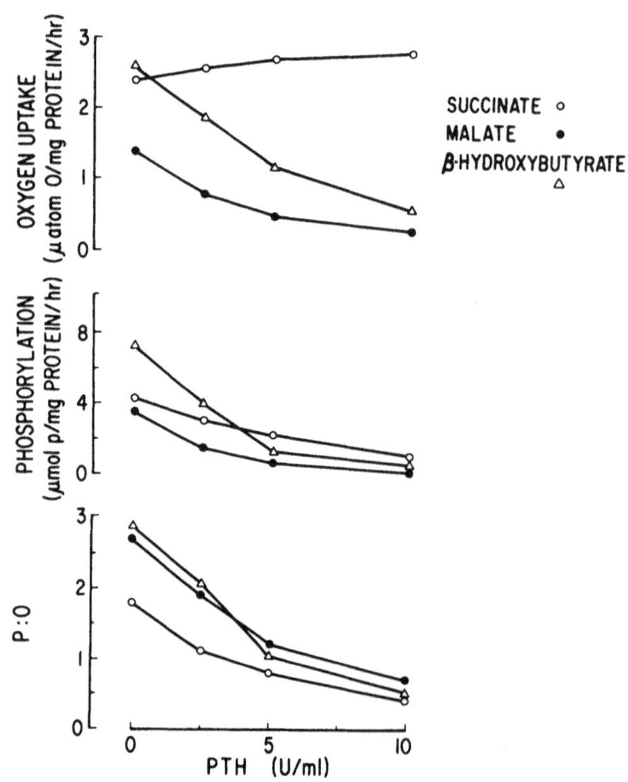

Figure 7. Effect of different doses of parathyroid hormone (PTH) on oxygen uptake and oxidative phosphorylation of isolated heart mitochondria in the presence of succinate, malate, or β-hydroxybutyrate as substrate.

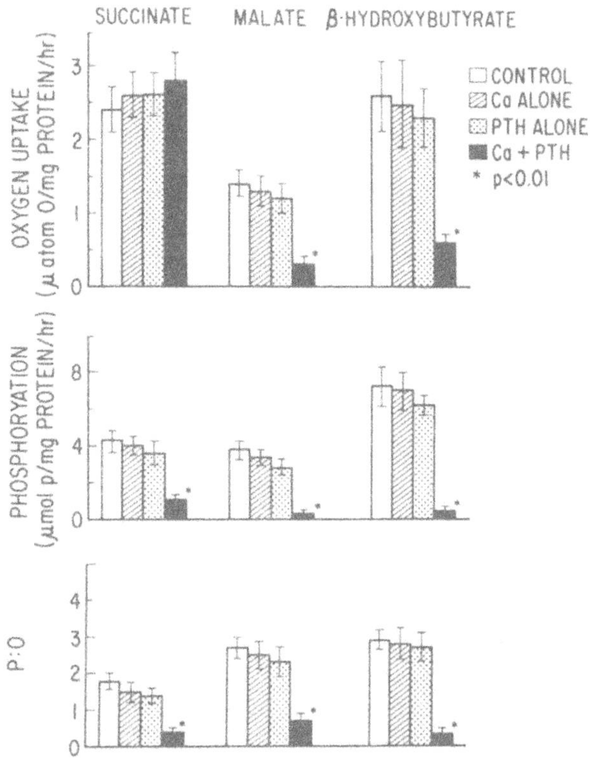

Figure 8. The effects of 1 mM calcium (Ca) or parathyroid hormone (PTH) alone and of calcium and PTH together on oxidative phosphorylation of isolated heart mitochondria. Data are presented as mean±SE of six experiments. By permission from (11).

We also examined the in vivo effect of PTH on myocardial energetics of rats receiving injectors of the hormone (17). PTH inhibited as in the in vitro studies oxygen uptake and phosphorylation by the heart mitochondria. Myocardial ATP and creatine phosphate were reduced in the PTH treated rats. The hormone also inhibited the activity of mitochondrial and myofibrillar creatine phosphokinase. Thus, PTH administration in vivo caused impaired energy production, transfer and utilization by the myocardium. These data further extend the in vitro observation and document the deleterious effect of PTH on the myocardium.

Others have confirmed our observation that the heart is a target organ for PTH. Lhoste et al (18) evaluated the effect of amino-terminal fragment of PTH on the isometric contractile force of isolated guinea pig auricles. They found that PTH inhibited the depressant effects of both l- and d-propranolol on the contractile force of the auricles. Since both of these agents have membrane-stabilizing activity and since the l-isomere has no adrenergic blocking effect, the influence of propranolol is, therefore, at least partly mediated by its membrane-stabilizing action which would result in decreasing calcium movement into the myocardial cell (19). These observations agree with our data and provide additional evidence for an interaction between PTH and the heart, with the hormone displaying an inotropic effect as well; their results also suggest that the action of PTH on the heart is mediated via movement of calcium into the heart cells. Other investigators (Katoh et al, in another paper in this book) utilizing isolated papillary muscle, also demonstrated an inotropic effect of PTH on the myocardium.

Our data are consistent with the notion that the elevated blood levels of PTH in uremia affects myocardial function by altering energy production, transfer and utilization. It is also possible that other compounds retained or produced in excess by the uremic patients have adverse effects on the heart as those of PTH. However, our studies of uremic sera with and without excess endogenous PTH clearly demonstrate that the uremic sera has no effect on the heart rate unless they contain PTH. The observation by Lhoste et al (18) also indicate that it is the PTH, and not other compounds in the uremic sera that affects myocardial contractile force.

Recently, Drueke et al (20) reported marked improvement in left ventricular function after parathyroidectomy in 22 dialysis patients with secondary hyperparathyroidism. These observations provide further support for the notion that the elevated blood levels of PTH in patients with uremia may adversely affect myocardial function and could, at least in part, be responsible for uremic myocardiopathy. Finally, the interaction between catecholamines and PTH on the heart, as demonstrated in our study, may expose patients with renal failure to double jeopardy, since these patients may have elevated blood levels of catecholamines (21-23) in addition to secondary hyperparathyroidism.

REFERENCES

1. S.G. Massry, Is parathyroid hormone a uremic toxin? Nephron, 19:125 (1977).

2. A. Arieff and S.G. Massry, Calcium metabolism of brain in acute renal failure, J. Clin. Invest. 53:387 (1974).

3. R. Guisado, A.I. Arieff, and S.G. Massry, Changes in the electroencephalogram in acute uremia. J. Clin. Invest. 55:138 (1975).

4. D.A. Goldstein, and S.G. Massry, Effect of parathyroid hormone administration and its withdrawal on brain calcium and electroencephalogram. Min. Elect. Metab. 1:84 (1978).

5. D.A. Goldstein, L.A. Chui, and S.G. Massry, Peripheral nerve calcium and motor nerve conduction velocity in acute renal failure, J. Clin. Invest. 62:88 (1978).

6. D.A. Goldstein, E.I. Feinstein, L.A. Chui, R. Pattabhiraman, and S.G. Massry, The relationship between the abnormalities in elecrroencephalogram and blood levels of PTH in dialysis patients. J. Clin. Endocrinol. Metab. 51:130, (1980).

7. M. Akmal, D.A. Goldstein, S. Multani, and S.G. Massry, Parathyroid hormone (PTH) and glucose (G) intolerance test in uremia, Proc. Amer. Soc. Nephrol. 13:87A (1980).

8. E. Bogin, S.G. Massry, and I. Harary, Effect of parathyroid hormone on rat heart cells, J. Clin. Invest. 67:1215 (1981).

9. D. Meytes, E. Bogin, A. Ma, P.P. Dukes, and S.G. Massry, Effect of parathyroid hormone on erythropoiesis, J. Clin. Invest. 67:1263 (1981).

10. E. Bogin, S.G. Massry, J. Levi, M. Djaldeti, G. Bristol, and J. Smith, Effect of parathyroid hormone on osmotic fragility of human red blood cells, J. Clin. Invest. In press (1982).

11. E. Bogin, J. Levi, I. Harary, and S.G. Massry, Effect of parathyroid hormone on oxidative phosphorylation of heart mitochondria. Min. Elect. Metab. 7:151 (1982).

12. C.C. Doherty, P. LaBelle, N. Brautbar, D. Moyer and S.G. Massry, Effect of intact parathyroid hormone and its fragments on human polymorphonuclear leukocytes, Clin. Res. In press (1982).

13. R.C. Pabico and R.B. Freeman, Pericarditis and myocardiopathy, In Clinical Aspects of Uremia and Dialysis, S.G. Massry and A.L. Sellers, eds., Charles C. Thomas, Springfield, Illinois, pp 69-99 (1976).

14. J. Seyle, The Pleuricausal Cardiopathies, Charles C. Thomas, Springfield, Illinois (1961).

15. D. Lehr, The role of certain electrolytes and hormones in disseminated myocardial necrosis, In Electrolyte and Cardiovascular Disease, E. Bajusz, ed., S. Karger, Basal, Switzerland, 1:248 (1966).

16. I. Harary and B. Farley, In vitro studies of heart cells in culture. I. Growth and organization, Exp. Cell Res. 29:451 (1963).

17. S.G. Massry, Effect of parathyroid hormone on energy metabolism of heart, Proc. Amer. Soc. Nephrol. 14:1A (1981).

18. F. Lhoste, T. Drueke, S. Larus, and J.R. Boissier, Cardiac interaction between parathyroid hormone, β-adrenoreceptor, and verapamil in the guinea pig in vitro. Clin. Exp. Pharmacol. Physiol. 7:377 (1980).

19. W.G. Nayler, Some factors involved in the maintenance and regulation of cardiac contractility, Circ. Res. 21 (Suppl III): 213 (1967).

20. T. Drueke, I. Fleury, Y. Toure, P. DeVernejoul, M. Fauchet, P. Lesourd, C. LePailleur and J. Crosnier, Effect of parathyroidectomy on left-ventricular function in haemodialysis patients, Lancet 1:112 (1980).

21. N.O. Atuk, C.J. Bailey, S. Turner, M.J. Peach and F.B. Westervelt, Red blood cell catechol-o-methyl transferase, plasma catecholamines and renin in renal failure, Trans. Am. Soc. Artif. Intern. Organs 22:195 (1976).

22. H.M. Brecht, W. Ernst and K.M. Koch, Plasma moradrenaline levels in regular hemodialysis, Proc. Eur. Dialysis Transplant Assoc. 12:281 (1975).

23. V.M. Campese, M.S. Romoff, D. Levitan, K. Lane and S.G. Massry, Reduced end-organ response to norepinephrine in uremia: a mechanism of autonomic dysfunction, Proc. Am. Soc. Nephrol. 12:181A (1979).

VASCULAR EFFECTS OF PARATHYROID HORMONE (PTH)

M. Rambausek, E. Ritz, W. Rascher, W. Kreusser,
J.F.E. Mann, V.A.W. Kreye, O. Mehls
Dpt. Internal Medicine, Pharmacology, Physiology and Pediatrics, Ruperto-Carola-University Heidelberg, Germany (FRG)

The effects of PTH on blood pressure (BP) are complex and many observations in literature on acute or chronic PTH excess or withdrawal are apparently contradictory. The present report reviews the information in literature and tries to provide a conceptual framework for the different vascular effects of PTH.

Blood pressure and primary hyperparathyroidism and hypercalcemia

Many authors observed a high prevalence of hypertension (HT) in patients with primary hyperparathyroidism. A review of 10 reports, bearing on a total of 1,102 patients, revealed a prevalence between 18 and 70% with an average of 39%.

Table 1

Hypertension (HT) in patients with primary hyperparathyroidism.

	No.of pat.	Percent HT
Hellstrom et al.,1958(ref.1)	105	70
Lemann,1964 (ref. 2)	46	35
Pyrah et al., 1966 (ref. 3)	62	28
Madhavan et al.,1970 (ref.4)	80	18
Rosenthal and Roy,1972(ref.5)	40	33
Johansson et al.,1972 (ref.6)	208	10
Romanus et al., 1973 (ref. 7)	274	60
Genant et al., 1973 (ref. 8)	65	40
Mallette et al., 1974 (ref.9)	57	53
Ohlsson, 1975 (ref. 10)	160	31
Total	n = 1102	39%

In our own experience, covering 77 patients seen in Heidelberg by Dr. Ziegler (Dpt. Endocrinology) or us, hypertension defined as BP above 140/90 mm Hg was also present in 42%. The proportion of patients with BP above the age and sex corrected 95% confidence interval was somewhat less (37.7%), but still markedly elevated. In a more recent study, Christensson et al. (11) analyzed BP in subjects with primary hyperparathyroidism detected because of hypercalcemia at a health screening program. Both systolic and diastolic pressure were significantly higher, even when subjects with impaired renal function, renal calculi or without surgical confirmation of adenoma were excluded. This finding indicates that PTH excess, or hypercalcemia, or some indirect consequences of either, cause hypertension.

Table 2

	Systolic BP (mmHg)		Diastolic BP (mmHg)	
	HPT	Controls	HPT	Controls
Total (n=48)	158±1.6	140±1.2	90.2±1.0	83.2±0.9
Ccr 85 ml/min (n=39)	157±1.7	136±1.4	90.3±0.8	80.2±0.7
No calculi (n=37)	158±1.5	138±1.4	90.1±0.8	80.1±0.8
Surgery of adenoma (n=32)	158±1.6	138±1.1	90.1±0.7	82.1±0.7

After Christensson et al. (ref. 11).

Acute hypercalcemia resulting from infusion of calcium (Ca) raises BP in man (12). More recently, Marone et al. (13) acutely raised serum Ca to 13.0 mg/dl by infusion of Ca (15 mg/kg in 3 h); concomitantly systolic (from 144 ± 10 to 184 ± 12 mm Hg.), mean and diastolic pressure rose. High BP occured despite a decrease of blood volume and was caused primarily by an increase of total peripheral resistance with no significant change of cardiac output. The mechanism of the vasoconstrictor action of Ca remains unclear. Acutely elevated Ca concentrations do not increase the sensitivity of vascular tissue to norepinephrine or other vasoconstrictor agents (14). Therefore, a direct effect of Ca on the contractile apparatus of vascular smooth muscle is possible, but potential effects of PTH withdrawal secondary to hypercalcemia are not excluded.

The acute vasodilatory effect of PTH

Circulatory effects of parathyroid extracts (PTE) and an increase of GFR were commonly observed with the early impure parathyroid extracts, as reviewed by Bartter (15). More recent studies, using parathyroid hormone or synthetic fragments, leave no doubt that the hormone itself has vasodilatory effects.

Vasodilatory action of PTH in various vascular beds

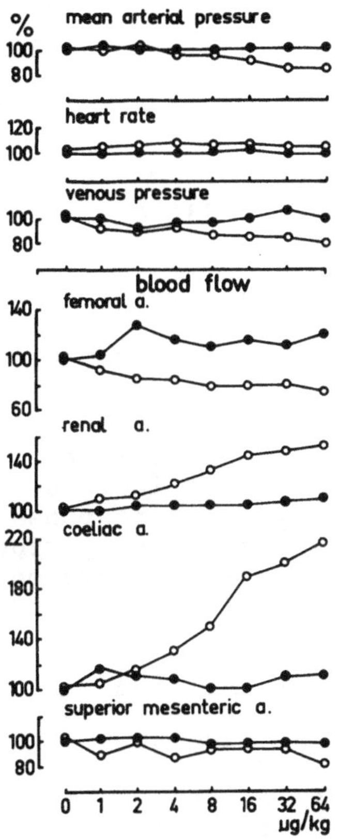

Fig. 1
Effect of PTE on hemodynamics

As shown in fig. 1, Charbon (16) observed a transient, dose dependent increase of renal and coeliac blood flow with supraphysiological doses of PTE, and later with synthetic PTH (17,18).

Lindner et al. (19) examined the effect of an intraarterial bolus of 1-34 bPTH into the renal artery of conscious dogs. As shown in table 3, a rapidly evanescent increase of renal blood flow (RBF), and an associated increase of the fraction of blood flow into the rapid vascular component (as evaluated by radioxenon washout) were associated with a sixfold increase of renin secretion rate (RSR). Stimulation of renin secretion with no change of systemic hemodynamics was also observed by Smith et al. (20) when citrate was infused into the parathyroid blood supply in order to release endogenous PTH.

An increase of coronary blood flow with PTH was observed by Crass and Pang (21) and more recently by Hashimoto et al. (22). The latter authors found an immediate increase (approx. 40%) of coronary blood flow after injection of 100 U 1-34 PTH into the left atrium of a canine heart lung preparation. This was associated with a transient increase of oxygen consumption and an inotropic effect. Vasodilatation was considerable, approximately 2/3 of the maximal increase induced by adenosine, and the authors argued that the increase was greater than expected for the observed inotropic action.

Table 3

	After PTH injection (15 μg bolus)			
	Control	5 min	15 min	30 min
Mean RBF (ml/min 100g tissue)	159±10	264±21	231±23	168±18
Fraction of RBF to rapid component	66± 3	74± 3	73± 4	71± 4
RSR (ng/min 100 g tissue)	551±252	3508±1469	1170±520	1510±577

Lindner et al. (ref. 19).

Although studies in chicken - with no measurement of BP - suggested an early decrease and late increase of blood flow (microsphere method) to bone in response to PTH (23), direct measurements in the isolated perfused tibia of the dog failed to show an effect of PTH on basal blood flow or the vasoconstrictor response to norepinephrine (24).

Effect of PTH on blood pressure in the intact animal
A hypotensive action of PTE, PTH and various synthetic PTH fragments was demonstrated in an elegant series of experiments by Pang et al. (25, 26, 27) and by Mc Carron (28). Such an effect is also evident from experiments (fig. 2) in the conscious rat which demonstrates hypotension and tachycardia (baroreceptor response or chronotropic effect of PTH or both).

A vasodepressor effect of PTH was observed by Pang in various species (e.g. south american lung fish, bull frog, water snake, chicken, rat and mongrel dog) and even in species (e.g. eel) in which PTH had no hypercalcemic effect. This may indicate that the vascular receptor for PTH is phylogenetically older than the bone receptor.

The vasodepressor response was demonstrable in the presence of propranolol, phentolamin, atropin and promethazin and does not appear to be mediated through alpha- and beta-adrenergic, cholinergic or histaminergic receptors. Definite, though less marked, vasodepressor actions were also observed with the 24-34 and 24-28 PTH fragments (27), although the latter fragment was not calcemic.

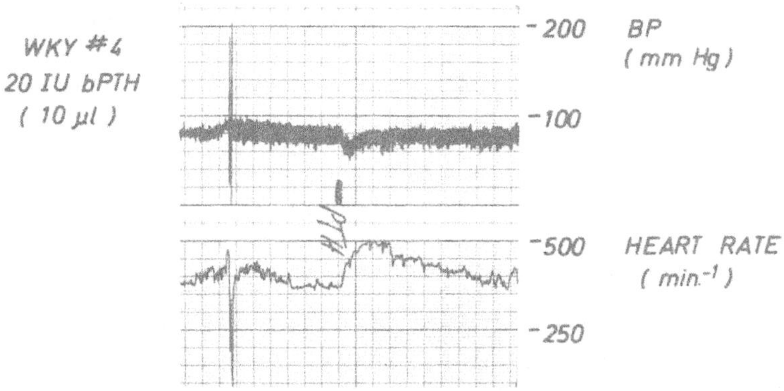

Fig. 2
Hemodynamic effects of 1-34 bPTH in the conscious rat (20 min. registration).

Effects of PTH on smooth muscle cells

The effect of PTH on vascular smooth muscle obviously raises the question, whether the vascular wall has the molecular machinery to respond to PTH and by which mechanism(s) the effect of PTH is mediated. These questions are currently addressed in this laboratory (29) and some preliminary concepts emerge from these studies. A dose dependent increase of cAMP (and cGMP) concentrations could be demonstrated in monolayer cultures of smooth muscle cells of the aortic media of newborn rabbits. Explants were grown in HEPES Dulbecco medium with 10% calf serum for 14 days and secondary cultures were subsequently established until monolayers were obtained. The material contained over 95% smooth muscle cells as evaluated by electronmicroscopy (courtesy Prof. Hoffmann, Heidelberg) and by immunofluorescence with antibodies specific for smooth muscle myosine (courtesy Prof. Groeschel-Stewart, Darmstadt). Some of the results are shown in table 4.

Table 4

Solvent control	0.794 ± 0.07	pmol cAMP/mg protein(8)
40 U 1-34 bPTH/ml	1.41 ± 0.19	pmol cAMP/mg protein(8)

$p < 0.05$

100,000 cells/culture, no theophylline, deproteinisation with TCA after 5 min incubation with PTH.

cAMP was also increased with norepinephrine (10^{-6}M) and glucagon (50 µg/ml). The effects did not appear to be additive to that of PTH, but further experiments are necessary to clarify this point. The cAMP response to PTH was not specific for vascular smooth muscle cells, as a similar increase of cAMP (and a depression of the contraction with norepinephrine)could also be observed, among others, in ductus deferens (control: 134 ± 53 pmol cAMP/mg protein; 5 U bPTH/ml: 230 ± 61; n=8; $p < 0.02$). In rat aorta, preincubation (5 U/ml; 5 min) with 1,34 bPTH also significantly increased phosphorylase b kinase activity as one index of a cAMP dependent protein kinase mediated event (control:32.8 ± 5.13 nmol/mg protein x min; bPTH 39.5 ± 4.40; n=10; measured at 37°C and pH 8.6 in homogenate; $p < 0.05$).

Effects of PTH on rat aortic strips

To further evaluate the mechanism of action, the relaxant effect of 1-34 was studied in isolated helical aortic strips of rats, precontracted with 10^{-7} M norepinephrine (30).

Influence of 1-34 bPTH on force generation in aortic strips

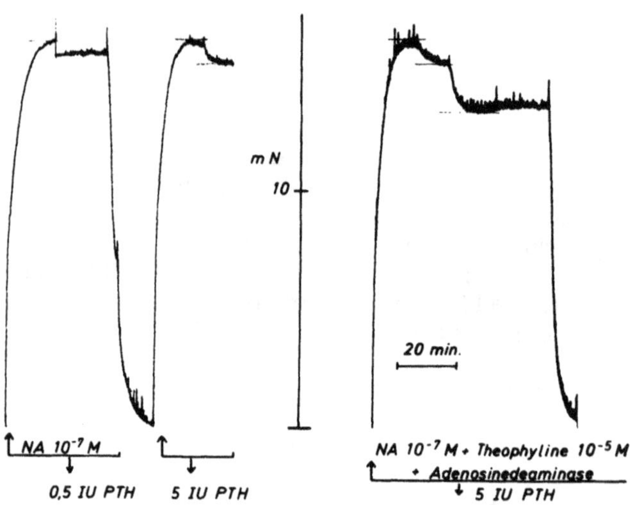

Fig. 3

As shown in fig. 3, 1-34 bPTH caused a modest, dose-dependent, transient relaxation of tonic contraction which amounted to approximately 7% at the dose of 20U/ml. Tachyphylaxis was observed but washing of the bath restored the susceptibility to PTH. The action of PTH was potentiated and prolonged by 10^{-5} M theophylline. PTH-induced relaxation was demonstrable in the presence of 20 mmol KCl; as cells are depolarized at this concentration, the result shows that PTH does not act through electromechanical coupling but through pharmacomechanical coupling. The relaxant effect of PTH was minor as compared with Na-nitroprusside and Na-nitroprusside (or isoprenaline) further relaxed strips exposed to maximal concentrations of PTH.

Effects of PTH on the isolated perfused rat hind limb

Because of the limited sensitivity of the aortic system and because of potential differences with resistance vessels, the effect of PTH was also studied in the isolated perfused hind limb of rats as an index of resistance vessels (31). After precontraction of the hind limb vasculature by constant infusion of norepinephrine ($3x10^{-6}$ M), PTH caused a dose-dependent decrease in vascular resistance. Since PTH stimulates cAMP generation in vessel wall, a cAMP mediated mechanism was considered.The mechanism(s) by which cAMP causes relaxation of smooth muscle has not been clarified. According to Adelstein et al. (32), cAMP stimulates the cAMP dependent protein kinase which phosphorylates the myosine light chain kinase, thereby inhibiting phosphorylation of the myosine light chain which is necessary for actin myosin interaction. Evidence in support of this mechanism is the demonstration of relaxation of skinned smooth muscle following preincubation with the catalytic subunit of cAMP dependent protein kinase (33). Alternative, and not mutually exclusive, mechanisms include enhanced calcium pumping into the sarcoplasmic reticulum (34) and cAMP dependent phosphorylation of Na, K-ATP'ase with consecutively enhanced Na/Ca-exchange, as suggested for beta adrenergic relaxation by Scheid et al. (35). To further evaluate these possibilities, experiments were performed on effect of ouabain on flow resistance. As shown in table 5, ouabain atteuated the vasodilator response of PTH.

Surprisingly, two inhibitors of cyclooxygenase also reduced the vasodilatory effect of PTH, suggesting that prostaglandins are involved in PTH-induced vasodilatation.

Table 5. Decrease in flow resistance after injection of 1-34 bPTH (x10^4 dyne x sec x cm^{-5})

dose (Units)			5	10	50
control		(9)	4.8±1.6	9.6±1.4	17.2±2.3
ouabain	(10^{-4}M)	(6)	2.8±0.7	3.0±0.6*	7.4±0.9**
indomethacin	(10^{-6}M)	(5)	3.0±1.2	5.9±1.8	7.4±0.8**
diclofenac sodium	(10^{-5}M)	(6)	2.2±0.6	3.4±1.0*	7.0±0.8**

* $p<0.05$
** $p<0.01$

Presently, one can only speculate about possible mechanisms by which PTH may affect prostaglandin production. PTH is known to increase Ca entry into cells and phospholipase A_2, a rate controlling step in the prostaglandin biosynthesis, is an enzyme activated by Ca (36). The assumption of a Ca mediated effect is attractive since Ca ionophores have been shown to stimulate prostaglandin production in platelets and renal papillary tissue (37). It is of note, that in chronic experimental uremia (31) hyporesponsiveness of resistance vessels to norepinephrine is reversible after administration of indomethacin and this may well be due to PTH excess.

The chronic effects of parathyroidectomy on blood pressure

The acute hypotensive action of PTH contrasts with the observation of hypertension in patients with primary hyperparathyroidism. This suggests that chronic excess of PTH has effects additional to, or even opposite to, its acute effects on blood pressure. Experimental observations are compatible with the permissive role of PTH for the development of high BP in DOCA (38-40) or genetic hypertension of rats, as shown in fig. 4. A similarly attenuated rise of BP was observed in SH-rats when dietary intake of Ca was increased and PTH secretion presumably suppressed (41).
Several possibilities could explain such a chronic effect of PTH promoting a rise in BP.
In the above experiments it cannot be absolutely excluded that the high Ca diets used were natriuretic, although a similar weight gain (fig. 4) argues against this possibility.

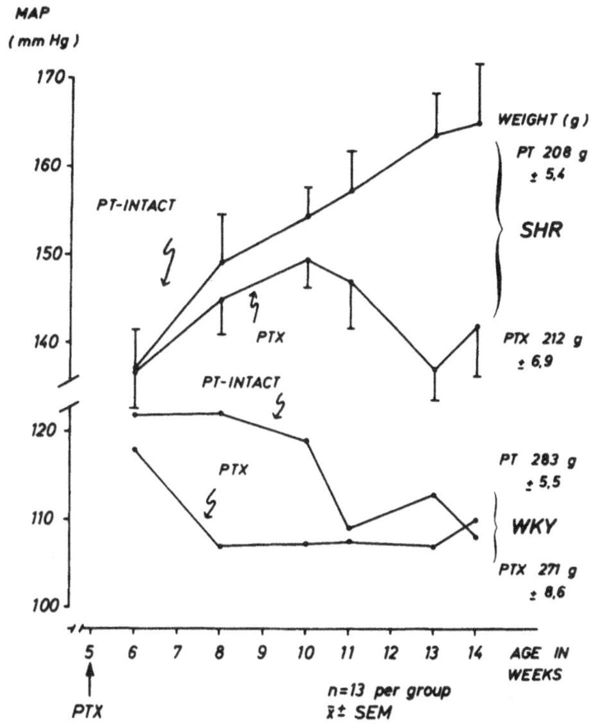

Fig. 4. Effect of parathyroidectomy (PTX) on BP in spontaneously hypertensive rats (SHR)

Surgical PTX, pairfeeding of sham operated controls, eucalcemia maintained by high Ca diet (1.2% Ca with S-Ca 4 weeks after PTX in SHR: 9.02±0.2 mg/dl; WKY 9.76±0.2 mg/dl).

Furthermore, polypeptide hormones may be taken up intracellularly and exert chronic effects which are different from the acute responses resulting from interaction with membrane receptors.
On the other hand, some central actions of PTH are conceivable, analogous to the contrasting peripheral and central effects on BP of some intestinal hormones (42). However, acute infusions of PTH into the cerebroventricle (osmotic minipump) failed to affect blood pressure in our own studies (unpublished).

Finally, PTH promotes Ca entry into cells. Effects of chronic PTH excess on vascular (aorta) Ca exchange and total (and lanthanum resistant) Ca content were demonstrated in this laboratory (table 6). Diminished availability of Ca in vascular smooth muscle cells may be responsible for the effects of PTX on BP development in rats.

Table 6. Effect of nutritional (0.04% Ca diet) hyperparathyroidism on aortic Ca content in rats

Control-pairfed (17)	257 ± 61 (10^{-5}mol Ca/g)
Experimental-low Ca (17)	316 ± 53; $\bar{x} \pm$ SEM; $p < 0.02$

The observations in PTX animals (suggesting a permissive role of PTH for the development of hypertension) do not exclude a chronic vasodilatory effect of PTH or chronic alterations of the pressor response to vasoconstrictor agents (31). Appropriate experiments must yet be carried out to exclude such a possibility.

Summary

PTH causes dose dependent transient vasodilatation in various vascular beds, specifically renal, coeliac, coronary, but not osseous. It has an acute dose-dependent hypotensive effect in the intact animal which is not mediated by alpha- or beta-adrenergic, cholinergic or histaminergic mechanisms.

Aortic medial smooth muscle cells respond to PTH with an increase of cAMP, cGMP and, presumably via protein kinase, with activation of phosphorylase B kinase. The acute vasodilatory effect of PTH is antagonised by indomethacin and diclofenac as well as by ouabain, suggesting that the membrane Na-K pump and prostaglandins are involved in PTH-induced vasodilatation.

Parathyroidectomy and a high calcium diet attenuate the rise of arterial pressure in experimental hypertension, pointing to some permissive effect of PTH for development hypertension. This is most likely due to long term effects of PTH on vessel wall calcium content and exchange. This chronic effect of PTH may explain the high prevalence of hypertension in patients with primary hyperparathyroidism.

References

1. Hellstrom, J., Brike, G., Edvall, C.A., 1958, Hypertension in hyperparathyroidism, Br.J.Urol., 30:13

2. Lemann, J., Donatelli, A.A., 1964, Calcium intoxication due to primary hyperparathyroidism, Ann. Int.Med. 60: 447
3. Pyrah, L.N., Hodgkinson, A., Anderson, C.K., 1966, Primary hyperparathyroidism. Critical review, Brit.J.Surg., 53: 245
4. Madhavan, T., Frame, B., Bloch, M.A., 1970, Influence of surgical correction of primary hyperparathyroidism on associated hypertension, Arch.Surg. 100: 212
5. Rosenthal, F.D., Roy, S., 1972, Hypertension and hyperparathyroidism, Brit.Med.J., 4: 396
6. Johansson, H., Thoren, L., Werner, I., 1972, Hyperparathyroidism. Clinical experiences from 208 cases, Uppsala J.Med.Sci., 77: 41
7. Romanus, R., Heimann, P., Nilsson, O., Hansson, G., 1973, Surgical treatment of hyperparathyroidism, Progr.Surg., 12: 22
8. Genant, M.K., Heck, L.L., Lanzl, L.M., Rossmann, K. van der Horst, J., Paloyan, E., 1973, Primary hyperparathyroidism, Radiology 109: 513
9. Mallette, L.E., Bilezikian, J.P., Heath, D.A., Aurfach, G.D., 1974, Primary hyperparathyroidism: clinical and biochemical features, Medicine, 53: 127
10. Ohlsson, L., 1975, Primär hyperparathyroidism. En studie av 160 patienter med särskild hänsyn till njurfunktion och stensjukdom efter operation. Academic thesis. Uno Lundgrens. Trykeri AB, Gothenburg
11. Christensson, T., Hellström, K., Wengle, B., 1977, Blood pressure in subjects with hypercalcemia and primary hyperparathyroidism detected in a health screening programm, Eur. J. Clin. Invest, 7: 109
12. Weidmann, P., Massry, S.G., Coburn, J.W., Maxwell, M.M., Atleson, J., Kleeman, C.R., 1972, Blood pressure effects of acute hypercalcemia, Ann.Int. Med. 76: 741
13. Marone, C., Beretta-Piccoli, C., Weidmann, P., 1980, Acute hypercalcemic hypertension in man: Role of hemodynamics, catecholamines and renin, Kidney Int., 20: 92
14. Frohlich, E.D., Scott, J.B., Haddy, F.J., 1962, Effects of cations on resistance and responsiveness of renal and forelimb vascular beds., Am.J. Physiol., 203: 582
15. Bartter, F.C., 1954, The parathyroids, Ann.Rev. Physiol. 16: 429
16. Charbon, G.A., 1964, Parathormone a relative vasodilator, in: "Parathyroid Hormoneand Thyreocalcitonin", R.V. Talmage, ed., Excerpta Medica, 475

17. Charbon, G.A., Hulstaert, P.F., 1974, Augmentation of arterial hepatic and renal flow by extracted and synthetic parathyroid hormone, Endocrinology, 95: 621
18. Hallberg, D., Werner, S., 1977, Circulatory and lipolytic effects of parathyroid hormone, Horm. Metab. Res. 9: 424
19. Lindner, A., Tremann, J.A., Plantier, J., Chapman, W., Forrey, A.W., Haines, G., Palmieri, G.M., 1978, Effects of parathyroid hormone on the renal circulation and renin secretion in unanesthesized dogs, MEM 1: 155
20. Smith, M.J., Mouw, D.R., Vander, A.J., 1979, Effect of parathyroid hormone on plasma renin activity and sodium excretion, Am.J.Physiol. 236 (3): 311
21. Crass, M.F., Pang, P.K.T., 1980, Parathyroid hormone: a coronary artery vasodilator, Science, 207: 1087
22. Hashimoto, K., Nakagawa, Y., Shibaya, T., Satob, M., Ushijima, T., Imai, S., 1981, Effects of parathyroid hormone and related polypeptides on the heart and coronary circulation of dogs, J.Cardiovasc. Pharm. 3: 668
23. Boellins, J.N., Mazurkiewicz, M., Mazur, P.E., Müller, W.J., 1976, Changes in blood flow to bones during the hypocalcemic and hypercalcemic phases of the response to parathyroid hormone, Endocrinology 98: 403
24. Driessens, M., Vanhoutte, P.M., 1981, Effect of calcitonin, hydrocortisone, and parathyroid hormone on canine bone blood vessels, Am.J.Physiol., 241: 91
25. Pang, P.K.T., Yang, M., Oguro, C., Phillips, J.G., 1980, Hypotensive actions of parathyroid hormone preparations in vertebrates, Gen.Comp.Endoc. 41: 135
26. Pang, P.K.T., Tenner, Th.E., Yee, J.A., Yang, M., Jansson, H.F., 1980, Hypotensive actions of parathyroid hormone preparations on rats and dogs, Proc. Natl.Acad.Sci.USA 77: 675
27. Pang, P.K.T., Yang, M.C., Tenner, Th., Chang, J.K., Shimiza, M., 1981, Hypotensive action of synthetic fragments of parathyroid hormone, J.Pharmacol. Exp.Ther. 216: 567
28. Anderson, S., McCarron, D.A., 1981, Enhanced sensitivity to parathyroid hormone administration in the SH rat, 4th Intern. Symp. Rats Spont. Hypertension, Heidelberg, Sept. 1981, a 58

29. Rascher, W., Rambausek, M., Kreusser, W., Ritz, E., 1982, Are prostaglandins and the sodium potassium pump involved in the vasodilations induced by parathyroid hormone? 9th Scient. Meeting Int. Soc. Hypertension, Mexico, Feb. 1982, abstr.
30. Kreye, V.A.W., Baron, G.D., Lüth, J.B., Schmidt-Gayk, H., 1975, Mode of action of sodium nitroprusside on vascular smooth muscle, Naunyn-Schmiedebergs Arch.Pharmacol., 288: 381
31. Rascher, W., Schömig, A., Kreye, V., Ritz, E., Diminished vascular response to norepinephrine in experimental uremia, Kidney Int. (in press)
32. Adelstein, R., Conti, M.A., Hathaway, D.R., 1978, Phosphorylation of smooth muscle myosin light chain kinase by the catalytic subunit of adenosine 3'5'-monophosphate-dependent protein kinase, J.Biol.Chem., 253: 8347
33. Rüegg, J.C., Sparrow, M.P., Mrwa, U., 1981, Cyclic AMP mediated relaxation of chemically skinned fibres of smooth muscle, Pflügers Arch., 390: 198
34. Namm, D.L., Leader, J.P., 1976, Occurence and function of cyclic nucleotides in blood vessels, Blood Vessels 13: 24
35. Scheid, C.R., Honeyman, T.W., Fay, F.S., 1979, Mechanism of ß-adrenergic relaxation of smooth muscle, Nature 277: 32
36. Cheung, W.Y., 1980, Calmodulin plays a pivotal role in cellular regulation, Science 207: 19
37. Oelz, O., Knapp, M.R., Robert, L.J., Oelz, R., Sweetman, B.J., Oates, J.A., Reed, W.P., 1978, Calcium-dependent stimulation of thromboxine and prostaglandin biosynthesis by ionophores, Adv. Prostaglandin Thromboxane Res. 3: 147
38. Berthelot, A., Gairard, A., 1980, Parathyroid hormone and deoxycorticosterone acetate induced hypertension in the rat, Clin. Science, 58: 365
39. Berthelot, A., Gairard, A., 1978, Effect of parathyroidectomy on cardiovascular reactivity in rats with mineralocorticoid-induced hypertension, Br.J. Pharmac., 62: 199
40. Bertholet, A., Gairard, A., Goyault, M., Pernot,F., 1980, Relation between calcium and cardiovascular reactivity in mineralocorticoid-induced hypertension in the rat, Br.J.Pharmac., 70: 301
41. Ayachi, S., 1979, Increased dietary calcium lowers blood pressure in the spontaneously hypertensive rat, Metabolism, 28;12: 1234
42. Ganten, D., Unger, Th., Simon, W., Schaz, K., Schölkens, B., Mann, J., Speck, G., Lang, R.,

Rascher, W., 1981, Contral peptidergic stimulation: Focus on cardiovascular actions of angiotensin and opioid peptides, in: "Perspectives in Cardiovascular Research", A.M. Katz, ed., Raven Press

ROLE OF PTH, METABOLIC FACTORS AND OTHER HORMONES IN EXTRA-RENAL ACID BUFFERING

Neil A. Kurtzman

Section of Nephrology
University of Illinois College of Medicine
Chicago, Illinois

INTRODUCTION

The maintenance of normal acid-base homeostasis is dependent on the renal excretion of acid (as well as the reclamation of bicarbonate) and extra-renal buffering of acid which originates either from normal metabolism or from exogenous sources. The factors influencing renal acid excretion have been well studied. Those events which control the buffering of an acid load are less completely understood (1). Since it is believed that the skeleton is a major source of buffer, events which influence the metabolism of bone may have a profound effect on extra-renal buffering. Fraley and Adler, as well as our own group, have demonstrated that parathyroid hormone (PTH) plays a major role in the buffering of acute acid loads (2,3). More recently we have had the opportunity to study the effects of a number of other hormonal and metabolic factors which influence extra-renal buffering (4). This paper reviews our work; it examines the effect of PTH and other metabolic regulators on extra-renal buffering.

PARATHYROID HORMONE

All the data referred to in this paper were obtained by infusing 5 mEq/kg/hr of hydrochloric acid to rats previously nephrectomized. As shown in the top panel of Figure 1, this maneuver caused a sharp decline in arterial pH and bicarbonate concentration when compared with the administration of an equal amount of sodium chloride. The bottom panel of this figure shows the effect of the same maneuver to rats subjected to thyroparathyroidectomy (TPTX) two hours before study. While there was no difference in the effect of acid infusion on blood pH in these two groups, the mortality

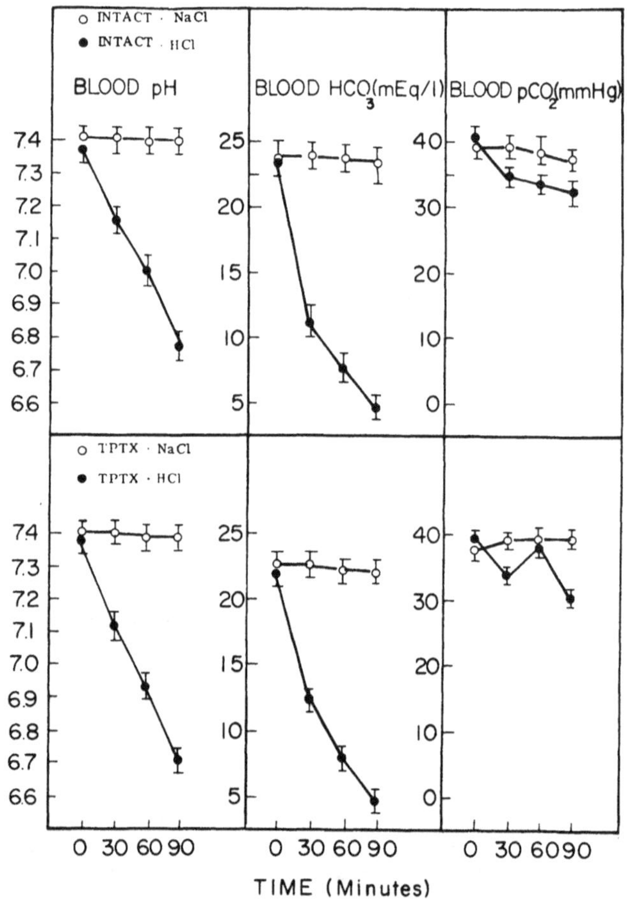

Fig. 1. Upper panel shows blood pH, HCO_3, and pCO_2 in intact rats infused with either NaCl (open circles) or HCl (filled circles). Lower panel shows same data in TPTX rats infused with either NaCl (open circles) or HCl (filled circles).

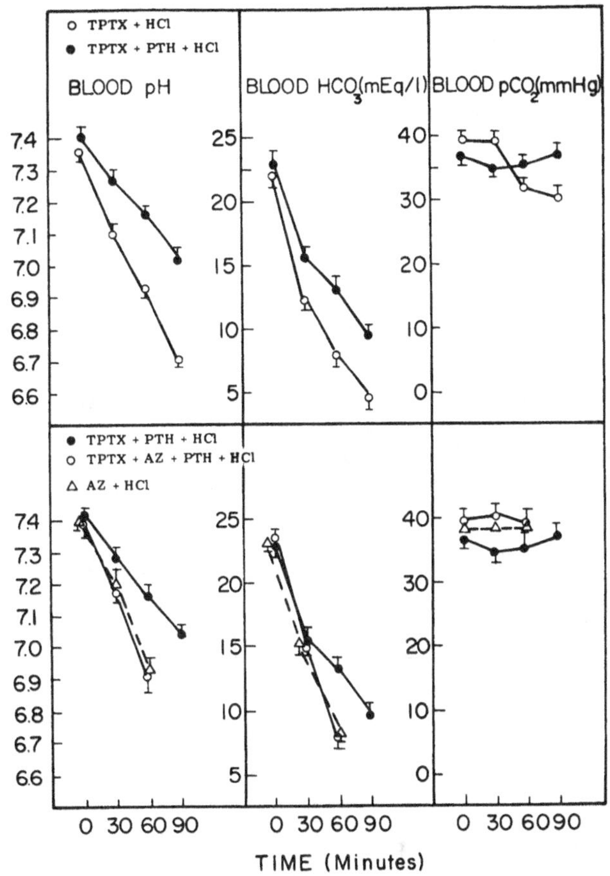

Fig. 2. Upper panel shows blood pH, HCO_3 and pCO_2 during HCl infusion in TPTX rats (open circles) and TPTX rats infused with PTH (filled circles). Lower panel depicts data of TPTX rats infused with PTH and acetazolamide (open circles). Data of TPTX rats infused with PTH (closed circles) from upper panel are displayed for comparison. Data of intact rats infused with acetazolamide (open triangles) are also shown.

rate at 90 minutes was more than three times greater in the TPTX animals. The top panel of Figure 2 shows the effect of the administration of parathyroid hormone in this model. The infusion of purified PTH at a dose of 5 units/kg/hr markedly attenuated the fall in pH induced by hydrochloric acid administration. Furthermore, as shown in the bottom panel of Figure 2, the administration of acetazolamide (20 mg/kg IV in a bolus followed by 5 mg/kg/hr) with parathyroid hormone completely obliterated the protective effect of PTH on blood pH. Thus, the inhibition of carbonic anhydrase activity totally abolished the protective effect of parathyroid hormone on blood pH.

Since the dose of PTH infused was large, it was necessary to ascertain whether endogenously released PTH would aid in the defense of blood pH. The top panel of Figure 3 shows that the administration of EDTA (250 mg/kg), which induced a significant decline in blood calcium concentration and thus stimulated PTH release, resulted in a marked protection of pH when hydrochloric acid was infused as compared to control animals. Furthermore, this protective effect was abolished when EDTA was infused to TPTX animals. This observation strongly suggests that endogenously reduced PTH was capable of exerting a protective effect similar in magnitude to that seen following the infusion of PTH. The bottom panel of the figure shows the effect of colchicine (0.2 mg two hours before HCl infusion) administration on extra-renal buffering. Colchicine exhibited a protective effect when administered to intact animals. This protective effect, however, was lost when the colchicine was given to TPTX animals. Colchicine has been shown to cause hypocalcemia by preventing osteoclastic bone resorption (5). Hypocalcemia, in turn, increases PTH release. Theoretically, colchicine either could increase buffering by releasing PTH or decrease buffering by blocking the action of PTH on bone (6,7). Our data demonstrate that colchicine in a dose capable of stimulating PTH release was associated with a significant increase in the capabity to buffer an acid load. The failure to demonstrate this effect in TPTX rats strongly suggests that this capacity was mediated by the release of PTH. The failure of colchicine to inhibit the action of PTH on extra-renal buffering suggests that this effect of PTH is not mediated by stimulation of osteoclasts.

Figure 4 demonstrates the effect of acid administration to animals with chronic renal failure. Chronic renal failure was induced by unilateral renal infarction with contralateral nephrectomy. As shown in the top panel of the figure, animals with chronic renal failure had enhanced capacity to buffer an acid load as compared to control animals or animals with chronic renal failure subjected to TPTX. A similar effect was noted in animals with acute renal failure produced by bilateral ureteral ligation. The lower panel of Figure 4 shows that ligation of both ureters 24 - 36 hours prior to study also protected blood pH during acid infusion.

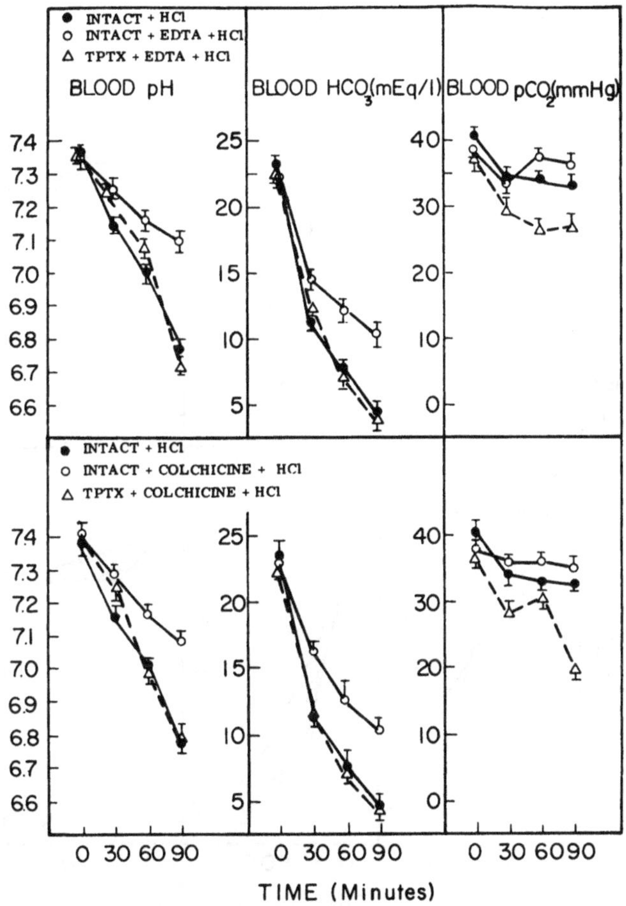

Fig. 3. Upper panel shows blood pH, HCO_3, and pCO_2 in intact (open circles) and TPTX (open triangles) rats treated with EDTA. Data of control rats (filled circles) from Fig. 1 are shown for comparison. Lower panel displays blood pH, HCO_3, and pCO_2 in intact rats (open circles) and TPTX (open triangles) colchicine-treated rats. Data of control rats from Fig. 1 (filled circles) are shown for comparison.

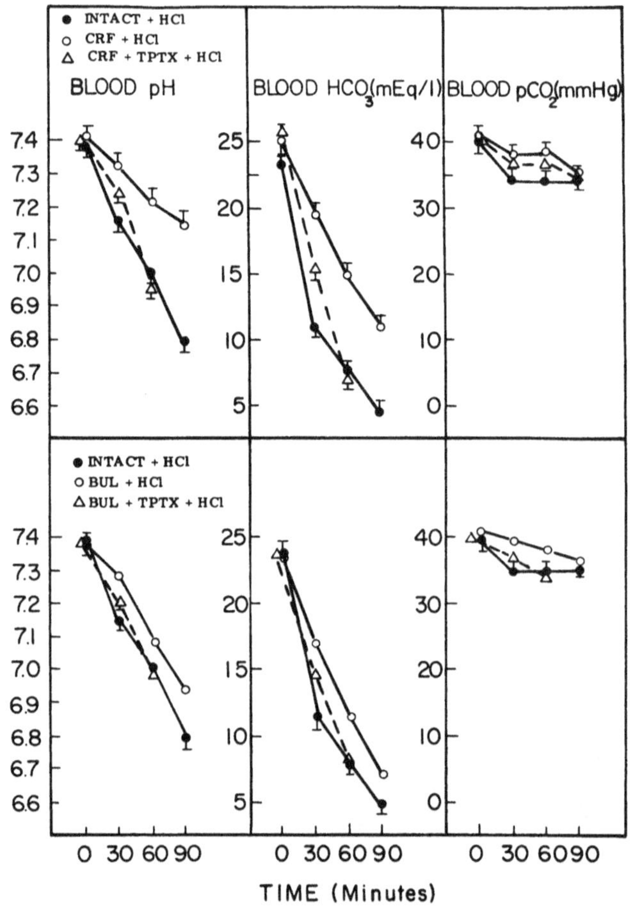

Fig. 4. Upper panel shows blood pH, HCO_3, and pCO_2 in rats with chronic renal failure (CRF) with (open circles) and without (open triangles) parathyroid glands. Data of control rats from Fig. 1 are shown for comparison (filled circles). Lower panel displays same data in rats with bilateral uretal ligation in presence (open circles) and absence (filled circles) of parathyroid glands.

This protective effect was lost when these animals were subjected to TPTX.

These studies clearly demonstrate that either exogenously administered PTH or endogenously released hormone is capable of mobilizing buffer into the extra-cellular fluid. This increased availability of buffer protects against the pH-lowering effects of acid infusion. While these studies cast no light on the source of this buffer, the most likely site of buffer release is bone. Because previous studies have demonstrated that acetazolamide inhibits PTH-mediated bone resorption (8-10) and since carbonic anhydrase inhibition with acetazolamide prevented the protective effects of PTH on blood pH, it seems reasonable to postulate that PTH releases buffer from the skeleton through an effect requiring carbonic anhydrase activity.

Although it is likely that PTH enhances acid buffering by mobilizing skeletal buffer, it is still possible that PTH may also affect the mobilization of extra-skeletal buffer. This possibility could explain the failure of colchicine to prevent the buffering effect of PTH while inhibiting its calcemic effect.

Although our observations demonstrate that PTH enhances buffering capacity under conditions of acute acid loading, it is not clear whether conditions associated with secondary hyperparathyroidism, such as chronic or acute renal failure, are associated with enhanced buffering capacity under clinical conditions. It is well known that patients with chronic renal failure are in positive acid balance for a prolonged time before they become acidotic. The role of PTH in this phenomenon has not been examined. It is possible that the effect of PTH in patients with uremia may be to protect blood pH. Thus, as regards acid-base homeostasis in chronic renal failure, PTH may exert a beneficial effect and in this limited area not function as a uremic toxin.

PHOSPHATE DEPRIVATION

Similar studies to those described above were performed to evaluate the effects of phosphate deprivation on extra-renal buffering. While it was previously demonstrated that prolonged phosphate deprivation increased extra-renal buffering capacity (11,12), the factors influencing such an effect of phosphate deprivation remained undefined. Since in previous studies, phosphate deprivation was of long duration, it was unclear as to whether short-term phosphate deprivation would also result in increased buffering capacity.

The animals described in this study were replaced on a low phosphate diet for 12 - 14 days prior to study. As shown in the upper panel of Figure 5, phosphate-deprived animals had a markedly

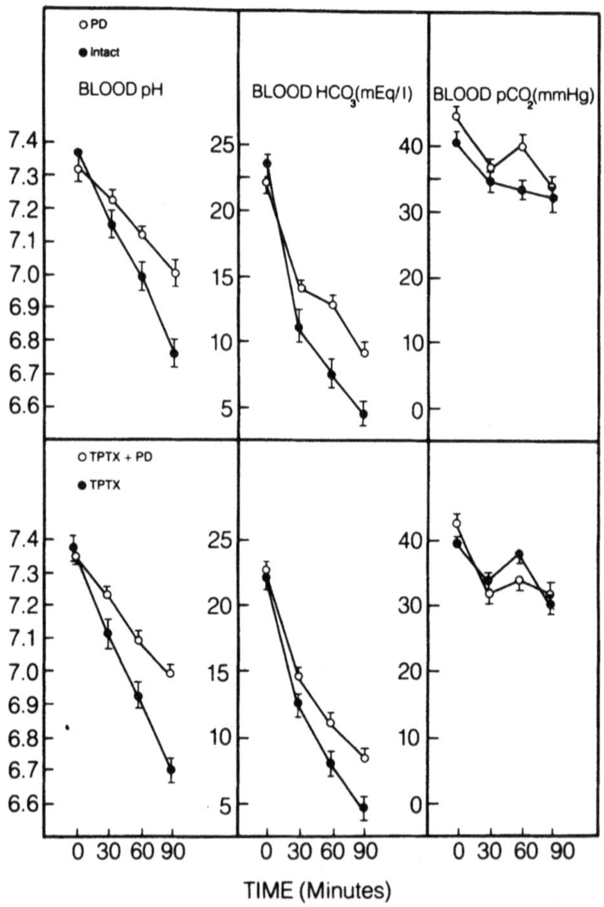

Fig. 5. Upper panel shows blood pH, HCO_3 and pCO_2 in control and phosphate-deprived rats. Lower panel depicts data of TPTX control and TPTX phosphate-deprived rats.

enhanced capacity to buffer exogenous acid load as compared to non-phosphate-deprived controls. Furthermore, as shown in the lower panel of this figure, TPTX had no effect on this enhanced buffering capacity. Thus, phosphate deprivation exerts an effect on extra-renal buffering which is independent of PTH release. The effect of phosphate deprivation is likely secondary to the enhanced bone resorption seen in this condition. Furthermore, Figure 6 shows

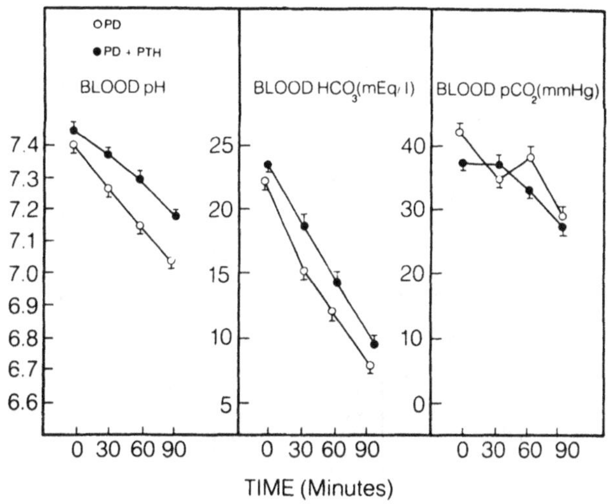

Fig. 6. Effect of PTH on blood pH, HCO_3, and pCO_2 in phosphate-deprived rats during acid loading. Also shown are the data of phosphate-deprived rats not infused with PTH.

that the effects of phosphate deprivation and exogenous PTH administration are additive. Note that at 90 minutes of acid loading the blood pH of phosphate-deprived animals receiving PTH is 7.2, a value that contrasts sharply with that of 6.7 observed in normal animals subjected to acid loading.

DIPHOSPHONATE

Diphosphonates inhibit bone resorption and therefore might be expected to inhibit bone buffering in both controls and in phosphate-deprived rats (13). The diphosphonate-treated rats received 20

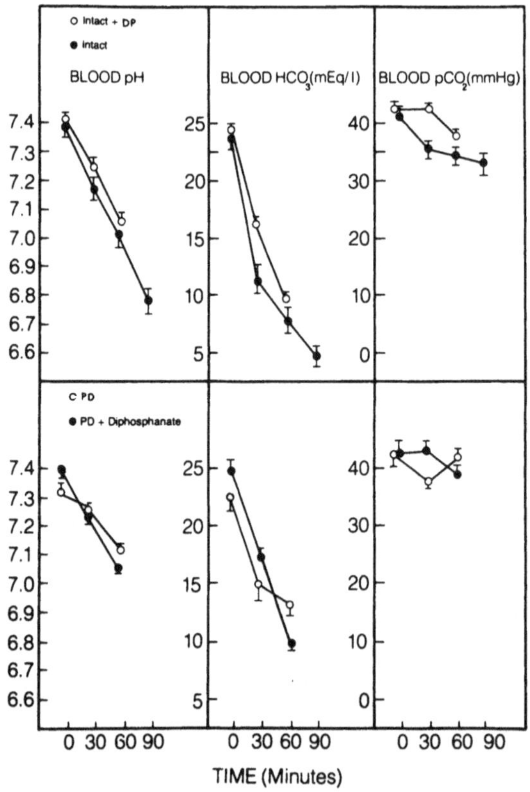

Fig. 7. Upper panel shows blood pH, HCO_3, and pCO_2 in control and di-phosphonate-treated rats. Lower panel shows blood pH, HCO_3, and pCO_2 in phosphate-deprived rats and phosphate-deprived rats pre-treated with diphosphonate.

mm/kg body weight per day subcutaneously for 6 days of diphosphonate. The upper panel of Figure 7 shows that chronic diphosphonate administration to normal rats did not significantly alter blood pH between control and treated rats at any period. At 30 minutes, the plasma-bicarbonate concentration was significantly higher in the diphosphonate group possibly as a consequence of the higher PCO_2 in the former group. The mortality rate at the end of 90 minutes was significantly higher in the diphosphonate-treated rats than in controls. The bottom panel of this figure shows that diphosphonate did not attenuate the enhanced capacity of phosphate-deprived rats to buffer an acid load. The mortality rate, however, in the diphosphonate-treated group was 80% at the end of 90 minutes, as compared to a 0% mortality rate in phosphate-deprived rats not receiving diphosphonate. Thus, the effect of diphosphonate on bone does not demonstrably inhibit the increased release of buffer into the circulation seen with phosphate deprivation.

VITAMIN D

In order to study the effect of vitamin D on extra-renal buffering, calciferol 200,000 units/day for 3 days was given to 8 rats. As is apparent in the top panel of Figure 8, vitamin D-treated animals had a markedly enhanced capacity to buffer an acid load when compared to controls not receiving the vitamin. Plasma calcium concentration was significantly higher in the vitamin D-treated rats than in the controls. Since vitamin D has an effect on bone (14), it was not surprising to demonstrate that it was capable of enhancing buffering capacity. Since the vitamin D-treated animals had a significantly higher calcium concentration, it is almost certain that the effect of vitamin D is not related to parathyroid hormone release.

VASOPRESSIN

Vasopressin (AVP) administration causes a rapid increase in plasma phosphate concentration. In addition, AVP administration in pharmacological doses is capable of eliciting effects which are similar to those of PTH (15-18) It is also capable of stimulating PTH release. For these reasons, we examined the effect of AVP on the buffering of acid load in TPTX rats. The bottom panel of Figure 8 shows that the administration of AVP at a dose of 50 milliunits/kg/hr has an effect on extra-renal buffering similar to that observed with parathyroid hormone. Since these studies were performed in TPTX rats, they indicate that AVP acts through a direct effect rather than by stimulating PTH release.

THYROCALCITONIN

To further examine the role of decreased bone resorption on extra-renal acid buffering, we infused thyrocalcitonin, a hormone

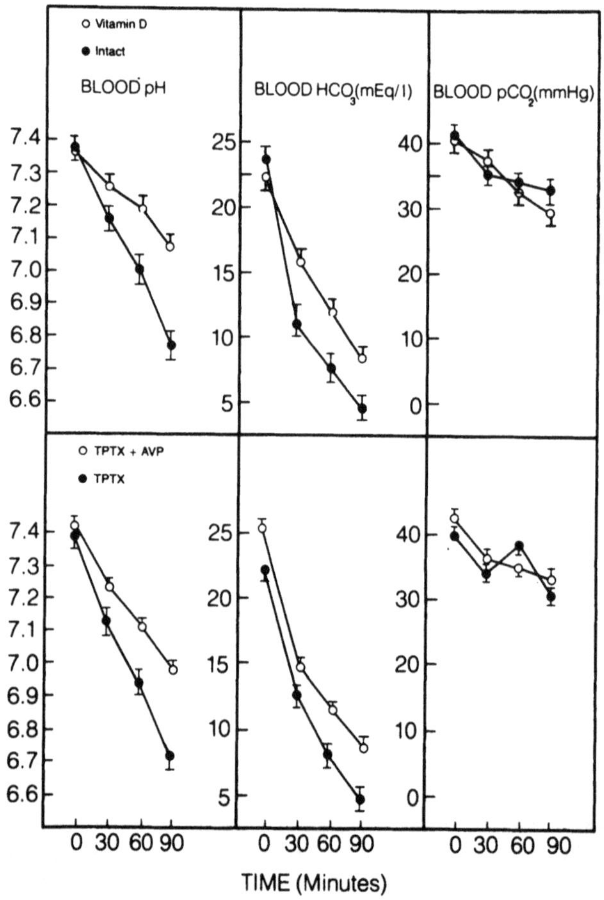

Fig. 8. Upper panel shows blood pH, HCO_3, and pCO_2 in control rats and in rats treated with vitamin D. Lower panel shows blood pH, HCO_3, and pCO_2 of TPTX rats and in TPTX rats infused with arginine vasopressin.

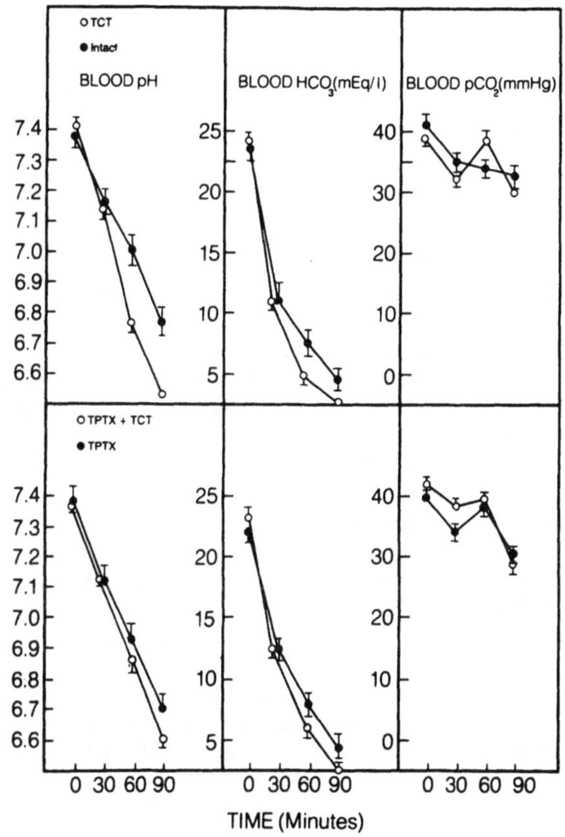

Fig. 9. Upper panel shows blood pH, HCO_3, and pCO_2 in control rats and in rats infused with thyrocalcitonin. Lower panel, the data of TPTX and TPTX rats treated with thyrocalcitonin are compared.

capable of producing hypocalcemia by inhibiting bone resorption (19). Salmon calcitonin was given at a rate of 60 mg/hr for 90 minutes. As shown in the top panel of Figure 9, the infusion of the hormone resulted in a significantly lower blood pH and plasma bicarbonate concentration than seen in control rats. The bottom panel of the figure shows that administration of thyrocalcitonin to TPTX animals had no significant effect on either blood pH or plasma bicarbonate concentration. Therefore, calcitonin administration to intact but not TPTX animals is capable of inhibiting extra-renal acid buffering. The effects of TPTX and calcitonin to impair extra-renal buffering are not additive. These observations suggest that calcitonin inhibits extra-renal buffering by blocking the effect of PTH on bone.

CONCLUSIONS

These studies demonstrate that parathyroid hormone markedly enhances the buffering capacity of nephrectomized animals subjected to acute acid loads. This is seen either with exogenous administration or endogenous release of the hormone. Furthermore, phosphate deprivation exerts a similar effect on extra-renal buffering which is additive to that seen with parathyroid hormone. The effect of parathyroid hormone on buffering is inhibited by acetazolamide administration, indicating that carbonic anhydrase activity is required for this effect. The effect of PTH however, is not inhibited by colchicine administration.

The effect of phosphate deprivation on extra-renal buffering of acid is not influenced by diphosphonate administration. AVP and vitamin D both enhance extra-renal buffering capacity to a degree similar to that seen with PTH or phosphate deprivation. Finally, thyrocalcitonin decreases the buffering capacity of normal animals; this effect of thyrocalcitonin is not seen in TPTX animals. These observations suggest that the calcitonin blocks the effects of PTH on bone.

ACKNOWLEDGEMENT

The studies described in this paper were supported in part by NIH Grant AM20170.

REFERENCES

1. N. Brautbar, Extrarenal factors in the homeostasis of acid-base balance, Seminars Nephrol., 1:232, (1981).

2. D.S. Fraley, and S. Adler, An extrarenal role for parathyroid hormone in the disposal of acute acid loads in rats and dogs, J. Clin. Invest., 63:985 (1979).

3. J.A.L. Arruda, V. Alla, H. Rubinstein, M. Cruz-Soto, S. Sabatini, D.C. Batlle, and N.A. Kurtzman, Parathyroid hormone and extrarenal acid buffering, Am. J. Physiol., 239:F533 (1980).

4. V. Alla, H. Rubenstein, M. Cruz-Soto, S. Sabatini, D.C. Batlle, J.A.L. Arruda, and N.A. Kurtzman, Metabolic and hormonal factors influencing extrarenal buffering of an acute acid load, Clin. Res., 28:434A (1980).

5. D.A. Heath, J.S. Palmer, and G.D. Aurbach, The hypocalcemic action of colchicine, Endocrinology, 90:1589 (1972).

6. C.V. Gay and W.J. Mueller, Carbonic anhydrase and osteoclasts: localization by labeled inhibitor autoradiography, Science, 183:432 (1974).

7. J. Chanard, R. Black, M. Purkerson, J. Lewis, S. Klahr, and E. Slatopolsky, The effects of colchicine and vinblastine on parathyroid hormone secretion in the rat, Endocrinology, 101:1792 (1977).

8. C. Minkin and J. Jennings, Carbonic anhydrase and bone remodeling: sulfonamide inhibition of bone resorption in organ culture, Science 176:1031 (1972).

9. L.C. Waite, Carbonic anhydrase inhibitors, parathyroid hormone and calcium metabolism, Endocrinology 91:1160 (1972).

10. L.C. Waite, W.A. Volkert and A.D. Kenny, Inhibition of bone resorption by acetazolamide in the rat, Endocrinology 87:1129 (1970).

11. M. Emmitt, S. Goldfarb, Z.S. Agus and R.C. Narins, The pathophysiology of acid-base changes in chronically phosphate depleted rats, Bone-kidney interactions J. Clin. Invest. 59:291 (1977).

12. J.A.L. Arruda, N. Julka, H. Rubenstein, S. Sabatini and N.A. Kurtzman, Distal acidification defect induced by phosphate deprivation, Metabolism 29:826 (1980).

13. U. Treschel, R. Schenk, J.P. Bonjour, R.G.G. Russell, and H. Rleisch, Relation between bone mineralization, Ca absorption and plasma Ca in phosphonate-treated rats, Am. J. Physiol., 232:E298 (1977).

14. E. Slatopolsky, K. Hruska, and W.T. Rutherford, Current concepts of parathyroid hormone and vitamin D metabolism: Pertubations in chronic renal disease, Kidney Internat., 7:S70 (1975).

15. J.A.L. Arruda, S. Stipanuk, R. Walter, and N.A. Kurtzman, Effect of vasopressin administration on sodium excretion and plasma phosphate concentration, Proc. Soc. Exp. Biol. Med., 155:308 (1977).

16. R. Rosenbaum, A. Greenwalt, J. Lewis, S. Klahr, and E. Slatopolsky, Evidence that ADH does not increase the release of parathyroid hormone directly, Proc. Am. Soc. Nephrol., New Orleans LA, p.8 (1978).

17. M. Martinez-Maldonado, G. Eknoyan, and W.N. Suki, Natriuretic effects of vasopressin and cyclic AMP: Possible site of action in the nephron, Am. J. Physiol., 220:2013 (1971).

18. N.A. Kurtzman, P.W. Rogers, S. Boonjarren, and J.A.L. Arruda, Effect of infusion of pharmacologic amounts of vasopressin on renal electrolyte excretion, Am. J. Physiol., 228:890 (1977).

19. H. Rasmussen, C. Anast, and C. Arnaud, Thyrocalcitonin, EGTA and urinary electrolyte excretion, J. Clin. Invest. 46:746 (1967).

EFFECT OF PARATHYROID HORMONE ON THE ISOLATED PAPILLARY MUSCLE OF THE RAT HEART

Kiyoshi Kurokawa and Yoichi Katoh

Medical and Research Services, Veterans Administration
Wadsworth Medical Center and the Department of Medicine
UCLA School of Medicine, Los Angeles, California

It has been well accepted that the bone and the kidney are the principal organs of parathyroid hormone (PTH) action. Several lines of evidence obtained during the last decade suggest that PTH directly acts on organs other than the bone and kidney; these include the brain, liver and blood cells (1-5).

Recent studies have shown that PTH also has significant effects on the cardiovascular system. Pang and associates showed that PTH causes peripheral vasodilation by its direct action on the vascular smooth muscle (6). Further, they showed that PTH increases coronary blood flow by directly dilating the coronary artery (7). In a more recent study, Bogin and associates (8) demonstrated a direct chronotropic effect of PTH in cultured rat heart cells. In a study of Crass and Pang (7) it was noted that PTH given directly into the coronary artery not only increased coronary blood flow more than 100%, but also increased the cardiac output by up to 46%. Since an increase in coronary blood flow itself is not likely to increase cardiac output, these observations suggested to us a possible inotropic action of PTH. To test this possibility, we examined the effect of PTH on the contractility of the isolated papillary muscle of the rat heart (9).

METHODS

An isolated papillary muscle of the right ventricle of rat heart was continuously perfused and its contraction properties were monitored using a standardized technique (10, 11). In brief, an isolated papillary muscle was placed horizontally in an incubation chamber (~60 μl capacity) with both the base and tendinous end of the muscle connected to steel hooks with 9-0 silk suture. It was perfused at 32°C at a flow rate of 2.5 ml/min with a buffer of the following composition (mM): NaCl 117, KCl 5.2, $NaHCO_3$ 25, $CaCl_2$ 1.0, $MgSO_4$ 1.2, and dextrose 5.6, pH 7.4, equilibrated with 95% O_2-5% CO_2 (v/v). The papillary muscle was allowed to contract isometrically for 90 min under electrical stimulation at a voltage 20% above threshold with a duration of 3 msec at a rate of 60 per min. During this period, the muscle length at which the developed tension became maximal was determined. Following this stabilization period, test agent(s) was added to the perfusate at concentrations specified. The developed tension or force development (DT), the maximal rate of tension rise (dT/dt), and time to peak tension (TPT) were measured continuously in a single papillary muscle before and after an addition of the test agent(s). For experiments with inhibitors, propranolol or methoxy-verapamil, the isolated papillary muscle was perfused with a perfusate containing an inhibitor for 10 min prior to perfusion with a perfusate containing the inhibitor with PTH (1-34 N-terminal amino acids, synthetic bovine PTH, Beckman, Palo Alto, California).

RESULTS

As depicted in Figure 1A, PTH caused an immediate increase in myocardial contractility which reached its peak within 60-90 sec; contractility then gradually fell over the following 5-6 min. As shown in the lower panel (B), isoproterenol also caused a similar increase in myocardial contractility which was sustained for the observation period of 5-20 min.

The dose-response curve for PTH is shown in Figure 2. Significant inotropic effects are observed at 10^{-12}M PTH and the maximal effects occurred at PTH concentrations greater than 10^{-11}M. Changes in DT, dT/dt, and TPT with 10^{-11}M PTH are summarized in Table 1. There was no change in myocardial contractility when the perfusate was changed to the one containing either vehicle of PTH (acetic acid, <0.01 mM) or PTH inactivated by H_2O_2.

Additional experiments were carried out to elucidate the mechanism underlying the inotropic action of PTH. As shown in Table 2, addition of propranolol partially blocked the effects of PTH. Moeover, the effect of PTH was suppressed in the isolated papillary muscle prepared from the heart of rats treated with reserpine 0.1 mg/kg/day given subcutaneously for two days prior to the experiments. This treatment has been shown to deplete the myocardial nonepinephrine content to less than 5% of normal (12).

The action of PTH on its target tissues is known to be associated with changes in Ca^{++} flux across plasma membranes as well as, in certain tissues, with adenylate cyclase activation.

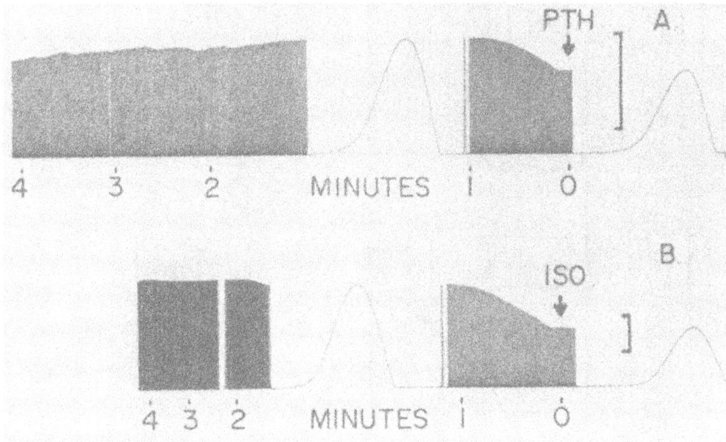

Figure 1. Representative tracings of positive inotropic effects of PTH, 10^{-11}M (A) and isoproterenol, 10^{-9}M (B). At time 0 the perfusate was switched to the one containing the agonist. Note both PTH and isoproterenol demonstrate positive inotropic effects. With PTH, however, a gradual decline in the increment in force development ensues. Vertical bars represent myocardial contractility of 2.0 g/mm^2. Reproduced from reference 9 with permission.

Therefore, the effects of PTH on myocardial adenylate cyclase activity and the effects of Ca^{++} on the inotropic action of PTH were examined.

As shown in Figure 3, PTH in a concentration range of 10^{-9}-10^{-7}M was without effect on myocardial adenylate cyclase activity while isoproterenol and sodium fluoride stimulated the enzyme activity. Increasing Ca^{++} concentration of the perfusate from 1.0 to 3.0 mM increased myocardial contractility as might be expected (Table 3). The addition of PTH further augmented the myocardial contractility at both 1.0 and 3.0 mM Ca^{++}. However, the percent increments in contractility by PTH were less at 3.0 mM than at 1.0 mM Ca^{++}. Though data are not shown here, methoxy-verapamil completely blocked the inotropic action of PTH.

DISCUSSION

The present study unequivocally demonstrates that PTH exerts a direct positive inotropic action on the myocardium. This effect was evident at PTH concentration as low as 10^{-12}M. The effect of PTH seems specific to the biologically active PTH since the biologically inactive PTH was without effect. The inotropic action

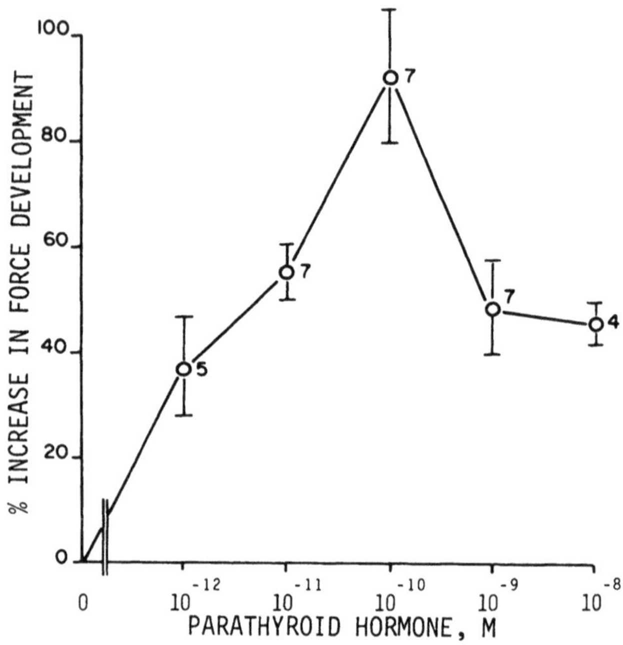

Figure 2. Dose response curve for PTH and percent increase in the force development of the papillary muscle. Values are the mean ± SEM, and the number of experiments is given beside each point. Effect of PTH at concentrations between 10^{-11}M and 10^{-8}M were not different but significantly different at 10^{-12}M and 10^{-10}M when analyzed by analysis of variance. Reproduced from reference 9 with permission.

of PTH appears to be mediated, at least in part, by release of endogenous norepinephrine from myocardium which stimulates β-adrenergic receptors. This interpretation is supported by the demonstration that the inotropic effect of PTH is markedly suppressed either by propranolol, a β-adrenergic blocking agent, or by depletion of endogenous myocardial norepinephrine store by reserpine. It is unlikely that PTH directly stimulates β-adrenergic receptors since PTH does not stimulate myocardial adenylate cyclase activity whereas isoproterenol, a known β-adrenergic agonist, stimulates the enzyme activity. A gradual decline in myocardial contractility following PTH may suggest depletion of myocardial norepinephrine.

It has been shown that actions of PTH on its target tissues are mediated by activation of membrane-bound adenylate cyclase and an increase in Ca^{++} influx across plasma membranes (14). The complete suppression of inotropic effects of PTH by methoxy-verapamil, an inhibitor of Ca^{++} transport across plasma membranes of the myocardium (15), and the attenuation of the hormone action by increasing Ca^{++} concentrations in the perfusate, observations similar to those reported in the renal tubules (16), together with the absence of PTH-sensitive adenylate cyclase in the myocardium, are consistent with the thesis that the PTH action on the myocardium is mediated by increased Ca^{++} influx across the plasma membranes independent of changes in adenylate cyclase activity. It

Table 1. Effects of Parathyroid Hormone on the Isolated Papillary Muscle Contracility

	Control[a]	With PTH[a]	%Change
N	7	7	
Cross-sectional area, mm^2	0.24±0.03	0.24±0.03	
Developed tension, g/mm^2	1.30±0.17	2.01±0.28[b]	+55±5
dT/dt, g/mm^2 sec.	22.1±2.3	28.9±2.9[b]	+32.2±6.1
Time to peak tension, msec.	84.1±4.5	92.9±6.5[b]	+8.4±1.9

Values are the man ±SEM. a) Determined prior to the addition of PTH, 10^{-11}M. b) vs. control, $p < 0.01$. Reproduced from reference 9 with permission.

Table 2. Isolated Papillary Muscle Contractility in Response to PTH in the Presence of Propranolol and in the Muscle Taken from Rats Pretreated with Reserpine.

	Prior to PTH	With PTH 10^{-11}M	%Incr.
I. Propranolol, 10^{-8}-10^{-5}M (n=9)			
DT, g/mm^2	1.20±0.13	1.37±0.16	
dT/dt, g/mm^2/sec	15.7±1.8	18.2±2.1	13±3.7[a]
TPT, msec	96.4±2.4	98.8±2.1	
II. Pretreatment with reserpine (n=7)			
DT	1.5-±0.22	1.90±0.27	
dt/dt	17.2±2.6	21.5±2.3	26±3.7[a]
TPT	98.0±7.2	106±7.3	

Values are the mean ±SEM. a) % increase in DT in response to PTH was significantly less than that seen in the absence of propranolol in normal rats (See Table 1).

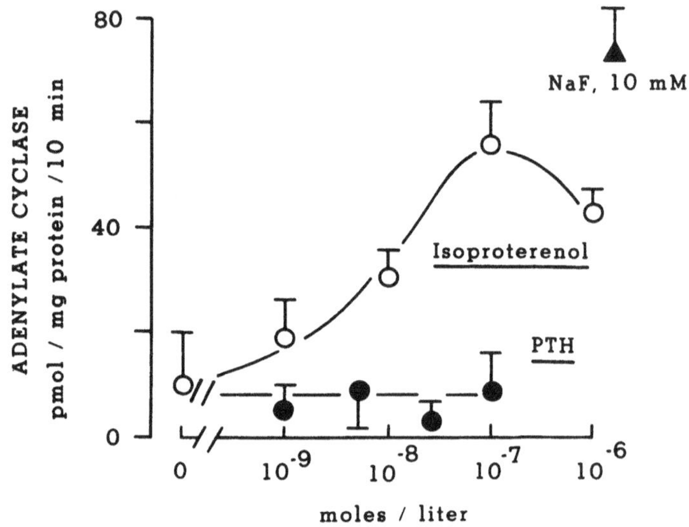

Figure 3. Effects of PTH, isoproterenol and NaF on adenylate cyclase activity of the rat ventricle. The enzyme activity was measured in the homogenate of the right ventricle using the method described by Levey and Epstein (14).

Table 3. Effects of Calcium and PTH on Force Development (DT) in Isolated Papillary Muscle

	-PTH	PTH, 10^{-11}M	%Incr.
Ca = 1.0 mM (n=7)	1.30±0.17	2.01±0.28	55±5
Ca = 3.0 mM (n=4)	2.31±0.21	2.87±0.26	24±3

Values are the mean ±SEM

is possible that the PTH-dependent Ca^{++} influx upon which Ca^{++} blockers might act may also be critical for norepinephrine release Alternately, Ca^{++} - dependent effects may be at the step of norepinephrine-dependent myocardial contraction. Measurements of cAMP contents in the intact papillary muscle preparations may provide information regarding steps or sites in which Ca^{++} play a role in the PTH-stimulated myocardial contraction. We did not measure cAMP contents in such preparations due to technical difficulties, and had to settle with assays of adenylate cyclase activity in the homogenates.

Whatever the exact cellular mechanisms of the PTH action on the myocardium, the present results may be of physiological significance. The inotropic effect of PTH was apparent at a PTH concentration of 10^{-12}M, the normal circulating level of the biologically active hormone (17), an observation suggesting that the physiological concentration of PTH may be of importance for "normal" cardiac function.

Based on the present and other studies it is now clear that PTH has the following acute cardiovascular effects; 1) inotropic effect, 2) chronotropic effect, 3) increase in coronary blood flow and 4) peripheral vasodilation.

ACKNOWLEDGMENTS

This study was supported by the Veterans Administration and by a grant from USPHS AM-21351, and by a grant-in-aid from the American Heart Association - Greater Los Angeles Affiliate.

REFERENCES

1. Arieff, A.I., and S.G. Massry, Calcium metabolism of brain in acute renal failure. J. Clin. Invest. 53:387-392 (1974).

2. Goldstein, D.A., L.A. Chui, and S.G. Massry, Effect of parathyroid hormone and uremia on peripheral nerve calcium and motor nerve conduction velocity. J. Clin. Invest. 62:88-93 (1978).

3. Maxley, M.A., N.H. Beel, S.R., Wazle, et al, Parathyroid hormone stimulation of glucose and urea production in isolated liver cells. Am. J. Physiol. 227:1058-1061 (1964).

4. Hruska, K.A., J. Blondin, R. Bass, et al, Effect of intact parathyroid hormone on hepatic glucose release in the dog. J. Clin. Invest. 64:1016-1023 (1979).

5. Meytes, D., E. Bogin, A. Ma, et al, Effect of parathyroid hormone on erythropoiesis. J. Clin. Invest. 67:1263-1269 (1981).

6. Pang, P.K.T., T.E. Tanner, Jr., J.A. Yee, et al, Hypotensive action of parathyroid hormone preparations on rats and dogs. Proc. Natl. Acad. Sci., USA, 77:675-678 (1980).

7. Crass, M.F., III., and P.K.T. Pang, Parathyroid hormone: A coronary artery vasodilator. Science 207:1087-1089 (1980).

8. Bogin, E., S.G. Massry, and I. Harary, Effect of parathyroid hormone on rat heart cells. J. Clin. Invest. 67:1215-1227 (1981).

9. Katoh, Y., K.L. Klein, R.A. Kaplan, et al, Parathyroid hormone has a positive inotropic action in the rat. Endocrinology 109:2252-2254 (1982).

10. Sonnenblick, E.H., Force-velocity relations in mammalian heart muscle. Am. J. Physiol. 202:931-939 (1961).

11. Sanborn, W.G., and B.L. Stremel, Ferrocyanide protection against uncoupling of excitation and contraction by maganese in rabbit ventricular myocardium. Circu. Res. 43:178-188 (1978).

12. Wennmalm, A., Maintenance of noradrenaline synthesis in rats after reserpine treatment. Acta Physiol. Scand. 73:523-526 (1968).

13. Levey, G.S., and S.E. Epstein, Activation of adenyl cyclase by glucagon in cat and human heart. Circu. Res. 24:151-156 (1969).

14. Rasmussen, H., P. Bordier, K. Kurokawa, et al, Hormonal control of skeletal and mineral homeostasis. Am. J. Med. 56:751-758 (1974).

15. Fleckenstein, A., Specific inhibitors and promoters of calcium action in the excitation-contraction coupling of heart muscle and their role in the prevention or production of myocardial lesions, in: "Caclium and the Heart," P. Harris and I.H. Opie, ed., Academic Press, London and New York (1971).

16. Kurokawa, K., T. Ohno, and H. Rasmussen, Ionic control of renal gluconeogenesis. II. The effects of Ca^{++} and H^{+} upon the response to parathyroid hormone and cyclic AMP. Biochim. Biophys. Acta. 313:32-41 (1973).

17. Goltzman, D., B. Henderson, and N. Loveridge, Cytochemical bioassay of parathyroid hormone. J. Clin. Invest. 65: 1309-1317 (1980).

EFFECT OF PARATHYROID HORMONE ON RAT ENTEROCYTE Na TRANSPORT IN VITRO

T. Drüeke, B. Lacour, E. Pierandrei, J. Chanard, J.L. Funck-Brentano

INSERM U 90, Hôpital Necker, Paris, and CHU Reims France

INTRODUCTION

Parathyroid Hormone (PTH) influences renal (1,2) and intestinal (3,4) handling of Na and water. In the intestine, it is not clearly established whether the observed effects are due to a direct action of the hormone or whether they are indirect via other mediators.

The purpose of this work was to investigate whether PTH exerted a possible direct effect on isolated rat enterocytes in vitro and if so, to get some insight into its mechanism of action.

MATERIAL AND METHODS

1. Animals and preparation of isolated cells.

Non fasted male Wistar AF rats weighing 100-150 g were used in all experiments. Animals were fed a standard laboratory diet containing : protein 24 %, cellulose 6.5 %, lipids 4.5 %, non-protein extract 45 %, mineral salt 8 %, vitamin D 200 IU %, and water 12 %. Calcium and phosphorus content were respectively 1.5% and 0.95 %. All animals had free access to tap water.

At the day of experiment animals received a blow on the head. After midline incision, a duodeno-jejunal segment of an approximately 20 cm length was entirely filled with icecold isotonic saline solution before excision. Then, the excised intestine was equilibrated during 20 min in a shaking water bath (shaking bath,

SB-4, Osi, Paris, France) at 37° C in a working medium of the following composition : NaCl 120, Tris 20, K_2HPO4 3.0, $MgCl_2$ 1.0, $CaCl_2$ 1.0, glucose 10 $mmol.l^{-1}$ containing also 1 $mg.ml^{-1}$ bovine serum albumin (pH 7.4 ± 0.1) with an osmolality of 295-305 mOsm. kg^{-1}. The epithelial cells were isolated from the everted jejunum by a mechanical vibration procedure (Vibro-Mischer El, Chemap AG, Switzerland) similar to that described by Levine and Weintraub (5) with the jejunum dived into the working medium (60 vibrations per sec, 1.0 mm amplitude during 20 min). No enzymatic digestion was performed.

2. Determination of sodium efflux rate constant ($^{\circ}K_{Na}$)

The measurement of Na efflux was performed using the method described by Gall et al (6).
In short, the isolated enterocytes were incubated at 37° C in the working incubation medium containing 10 µCi of $^{22}Na^{+}$ (NEN, Dreieick, Germany) for 20 min ("loading period"). The cell suspension was then centrifuged at 1000 g and the cells rapidly washed twice with ice-cold $MgCl_2$ - Tris buffer solution (respectively 110 and 2.0 $mmol.l^{-1}$, pH 7.4) at + 4°C. The cells were finally returned to fresh tracer-free working medium at a final dilution of 1/30 by volume and $^{22}Na^{+}$ efflux was determined ("efflux period"). $^{\circ}K_{Na}$ was calculated as reported by Gall et al (6). PTH and its vehicle solution ("vehicle") were added to the incubation medium during the loading and efflux periods, at identical concentrations.

3. Sodium uptake studies

The cell pellet obtained after vibration was divided into two parts. Each part was suspended in 6 ml of working buffer solution and maintained in constant agitation during 20 min at 37°C in a shaking water bath. Then PTH was added to one cell suspension and its vehicle to the other. Two samples of 1000 µl from each suspension were pipeted into a vial containing 5.0 ml ice-cold washing solution. Then 80 µl of a $^{22}NaCl$ solution were added (corresponding to 8 µCi ^{22}Na, specific activity 0.087 mCi/mg NEN, Dreieick, Germany). Aliquots of 500 µl each were obtained from both suspensions maintained and stirred at 37°C, at following time points : 30,60,90,120 sec, 3,4,5 and 15 min after ^{22}Na addition. Each sample was immediately distributed into its respective vial containing 5.0 ml ice-cold washing solution. Ten µl of the $^{22}NaCl$ solution (1 µCi ^{22}Na) were added at the end of experiment to the two samples obtained before ^{22}Na addition. These two samples were used to determine the value for nonspecific retention of radioactivity. All vials were thus centrifuged at 1000 g for 1 min at + 4°C. The supernatant was discarded and the pellets washed twice with 10 ml ice-cold washing buffer. Finally, 1.0 ml 10 % trichloroacetic acid solution was added to the last pellet, the pellet was vibrated with a Vortex (Bioblock, Paris, France) during 2 min., and the vials were kept at + 4°C during 15 min. After centrifugation, a 500 µl aliquot of supernatant was measured for its radioactivity using a liquid scintillator counter (S.L. 30, Intertechnique, Plaisir, France). The other 500 µl containing the disrupted cells were added to 5.0 ml of a 1.0 mol. 1^{-1}NaOH solution to solubilize the proteins, which were determined using the method described by Lowry et al (7) using bovine serum albumin as standard.

4. Study of cyclic nucleotide formation during PTH action

These studies were performed using isolated jejunal cells of the rat as described previously (4).

5. PTH and other substances

a) For the studies concerning Na uptake and efflux, the concentration of bovine (b) PTH used in the incubation medium was 1.2 I.U. ml^{-1}. Prior to experiments, b.PTH (highly purified b.PTH, Wilson Laboratoires, Flobio, Courbevoie, France) was maintained in a frozen vehicle stock solution (6.0. I.U. per 5.0 µl total volume) containing 1.0 mmol.1^{-1} cysteine chloride and 5.0 mmol. 1^{-1}acetic acid in a 154 mmol.1^{-1} sodium chloride solution.

The effect of ouabain (Boehringer, Mannheim, Germany) on $°K_{Na}$ was tested at a final concentration of 1.0 or 4.0 mmol.1^{-1}. Addition took place just at the start of ^{22}Na loading period. When the effect of b.PTH on enterocytes was studied in the presence of ouabain, ouabain was added to the incubation medium at a concentration of 4.0 mmol.1^{-1} during loading and efflux periods. The effect of b.PTH on epithelial cells was also studied when incubated in the working medium in the absence of calcium and the presence of 0.1 mmol.1^{-1} EGTA (bis-(aminoethyl)-glycolether N, N, N',N'-tetracetic acid, Merck, Darmstadt, Germany) during efflux period.

b) For the studies concerning cyclic nucleotide formation the hormones or vehicle studies were b.PTH at a final concentration of 1.0. I.U. ml^{-1} and prostaglandin E1 (PGE1, Upjohn Company, Kalamazoo, Michigan, USA) at a final concentration of 10 µg.ml^{-1}. The stock solution of PGE1 was prepared in 80 % (v/v) alcohol and stored at -20°C. This solution was diluted at 1:100 in cell suspension solution to obtain 10 µg.ml^{-1}. Thus alcohol concentration in incubation medium was 0.8 %. In the control experiment for PCE1, alcohol without PGE1 was added to the medium to obtain a final concentration of 0.8 %.

Theophylline (anhydrous crystal, Sigma Chemical Company, St-Louis, USA) at a concentration of 0.01 mol.1^{-1} was also added to some experiments done with b.PTH.

6. Statistical analysis of results

Results of enterocytes flux and nucleotide formation studies were expressed as means ± standard error of the mean (S.E.M.). Student's paired t test was performed when comparing values obtained with PTH to that obtained with its vehicle, since in each experiment the suspension of cells was divided into two parts, one treated with the hormone and the other with its vehicle only.

RESULTS

1. Effect of ouabain on sodium efflux rate constant ($^{\circ}K_{Na}$)

The validity of the model was appreciated by the inhibitory effect of ouabain on $^{\circ}K_{Na}$ of enterocytes. The mean inhibition of $^{\circ}K_{Na}$ for all experiments was 44 per cent for 1.0 mmol.l^{-1} ouabain (3.15 ± 0.30 S.E.M. versus control 5.63 ± 0.053 hr^{-1}, n = 10, $p < 0.005$) and 45 per cent for 4.0 mmol.l^{-1} (2.55 ± 0.56 versus control 4.65 ± 0.59 hr^{-1}, n = 3).

2. Effect of PTH on $^{\circ}K_{Na}$

Fig. 1 shows the effect of b.PTH (1.2 I.U. ml^{-1}) on $^{\circ}K_{Na}$ of a typical experiment using isolated enterocytes. A 28 per cent inhibition of $^{\circ}K_{Na}$ is observed in the presence of the hormone when compared to the control experiment containing the vehicle only. Sixteen such experiments have been performed (Table I). A mean inhibitory effect of b.PTH (1.2 I.U. ml^{-1}) on $^{\circ}K_{Na}$ of 26 per cent was observed when compared to control vehicle experiments (3.01 ± 0.19 versus 4.06 ± 0.36 hr^{-1}, $p < 0.02$). To further investigate the site of b.PTH inhibitory action on $^{\circ}K_{Na}$, studies with b.PTH were conducted in the presence of 4.0 mmol.l^{-1} ouabain. No effect of b.PTH (1.2 I.U. ml^{-1}) on ouabain-independent $^{\circ}K_{Na}$ of enterocytes was observed when compared to ouabain-exposed enterocytes incubated with the hormone's vehicle only. Table I shows the mean $^{\circ}K_{Na}$ values in response to b.PTH or its vehicle in the absence of ouabain (total $^{\circ}K_{Na}$) and in the presence of ouabain (ouabain-resistant $^{\circ}K_{Na}$). It furthermore indicates the calculated inhibitory effect of b.PTH on the ouabain-sensitive sodium transport site obtained by substracting ouabain-resistant from total $^{\circ}K_{Na}$. This yields an inhibition of 73 per cent.

3. Effect of PTH on Na uptake

The net uptake of ^{22}Na by isolated jejunal cells was comparable in the presence or the absence of b.PTH (1.2 I.U. ml^{-1}) in the incubation medium, at least during the time period of 15 min studied (Fig 2).

Table 1. Effect of b.PTH on sodium efflux rate constant $°K_{Na}$

Experimental conditions	b.PTH ($1.2\ I.U.ml^{-1}$)	Vehicle	P
Total $°K_{Na}$	3.01 ± 0.19 (n = 16)	4.06 ± 0.37 (n = 16)	< 0.02
Ouabain resistant $°K_{Na}$	2.56 ± 0.27 (n = 7)	2.37 ± 0.21 (n = 7)	N.S.
Ouabain sensitive $°K_{Na}$	0.45	1.69	—

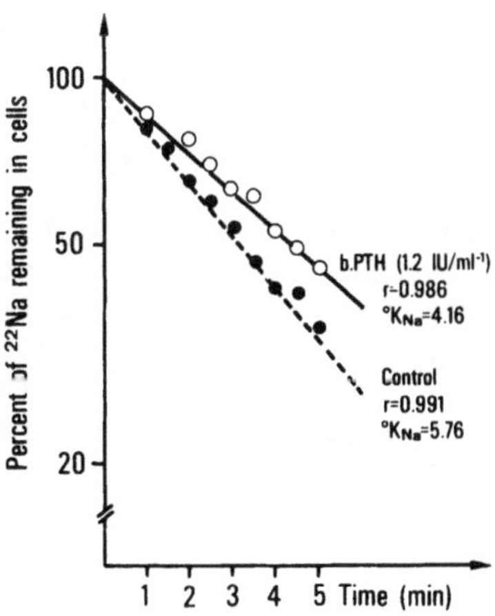

Fig. 1. Representative experiment with isolated enterocytes from one animal.

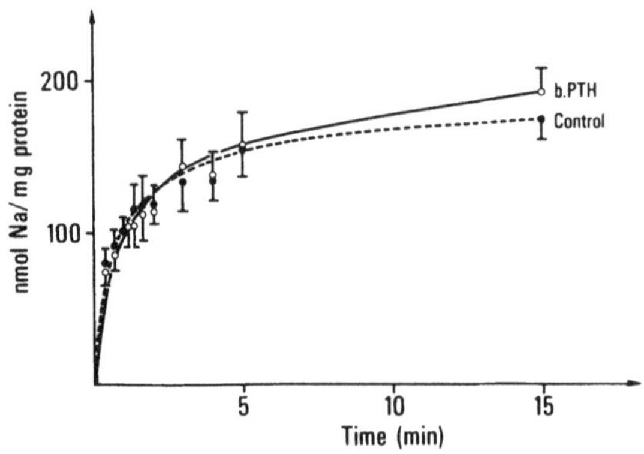

Fig. 2. Sodium uptake by isolated enterocytes. Values are means $\pm$ SEM.
Number of experiments = 13, p = N.S. for all time points studied.

4. Effect of PTH on cyclic nucleotide formation

The formation of cAMP was not significantly altered in the presence of b.PTH (1.0. I.U. ml^{-1}) when compared to control : 327 $\pm$ 55 vs 347 $\pm$ 43 pmoles/mg DNA for b.PTH (n = 5), 0 vs 2 min, and 265 $\pm$ 72 vs 258 $\pm$ 33 pmoles/mg DNA for control (n = 5), 0 vs. 2 min. The addition of theophylline led to comparable results. However, cAMP formation was significantly increased in the presence of PGE1 (10 $ug.ml^{-1}$) : 253 $\pm$ 66 vs 682 $\pm$ 174 pmoles/mg DNA (n = 5), 0 vs 2 min, $p < 0.05$. Similarly to the formation of cAMP, that of cGMP was also not altered in the presence of b.PTH (1.0 I.U. ml^{-1}) when compared to control.

5. Calcium-mediated effect of PTH on $°K_{Na}$

In additional experiments the effect of b.PTH was tested on enterocytes incubated in a solution containing no calcium and an additional 0.1 $mmol.l^{-1}$ EGTA concentration. In this setting, b.PTH exerted no inhibitory effect on $°K_{Na}$ (3.43 $\pm$ 0.45 hr^{-1}) when compared to b.PTH vehicle (4.16 $\pm$ 1.31 hr^{-1}, n = 7, p = N.S.) It should be noted that $°K_{Na}$ in the calcium-free sodium was comparable to that in the standard calcium-containing solution used in the former experiments (4.06 $\pm$ 0.37 hr^{-1}) whereas $°K_{Na}$ in this Ca^{2+} containing solution was depressed by b.PTH (3.01 ± 0.19 hr^{-1}) as demonstrated above.

DISCUSSION

The purpose of the present study using isolated rat enterocytes was to investigate a possible direct action of PTH on Na transport, and if so, the mechanism of its action.

At a concentration of 1.2 I.U. ml^{-1} PTH induced a 26 per cent decrease in the enterocyte efflux rate constant $°K_{Na}$ when compared to control values. This corresponded to roughly half the decrease (45 per cent) in $°K_{Na}$ induced by 4.0 $mmol.l^{-1}$ ouabain. The inhibitory action of b.PTH on the Na efflux rate constant of isolated enterocytes appeared to be directed at the ouabain-sensitive Na pump site since b.PTH exerted no effect on $°K_{Na}$ in the presence of ouabain. The calculated inhibition of the ouabain-sensitive $°K_{Na}$ by b.PTH was therefore approximately 73 per cent. In the isolated renal tubule, ouabain has also recently been shown to interfere with the action of PTH in that the former blunted the effect of the latter on phosphate uptake (8). Moreover, ouabain was also capable of inhibiting the bone resorbing effect of PTH in mouse calvaria (9). Thus, the cellular action of PTH appears to involve directly or indirectly the pump responsible for the active extrusion of Na from the cell interior directed outward. One could expect that Na entry into the cell would also be altered. However, b.PTH exerted no effect on enterocyte Na uptake under the experimental conditions studied. It must be stressed that the examined Na uptake represented not an influx of the ion but its net accumulation by the cells resulting from the difference between unidirectional influx and outflux. Therefore, a decrease in passive sodium permeability of the epithelial cell could well have ocurred in the presence of b.PTH but which remained undetected due to the experimental design of the Na uptake experiments.

In the present study, the inhibitory action of b.PTH on the ouabain-sensitive Na pump was independent of a measurable change in enterocyte cAMP or cGMP formation. Conversely, b.PTH lost its capacity of inhibiting $°K_{Na}$ when the incubation medium was Ca^{2+}-free. A comparable dependence on the presence of Ca^{2+} in the incubation solution has been recently reported for the effect of PTH on phosphate uptake by renal cortical slices (10). Therefore, we speculated that b.PTH inhibition of enterocyte $°K_{Na}$ must involve Ca^{2+}, possibly via an increase in cytosolic Ca^{2+} activity similary to the hormone's action in other epithelia (11,12). Furthermore, it has been shown in renal tubular epithelium that an increase in cytosolic Ca^{2+} activity was associated with a decrease in Na transport (13,14). It is thus possible that cytosolic Ca^{2+} activity, regulated in part through a process of Na-Ca exchange across the basolateral cell membrane, is important in the physiological regulation of Na transport across epithelial tissues.

The effect of b.PTH on enterocyte $^{o}K_{Na}$ observed in the present study could, therefore, be theoretically explained solely by a modulation of cytosolic Ca^{2+} activity, in the absence of detectable changes of intracellular cAMP or cGMP concentrations, leading to a decrease in the velocity of Na extrusion from the cell according to the recently proposed model by Taylor and Windhager (13).

SUMMARY

In the presence of b.PTH (1.2 I.U./ml) in the incubation medium, the Na efflux rate constant ($^{o}K_{Na}$) of isolated rat enterocytes was significantly reduced when compared to control experiments. The mean depression of $^{o}K_{Na}$ induced by b.PTH was 26% as compared to control (100%). No depressant effect of b.PTH on $^{o}K_{Na}$ was observed when the isolated enterocytes were incubated with ouabain (4.0mM). Thus, b.PTH appeared to inhibit the ouabain-sensitive Na pump. When incubating the isolated epithelial ce-ls in an EGTA-containing Ca free medium, b.PTH lost its capacity to inhibit $^{o}K_{Na}$. Thus, the presence of extracellular Ca appeared necessary for the inhibitory effect of b.PTH. In contrast to its effect on $^{o}K_{Na}$, b.PTH induced no change of net Na uptake by isolated enterocytes. Moreover, b.PTH did not induce significant changes in enterocyte cAMP or cGMP concentations.

It was concluded that b.PTH exerted a direct inhibitory effect on the ouabain-sensitive Na efflux rate constant of isolated rat enterocytes. The effect of b.PTH occurred without a measureable activation of the cyclic nucleotide system but needed the presence of Ca in the incubation medium to be operative.

REFERENCES

1. Amiel, C., Kuntziger, H. and Richet, G., Phosphate by proximal and distal nephron in normal and parathyroidectomized rats. Evidence for distal reabsorption, Pflugers Arch. 317:93 (1970).

2. Dennis, V.W., Influence of bicarbonate on parathyroid hormone-induced changes in fluid absorption by the proximal tubule, Kidney Int. 10:373 (1976).

3. Drueke, T., LaCour, B., and Chanard, J., Acute inhibitory effect of parathyroid hormone and calcitonin on jejunal electrolyte and water transport in normal and thyroparathyroidectomized rats, Miner. Elect. Metab. 4:68 (1980).

4. Lacour, B., Drueke, T. and Chanard, J., Effect of parathyroid hormone on jejunal electrolyte and water transport and cyclic nucleotide formation in the rat, Horm. Metab. Res. 12:624 (1980).

5. Levine, P.H. and Weintraub, L.R., Preparation of suspensions of small bone mucosal epithelial cells, J. Lab. Clin. Med. 75: 1026 (1970).

6. Gall, D.G., Butler, D.G., Teppermann, F.S. and Hamilton, J.R., Sodium ion transport in isolated intestinal epithelial cells. The effect of actively transported sugars on sodium ion efflex. Biochim. Biophys. Acta. 339:291 (1974).

7. Lowry, O.H., Rosebrough, N.J., Farr, A.L. and Randall, R.J., Protein measurement with the Folin phenol reagent, J. Biol. Chem. 193:265 (1951).

8. Rosenberg, E.M., Lee, S.W., Chase, L.R. and Avioli, L.V., Phosphate accumulation by the isolated renal tubule and the effects of parathyroid hormone and cyclic adenosine monophosphate, J. Lab. Clin. Med. 96:24 (1980).

9. Krieger, N.S. and Tashjian, A.H. Jr., Parathyroid hormone stimulates bone resorption via a Na-Ca exchange mechanism, Nature 287:843 (1980).

10. Rosenberg, E.M. and Fogel, A.J., Role of cyclic 3',5'-GMP in modulation of cellular uptake of phosphate, Am. J. Physiol. 233:E203 (1977).

11. Rasmussen, H. and Goodman, D.B.P., Relationship between calcium and cyclic nucleotides in cell activation, Physiol. Rev. 57:421 (1977).

12. Borle, A. and Uchikawa, T., Effects of parathyroid hormone on the distribution and transport of calcium in cultured kidney cells, Endocrinology 102:1725 (1978).

13. Taylor, A. and Windhager, E.E., Possible role of cytosolic calcium and Na-Ca exchange in regulation of transepithelial sodium transport, Am. J. Physiol. 236:F505 (1979).

14. Lee, C.O., Taylor, A. and Windhager, E.E., Cytosolic calcium ion activity in epithelial cells of Necturus kidney, Nature 287:859 (1980).

COMPARISON OF PROPRANOLOL AND ATENOLOL IN THE CONTROL OF HYPERPARATHYROIDISM IN UREMIA

R. Makdassi[1], M. Andrejak[1], Ph. Morinière[1], J.L. Sebert[1], S. Decourt[2], J. Guéris[3], B. Coevoet[1], A. Fournier[1]

CHU Amiens(1),Hop.A.Paré(2), Hop.Lariboisière (3) Paris
Service de Néphrologie - Hôpital Nord
80000 Amiens France

INTRODUCTION

Secondary hyperparathyroidism is a constant and not yet resolved complication of chronic renal failure. Current therapeutic methods for parathyroid gland suppression in uremic patients are mainly based on the use of phosphate binders, oral calcium supplementation and eventually on administration of vitamin D metabolites (1). Since these measures are not always quite successful, it is interesting to evaluate other measures suggested by recent physiological data on the regulation of PTH secretion. As a matter of fact, beside the circulating levels of ionized calcium and magnesium (2), PTH secretion appears to be regulated by substances such as dopamine, histamine (via H2 receptors), secretine, glucagon, PgE2 and catecholamines (3).

Catecholamines modulate PTH secretion possibly via alpha-receptors (3), and with more certainty via beta-adrenoreceptors (4). Presence and functional role of betaadrenoreceptors have been proved by in vitro (4), and in vivo (5,6) studies. In man with normal renal function, propranolol, a non selective beta-adrenoreceptor blocking agent has given conflicting results as regards the suppression of PTH secretion (7,8). In uremic patients on dialysis, retrospective (9,10,11), and prospective (12,13) studies have shown that chronic oral administration of propranolol could suppress PTH hypersecretion.

Recently, we pointed out the fact that in patients

with moderate renal insufficiency, acute i.v. injection of propranolol reduced PTH secretion whereas metoprolol a B1 selective betablocker given similarly at a dosage leading to the same B1 blocking activity, was without effect on PTH levels (14).

This results could be considered as an argument in favour of the exclusive role of B2 adrenoreceptors in the modulation of PTH secretion suggesting that cardio-selective betablocker would not be appropriate to control hyperparathyroidism. Therefore, in this study, we compared the effect on PTH secretion of the chronic administration of propranolol and of another B1 selective betablocker, atenolol, in hypertensive uremic patients not yet on dialysis.

PATIENTS AND METHODS

Patients

Twenty four hypertensive patients (18 men and 6 women, 21 to 69 years old) with chronic renal failure (serum creatinine $3.6 \pm .5$ mg/dl) were selected on the basis of their willingness to cooperate. Their renal failure was secondary to chronic glomerulonephritis in 6 cases, interstitial nephritis in 5 cases, nephroangio sclerosis in 8 cases, segmental hypoplasia in 3 cases, polycystic disease in 2 cases. Mean duration of renal function impairment (blood urea constantly higher than 50 mg/dl) was 5.5 years (from 2 to 13 years). None had radiological osteodystrophy or increase of serum alkaline phosphatase before and during the study. Most of them were already treated for their hypertension with various drugs (diuretics in 17 cases, small doses of clonidine in 4 cases, betablocking drugs in 10 cases).

Design of the study

In a cross-over randomized fashion, these patients received propranolol (125 ± 52 mg/day) or atenolol (155 ± 75 mg/day). The dose was titrated in order to achieve the same blood pressure control under the two drugs (diastolic blood pressure < 95 mmHg). In ten cases, propranolol was used as the first drug.

Other therapeutic measures (i.e. oral calcium supplement, phosphorus binders, other anti-hypertensive drugs) were maintained constant throughout the study, No patient was taking vitamin D supplement.

At the end of the 2 therapeutic periods, the following parameters were measured : body weight ; supine and standing blood pressure and heart rate ; plasma concentrations of calcium, phosphate, bicarbonate, proteins, alkaline phosphatase, PTH, calcitonin and 25 OH vitamin D, as well as the concentration of propranolol or atenolol.

To appreciate the cardioselectivity, we performed in 9 cases, a glucagon tolerance test with measurement of blood glucose : before and 15,30,45,60,120 and 180 min. after i.v. injection of 1 mg of glucagon.

Analytical methods

Plasma concentrations of phosphate, calcium, creatinine, proteins and bicarbonate were determined by auto-analyzer techniques (SMA 9).

Plasma PTH was measured by radioimmunoassay using C terminal (15), and N terminal specific antibodies (16). Normal values are 4-8 ng/ml of protein of a parathyroid culture medium for C terminal PTH and 0-0.45ng /ml for the N terminal PTH. Biological significance of these assays was proved by significant positive correlations with histomorphometric parameters of resorption (17,18).

Plasma calcitonin was measured with the homologeous radioimmunoassay of MOUKTHAR (19). Normal values are 0-0.30 ng/ml.

Plasma 25 hydroxy-vitamin D was determined by the protein binding assay of PREECE (20).

Atenolol and propranolol plasma concentrations were determined respectively by high performance liquid and gas chromatography (21).

Statistical methods

Comparison of clinical and biological parameters was performed with the non parametric test of Wilcoxon for paired data.

RESULTS (Table 1)

At the end of the two therapeutic periods, there was no difference in supine mean arterial blood pressure (126±2 mmHg with propranolol vs 123±3 mmHg with atenolol) and heart rate (67±2 beats/min with propranolol vs 63±2 with atenolol). Serum creatinine was also comparable as well as plasma concentration of calcium, phosphate, proteins, C and N terminal PTH, calcitonin , 25 OH vitamin D. The only significant difference was in the bicarbonate concentration which was significantly higher during propranolol treatment (28.8±1.3 vs 27.1± 1.8 mEq/l).

Figure 1 shows the results of glucagon tolerance test. There was no significant difference between the 2 drugs in the fasting blood glucose concentrations nor in the peak observed 30 min after glucagon injection.

Table 1 - Plasma concentrations of the various parameters at the end of the two therapeutic periods (mean ± SEM)

Plasma concentrations		Propranolol	Atenolol
- drugs	ng/ml	129 ± 25	722 ± 130
- creatinine	mg/dl	3.6 ± .1	3.5 ± 1.1
- calcium	mg/dl	9.5 ± 0.2	9.5 ± 0.2
- phosphate	mg/dl	3.8 ± 0.4	3.7 ± 0.4
- proteins	g/dl	7.1 ± 0.2	7.1 ± 0.2
- bicarbonates	mEq/l	28.8 ± 1.3	27.1 ± 1.8*
- PTH C terminal	ng/ml	18.0 ± 4.5	18.5 ± 4.5
- PTH N terminal	ng/ml	0.14± 0.04	0.12± 0.04
- Calcitonin	ng/ml	0.01± 0.01	0.02± 0.01
- 25 OH vitamin D	ng/ml	35 ± 18	29 ± 14

* significance of the difference between propranolol and atenolol : $p < .05$.

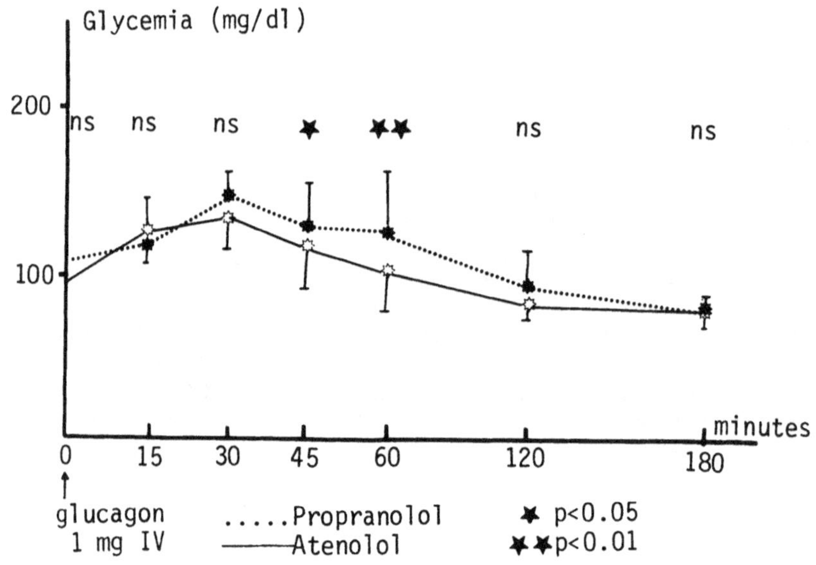

Figure 1. Results of glucagon tolerance test.

45 and 60 min after the injection, blood glucose was however significantly higher with propranolol.

DISCUSSION

This study fails to find a difference in the plasma concentrations of N and C terminal PTH levels after chronic oral administration of propranolol and atenolol a new cardioselective betablocker, given to uremic patients not yet on dialysis at a dosage equally effective on their blood pressure and heart rate. This is apparently in contradiction with the results of COEVOET et al (14) who found that i.v. administration of metoprolol, an other cardioselective betablocker, was not able, as i.v. propranolol, to decrease high levels of N terminal PTH. However the fact that plasma bicarbonate concentration were significantly higher with propranolol in this chronic study (in contrast to their lack of change in the acute study of COEVOET et al), suggests that parathyroid secretion is actually more efficiently suppressed by propranolol than by atenolol since it may be assumed that plasma ionized calcium was lower with propranolol. This assumption is made on the fact that there was no difference in plasma concentrations of total calcium, proteins, and phosphate and that none of these patients had cardio-pulmonary disorders susceptible to affect primarily the acid-base metabolism so that the small increase in bicarbonate concentration may be considered as a small degree of alcalosis, which is known to decrease ionized calcium.

The higher plasma concentration of bicarbonate with propranolol may be explained by an initially greater suppressive effect of propranolol on PTH secretion since PTH is known to decrease bicarbonate reabsorption (22). The fact that there was no difference between the plasma levels of PTH actually observed under the 2 drugs, may be explained by the secondary stimulation of PTH secretion by the lower ionized calcium since FISCHER and BLUM (6) have shown in cow that propranolol was unable to prevent the increase of PTH secretion due to hypocalcemia. In hemodialysed patients, with very low residual clearance, it is expected that changes in plasma bicarbonate by changes in tubular reabsorption of bicarbonate will be negligible. Therefore the greater suppressive effect of propranolol will not be counterbalanced and lower plasma PTH levels may be anticipated in those patients.

The fact that the long term control of hyperparathyroidism is comparable with atenolol and propranolol but that this latter probably has a greater initial suppressive effect on PTH secretion, is compatible with the demonstration by BROWN (23) of the presence of both B1 and B2 receptors on the parathyroid cells coming from patients with primary hyperparathyroidism.

The plasma concentrations of propranolol and atenolol found in this study are comparable to those usually observed in efficiently treated hypertensive patients (24,25). The levels of atenolol observed in this study are however in the range of those observed in non uremic patients treated with 300 mg/day (25). They are obtained in our patients with lower doses because renal failure increases the half life of atenolol (25). At this high plasma levels the persistence of the B1 selectivity of atenolol may be questioned. Therefore the glucagon tolerance test was performed to look for differences in the decrease of blood glucose after the hyperglycemic peak, since this decrease is related to the importance of the insulin secretion which is itself dependent on beta 2 receptor activity (26). The hyperglycemic peak is, on the other hand, independent of betareceptor activity, since it is secondary to glycogenolysis induced by stimulation of specific glucagon receptors of the hepatocytes. The greater decrease of blood glucose in the atenolol treated group suggests that insulin secretion is less suppressed in this group and therefore that the B1 selectivity of atenolol is still present at these relatively high plasma levels.

Since the patients were before starting the trial on various antihypertensive drugs including various betablockers, it was not possible to have an interpretable base-line measurement of the PTH levels.Therefore it can not be claimed with certainty that atenolol and propranolol have decreased PTH hypersecretion in our patients. It can only be stated that the levels of PTH under both drugs were comparable and satisfactory. N terminal PTH levels were even in the normal range whereas C terminal PTH were only twice the upper limit of normal. Histomorphometric studies by SEBERT et al (17) for the C terminal assay and by VIGO et al (18) for the N terminal assay have shown that these levels of PTH were associated with normal active resorption surface. The persistent elevation of the C terminal PTH levels is explained by the previous hyperparathyroid state and the longer half life of the C terminal inactive fragments which are no more as efficiently degradated in failing kidneys (28).

The clinical significance of PTH suppression by betablockers in uremia has been suggested up to now only by retrospective studies comparing two groups of patients on chronic hemodialysis which differed only by the use of propranolol. In the studies of CARO (9), and BRANCACCIO (10), the propranolol group had not only lower PTH levels but had also lower alkaline phosphatase levels and less severe bone disease ; in the studies of SURIAN et al (11) the PTH levels were comparable but the alkaline phosphatase levels were lower in the propranolol group. Therefore, prospective studies are still needed to prove the clinical usefulness of controlling hyperparathyroidism in uremia by beta-blockers in addition to the other most important measures aiming at counterbalancing the tendency to ionized calcium decrease.

ACKNOWLEDGEMENT
The authors thank Pr MILHAUD, Dr CALMETTES C., and Mr BOCCARD B. for performing the dosages of N terminal PTH and calcitonin and Mrs LAVAL for typewriting.

REFERENCES

1 - A. Fournier, Ph. Morinière, B. Coevoet, R. Makdassi A. Roussel,P.H. Decourcelle, J. Kassouf, G. Lambrey J.F. de Fremont,J.L. Sebert."Prevention and medical treatment of secondary hyperparathyroidism of chronic renal failure in the adult in "Advances in Nephrology from the Necker Hospital"ed. by GRUNFELD J.P.,M.H.MAXWELL Year Book Medical Publisher Chicago 1981 (in print).

2 - J.H. Targovnik,J.S. Rodman,L.M. Sherwood."Regulation of parathyroid hormone secretion in vitro:quantitative aspects of calcium and magnesium on control".Endocrinology, 88 : 1477-1482 (1971).

3 - E.M.Brown,D.G.Gardner,R.A.Windeck,S.Hurwitz,M.F. Brennan,G.D. Aurbach."B adrenergically stimulated 3,5-monophosphate accumulation in and parathyroid hormone release from dispersed human parathyroid cells". J. Clin. Endocrinol. Metab. 48:618-626 (1979)

4 - G.D.Aurbach,E.M.Brown,S.J.Marx, "Receptors and cyclic nucleotides in secretion of parathyroid hormone". Calcif. Tiss. Res. Supp 22:117-126 (1977).

5 - G.A.Williams, G.K.Hargis, E.M.Bowser,W.J. Henderson N.J.Martinez,"Evidence for a role of adenosine 3'5' monophosphate in parathyroid hormone release". Endocrinology, 92 : 687 - 691 (1973).

6 - J.A. Fischer, J.W. Blum. "Non calcium control of parathyroid hormone secretion" Mineral Electrolyte Metab. 1 : 158-166 (1980).

7 - S.C. Kukreja, G.K.Hargis, E.N.Bowser, W.J.Henderson E.W. Fisherman, G.A.Williams. "Role of adrenergic stimuli in parathyroid hormone secretion in man. J. Clin. Endocrinol. Metab. 40 : 478-481 (1975).

8 - M.S.Christensen, O.Brandsborg, N.J.Christensen. Inhibition of parathyroid hormone secretion by isoproterenol. In "Phosphate metabolism"ed. by Massry E.Ritz, Plenum Press,New York,London:363-368 (1977)

9 - J.F. Caro, A. Besarab, J.F. Burke, J.A. Glennon. "A possible role for propranolol in the treatment of renal osteodystrophy". Lancet,ii : 451-453(1978)

10- D. Brancaccio, C. Gacnozzi, S. Casati, D. Rurale, S. Belloli, A. Aroldi, G. Graziani, C. Ponticelli. "Propranolol and uremic osteodystrophy".EDTA Proceeding, Abstract 12 (1979).

11- M. Surian, G. Colussi, G. Civati, S.Masi, B.Corradi F. Malberti,H. Barbiano, G. di Belgiojoso,L.Minetti "No effect of chronic propranolol therapy in lowering plasma parathyroid hormone and in reducing osteodystrophy incidence in hemodialysis patients". EDTA Congress, Abstract 95 (1980).

12- K. Farrington, J. Hamzeh, Z.Varghese,J.F. Moorhead "Effect of oral propranolol on parathyroid hormone secretion in chronic renal failure". Brit. Med. J. 281 : 1320 (1978).

13- A. Bessarab, J.F. Carro, B.V. Ihle, J.F. Burke, J.A. Glennon, J.A. Fischer. "Suppression of secondary hyperparathyroidism by propranolol in renal failure patients". Nephron, 27 : 127-133 (1981).

14- B. Coevoet, C. Desplan, J.L. Sebert, R. Makdassi, M. Andrejak, J.D. Gheerbrant, M. Tolani,C.Calmette, M.S. Moukthar, A. Fournier. "Effect of propranolol and metoprolol on parathyroid hormone and calcitonin secretion in uremic patients". Brit. Med. J. 280 : 1344-1346 (1980).

15- J. Guéris, C. Ferrière. "Hétérogénéité de la parathormone plasmatique chez l'homme". Path. Biol. 23 : 821-826 (1975).

16- G. Desplan, A. Jullienne, M.S. Moukthar,G. Milhaud "Sensitive assay for biologically active fragment of human parathyroid hormon".Lancet ii:198-199(1977)

17- J.L.Sebert, A.Fournier, J.Guéris, G.Lambrey, J.F. de Fremont, P.Marié, R.Makdassi, A.Smadja, A.Marié, D.Kuntz, A.Ryckewaert, J.Quichaud, P.Meunier."Limit by phosphatemia of the usefulness of vitamin D metabolites (1αhydroxycholecalciferol and 25 hydroxycholecalciferol) in the treatment of renal osteodystrophy." Metab. Bone Dis. and Rel. Res. 2 : 217-222 (1980).

18- J.L. Vigo, E.E. Polli, G. Milhaud, M.S. Moukthar, C. Desplan, J. Duriez."Amino terminal parathyroid hormone radio-immunoassay to evaluate bone status in renal failure". Lancet,i, : 443-444 (1981).

19- M.S. Moukthar, A. Jullienne, P. Rivaille,G.Milhaud "Dosage radio-immunologique de la calcitonine humaine". In Radio-immunoassay and Related Procedures in Medicine. Vienne : International Atomic Energy Agency, 379-397 (1974).

20- M.A. Preece, J.L.M.O'Riordan, M. Lawsonde,K.Kodicek "A competitive protein binding assay for 25 hydroxy cholecalciferol and 25 hydroxyergocalciferol". Clin. Chem. Act. 54 : 235-242 (1974).

21- S. Decourt, B. Flouvat. "Dosage dans les milieux biologiques d'un nouveau bétabloquant l'atenolol par chromatographie liquide à haute performance". J. Chromatography. 174 : 258-263 (1979).

22- C.K. Grumb, M. Martinez Maldonado, Garabede,W.N. Suki. "Effects of volume expansion,purified parathyroid extract and calcium on renal bicarbonate reabsorption in the dog". J. Invest. 54 : 1287 - 1290 (1974).

23- E.M. Brown, S. Hurwitz, G.D. Aurbach. "Beta-adrenergic stimulation of cyclic AMP content and parathyroid hormone release from isolated bovine parathyroid cells". Endocrinology 100:1696-1702(1977).

24- G. Leonetti, G. Mayer, A. Morganti, L. Terzauli, A. Zanchetti, C.A. Chidsey. "Hypotensive and renin suppressing activities of propranolol in hypertensive patients. Clin. Sci. Mol. Med. 48, 491-499 (1975).

25- A. Amery, J.F. de Plaen, P. Lijnen, J. Mc Ainsh, T.Reybrouck. "Relationship between blood level of atenolol and pharmacologic effect". Clin. Pharmacol. Therap. 21, 691-699 (1977).

26- A. Kaneto, E. Miki, K. Kosaka. "Effect of B1 and B2 adrenoreceptor stimulant infused intrapancreatically on glucagon and insulin secretion". Endocrinology 97 : 1166-1173 (1975).

27- A. Luyck. "Le rôle du glucagon dans l'hyperglycémie" Diabète et Métabolisme i : 201-208 (1975).

28- J. Freitag, K.J. Martin, K.A. Hruska, C. Anderson, M. Conrades, E. Slatopolsky". Impaired parathyroid hormone metabolism in patients with chronic renal failure". New England J. Med. 208 : 29-32 (1978).

EFFECTS OF ORAL CIMETIDINE ON PARATHYROID HORMONE AND CALCITONIN PLASMA LEVELS IN UREMIC PATIENTS

J.L. Sebert*, P.H. Decourcelles*, Ph. Moriniere*, J.F. de Fremont*, J. Gueris**, R. Makdassi*, J. Khassouf*, M. Andrejak*, A. Fournier*

* Centre Hospitalier et Universitaire - 80030 Amiens
** Laboratoire de Radioimmunologie, Hôpital Lariboisiere 75010 Paris, France

INTRODUCTION

Reports concerning the effects of cimetidine on parathyroid hormone levels in primary hyperparathyroidism (1-4) and in secondary hyperparathyroidism of renal failure (5-8) are increasing in number, but lead to disagreeing conclusions. These discrepancies are unclear and could be possibly explained by : 1) a variable compliance to treatment, since no measurement of plasma levels of cimetidine has been made in these reports, 2) differences in specificity of parathyroid hormone immunoassays, since, in a studied group of hemodialysed patients, the lowering effect of cimetidine on parathyroid hormone levels previously observed using a carboxyterminal antiserum (5), was not confirmed when the same samples were assayed a second time using an aminoterminal antiserum (9). It has also been suggested (8) that cimetidine could act on the metabolic fate of circulating parathyroid hormone rather than on its secretion, thus explaining differences between results derived from either carboxy or aminoterminal immunoassays.

These conflicting observations led us to evaluate the effects of oral cimetidine on parathyroid hormone levels in a group of patients on chronic hemodialysis. Both carboxy - and aminoterminal antiserums were used for parathyroid hormone assay and compliance to treatment was checked by monitoring plasma cimetidine concentration. Furthermore, since calcitonin has been implied (10) in the pathogenesis of uremic osteitis fibrosa, plasma levels of calcitonin were also simultaneously measured.

PATIENTS AND TREATMENT PROTOCOL

12 uremic patients (6 males, 6 females, aged 21-71 years) who had been on regular hemodialysis for more than 12 months were studied. These patients had been previously treated as follows : 1) a dialysis schedule of 4 hours 3 times weekly with a dialysate calcium concentration of 1.75 mmol/L and a magnesium concentration of .74 mmol/L, 2) an oral supplement of calcium carbonate (3g/day) given to 7 of them, 3) aluminium hydroxide (4g/day) given to 11 of them in order to correct hyperphosphatemia. None of them had been treated with vitamin D and its derivatives or betablockers. During the period of the study, this basic treatment was maintained unchanged.

Patients were studied on 3 successive periods of 1 month duration each, before, during and after treatment with oral cimetidine 200 mg twice daily. Compliance to treatment was checked by monitoring plasma cimetidine concentrations on 2 occasions during treatment. Post treatment evaluation was not possible in one patient who kept on taking cimetidine after discontinuation had been ordered. Blood samples were taken before the first dialysis of the week on 3 occasions during the control period and then, at the middle and at the end of the 2 following periods. Blood was immediately centrifugated and plasma was stored deep-frozen. Hormonal measurements were carried out, within a single assay, at the end of the study.

METHODS

Parathyroid hormone was measured using 2 distinct antiserums. Carboxyterminal parathyroid hormone (C-terminal PTH) was measured using antiserum CH9S raised against bovine parathyroid hormone, as previously described (11). The standard was a human adenoma parathyroid extract (kindly provided by Dr. C. ARNAUD, San Francisco) approximatively 10% pure. The sensitivity was .5 ng/ml and the upper limit of the normal range 8 ng/ml. Aminoterminal parathyroid hormone (N-terminal PTH) was measured with a previously described radioimmunoassay (12) using an antiserum directed against the synthetic 1-34 fragment of human parathyroid hormone (sensitivity : .07 ng/ml, upper limit of the normal range : .45 ng/ml). The biological significance of both carboxy - and aminoterminal assays has been proved (13,14) on the basis of positive correlations with active resorption surfaces in bone histomorphometric studies of hemodialysed patients.

Calcitonin was measured with a previously described homologous radioimmunoassay (15) which had a sensitivity of .07 ng/ml (upper limit of the normal range : .30 ng/ml).

Calcium, phosphate, bicarbonates were measured on a Technicon Auto-Analyizer. Corrected calcium was calculated according to PARFITT's formula (16).

Plasma concentration of cimetidine was determined by a liquid chromatographic method (17). The lower limit of detection was .02 mg/L.

Statistical methods : data are expressed as means ± SEM. For statistical purposes, individual pre-, during and post-treatment values were expressed as the individual average values of each considered period. Statistical analysis was performed with the Wilcoxon test for either paired or unpaired data.

RESULTS

Plasma concentrations of cimetidine : they were always above .30 mg/L in 7 patients, with mean individual values during treatment ranging from .30 to 4.10 mg/L. The mean cimetidine plasma level (± SEM) of this group of 7 patients who adequately adhered to treatment was 1.50 ± .50 mg/L. On the other hand, plasma cimetidine was constantly undetectable (<.02 mg/L) in 5 patients who therefore were considered as having not taken properly the prescribed treatment, since intestinal malabsorption of this drug has not been reported.

Biochemical and hormonal results : data concerning the 7 patients with measurable plasma cimetidine concentrations during treatment are reported in Table I and Figure 1.

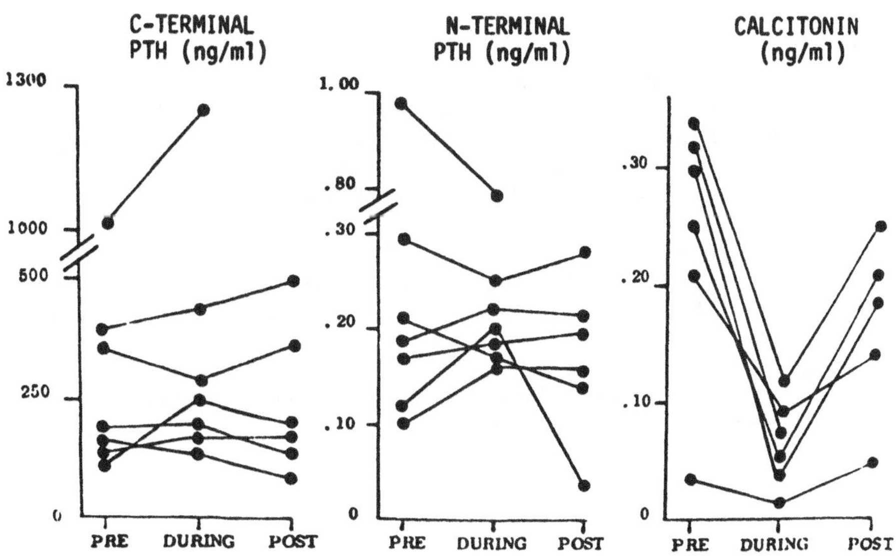

Figure 1. Evolution of hormonal parameters.

Table I. Evolution of biochemical and hormonal parameters in treated patients with measurable plasma concentrations of cimetidine during treatment.

	BEFORE	DURING	AFTER
CORRECTED PLASMA CALCIUM (mmol/L)	2.50 (±.09)	2.45 (±.08)	2.34 (±.04)
PLASMA PHOSPHATE (mmol/L)	1.63 (±.12)	1.82** (±.14)	1.51 (±.08)
PLASMA BICARBONATES (mmol/L)	23.9 (± 1)	21.9* (±1.1)	24.3 (±.5)
PLASMA C-TERMINAL PTH (ng/ml)	355 (±120)	402 (±149)	259 (±62)
PLASMA N-TERMINAL PTH (ng/ml)	.30 (±.11)	.29 (±.08)	.17 (±.03)
PLASMA CALCITONIN (ng/ml)	.23 (±.04)	.06** (±.01)	.16 (±.03)

Wilcoxon test for paired differences with during and after treatment values compared to before treatment values :
* $p < .10$, ** $p < .05$

The plasma levels of corrected calcium and either C- or N-terminal PTH did not change significantly. Plasma phosphate increased significantly but weakly in all patients during treatment and returned pre-treatment values after cimetidine discontinuation. Plasma bicarbonates showed a small but not significant trend to decrease during treatment. Plasma calcitonin was initially undetectable in one patient and remained undetectable thereafter. In the 6 other patients plasma calcitonin decreased dramatically during treatment, with a mean 75% fall from initial values, and returned to pre-treatment values, after cessation of therapy.

Results observed in these 7 patients with measurable cimetidine concentration during treatment were compared to those obtained in the 5 patients with undetectable plasma cimetidine. In this group of 5 patients, none of the biochemical and hormonal parameters changed significantly throughout the study. As shown in Table II, these 2 groups of patients only differed as regards variations of plasma phosphate and calcitonin levels.

DISCUSSION

No consistent effect of oral cimetidine on parathyroid hormone levels was observed in spite of simultaneous use of 2 immunoassays with either carboxy or aminoterminal specificity.

Table II. Comparison of the biochemical and hormonal changes with cimetidine administration and discontinuation, between patients with measurable plasma concentrations of cimetidine (n = 7) and patients with undetectable plasma cimetidine (n = 5).

	DURING minus BEFORE DIFFERENCES PLASMA CIMETIDINE		AFTER minus DURING DIFFERENCES PLASMA CIMETIDINE	
	< .02mg/L	> .30mg/L	< .02mg/L	> .30mg/L
CORRECTED PLASMA CALCIUM (mmol/L)	- .01 (±.04)	.04 (±.04)	.03 (±.05)	- .06 (±.04)
PLASMA PHOSPHATE (mmol/L)	- .15 (±.171)	.19* (±.09)	.51 (±.12)	- .25** (±.08)
PLASMA BICARBONATES (mmol/L)	- .80 (±.50)	-2.01 (±.67)	1.53 (±.96)	1.3 (±.68)
PLASMA C-TERMINAL PTH (ng/ml)	- 9 (± 41)	47 (± 35)	27 (± 59)	2 (± 24)
PLASMA N-TERMINAL PTH (ng/ml)	.02 (±.02)	- .01 (±.03)	.04 (±.13)	- .03 (±.03)
PLASMA CALCITONIN (ng/ml)	.09 (±.09)	- .16** (±.03)	- .06 (±.05)	.10** (±.02)

Significance of the comparison between the 2 groups of patients (Wilcoxon test for unpaired data) : * $p < .10$, ** $p < .05$

These results do not agree with other studies (5,6,8) reporting a significant fall of parathyroid hormone measured with a carboxy-terminal specific antiserum in hemodialysed patients treated with oral cimetidine. In one of these previous studies (8), it was noted that circulating parathyroid hormone levels decreased when parathyroid hormone was assayed with a carboxyterminal specific antiserum but increased when using an aminoterminal antiserum, suggesting a possible role of cimetidine on peripheric metabolism of parathyroid hormone. The present results do not support this concept. These discrepancies cannot be explained by a too short duration of cimetidine administration since previously reported (8) significant changes have been observed after only 15 days of treatment. A possible explanation could be the use of a daily dosage of cimetidine (400 mg/day) lower than that previously applied (600-1000 mg/day), since it has been suggested (5) that cimetidine-induced parathyroid suppression may be dose-related. The reason why the daily dosage of 400 mg was chosen is that it has been demonstrated (18) that this dosage, given to hemodialysed patients, resulted in durable plasma concentrations well above .50 mg/L, a level which adequately suppresses gastric acid secretion in healthy subjects. In fact, the mean plasma cimetidine concentration of the 7 patients who adhered to treatment was 1.50 ± .50 mg/L, a level largely above this threshold of antihistaminic activity. Since mental confusion has been related (19) to trough plasma concentration of cimetidine higher than 1.25 mg/L in uremic patients treated with 1200 mg of cimetidine, we felt not justified to give doses higher than 400 mg/day.

At contrast with the absence of change in parathyroid hormone levels, plasma calcitonin fell dramatically during treatment, in patients with therapeutically significant plasma cimetidine concentration. This fall cannot be explained by a simultaneous decrease in plasma calcium concentration since this latter did not change significantly during treatment. Since, gastrin is an important stimulator of calcitonin secretion, and since cimetidine therapy for duodenal ulcer in hemodialysed patients led to enhanced gastrin secretion (20), the observed decrease in plasma calcitonin levels is still more conspicuous. It is therefore suggested that oral cimetidine may directly suppress calcitonin secretion in hemodialysed patients, as previously reported (21) during acute intravenous administration in normal human subjects.

From a practical point of view, the absence of consistent suppression of parathyroid hormone secretion makes the use of cimetidine of no value in the treatment of uremic osteodystrophy. Moreover, the fact that cimetidine may decrease calcitonin secretion appears to be inopportune, since lack of calcitonin is considered (10) as a potential aetiological factor of bone disease in hemodialysed patients.

ACKNOWLEDGMENTS

The authors thank Pr. A. MILHAUD, Dr. C. CALMETTE and Mr. B. BOCCARD for performing the dosages of N-terminal PTH and calcitonin. They thank Smith Klein and French Laboratories for measuring plasma cimetidine concentrations.

REFERENCES

1. J.C. Sherwood, F.W. Ackroyd, M. Garcia. Effect of cimetidine on circulating parathyroid hormone in primary hyperparathyroidism. Lancet i : 616 (1980).
2. F.J. Palmer, T.M. Sawyers, S.J. Wierzbinski. Cimetidine and hyperparathyroidism. Lancet i : 692 (1980).
3. S. Ljunghall, G. Akerstrom, C. Rubberg, L. Wide, H. Johansson. Cimetidine in primary hyperparathyroidism. Lancet ii : 480 (1980).
4. M.F. Robinson, A.B. Hayles, H. III. Heath. Failure of cimetidine to affect calcium homeostasis in familial primary hyperparathyroidism (Multiple endocrine neoplasia, Type I). J. Clin.

Endocrinol. Metab. 51 : 912 (1980).
5. A.I. Jacob, D.Jr. Lanier, J. Canterbury, J.J. Bourgoignie. Reduction by cimetidine of serum parathyroid hormone levels in uremic patients. N. Engl. J. Med. 302 : 671 (1980).
6. C.J. Beehler, J.R. Beckner, C. Rosenquist, S.W. Shankel. Parathyroid hormone suppression by cimetidine in the uremic patients. Ann. Inter. Med. 93 : 840 (1980).
7. J.L. Vanherweghem, N. Bourgeois, M. Fuss. Cimetidine and parathyroid hormone levels. N. Engl. J. Med. 303 : 395 (1980).
8. C.E. Fiore, L.S. Malatino, J.A. Kanis. Effects of cimetidine on parathyroid hormone metabolism. Lancet i : 501 (1981).
9. A.I. Jacob, J.F. Bourgoignies. Cimetidine and parathyroid hormone levels. N. Engl. J. Med. 303 : 396 (1980).
10. J.A. Kanis, M. Earnshaw, G. Heynen, J.G.G. Ledingham, D.O. Oliver, G.G. Russell, C.G. Woods, P. Franchimont, S. Gaspar. Changes in histologic and biochemical indexes of bone turnover after bilateral nephrectomy in patients on hemodialysis. Evidence for a possible role of endogenous calcitonin. N. Engl. J. Med. 296 : 1073 (1977).
11. J. Gueris, C. Ferriere. Hétérogénéité de la parathormone plasmatique chez l'homme. Pathol. Biol. 23 : 821 (1975).
12. C. Desplan, A. Jullienne, M.S. Moukhtar, G. Milhaud. Sensitive assay for biologically active fragment of human parathyroid hormone. Lancet ii : 198 (1977).
13. J.L. Sebert, A. Fournier, J. Gueris, G. Lambrey, J.F. de Fremont, P. Marie, R. Makdassi, A. Smadja, A. Marie, D. Kuntz, A. Ryckewaert, J. Quichaud, P.J. Meunier. Limit by hyperphosphatemia of the usefulness of vitamin D metabolites (1 - hydroxycholecalciferol and 25 hydroxycholecalciferol) in the treatment of renal osteodystrophy. Metab. Bone. Dis. and Rel. Res. 2 : 217 (1980).
14. P.L. Vigo, E.E. Polli, G. Milhaud, M.S. Moukhtar, C. Desplan, J. Duriez. Aminoterminal parathyroid hormone radioimmunoassay to evaluate bone status in renal failure. Lancet i : 443 (1981).
15. M.S. Moukhtar, A. Jullienne, P. Rivaille, G. Milhaud. Dosage radioimmunologique de la calcitonine humaine. Etude immunochimique et comparaison avec le dosage biologique. In : Radioimmunoassay and related procedures in clinical medicine and research p. 381, International Atomic Energy Agency, Vienna (1973).
16. A.M. Parfitt. Correction of plasma calcium measurements. Br. Med. J. 1 : 520 (1974).
17. W.C. Randolph, V.L. Osborne, S.S. Walkenstein, A.P. Intoccia. High-pressure liquid chromatographic analysis of cimetidine, a histamine H_2 - receptor antagonist in blood and urine. J. Pharm. Sci. 66 : 1148 (1977).
18. R. Larsson, G. Bodemar, B. Norlander. Oral absorption of cimetidine and its clearance in patients with renal failure. Eur. J. Clin. Pharmacol. 15 : 153 (1979).

19. J.J. Schentag, F.B. Cerra, G. Càlleri, E. Deglopper, J.Q. Rose, H. Bernhard. Pharmacokinetic and clinical studies in patients with cimetidine associated mental confusion. Lancet i : 177 (1979).
20. C.C. Doherty, F.A. O'Connor, M.G. Mc Geown. Cimetidine for duodenal ulceration in patients undergoing hemodialysis. Br. Med. J. 2 : 1506 (1977).
21. R.S. Longley, G.K. Hargis, E.N. Bowser, S.C. Kukreja, P.A. Johnson, B.L. Jackson, W.J. Kawahara, G.A. Williams. Parathyroid hormone and calcitonin secretion : role of histamine H_2 receptors. Clin. Res. 28 : 398 A (1980).

INDEX

www.ingramcontent.com/pod-product-compliance
Lightning Source LLC
Chambersburg PA
CBHW081123180926
51611CB00004B/35

9781468442618